P9-BYF-364

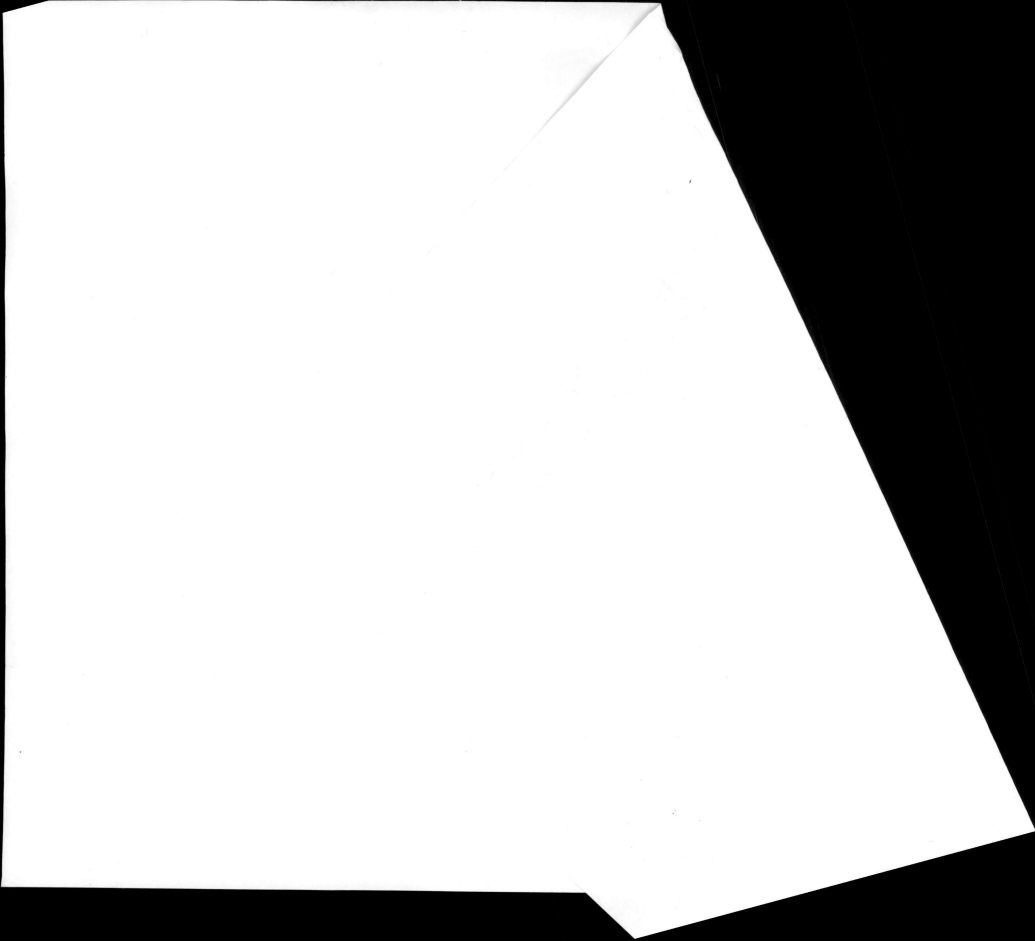

THEORETICAL NURSING
Development and Progress

THIRD EDITION REVISED REPRINT

Afaf Ibrahim Meleis, PhD, DrPS (hon), FAAN
Margaret Bond Simon Dean of Nursing
Professor of Nursing and Sociology
University of Pennsylvania
Philadelphia, Pennsylvania

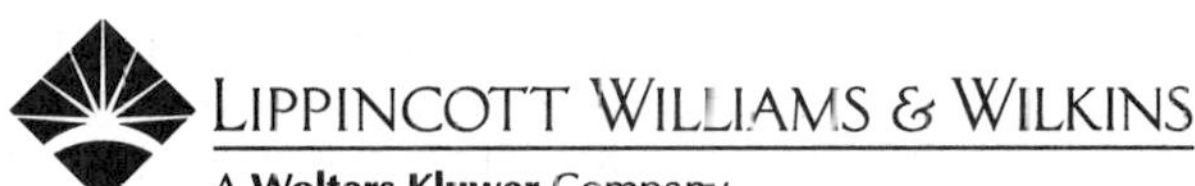

LIPPINCOTT WILLIAMS & WILKINS
A **Wolters Kluwer** Company
Philadelphia • Baltimore • New York • London
Buenos Aires • Hong Kong • Sydney • Tokyo

Acquisitions Editor: Margaret Zuccarini
Managing Editor: Helen Kogut
Editorial Assistant: Carol DeVault
Senior Production Editor: Tom Gibbons
Director of Nursing Production: Helen Ewan
Managing Editor / Production: Erika Kors
Design Coordinator: Brett MacNaughton
Senior Manufacturing Coordinator: Michael Carcel
Senior Manufacturing Manager: William Alberti
Indexer: Ann Cassar

Third Edition, Revised Reprint

9 8 7 6 5 4 3 2 1

Library of Congress Cataloging-in-Publication Data
Meleis, Afaf Ibrahim.
Theoretical nursing : development and progress / Afaf I. Meleis.—3rd ed., rev. reprint.
p. ; cm.
Includes bibliographical references and index.
ISBN 0-7817-5767-3 (hardcover : alk. paper)
1. Nursing—Philosophy. I. Title.
[DNLM: 1. Nursing Theory. WY 86 M519t 2005]
RT84.5.M45 2005
610.73'01—dc22

2004009911

Care has been taken to confirm the accuracy of the information presented and to describe generally accepted practices. However, the authors, editors, and publisher are not responsible for errors or omissions or for any consequences from application of the information in this book and make no warranty, express or implied, with respect to the content of the publication.

The authors, editors, and publisher have exerted every effort to ensure that drug selection and dosage set forth in this text are in accordance with the current recommendations and practice at the time of publication. However, in view of ongoing research, changes in government regulations, and the constant flow of information relating to drug therapy and drug reactions, the reader is urged to check the package insert for each drug for any change in indications and dosage and for added warnings and precautions. This is particularly important when the recommended agent is a new or infrequently employed drug.

Some drugs and medical devices presented in this publication have Food and Drug Administration (FDA) clearance for limited use in restricted research settings. It is the responsibility of the health care provider to ascertain the FDA status of each drug or device planned for use in his or her clinical practice.

LWW.com

To Soad Hussein Hassan, R.N., Ph.D.—

a maverick—for exemplifying humanism and commitment, for encouraging feminism and autonomy, for accepting challenge and diversity, for tolerating rebellion, for sponsoring inquisitiveness, and for being my mother.

And

To Mahmoud Meleis, Ph.D.:

for caring without knowing; for knowing and challenging without understanding; and then, for understanding and supporting.

Preface to the Third Edition Revised Reprint

Theoretical thinking is not a luxury reserved only for academicians, doctoral students, or philosophers. With the recent changes in the health care system, the shortage of nurses, and the proliferation of global events, it is more imperative to ensure that nursing assessments and interventions are driven by nursing thought, mission, and research evidence. The content of this book is provided to stimulate nursing thought about mission, goals and actions. It is also provided to stimulate clinicians as well as thought leaders to question Eurocentric theories, to critique biomedical frameworks, and to analyze the influence of gender, class, race, culture, and religion in understanding responses to health care and in testing the evidence underlying the practices used for providing nursing care.

By stimulating and reinforcing interest in theoretical thought, a next generation of theorists may develop theories that are culturally sensitive and research that is culturally competent. The revised printing of the third edition is intended to provide continuity of and consistency with the third edition, which is deemed highly relevant and useful by faculty and students. New to this printing is the updating of Chapter 21, which now includes most of the new, relevant writing that is published up to the printing of this edition.

The nursing profession is being taken more seriously by legislators, the public, and other health care professionals. Articulating the theoretical thoughts that drive nursing action makes a major contribution to how nurses are viewed, the quality of care that is provided, and the outcomes of care evaluated.

As you use this book for teaching, for research, and for practice, keep in mind that you are a critic, a utilizer, and a developer of theory.

Preface to the Third Edition

This third edition celebrates the progress we have witnessed in the development of the knowledge base of the discipline. It is written in tribute to the theorists and the metatheorists who dare to dream and who go the extra mile in reflecting the mission of the discipline. I have revised the book to capture this growth, and I have maintained those features that have been most helpful to my colleagues in their teaching, research, theory development, and/or clinical practice. I have taken seriously the reviews, recommendations, comments, and spontaneous feedback by the readers of earlier editions, and I have made appropriate revisions to reflect them.

First-generation theorists will continue to hold a special place in our Theoretical Halls of Fame; however, the emergence of second- and third-generation theorists has been instrumental in providing us with strategies for knowledge development and theoretical analyses that have made major contributions to the discipline. It is because of this extraordinary theoretical productivity that this edition provides a more polished view of the structure of the discipline and a more discipline-congruent approach to its theoretical development. This contemporary analysis reflects a more current view of the stage of development of our discipline, represents the degree to which many scholars have come to accept our discipline's focus and mission, and provides a critical analysis of the strategies that are more friendly to the nature of a nurse's daily practice. I also join many of my colleagues in providing a future-oriented analysis of the theoretical structure of the discipline. These futuristic projections are inspired by the caliber and the sophistication of the emerging generations of clinicians, graduate students, and academicians.

For both previous editions, I worked with a different editor, and invariably I approached the revising, rewriting, and the updating project with concerns about mutual expectations and varied levels of understanding of the role of theory in the development of the discipline. The working relationship that evolved with the editors was phenomenal, and for this one it is exceptional. I am grateful to my current editor, Margaret Zuccarini, for her commitment to the project, but more importantly for her expertise and tangible support throughout the process. Her gentle approach, flexibility, and resourcefulness contributed greatly to the timeliness in completing this edition.

Completing a project such as this requires the commitment, assistance, and expertise of many individuals. I am appreciative of Kathleen Zvanovec's word processing and organizational skills and her willingness to adjust her schedule to accommodate my demanding professional life. Tom Gibbons' superb editing skills and amazing flexibility in following me around the globe with edited copies and galleys made this project even more pleasurable to complete.

My immediate extended family continues to provide me with new, challenging demands that help me to maintain a balance in my life. The inspiring and challenging questions of my sons, Waleed and Sherief, now reflect their graduate education and their different life experiences. They, along with my students, manage to sharpen my debating abilities and keep me on my toes!

A special word of appreciation to Mahmoud for assuming more and more responsibilities in our daily lives (vive early retirement!) and for his patience in the meticulous review of the references and citations in this edition.

Preface to the Second Edition

The rationale for writing the first and the second editions of *Theoretical Nursing: Development and Progress* parallels some developmental phases in my career. I wrote the first edition because I was inspired by nurses who have dared to conceptualize and theorize in a practice discipline and because I was privileged to have worked with some significant mentors who have, knowingly or unknowingly, supported my evolving ideas and showed me the ropes.

The writing of the second edition, however, was inspired by a completely different group of mentors and supporters: the readers of my writings in general and of the first edition in particular. They are the students who thought the book helped them to demystify theory; the clinicians who shared with me the ways by which they were able to connect their expertise and their practice with theoretical nursing; the colleagues who have taken the time to write or call analyzing, critiquing, and extending the ideas I have presented; the conference audiences who persisted in their attempts to meet with me and to discuss and debate ideas; and others who through serendipitous meetings were ready with comments, examples, and recommendations. One particularly significant comment I have heard repeatedly was that the ideas conveyed in the first edition have *"touched their lives in a meaningful and profound way."* My response to these readers is *"not as much as your comments have touched mine."* All these comments were thoughtful, stimulating, and challenging. In short, the intense interactions with nurses (national and international educators, students, administrators, clinicians, researchers, theoreticians), my international research on women, and my research on immigrants in the United States have all helped in shaping the modifications and changes reflected in this second edition.

For those who understood, those who did not understand, those who challenged me, those who supported my arguments, as well as those who provided counterarguments, I have learned a great deal from you and I have attempted to reflect all that in this edition.

Once again, here is a synthesis that reflects a pride in our discipline, a respect for our heritage, a concern about health care for those who need it the most, a belief in our abilities to develop knowledge, and a belief in the potential of knowledge development in empowering our profession as well as our clients. I share these ideas with you, claiming neither finality nor closure. I only share them to initiate, maintain, and support dialogues about theoretical nursing. If you are moved to discuss, challenge, refute, critique, support, extend, or discard any of the ideas presented here, I will consider that writing the second edition was a worthwhile endeavor.

Many people helped me to accept the challenge of writing the second edition. David Carroll, my editor at J.B. Lippincott Company, proposed the second edition and encouraged and supported my efforts with advice and prompt responses. Barbara Mow, reluctant at first to undertake typing this project, then tackled it with enthusiasm and zeal, demonstrating throughout a commitment to perfection and deadlines.

There is no project of this magnitude that does not attract questions, discussions, and solicited or unsolicited advice from family members and friends. These daily subtle or unsubtle inquiries ("How far along are you in writing the second edition?" "Aren't you finished yet?") from many continents in the world kept me focused and ensured progress. It is much easier to maintain deadlines than to attempt to justify delays to all these interested family members and friends. Therefore, they all have played a significant role in my accepting to do the second edition and in completing it.

The attention given my work by my sons, Waleed and Sherief, and their constant attempts to understand my perspective have been enormously valuable at many more levels than could be given justice here. To them I offer my special appreciation for their intellectual support.

Mahmoud, my friend and husband, continues to give of himself, his time, and his energy, in supporting all aspects of my professional, academic, and personal life, as well as such tangible ways as reviewing and verifying references, citations, tables, and figures.

Afaf Ibrahim Meleis, R.N., Ph.D., F.A.A.N.

Preface to the First Edition

"How long did it take you to write your book?" is perhaps the most frequently asked question of a writer. It is not a question that can be answered with any degree of precision. Thoughts, ideas, and analyses exist long before they ever become written and translated into an articulate whole. If there is an answer to the question above, maybe it could be that it all started in 1969 when Dorothy Johnson asked me to teach her theory classes while she was on sabbatical leave. I owe a great deal to her and I learned a great deal from her. Not only did she leave an indelible impression upon me, but she provided me with the first opportunity to test my ideas about theory; I have been teaching theory ever since.

However, it is possible that I began this book even earlier. When I started my graduate work at UCLA in 1964, the late Burton Meyer challenged me to identify the theoretical underpinnings for my research and practice. His questions—incomprehensible at the beginning—were the impetus for my interest in theory, an interest that was then fostered by many others. Ralph Turner continued to challenge me with his critiques of my research, continued to help me by smoothing the rough edges of my conceptualizations, and continued to provide for me, in his presence, a model of scholarliness. To both of these men I am indebted for their profound influence. I am also grateful to Martha Rogers and Abe Kaplan, who managed to ignite my interest in both philosophy and humanism.

The discussion, analysis, and debates with students over the past years while teaching theory in the United States, Europe, and the Middle East have sharpened my ideas and have challenged me to further develop my thoughts and to refine the focus contained in this book. My students have been among my staunchest supporters and my best critics; I greatly value the impetus to ideas and insights that these ongoing dialogues have provided.

I would like to acknowledge the anonymous reviewers of this manuscript. Their exhaustive and extensive reviews and critiques have been pivotal in the development of the book. I hope I have done justice to their recommendations and that I have matched their seriousness in criticism with equal seriousness in revision. *Vive la* collegial skepticism!

Cheyney Johansen is a true author's companion. She typed and edited the numerous drafts, starting from a prospectus to a completed manuscript. I have appreciated her striving for perfection, her involvement and sense of pride in the book, and, most of all, the energy and dedication with which she approaches her work.

I am grateful to the J.B. Lippincott Company staff for their support from inception to completion. John Connolly's innovative approach and Paul Hill's unwavering support have helped immensely to bring the book to fruition.

It is nearly impossible to express in words the appreciation I feel toward my friend and husband, Mahmound. He provides joy, insights, wisdom, challenge, and support to my life that is reflected in all of its facets, including this book. He and my sons, Waleed and Sherief, actively participated in the thinking and writing process by asking questions, participating in discussions, and assuming more family responsibilities. What I have learned from them is incalculable, and my debt to them is enormous.

Afaf Ibrahim Meleis, R.N., Ph.D., F.A.A.N.

Contents

PART FOUR
Our Scholarship 165

PART FIVE
Our Epistemology 201

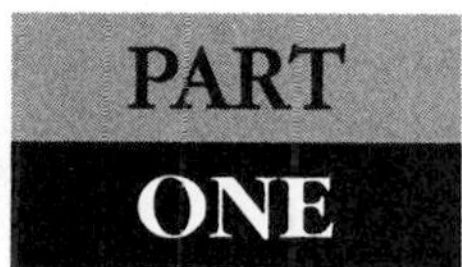

Our Theoretical Journey

Uncovering the role that theory plays in our daily experiences as nurses is the first step in the theoretical journey proposed in this book. In the two chapters in Part I, the journey and its destinations are described. In Chapter 1, you will find assumptions on which the journey is planned, the organizational plan for the journey, and some of the supporting material. The context for the journey is set in Chapter 2, where the key definitions of theoretical terms are provided.

CHAPTER 1

Introduction

By unfolding the development of our theoretical past, we gain insights that improve our understanding of our current progress, and we are empowered to achieve our disciplinary goals. By looking at our theoretical present, we see shadows of our past as well as visions of our future. Reconstructing our theoretical heritage is a process that involves reconstructing our present reality. The intent of the journey proposed in this book is to demonstrate the progress of nursing through analyses of the philosophical assumptions, the theoretical methods, and the theoretical threads that have influenced the development of the discipline. We will perform these analyses in ways that value our experiences as nurses, in ways that support and enhance our progress, and in ways that allow us to proactively develop abstractions, exemplars, conceptualizations, and theories that reflect and guide our nursing assessments and actions. Synthesizing insights of the past with visions of the future can enhance creativity in the discipline of nursing, significantly furthering its development and progress.

This book is designed to unfold the thought processes inherent in nursing, to analyze the origins of nursing ideas, and to contribute to the ongoing dialogue about the role of theory in the development of the discipline of nursing. Its intent is to provide the reader with the knowledge base necessary to understand the theoretical present of nursing and to begin to formulate ideas for the future.

The development of the discipline of nursing has progressed by leaps and bounds during the last 30 years of the 20th century. Few would dispute the notion that theory in general has been responsible for this development; yet some still question its specific role in the development of the discipline and its effects on clinical practice. The thesis of this book is that the evolution of the discipline of nursing and its scholarliness is greatly intertwined with its focus on theory and theory development. The discussions go beyond this thesis to delineate boundaries of nursing knowledge, origins of knowledge, ways and approaches to knowing, theories that guided the development of nursing's scientific base, and criteria of truth that the discipline may or may not use. Although the book intends to provide the reader with a sense of history, the process itself helps to unfold a futuristic course.

The ideas contained in this book are articulated to compete vehemently with any work that denigrates the theoretical history of nursing—past, present, or future. At the same time, the ideas complement and are intended to collaborate with all other writings of colleagues on theory and metatheory. When I provided critique, I attempted to voice it from a nursing perspective, to place the critique within an historical context, and to analyze the contributions allowing for the contextual forces and constraints.

This book is not intended to promote a certain epistemological perspective, a certain theory, or a certain set of ontological propositions over any others. Instead, this book explores, discusses, analyzes, critiques, compares, and contrasts different epistemologies, theories of truth, and nursing theories. It delineates components of theory and criteria for theory critique. It describes different strategies used in the development of nursing theories and the consequences of each strategy. This book is intended to be used by those who want to understand a significant aspect of the nursing discipline that has been dichotomized with practice and shadowed by an emphasis on education of nurses. It attempts to promote understanding, not by dissecting the discipline of nursing into separate compartments, but rather by emphasizing nursing as a discipline that is based on philosophy, theory, practice, and research. Although the focus is on nursing theories, the relationships and interdependence among research, art, philosophy, and practice are highlighted and explicated.

This book is based on several assumptions:

- Understanding theory and its role is enhanced by exploring the origin of ideas and the processes by which ideas develop into theories.
- Pluralism in nursing theories is desirable and inevitable; therefore, an exploration of existing theories is essential for improving the utility of theory and for continuing the development and progress of the discipline.
- A critical assessment of the history of theoretical thought will pave the way for development of theories that further describe and prescribe nursing practice. This understanding will help delineate issues that could be resolved in the future.

Theory is no longer a luxury in nursing. At one time using theory was equated with developing a conceptual framework to be used only as a guide to curriculum development. Theory now is part and parcel of the nursing lexicon in education, administration, and practice. We need to understand its role in the discipline, the processes and strategies used to develop it, the most accepted criteria used to analyze and critique it, and how to use it to enhance the discipline.

The Theoretical Journey

Like all journeys, the journey proposed for you, the reader, could be short or long, detached or involved, superficial or profound, simple or complex, preplanned or spontaneous, and structured or discovered. Like all journeys, this one has maps, destinations, lampposts, detours, setbacks, surprises, disappointments, and insights. Like all journeys, you will get out of it what you put into it. It has been my experience in sharing this journey with others through teaching, research, or practice that the insights gained and advancements in knowledge made depend on complete openness to the journey, on true involvement in all its aspects, and on synthesizing this journey with personal experiences.

Therefore, you are invited to embark on a long journey that spans the theoretical past, present, and future of our discipline. You are also encouraged to reflect on your own theoretical journey and to compare and contrast your journey with that of the discipline. Both journeys will take on different meanings—the insights from one journey will enhance the insights from the other.

The following are some questions to guide a reflective approach to your journey:

- How did you come to define theory nursing, human beings, and health? What values and assumptions do these definitions hold, and what courses of action are dictated by those values?
- What theories guided you in your assessment of your patients, in your research projects, and in your teaching methods? Why did you select these theories? How congruent are the ontological beliefs of these theories with your own? With those of the discipline of nursing?
- What criteria did you use in selecting or rejecting theories to guide your actions? Are these the same as or different from those criteria used in selecting or rejecting nursing theories?
- In what ways do you demonstrate your critical assessment of progress in theoretical and scientific nursing? Are these critiques illuminated by a true understanding of daily experiences of members of the discipline? Are these critiques guided by a nursing perspective?

Organization of the Book

To improve the potential of achieving the goals of understanding the role of theory in the development and progress of the discipline and understanding the role of members of the discipline in developing and constructing theory, this book is organized in parts and chapters according to potential illuminations throughout the journey. It is divided into seven major parts.

Part One describes terms of the journey into the past and the future; it includes this introduction, assumptions to guide the journey, and the lampposts that define key elements of the journey.

Part Two presents a historical analysis of the discipline's progress toward its present theoretical perspective. Stages of development and milestones leading to the next phase are discussed. A proposed pattern of progress unique to the discipline of nursing is explored. Forces and barriers are discussed that may have affected theory development and therefore indirectly affected the scholarly evolution of the discipline of nursing. Different theories of progress are explored, and the course of development of nursing knowledge is traced, compared, and contrasted with the development of other sciences.

Part Three focuses on an analysis of the discipline as it is perceived by its members at the beginning of the 1990s. It is devoted to a description of the nursing perspective, the domain of nursing, its central problems, and its human and caring properties. This part includes discussions of the sources and resources for the theoretical development of the discipline and of the major historical issues related to nursing theory and the debates about the nature of nursing and its underpinnings. The debates about whether nursing is basic or applied science, whether its theories are unique or borrowed, and whether its theories are conceptual models or applied theories are reflected in the discussions. Part Three also includes analyses and discussions of the different ways and patterns of knowing in nursing.

Part Four evolves from the analysis provided in the first three parts, and it focuses on the agents and producers of knowledge, the scholars in the discipline. Different frameworks for scholarship are analyzed, and scholarship is defined within the context of the practice properties of the discipline. Scholarship inlcudes giving careful attention to the development of nursing theories and to ways in which nursing theories are viewed and analyzed. The many ways by which nursing theories may be considered and viewed are presented and discussed in this part. Nursing theories are classified in terms of their paradigmatic origins and in terms of central domain concepts. How such classifications may determine the different properties in theories should motivate the reader to consider other possible ways to analyze the theories.

In Part Five, the different strategies for the development and analysis of theories are provided. The first chapter in Part Five delineates several major strategies for concept development. The second chapter focuses on strategies, processes, and tools essential to the development of theories. Several major strategies are considered and exemplars are included. Part Five concludes with a model for the description, analysis, critique, and testing of theory.

Part Six focuses on our theoretical present. This part is devoted to the use of the model for theory description, analysis, critique, and testing that was proposed in the previous part for analyzing selected theories in nursing. The selections, based on the theories' central questions, are matched with domain concepts.

Part Seven discusses conclusions and future directions. A future course is charted, and means for achieving that course are proposed.

Part Eight contains two chapters. The first presents an abstracted analysis of selected central writings on metatheory and nursing theory. It is not intended as a comprehensive compilation of abstracts of everything that has been written about metatheory and theory; rather, it is intended as a beginning—but central—collection that you are encouraged to use as a model for your own collection of analytical abstracts. The analyses are intended to provide a beginning point for discussion and debate. The last chapter of the book contains an extensive and considerable bibliography on metatheory, on paradigms that have been used in nursing, and on nursing theory.

Sections 1 through 12 of the final chapter, containing the metatheory literature, are organized around common themes in nursing and theory, such as philosophy and methods, theory development in nursing, forces and constraints in theory development, theory and science, theory and research, theory and practice, theory and education, and theory analysis and critique. Sections 13 through 36 contain writings about nursing theories by theorists or by others who have used the theories for research practice, education, or administration. You can find all the writings related to a theory—to the best of my knowledge—by looking under the theorist's last name in this section. Asterisked citations in this entire chapter indicate citations that have been abstracted and analyzed in the previous chapter under metatheory or theory. Sections 37 through 47 contain writings on several central paradigms that have influenced the discipline of nursing, including psychoanalytical theory, symbolic interaction, developmental systems, adaptation, and role theories. Sections 48 through 52 provide a descriptive list of audiotapes and videotapes that have been created to explicate theorists' ideas.

This book is designed to be used sequentially or nonsequentially. This free use of each chapter and each part necessitates a slight repetitiveness of ideas. The repetitions emphasize and expand on significant themes and present the same or similar ideas with a different analytical posture. This book ideally should be used in five teaching/learning units: the first focusing on Part One and Part Two, the second on Part Three, the third on Part Four, the fourth on Part Five, and the fifth on Part Six and Part Seven. Part Eight provides the necessary supportive material for each of the parts.

On a Personal Note

Writing and reading books are both existential experiences and ongoing, evolving processes. Neither the reader nor the writer is the same person after reading or writing a book, nor are their ideas and viewpoints the same. A book is never complete because ideas are never complete. Yet at some point a project needs to be abandoned so that others can explore its ideas to modify, extend, affirm, refine, or refute their own—all of which, if shared with the author, will allow her to do the same.

I urge you to consider this book complete as well as incomplete, a temporarily abandoned project that represents my own thinking and analysis. It incorporates my past, present, and future, intermingled with the past, present, and future of nursing and of nurse theorists. It is from all of this that my present interpretation of theoretical nursing has evolved, but this continuous, evolving process is presented here with temporal boundaries. Therefore, if I misinterpreted any theorists' or metatheorists' admonitions, it was unintentional, and my critique should be viewed as an honest epistemological interpretation bounded by cognitive, historical, and sociocultural meanings of the time.

I firmly believe that without the theorists and metatheorists and their writings, this book would not have been written, nor would it have been necessary. Interpretations and selections of theorists and metatheorists and their ideas were not guided by desire for omission but rather by limitations imposed by time and space. The conceptualizations of all theorists and all the analyses of the metatheorists, whether included in this text or not, provide the tapestry that depicts the future of theoretical nursing.

Finally, I have tried to avoid language that suggests stereotypical views of the nurse, patient, and physician, but at times comprehension, clarity, and simplicity took precedence. Because the majority of nurses are women, I have used "she" to encompass both "she" and "he." I have done the same elsewhere with "he."

CHAPTER 2

Theory: Who Needs It . . . What Is It?

The Destination: Theory and Theoretical Thinking

The destination of our theoretical journey is to achieve a useful level of theoretical thinking and to further the development of theoretical nursing and to provide quality theory-based care to populations.

Theory is the goal of all scientific work; theorizing is a central process in all scientific endeavors; and theoretical thinking is essential to all professional undertakings. This book is about theory, theorizing, and theoretical thinking. Critical thinking is essential for theoretical thinking. It is about these theoretical activities that clinicians, theoreticians, and researchers use in their work. It is about how we have been theorizing and using theory, perhaps without attaching the label of theory to these activities. It is also about how we can continue to advance the discipline of nursing through knowledge development, how we can enhance professional nursing through the processes that nurses use in conceptualizing their actions, and how we can facilitate better care for clients through theory-based policies and theory-driven practices. This book does not provide recipes for achieving these goals; instead, it provides ideas, questions, processes, and some strategies to enable you to pursue your own goals, to develop your own action plans, and to share your own insights and wisdom with your colleagues.

Despite the tremendous progress made in the theoretical development of the discipline of nursing, as demonstrated in the explosion of theoretical writing, some confusion remains regarding the role of theory in the development of knowledge and the role of researchers and clinicians as theorists. It is natural and expected for some nurses to declare themselves only clinicians, only theoreticians, or only researchers. Yet it is cause for concern when theorization, theory development, and theory utilization are seen as "ivory tower" activities, removed from other scientific and professional processes. It is of concern because these are activities that clinicians and researchers perform in some form or other, with varying degrees of intensity, throughout their careers; otherwise we could not be claiming expert and advanced clinical practice or sound research trajectories.

Nurses are demonstrating more commitment to the activities associated with theory, as manifested in the language nurses use to describe the activities that occupy them. One example is the use of criteria-based adjectives to describe theory utilization (Cormack and Reynolds, 1992) in nursing such as scope, usefulness, or goodness of fit of theory with one's own values or with clients' clinical problems. Skepticism and non–criteria-based critiques founded on limited knowledge and a paucity of criteria are not helpful in making changes or in developing knowledge. However, healthy skepticism and criteria-based critiques that are based on knowledge are essential to the development of knowledge.

Theory and theoretical thinking are not limited to theoreticians in the discipline. Theoretical thinking is integral to all the roles played by nurses, including those of researcher, clinician, consultant, and administrator. In research, for example, theoretical thinking could be demonstrated in all aspects of the research process. First, it is demonstrated in identifying the phenomenon within the domain of nursing, in differentiating between relevant and irrelevant phenomenon, and in deciding how the research questions are related to the theoretical domain of nursing and to the focus of nursing practice. In a human science, theoretical thinking is also demonstrated when and if the researcher attempts to determine the importance of the research questions for the discipline of nursing as well as to society at large. Theoretical thinking helps in raising questions about the meaning of the investigation to the researcher personally and the researcher's personal commitment to the research process. When these questions are asked, discussed, and answered, a process of theoretical thinking has already occurred.

Second, after defining a phenomenon, theoretical thinking continues to guide the process of research (Quinn, 1986). The researcher seeks theories that can help in describing the phenomenon or its relationships to other phenomena, or that can prescribe a nursing action for it. If theories are available, then the researcher evaluates them to determine the most useful theory for the research process—one that will expand knowledge. Evaluation of theories is as much the business of the theoretician as it is the business of the researcher and clinician. The researcher evaluates whether a theory should be tested as well as whether and in which ways the findings of the research can help refine and extend the theory. The clinician evaluates theories for use in practice. This evaluation of a theory, for research or practice, is integral to the whole process of theorizing and demonstrates another aspect of theoretical thinking.

Third, after evaluation, a hunch may evolve and propositions may be developed to guide the research process or to test the theory. Fourth, after testing a theory or propositions of a theory, the researcher may complete the task by simply describing the findings or by interpreting those findings in relationship to the original theory, perhaps choosing to refine, extend, or modify the original theory. Each of these activities is theoretical in nature and represents theoretical thinking and theory building; each of these activities should be acknowledged as an aspect of engaging in the work needed to develop theoretical nursing.

The professional clinician goes through a similar process in deciding what to assess in her clients, the timing of assessment, how she defines the needed actions, and what interventions are best for the situation. She develops hunches, pursues some, and refutes others. She develops priorities, she modifies them, and reorders them in the process. She makes some "automatic" decisions and others that require careful consideration and deliberation. Some of these decisions are based on theory; others could be the impetus for theoretical development. These processes reflect activities of theoretical analysis and development that are described in this book. In engaging in any or all of these processes, a clinician is experiencing theoretical thinking, but she may not be aware of the process, she may not label it as such, or she may not allow the theoretical process to move far enough to culminate in knowledge development progress. To understand these processes and to use them to the fullest, definitions of some key concepts are first proposed as a baseline.

Definitions

Each concept used in developing, evaluating, and operationalizing theories can be defined in many ways. I encourage you to become knowledgeable about the different definitions and to select the options that are most congruent with your own philosophical values. The following definitions (Meleis, 1997) are influenced by my feminist perspective, which shapes the fabric of my tentative realities (Bleier, 1990). Another major influence on my thinking and writing about theory is the tradition of symbolic interactionism (Mead, 1934). The definitions are limited in depth and scope and are provided only as guidelines for your refinements and extensions.

Philosophy

Philosophy is a distinct discipline in its own right, and all disciplines can claim their own philosophical bases that form guidelines for their goals. Philosophy is concerned with the values and beliefs of a discipline and with the values and beliefs held by members of the discipline. An individual's values and beliefs may or may not be congruent with those of the discipline. Philosophy focuses on providing the framework for asking both ontological and epistemological questions about central values, assumptions, concepts, propositions, and actions of the discipline. It also provides the assumptions inherent in its theoretical structure.

The philosophy of a science deals with the values that govern the scientific development and the justification of the discipline. It helps in defining or questioning priorities and goals. Philosophical inquiries help members of the discipline uncover issues surrounding priorities and analyze these priorities against societal and humanistic priorities.

Science

Science is a unified body of knowledge about phenomena that is supported by agreed-on evidence. Science includes disciplinary questions and provides answers to questions that are central to the discipline. These answers represent wisdom based on the results of data that have been obtained through the different designs and methodological approaches. These answers are also the seeds from which science evolves and develops. There are different approaches to evaluating and judging scientific findings: support of truth through repeated findings, tentative consensus among a community of scholars supporting aspects of evidence, tentative consensus among other subcommunities attesting to descriptions of reality, and the use of objective criteria by members of the community (Brown, 1977; Kuhn, 1962; Popper, 1962).

Paradigm

The definition of paradigm is closely associated with Kuhn (1970), who introduced the concept to members of the scientific community interested in philosophical analyses of disciplines and their development. Critics and supporters of Kuhn's work have created a multitude of meanings for paradigm, which were further confused by the many usages of the term that Kuhn demonstrated in his own writings. Kuhn reported a critic's finding of "twenty-two different" usages of paradigm in his writings (Kuhn, 1977, p. 294). *Paradigm* is defined as those aspects of a discipline that are shared by its scientific community. To dispose of the confusion created by his multiple use of paradigm, Kuhn (1977, p. 297) proposed to replace it with "disciplinary matrix." A *disciplinary matrix* includes the shared commitments of the community of scholars, the shared symbolic generalizations, and the exemplars, which are the shared problems and solutions in the discipline. The varied and at times conflicting definitions of paradigm within and among disciplines makes its use in nursing problematic. (See Chapter 5 for further discussion of paradigms.)

Domain

Domain is the perspective and the territory of the discipline. It contains the subject matter of a discipline, the main agreed-on values and beliefs, the central concepts, the phenomenon of interest, its central problems, and the methods used to provide some answers in the discipline. A domain includes the players and the actors who help ask and answer the questions. The actors for the domain of nursing are the clinicians, the researchers, the theorists, the metatheorists, the philosophers, the teachers, the consultants, and the ethicists. Domains are discussed further in Chapter 7.

Phenomenon

A phenomenon is an aspect of reality that can be consciously sensed or experienced. Phenomena within a discipline are the aspects that reflect the domain or the territory of the discipline. A phenomenon is the term, description, or label given to describe an idea about an event, a situation, a process, a group of events, or a group of situations. A phenomenon may be temporally and geographically bound. Phenomena can be described from evidence that is sense based (eg, something seen, heard, smelled, or felt) or from evidence that is grouped together through thought connections (eg, the observation that more children die in pediatric intensive care units during the 3:00 to 11:00 pm shift than on other shifts). In this example, simply observing the deaths does not make the phenomenon; it is grouping them and considering a connection between them, or it is considering a connection between the deaths and the specific staff shift that makes it a phenomenon. As another example, taking a certain amount of time to adjust to new time zones, having trouble remembering, experiencing foggy thinking, and being indecisive may all be part of the phenomenon related to flying, or flying across time zones. Another discussion of phenomena appears in Chapter 12.

Assumptions

Assumptions are statements that describe concepts or connect two concepts that are factual, accepted as truths, and represent values, beliefs, or goals. These statements represent the thread that holds different aspects of knowledge together. Assumptions are the taken-for-granted statements of the theory, the concept, or the research that preceded. When assumptions are challenged, they become propositions. Assumptions emanate from philosophy; they may or may not represent the shared beliefs of the discipline.

Concept

Concept is a term used to describe a phenomenon or a group of phenomena. Concept denotes some degree of classification or categorization. A concept provides us with a concise summary of thoughts related to a phenomenon; without such concise labeling, we would have to go into great detail to describe the phenomenon. Notice the difference between describing the phenomenon of what happens to individuals who travel from one time zone to another through detailing their sleep disturbances, the changes in their moods and eating habits, and so forth, and summarizing all those details through the concept of "jet lag." The latter is a more concise and a more efficient way of communicating the ideas contained in and related to "jet lag." Labeling a concept may make it more feasible to continue to analyze and develop it.

Theory

Theory is an organized, coherent, and systematic articulation of a set of statements related to significant questions in a discipline that are communicated in a meaningful whole. It is a symbolic depiction of aspects of reality that are discovered or invented for describing, explaining, predicting, or prescribing responses, events, situations, conditions, or relationships. Theories have concepts that are related to the discipline's phenomenon. These concepts relate to each other to form theoretical statements.

Nursing Theory

Nursing theory is defined as a conceptualization of some aspect of nursing reality communicated for the purpose of describing phenomena, explaining relationships between phenomena, predicting consequences, or prescribing nursing care. Nursing theories are reservoirs in which findings related to nursing concepts, such as comfort, healing, recovering, mobility, rest, caring, enabling, fatigue, and family care, are stored. They are also reservoirs for answers related to significant nursing phenomena, such as levels of cognition after a stroke, process of recovery, refusing a rehabilitation regimen for myocardial infarction patients, and revolving admissions.

The definition of nursing theory has been most problematic as demonstrated by many exchanges in the nursing literature. Many concepts have been used interchangeably with theory, such as conceptual framework, conceptual model, paradigm, metaparadigm, theorem, and perspective. The multiple use of concepts to describe the same set of relationships has resulted in more confusion and perhaps in less use of nursing theory.

There are several types of theory definitions, the first four of which were identified by Chinn and Jacobs (1987) and Chinn and Kramer (1991):

1. The first type of definition focuses on the structure of theory, as exemplified by McKay (1969), who defined theory as "logically interrelated sets of confirmed hypotheses" (p. 394). This definition incorporates research as a significant step in theory development and discounts conceptualizations that are based only on mental processes. Therefore, using this definition would not allow for consideration of any of the current nursing theories as theories.
2. The second type of definition focuses on the goals on which the theory is based. Different theorists, such as Dickoff and James (1968), define nursing theory as "a conceptual system or framework invented for some purpose" (p. 198). Not only do they focus on outcomes and consequences because of their premise that prescriptive theory should be the ultimate goal for all theory activities in nursing, but they also do not distinguish between conceptual framework and theory. Indeed, theory is defined in terms of a conceptual framework. This definition also brings to our attention the potential for inventing nursing reality (Chinn and Jacobs, 1987, p. 65); mental images are therefore not restricted to the discovery of reality but to the construction of reality.
3. The third type of definition alludes to the tentative nature of theory, as exemplified by Barnum (1990). Barnum defines theory as "a statement that purports to account for or characterize some phenomenon" (p. 1). Barnum emphasizes that the source of nursing theory is not "what is" but what "ought to be" and that existing conceptualizations are indeed nursing theories because, she asserts, quibbling over labels of theory, concept, framework, and so forth only "leads one to worry over labels rather than to look at the substance of the given thesis" (p. xi). Barnum's definition is significant in a number of ways. It acknowledges that theories are always in the process of development (Chinn and Jacobs, 1987), that existing conceptualizations are theories, and that invention is as much an arena for theory development in nursing as discovery is.
4. The fourth type of definition focuses on research and is exemplified by Ellis (1968). Ellis defines theory as "a coherent set of hypothetical, conceptual, and pragmatic principles forming a general frame of reference for a field of inquiry" (p. 217). Ellis' definition reminds us that theory is developed for the purpose of guiding research. This definition assumes that practice guides theory development, theory guides research, and research guides theory.

5. A fifth definition emerged from the first four and was articulated by Chinn and Jacobs (1987). They define theory as:

> A set of concepts, definitions, and propositions that projects a systematic view of phenomena by designating specific interrelationships among concepts for purposes of describing, explaining, predicting, and/or controlling phenomena (p. 70).

According to this definition, when concepts are defined and interrelated in some coherent whole for some purpose, we have a theory. The definition leaves the door wide open for using theory in practice and research and does not restrict theory to research-verified propositions. This definition exemplifies the multiple usages of theory.

6. A sixth type of definition focuses on nursing phenomena and is exemplified by Fawcett (1989). Nursing theories "are made up of concepts and propositions," they address "phenomena with much greater specificity than do conceptual models" (p. 17), and they address "the metaparadigm phenomenon of person, environment, health, and nursing by specifying relationships among variables derived from these phenomena" (p. 22). This type of description adds a new dimension to the definition of nursing theory: the specific, agreed-on nursing concepts. Table 2-1 summarizes these different types of definitions for nursing theory.

The definition of nursing theory adopted in this text was based on the work and the definitions of previous theorists. I have considered the common themes that evolved from these definitions and incorporated them in the definition offered in this text. Theorists and utilizers used labels interchangeably to describe their conceptualizations and sometimes different labels were used to describe the same structures. The criteria for the selection of the different labels (model, paradigm, science, theory, framework) are not always entirely clear. For example, the utilizers of theory have used "models" and "theories" interchangeably; although some usage differentiated between models and theories, such differentiation was not completely clear. For some, models are considered structures of concepts that precede the development of theory. They are also used as structures of concepts evolving from theories. (Refer to Chap. 21, where a cursory review of article titles will document this multiple usage).

A deliberate decision was made to avoid the fine-line debates about what to label existing conceptualizations about nursing. These differences are tentative at best and

Table 2-1 ***Types of Theory Definitions***

Chinn and Jacobs (1987) identify four types:

1. Definitions focusing on structure
2. Definitions focusing on practice goals
3. Definitions focusing on tentativeness
4. Definitions focusing on research

From these, Chinn and Jacobs (1987) present a fifth type:

5. Definitions focusing on concepts and the use of theory in practice as well as research

Fawcett (1989) provides a sixth type:

6. Definitions focusing on nursing phenomena

hair-splitting, unclear, and confusing at worst. Some theorists who differentiate between theory, metaparadigm, conceptual framework, and model have provided analyses that tend to overlap the properties of each of these concepts. If, indeed, conceptual models are more abstract, less specific, and contain fewer defined concepts and testable propositions, then their linkages with research and practice should not be expected. Because the utility of these models in practice and research has in fact been evaluated, and the linkages between theory and practice, research, education, and administration have been addressed by the utilizers, the properties of the existing conceptualizations do not lend themselves to the label "conceptual models." (See Chap. 8 for specific examples.) Therefore, the differences between the different labels (theory, metaparadigm, conceptual frameworks, and so forth) are differences in emphasis rather than substance and may not be worth continued debate or the creation of new esoteric entities to describe the mental images of nurse theorists. There is limited support that the use of one label over another has helped in the differentiation of the type of knowledge developed and that it may have managed to create more ambiguity for the novice and the experienced alike. Perhaps we need to debate *more substance and less form*!

When comparing nursing theories with theories in other fields, such as role theory in sociology or psychoanalytical theory in psychology, we often find that some of our nursing theories may be as specific or as nonspecific as those theories, or as abstract or as concrete—so why did we continue to unwittingly downgrade nursing theory by relegating it to a conceptual framework status when other conceptualizations have been called theory? The early reluctance of nurses to designate their work or others' as theories has changed in the mid-1990s (Lenz, Suppe, Gift, Pugh, and Milligan, 1995).

Theories are always in the process of development. Therefore, a theory in process should not be considered a conceptual framework just because it is in progress or in process. It is simply in an expected stage in the process of development and in a human science it will always be in process and in progress.

Some theorists and theory utilizers may prefer to use one particular label over another; however, they may find that they may use the same conceptualization differently and for different purposes. Theories could be used as conceptual frameworks when concepts from different theories are linked together to form a new whole. They could be used as theoretical frameworks when concepts from one theory are given new meanings or when they are linked with another theory to form a new structure that will be tested. They could be labeled a conceptual model when a theory is used as a prototype and is modeled in form or structure

Nurse theorists (such as Rogers, Johnson, and Henderson) developed coherent, systematic, and organized visions of what nursing is and what the nursing mission ought to be. To consider the conceptualizations as models and frameworks for nursing as a whole is to convey the idea that nursing is conceptualized in one way and according to one model. Therefore, other conceptualizations may be excluded prematurely by the one-particular-model advocate. Proponents may ask: How can we see the world through different pairs of glasses simultaneously? (Further development of these ideas can be found in Chaps. 8 and 11.)

The position taken in this book is that existing nursing conceptualizations are theories that could be used to describe and explain different aspects of nursing care. They are not competing models; they are complementing theories that may provide a conceptualization of different aspects, components, or concepts of the domain. They reflect and represent different realities. They also address different aspects of nursing. **Nursing theory is then defined as a conceptualization of some aspect of reality (invented or discovered) that pertains to nursing. The conceptualization is articulated for the purpose of describing, explaining, predicting, or prescribing nursing care**. Therefore, not only is nursing theory an articulation of phenomena and their relationships, but such articulation has to be communicated to colleagues.

Nursing theories evolve from extant nursing reality as seen through the mind of a theorist who is influenced by certain historical and philosophical processes or events. They also may evolve from a perception of ideal nursing practice, tinted by one's history (personal, professional, and disciplinary) and philosophy. They also may reflect a coherent representation of the dailiness of nurses' work. Theory is a tool for the development of research propositions (see the left side of Fig. 2-1). Theory is also a goal, a

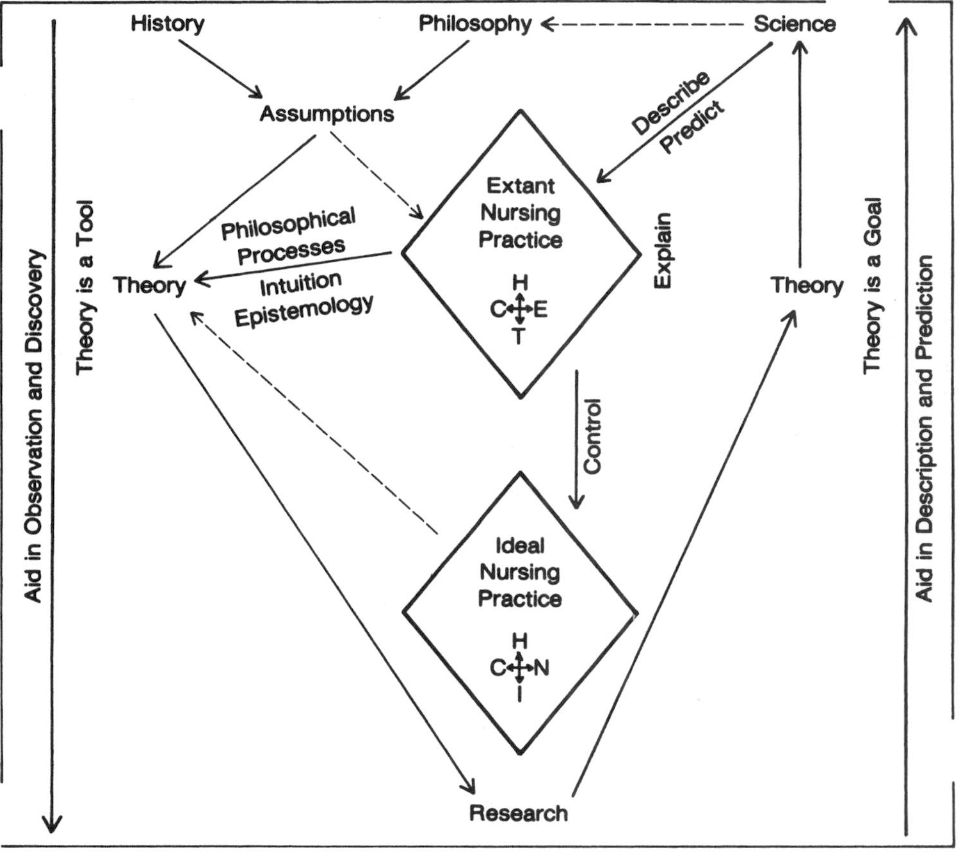

Figure 2–1 Knowledge base for nursing theory (H, health; C, client; T, transitions; E, environment; ↔, interactions and process).

reservoir in which findings (both quantitative and qualitative) become more coherent and meaningful. The cyclical nature of theory, practice, philosophy, history, research, and science is depicted in Figure 2-1. Taken together, and in relationship to each other, they constitute the knowledge base for the discipline of nursing.

Examples of phenomena and relationships depicted in nursing theories are:

- A nursing client is conceptualized as a self-care agent.
- A nursing client is a biopsychosocial and cultural being.
- A nursing client is a system with a number of behavioral subsystems.
- A nursing client is conceptualized as a conglomerate of needs.
- A nursing client is a system of such modes as interdependence, self-concept, roles, and psyche, among others.
- Person–environment interactions are the focus of nursing care.
- Health and illness behavior is a product of person–environment interactions.
- Communication is a tool for diagnosis and intervention in nursing.
- An efficient, functional, productive interaction has several components: sensing, perceiving, conceiving.
- A goal of interaction is to develop rapport, which in turn enhances patient care.
- The focus of intervention is the client's environment.
- Environment is a composite of energy fields.
- Nursing care deals with manipulation of environment.
- Nursing provides self-care needs only until the client or a significant other is capable of providing self-care.
- A nurse is conceptualized as performing a number of functions designed to meet the patient's needs.

Types of Theories

Theories are reservoirs in which related knowledge is articulated and organized in meaningful wholes. Theories answer significant questions and help investigators and clinicians to focus on raising questions in a systematic and a coherent way. Tentative theories reflect growth in disciplines. They reflect the wisdom of articulating disparate facts in a meaningful whole and the challenge of answering new questions as they arise. To accomplish its goals of optimum health for its clients, the discipline of nursing must have theories to describe its phenomena, to explain relations, to provide a framework for interventions, and to predict outcomes.

Level of Abstraction

Theories may be described in terms of their levels of abstraction or in terms of their goals. When considered in terms of their levels of abstraction, three types of theories emerge in nursing: grand theories, mid-range theories, and situation-specific theories. Each is described below.

Grand Theories

Grand theories are systematic constructions of the nature of nursing, the mission of nursing, and the goals of nursing care.

Mid-Range Theories

Theories that have more limited scope, less abstraction, address specific phenomena or concepts, and reflect practice (administrative, clinical, or teaching) are considered mid-range theories. The phenomena or concepts tend to cross different nursing fields and reflect a wide variety of nursing care situations. Examples are uncertainty, incontinence, social support, quality of life, and health as empowerment.

Situation-Specific Theories

Theories that focus on specific nursing phenomena that reflect clinical practice and that are limited to specific populations or to a particular field of practice are situation-specific theories. These theories are socially and historically contexted; they are not developed to transcend time, a socially constraining structure, or a politically limiting situation. Therefore, their scope and the questions driven by them are limited.

Goal Orientation

Theories can also be classified in terms of their goals. As such, there are *descriptive* and *prescriptive* theories. Descriptive theories describe relationships between phenomena, describe nurses' and patients' relationships, and describe guidelines for interventions. Processes of assessing, diagnosing, and intervening must be considered in the development of nursing theories (Kritek, 1978). To accomplish their goals of supporting and promoting optimum health and well-being, nurses also need theories to capture efficient and effective clinical therapeutics to use in their practices.

Descriptive Theories

Descriptive theories are ones that describe a phenomenon, an event, a situation, or a relationship; identify its properties and its components; and identify some of the circumstances under which it occurs. Although descriptive theories have an element of prediction (eg, predicting when a phenomenon may occur and when it may not occur), their contribution to knowledge is mainly to help sort out observations and meanings regarding the phenomenon. Descriptive theories describe a phenomenon, speculate on why a phenomenon occurs, and describe the consequences of that phenomenon; therefore, they have explanatory, relating, and predicting utility. Descriptive theories are complete theories and have the potential for guiding research.

There are two types of descriptive theories. The first type is the *factor-isolating, category-formulating,* or *labeling theory.* This theory describes the properties and dimensions of phenomena. The second type is the *explanatory theory,* which describes and explains the nature of relationships of certain phenomena to other phenomena. Examples of descriptive theories are the descriptions of the life processes of a nursing client, person–environment interactions in health and illness, health status, ways of assessment, types of diagnosing, disruptions of life processes, and interventions. Descriptive nursing theories are those that help describe, explain, and predict nursing phenomena and relationships between nursing phenomena. Descriptive theories are not action oriented and do not attempt to produce a situation.

Types of descriptive theories in nursing include:

Life processes
Person–environment interactions
Assessment
Diagnosis
Descriptions of alterations in life processes
Clinical therapeutics

Prescriptive Theories

Prescriptive theories are those addressing nursing therapeutics and the consequences of interventions. A prescriptive theory includes propositions that call for change and predict the consequences of a certain strategy of nursing intervention. A prescriptive theory should designate the prescription and its components, the type of client to receive the prescription, the conditions under which the prescription should occur, and the consequences. It articulates the conditions in the life process, person–environment interactions, and health status that need the prescription and the effect on the client's life process, health status, and interaction with the environment. Prescriptions may also be focused on the environment.

In summary, all theories used in nursing to understand, explain, predict, or change nursing phenomena are nursing theories, whether or not they evolved out of other theories, other paradigms, other disciplines, nursing experiences, diagnoses, nursing processes, or nursing practices, and whether or not they were developed by nurses. If we must differentiate between different types of theory, then such differentiation is meaningful only in terms of the levels and the goals, not the source of the theory. Theories that are developed to understand and explain human processes in health and illness are pure or basic theories. In other words, they are theories with a descriptive focus. Theories that are developed to control, promote, and change are nursing practice theories or prescriptive theories (Crowley, 1968).

Theory Components

Theories are made up of assumptions, concepts, narrative descriptions, propositions, and exemplars. The structural components of descriptive and prescriptive theories differ somewhat.

Structural components of descriptive theories include:

Clients' state or condition
Patterns of responses to conditions, situations, or events

Analyses of contexts of conditions and responses
Analyses of promoting and inhibiting contexts

Structural components of prescriptive theories include:

Definition of clients' situation
Nursing therapeutics
Process by which therapeutics is implemented
Patterns of desired status or consequences
Context for desired/undesired status and for therapeutics

Uses of Theory

Theory and Research

The objective of theory is to formulate a minimum set of generalizations that allow one to explain a maximum number of observable relationships among the variables in a given field of inquiry. The theory sets limits on what questions to ask and what methods to use to pursue answers to the questions. The relationship is cyclical in nature; the results of the research can then be used to verify, modify, disprove, or support a theoretical proposition. Nursing theories have provided nurse researchers with many new propositions for nursing research. Nursing research has been driven in the past by educational, sociological, and psychological theories and less by nursing theories. Nursing theories stimulate nurse scientists to explore significant problems in the field of nursing. In doing so, the potential for the development of nursing knowledge increases.

Theory and Practice

The primary uses of theory are to provide insights about nursing practice situations and to guide research. Through interaction with practice, theory is shaped and guidelines for practice evolve. Research validates and modifies theory. Theory then guides practice. Until empirical validation, modification, and support are completed, theory can be given support through clinical utilization and validation and can therefore be allowed to give direction to practice.

Theory provides the nurse with the goals for assessment, diagnosis, and intervention. A nurse working as part of a health care team focuses on those aspects of care that are delineated in theory for a more effective assessment of a health care client. If the goals are health maintenance, promotion of self-care, and enhancement of stability during the illness, then the nurse has an intellectual checklist by which the levels of health, self-care needs and abilities, and stability are assessed. Diagnosis is related to those areas in which the nurse plans an intervention.

Theory is a tool that renders practice more efficient and more effective. Just by being goal directed, our energies in assessing extraneous areas are minimized. If no nursing goals exist, the nurse might use her energy and her time inefficiently. By considering areas of assessment or intervention that may be handled more efficiently and expertly by other members of the health care team, the nurse conserves her own energy, time, and talent for the areas and phenomena for which she is well prepared.

Theory has other uses. Language of theory provides us with common grounds for communication and with labels and definitions for phenomena; therefore, nursing practice could be described and explained by common concepts. These common concepts allow us to communicate succinctly with each other. More effective and efficient communication can eventually lead to further theory development as concepts are refined, sharpened, extended, and validated. Well defined concepts with conceptual and construct validity enhance the cyclical communication among practitioners, theorists, clinicians, and educators. The world of nursing can become more coherent, more goal oriented, and more efficient.

Professional autonomy and accountability are enhanced by theory use in practice. Being able to practice by scientific principles allows nurses the opportunity to accurately predict patterns of response that are consequences of care. Articulation of actions, goals, and consequences of actions enhances nurses' accountability. If we can clearly talk about our purpose and what we hope to accomplish, perhaps other professionals and patients are also able to describe or articulate nurses' actions and goals more accurately and comprehensively. Defining the focus and the means to achieving that focus and being able to predict consequences increase our control of our practice and therefore increase our autonomy. As stated by Fuller (1978),

> The autonomy of a profession rests more firmly on the uniqueness of its knowledge, knowledge gathered ever so slowly through the questioning of scientific inquiry. Nursing defined by power does not necessarily beget knowledge. But knowledge most often results in the ascription of power and is accompanied by autonomy (p. 701).

In summary, theory helps to identify the focus, the means, and the goals of practice. Using common theories enhances communication, increasing autonomy and accountability to care. Theory helps the user gain control over subject matter (Barnum, 1994). All these in turn help bring about further refinements of theory and better relationships among theory, research, and practice. Figure 2-1 identifies the relationships among theory, research, practice, and philosophy.

REFERENCES

Barnum, B.J. (1990). *Nursing theory: Analysis, application, and evaluation* (3rd ed.). Boston: Little, Brown.

Barnum, B.J.S. (1994). *Nursing theory: Analysis, application, and evaluation* (4th ed.). Philadelphia: J.B. Lippincott.

Bleier, R. (1990). *Feminist approaches to science.* New York: Pergamon Press.

Brown, N.H. (1977). *Perception, theory and commitment: The new philosophy of science.* Chicago: University of Chicago Press.

Chinn, P.L., and Jacobs, M.K. (1987). *Theory and nursing: A systematic approach.* St. Louis: C.V. Mosby.

Chinn, P.L., and Kramer, M.K. (1991). *Theory and nursing: A systematic approach* (3rd ed.) St. Louis: C.V. Mosby.

Cormack D.F.S., and Reynolds, W. (1992). Criteria for evaluating the clinical and practical utility of models used by nurses. *Journal of Advanced Nursing*, 17, 1472–1478.

Crowley, D.M. (1968). Perspectives of pure science. *Nursing Research*, 17(6), 497–501.

Dickoff, J., and James, P. (1968). A theory of theories: A position paper. *Nursing Research*, 17(3), 197–203.

Ellis, R. (1968). Characteristics of significant theories. *Nursing Research*, 17(3), 217–222.

Fawcett, J. (1989). *Analysis and evaluation of conceptual models of nursing* (2nd ed.). Philadelphia: F.A. Davis.

Fuller, S. (1978). Holistic man and the science and practice of nursing. *Nursing Outlook*, 26, 700–704.

Kritek, P. (1978). The generation and classification of nursing diagnosis: Toward a theory of nursing. *Image*, 10(2), 33–40.

Kuhn, T.S. (1962). *The structure of scientific revolutions.* Chicago: University of Chicago Press.

Kuhn, T.S. (1970). *The structure of scientific revolutions* (2nd ed.). Chicago: University of Chicago Press.

Kuhn, T.S. (1977). *The essential tension.* Chicago: University of Chicago Press.

Lenz, E.R., Suppe, F., Gift, A.G., Pugh, L.C., and Milligan, R.A. (1995). Collaborative development of middle-range nursing theories: Toward a theory of unpleasant symptoms. *Advances in Nursing Science*, 17(3), 1–13.

McKay, R. (1969). Theories, models and systems for nursing. *Nursing Research*, 18(5), 393–399.

Mead, G.H. (1934). *Mind, self, and society.* Chicago: University of Chicago Press.

Meleis, A.I. (1997). Theoretical nursing: Definitions and interpretations. In J. Fawcett and I.M. King (Eds.), *The language of nursing theory and metatheory.* Indianapolis: Sigma Theta Tau.

Popper, K. (1962). *Conjecture and refutations.* New York: Basic Books.

Quinn, J.F. (1986). Quantitative methods: Descriptive and experimental. In P. Moccia (Ed.), *New approaches to theory development.* New York: National League for Nursing.

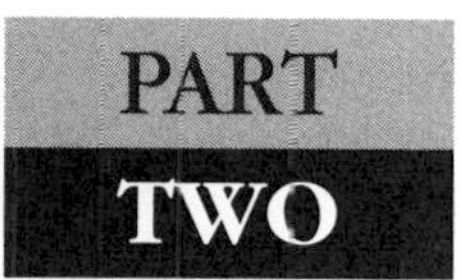

Our Theoretical Heritage

The discipline of nursing has established itself as a practical field with a theoretical base. The process of the evolution of the discipline and its theoretical base follows a unique path, a path that may not be clearly understood by those who attempt to measure progress and development of the discipline by the same criteria used to measure progress of the physical and natural sciences. The origins of the development path for nursing can be traced through an analysis of both its research tradition as well as its theory traditions. This part, which includes Chapters 3, 4, and 5, traces the historical development of nursing theory and theoretical nursing. The course of the evolution of nursing as a theoretical discipline is mapped and discussed. Forces and constraints that nurses confronted in their quest to establish theoretical nursing are analyzed.

The development of the discipline of nursing is conceptualized as evolving in stages. The premise on which the discussion proceeds is that all stages preceding the most current stage made major contributions to the maturity of the discipline. Milestones in every stage are delineated, and the influence of each milestone on nursing theory is explored. The relationships between theory, science, practice, and philosophy are also explored.

Forces and barriers in the development of theory in nursing are identified. The roles of nurses—as nurses, as predominantly women, and as nurse theorists in the development of nursing theory against many odds—are explored and discussed. Different theories are proposed to analyze the levels of the progress and development of the discipline. The meaning of each of these theories and the contribution they make to the discipline and its scientific base are discussed. Different theories of "truth" are examined and the impact of each of these theories on progress and development in nursing is also discussed. Part Two concludes with propositions that reject the idea that the development of the discipline of nursing follows either a revolutionary or an evolutionary path. An integrative process is proposed to describe the unique nature of progress in nursing.

CHAPTER 3

On the Way to Theoretical Nursing: Stages and Milestones

Ever since nurses started to care for human beings in an orderly and organized way, they have been involved in some form of theorizing. Concepts of care, comfort, communication, protection, healing, and health, among others, were used to guide clinical practice before they were labeled as concepts and before they were linked together to form nursing theories. They were not communicated in articulated wholes to describe nursing and nursing care actions. A process of serious labeling and a more systematic communication of concepts and theories occurred in nursing between 1950 and 1980. This process continues to enrich the discipline of nursing.

First attempts in theoretical nursing were made by Florence Nightingale in the late 19th and early 20th centuries to describe nursing focus and action in the Crimean War. Nightingale was prompted to articulate her ideas in numerous publications for different goals. Among these goals were gaining support for a national need for nurses, achieving acceptance for the development of educational programs for nurses, and exposing the unhealthy environmental conditions that were endured by English soldiers during wars.

Subsequent attempts in theorizing were published by American nurse educators in the mid-1950s, prompted by the need to justify different educational levels for nurses and the need to develop curricula for each of the educational levels in nursing. To differentiate between curricula, and to enhance the quality of education in each curriculum, a few pioneer nurses combined their clinical expertise with forward visions to answer such questions as "What are nursing goals?" and "What ought to be the aims of nursing?" These early theorists were aware that by developing programs that represented a nursing perspective, they would help nursing students, that is, future clinicians, to focus on nursing phenomena and problems rather than on medical phenomena and problems. Groups were formed in different parts of the United States (and subsequently or simultaneously in other parts of the world) and committees were formed to discuss the nature of nursing, the nature of nurses' work, and the unique aspects of nursing. The goals of these early efforts were also focused on differentiating nursing from other health science disciplines. These dialogues went further to explore the nature of nursing knowledge.

Perhaps the best way to consider the history of nursing theory and to analyze nurses' current interest in theory in perspective is to consider dominant themes in the different stages of the development of nursing knowledge. The implicit assumption here is that the themes discussed in the literature are indicative and representative of what members of the discipline were interested in at different times during the process of its development. In addition to delineating these themes, an analysis of the theory literature provides us with specific milestones that may have helped the development of theoretical nursing. Both approaches provide insights into how nursing evolved into its current status.

In this chapter, the stages that have influenced knowledge development are traced and defined. The central themes are:

- Stages that mark the development of theoretical nursing
- Milestones in the development and use of theoretical nursing

These stages and milestones helped achieve the current level of progress in the discipline.

Stages in Nursing Progress

Since the time of the Crimean War, nursing has gone through many stages in its search for a professional identity and in defining its domain. It is interesting to note that our analysis and evaluation of nursing's theoretical thought, the patriarchal societies we live in, and the view and status accorded nurses and nursing may make it appear as if each of these stages was a deviation from the goal of establishing the discipline of nursing. However, each of these stages has indeed sharpened and clarified the dimensions needed for the establishment of the scientific aspects of the discipline, promoting or leading to a scholarly evolution of the nursing discipline. Each stage has helped nurses come closer to identifying the domain of nursing, defining its mission, and defining its theoretical base. Progress in the development of theoretical nursing is definable in terms of five stages: practice, education and administration, research, theory, philosophy, and integration.

Stage of Practice

The Western version of nursing as an occupation dates from the late 19th century and the early 20th century, a product of the Crimean War. From the need to care for wounded soldiers, Florence Nightingale organized a group of women to deliver care under her supervision and that of the war surgeons. Nightingale focused on hygiene as her goal and environmental changes as the means to achieve that goal.

The Eastern version of the beginning of nursing gives credit to Rofaida Bent Saad Al-Islamiah (also referred to as Koaiba Bent Saad), who accompanied the prophet Mohammed in his Islamic wars. She, too, organized a group of women and focused on hygiene and environment in caring for the wounded. She established special moving tents to attend the sick, the wounded, and the disabled. She modeled first aid, emergency care, and long-term healing and caring. She cared for patients and trained women in the art of first aid and nursing (Fangary, 1980; S.H. Hassan, personal communication, 1990). In both Eastern and Western versions of the beginnings of nursing, a woman saw the need for organizing other women to care for the wounded in wars; in both they provided emergency care as well as long-term care. They both focused on caring, healing, promoting healthy environments, and on training other nurses.

During this stage, the mission of nursing was defined as providing care and comfort to enhance healing and a sense of well-being and to create a healthy environment that helps decrease suffering and deterioration. Nurses defined their domain to include the patient and the environment in which the care is offered. Both Nightingale and Al-Islamiah created and monitored the environment in which the care was being given. The stage of practice gave nursing its *raison d'etre*, its focus, and its mission. Theoretical writings by Nightingale (1946) describing the care goals and processes are testimony to the potential for nurses to articulate practice activities theoretically. These writings also point to the potential for nursing as a field of practice to be articulated theoretically.

Stage of Education and Administration

From that early focus on practice and the concomitant traditions of apprenticeship and service, there was a shift to questions related to training programs and nursing curricula. The "how to" of practice eventually was translated into what curriculum to develop and how to teach it. Almost three decades were spent experimenting with different curricula, ways of preparing teachers, modes of educating administrators for schools of nursing and for service, and ways of preparing nurse practitioners. During this stage the focus was on the development of functional roles for nurses. The dominant themes of this stage evolved from the educational and administrative roles of nurses.

The significance of this stage in the theoretical development of the discipline lies in the impetus it provided nurses to ask questions related to the domain of nursing. In developing curricula that are geared toward preparing nurses for different educational levels, nurses asked such questions as: What is nursing? How different is nursing care as provided by a diploma graduate, an associate degree graduate, a bachelor of science graduate, or a master's degree graduate? These questions prompted nurses to articulate the core of nursing theory (Henderson, 1966). In a curious way, it is during this stage that the theoretical ideas of the pioneering American nurse theorists were born. A focus on teaching and education, therefore, may have paved the way for the further development of theoretical nursing.

Stage of Research

The focus on education, curriculum, teaching, learning strategies, and administration led educators to an interest in research. Experts in nursing curricula recognized that without research and a systematic inquiry into, for example, the different teaching/learning modalities and the teaching/learning milieu on outcomes, education of nurses could not be improved. Therefore, the research interest emerged from and focused on questions related to educational and evaluative processes.

How to teach, how to administer, how to lead, and which strategies would be more effective in teaching and administering were the questions that led to the development and expansion of nursing research (Gortner and Nahm, 1977). The first nursing research journal—titled *Nursing Research*—in the United States (and in the world) was established in 1952, and the Southern Regional Educational Board (SREB) and the Western Council for Higher Education in Nursing (WCHEN) were developed in the mid-1950s and mid-1960s, respectively. Their objectives called for improving nursing education, enhancing nursing research productivity, and raising the quality of research. The journal and the meetings of the SREB and WCHEN helped nursing develop its scientific norms—that "set of cultural values and mores governing the activities termed scientific" (Merton, 1973, p. 270).

Criteria for reviewing scientific papers were established, based on the assumption that scientific inquiry must be judged by peers. Thus, nurse researchers began to abide by Merton's norm of universalism, the impersonal evaluation of a research product by some objective criteria (Merton, 1973, p. 270). Universities also held the same expectations for nursing faculty that they held for other faculty; specifically, members of faculty in schools of nursing were required to develop their ideas and communicate them in the scientific arena through publications in refereed journals and scholarly presentations in meetings. Therefore, when seen in the context of science, the "publish or perish" dogma was not unrealistic but was rather another norm governing nursing science. Nurses were now involved in that communality—the sharing of ideas—and their research was subjected to the scrutiny of their peers and anonymous critics (Gortner, 1980; Merton, 1973).

Nursing's initial attempts at introducing ideas and sharing research results were met with severe and, at times, devastating criticisms by other nursing colleagues. (Those who participated in the early research conferences may remember the lengthy and severe research critiques that may not have considered the stage of nursing research development and that traumatized researchers and audience alike.) As a result, and in addition to universality and communality, two other norms evolved: objectivity and detached scrutiny. Objective criteria for research evaluation, which were identified and shared, provided a turning point—a scholarly medium for research refinement and further development (Leininger, 1968).

The stage of research development made major contributions to contemporary scholarly nursing. It was also the stage in which tools of science left a major mark on curricula through the new offerings of research classes and statistics courses and through the several publications in which major research tools and instruments were compiled and combined.

These, then, were the beginnings of nursing inquiry and science. During this stage, as in other sciences, researchers emphasized scientific syntax—the process rather than the content of research (Kuhn, 1970). The binding frameworks or depositories of collected facts were still lacking. Nevertheless, the syntax of the discipline had been formulated.

Stage of Theory

Eventually, the fundamental questions about the essence of nursing—its mission and its goals—began to surface in a more organized way. An incisive group of leaders, nurses who believed that theory should guide the practice of nursing, wrote about the need for theory, the nature of nursing theory, philosophers' views of theory, and how nursing theory ought to be shaped. Although nurse theorists' conceptual schemata for the discipline of nursing appeared during the education and administration stages of the discipline, it was not until the stage of theory emerged that they were taken seriously.

During this stage, arguments arose about whether nursing was merely a chapter of medicine or whether it was part of the biologic, natural, or physical sciences (analogous to the earlier Cartesian concept that biology is simply a chapter of physics). The Cartesian concept was rejected (biology is indeed a distinct and autonomous science), and nursing continued to resist the implication that it was a part of medicine. It became clear to a new breed of nurse leaders—the philosophers and the theorists (or conceptualists, as some referred to them)—that nursing could not be reduced to a single science that inquires into just one aspect of man just as biology is not reducible to physics. Nursing is complex, necessitating its intrinsic autonomy in content and methods.

The search for conceptual coherence evolved from a preoccupation with syntax to the disciplined and imaginative study of the realities of nursing and the meaning and truths that guide its actions (Table 3-1). The development from preoccupation with scientific method to speculation and conceptualization in nursing is reminiscent of the development of philosophical thought in the 18th and 19th centuries. The 18th century was greatly influenced by Newton and by Bacon, who was in turn influenced by Descartes. The 19th century was dominated by Kant, whose hypothetical, deductive, and metaphysical approach encouraged the speculative nature of science. The speculators in nursing began to construct realities as they saw them, and their imaginative constructs evolved from their philosophical backgrounds and from their educational inclinations.

It was natural for theory development to be influenced by the paradigms of other disciplines, by the educational background of nurse theorists, and by the philosophical underpinnings of the time. Therefore, we find premises stemming from existentialism, analytical philosophy, and pragmatism guiding the development of those theories, sometimes explicitly and often implicitly. Nurses also adopted concepts and propositions from other paradigms, such as psychoanalysis, development, adaptation, and interaction, as well as from humanism, to guide its assessment and its action. Theories were developed in response to dissatisfaction with isolated findings in research. The emerging theories addressed the nature of the human being in interactions and transactions

Table 3-1 **Characteristics of the Beginning of the Stage of Theory Development**

- Use of external paradigms to guide theory
- Uncertainty about discipline phenomena
- Discrete and independent theories
- Separation between research, practice, and theory
- Search for conceptual coherence
- Theories used for curricula
- The goal of a single paradigm prevails

with the health care system as well as the processes of problem solving and decision making for assessment and intervention.

Although certain theoretical concepts were synthesized from diverse paradigms, most nursing theories, such as subsystems of behavior, role supplementation, therapeutic touch, and self-help, were definable and analyzable only from the nursing perspective. Theories offered a beginning agreement on the broad intellectual endeavors and the fundamental explanatory tasks of nursing. This stage offered knowledge of relevant phenomena, but there was continued uncertainty about the discipline of nursing and its intellectual goals. Just as in nuclear physics, when the first achievement was not one of observation or mathematical calculation but one of intellectual imagination, conceptual schemata evolved before there was any clear recognition of nursing's empirical scope. In nursing, the theories helped the discipline to focus on its concepts and problems.

Rogers (1970) offered a conception of nursing that focused on the constant human interaction with the environment. Johnson (1980) developed the notion that a human being—a biologic system—is also an abstract system of behavior centered on innate needs. Levine (1967) and Orem (1971) proposed guidelines for nursing therapeutics that preserve the integrity of the human being, the psychology, the community affiliation—in short—the entire person. Orem (1985) reminded us that the human being is perfectly capable of self-care and should progress toward that goal.

Because of the earlier focus on education and professional identity, because the National League for Nursing stipulated a conceptual framework for curricula, and because the truth of a theory had not yet been established using the empirical positivists' criteria of corroboration, emergent theories were not used to guide practice or research but were instead used to guide teaching. Consequently, scientific energies were dissipated in developing curricula that corresponded to these theories.

Although theories may have influenced practice through students, such influence was not documented in the literature that focused more on theory in educational programs. As an educator who was a member of a school that used nursing theory (also called a model) as a framework for the curriculum, I experienced first hand, in the mid-1960s, the conflicts that graduates of the program encountered when they wanted to use a nursing framework, one that they studied and experienced in their educational program, in practice and were unable to do so because of its novelty and its esoteric concepts. Whether the use of nursing models in education rendered nursing care more effective and efficient is a matter left to speculation and was evidenced only in isolated incidents and through experiential narrative analyses that were discounted for their lack of universality and generalization. The graduates of programs based on nursing theories in the early and mid-1960s should be encouraged to write the stories of their experiences with these theoretically based programs and ways by which their practice was informed or not informed by these programs.

The nagging questions continued:

- What fundamental process does nursing represent?
- Which are its units of analysis?
- What are the goals of nursing?
- What are the desired outcomes?
- How do nursing interventions relate to desired outcomes?

These questions continued to lead to one type of answer. That is, let us find a guiding paradigm or search for a universal theory with explanatory power for all dimensions of nursing. Once we find this all-encompassing theory, we will be able to answer questions related to the discipline. This approach reminds us that Galileo and Descartes talked of the scientist's task as that of being able to decipher once and for all the secrets of nature and to arrive at the "one true structure" of the nature of the world. However, that was a Platonic ideal rather than a plain description of the task of scientific research. Later, scientists began to discard this line of pursuit. Physicists and physiologists "now believe that . . . we shall do better in these fields by working our way toward more general concepts progressively, as we go along, rather than insisting on complete generality from the outset" (Toulmin, 1977, p. 387). Toulmin proposed that "human behavior in general represents too broad a domain to be encompassed within a single body of theory" (p. 387). When scientists accept the need for multiple theories, and when they accept the process nature of science, it will be a "sign of maturity rather than defeatism" (p. 387) within the discipline.

Because nurse scientists searched for one theory for the entire discipline, the task was either overwhelming and too highly abstract (Rogers, 1970) or too simplistic and reductionist (Orem, 1971). The sentiment of practitioners was to question the possibility and usefulness of an encompassing theory, as evidenced by the meager literature throughout the 1960s and 1970s on nursing practice using nursing theory. The desire for a single conceptual framework to guide the nursing curriculum was carried to nursing practice. Nurse practitioners believed that there was also a movement toward making a choice between theories and adhering to that one particular theory. Because none of the theories addressed all aspects of nursing, nurse practitioners avoided nursing theory, ignored it, or refused to use it. A myth was being formed. However, many nurses were beginning to abandon the notion of a universal theory to describe and explain nursing phenomena and units of analysis and to guide nursing practice, just as physicists did when they abandoned the 17th century hope that a universal science of nature could be developed within the framework of fundamental ideas of classical mechanics.

Three themes in nursing that evolved during this stage were: acceptance of the complexity of nursing and the inevitability of multiple theories; acceptance of the need to test and corroborate major propositions of differing theories before dismissing any of them; and the idea that concepts or theories remaining in the field, through a cumulative effect, become the basis for the development of a specific perspective. Dualism and pluralism were the norms of the stage of theory. It was also during this stage that nursing developed the boundaries necessary to focus its inquiry and the flexibility necessary to allow expansion through creative endeavor.

Stage of Philosophy

As nurses began reflecting on the conceptual aspects of nursing practice, on defining the domain of nursing, and on the most appropriate methods for knowledge development, they turned to philosophical inquiries. The focus during this stage was on raising and answering questions about the nature of nursing knowledge (Carper, 1978; Silva, 1977), the nature of inquiry (Ellis, 1983), and the congruency between the essence of nursing knowledge and research methodologies (Allen, Benner, and Diekelman, 1986). During this stage, philosophy was considered an attempt to understand philosophical premises underlying nursing theory and research (Sarter, 1987) and an attempt to develop philosophical inquiry as a legitimate approach to knowledge development in nursing (Fry, 1989).

This stage influenced profoundly the intellectual discourse in nursing literature. During this stage epistemological diversity was accepted and the need for ethical, logical, and epistemological inquiries was legitimized, as evidenced in the numerous philosophically based manuscripts accepted for publication (Ellis, 1983).

This stage was also marked by a scholarly maturity in the discipline, as its members acknowledged the limitation of appropriate tools to investigate fundamental and practical issues. Assumptions about wholeness of human beings, contextual variables, and holism of care called for congruent investigative tools, and nurse scholars acknowledged the complexity of capturing nursing phenomenon using existing tools (Newman, 1995; Stevenson and Woods, 1986). Accepting limitations while maintaining the reality of the contextuality and complexity of the phenomenon represents a marked scholarly maturity and the potential to focus on the development of appropriate tools.

Earlier during this stage discussions encompassed the different "ways of knowing" in nursing and a call for going beyond the empirical (Carper, 1978). These epistemological discussions focusing on the structure of knowledge, nature of theory, criteria for analysis, and justification of particular methodologies for knowledge development significantly contributed to the discovery and construction of an identity for the discipline of nursing. As theorists and metatheorists discussed the philosophical bases that shaped nursing knowledge (Allen, Benner, Diekelman, 1986; Roy, 1995), a new set of questions emerged. These questions reflected more the values and meaning of the knowledge that is being developed, and consequences of this knowledge on nursing practice and less on the structure and justification of knowledge (Bradshaw, 1995; Silva, Sorrell, and Sorrell, 1995).

The emphasis on knowing was complemented with another emphasis on "being." The being was not limited to the nurse, or to the patient, but to each separately and to both joined in caring interactions (Benner, 1994; Newman, 1995). This philosophical stage encompassing both components of epistemology and ontology provided nurses with the legitimacy to ask and answer questions related to values, meanings, and realities using multiple philosophical and theoretical bases.

Stage of Integration

A first characteristic of this stage is substantive dialogues and discussions focused on identifying coherent structures of the discipline of nursing at large and of the specific areas of specialization (Schlotfeldt, 1988). The structures include nursing, scientific, theoretical, philosophical, and clinical knowledge that is focused on the nursing domain and its phenomena. These dialogues take place in conferences, think tanks, and theme journal editions devoted to the development of middle-range and situation-specific theories focused on an aspect of nursing.

A second characteristic of this stage is the development of educational programs that are organized around substantive areas through the integration of theory, research, and practice—such as environment and health, symptom management, or transitions and health. It is also manifested in the ease by which nursing administrators, clinicians, and educators use theoretical nursing, and in the increasing dialogue among members of the discipline regarding matters related to knowledge, discovery, and development that is focused on and emanates from the domain of nursing.

A third characteristic of this stage is the evaluation of different aspects of theoretical nursing by members of the discipline representing nursing clinicians, teachers, administrators, researchers, and theoreticians. Evaluation is not limited to theory testing; it includes description, analysis, and critiques as well. Each of these processes is important in the development and progress of our discipline because of its diverse philosophical bases.

A fourth characteristic of this stage is the attention that members of the discipline give to the strategies of knowledge development that are congruent with the discipline's shared assumptions and that consider the conditions of holism, patterning, experience, and meaning (Newman, 1995).

A fifth characteristic is the involvement of members of specialty fields in developing theories that are pertinent to the phenomena of that particular field. This involvement does not preclude similar attention to theories related to phenomena of the domain of nursing at large.

A final characteristic is the systematic reappraisal of philosophical and theoretical underpinnings that have guided the definitions and the conceptualizations of the central concepts of the domain of nursing. An example of such discourse is the reappraisal of the definition of client in the nursing literature and the congruency of these definitions with domain assumptions (Allen, 1987).

Milestones in Theory Development

The progress and development of theoretical nursing is marked by several milestones, which are identified through an analysis of theoretical literature that appeared in selected nursing journals between 1950 and 1995. These milestones substantially changed the position of theory in nursing and profoundly influenced the further development of theoretical nursing. Each milestone is defined and briefly described here (Table 3-2). Identifying and defining these milestones challenges others to explore the impact each milestone may have had on the progress and development of nursing knowledge.

Prior to 1955—From Florence Nightingale to Nursing Research

The significant milestone of the period before 1955, which has influenced the subsequent development of all nursing science, was the establishment of the journal, *Nursing Research*, with the goal of reporting on scientific investigations for nursing by nurses

Table 3-2 ***Theory Development in Nursing: Milestones***

Prior to 1955	From Florence Nightingale to nursing research
1955–1960	Birth of nursing theory
1961–1965	Theory: A national goal for nursing
1966–1970	Theory development: A tangible goal for academics
1971–1975	Theory syntax
1976–1980	A time to reflect
1981–1985	Nursing theories' revival: Emergence of the domain concepts
1986–1990	From metatheory to concept development
1990–1995	Mid-range and situational theories

and others (Fig. 3-1). The journal's most significant goal was to encourage scientific productivity. The establishment of the journal confirmed that nursing is indeed a scientific discipline and that its progress will depend on whether or not nurses pursue truth through an avenue that respectable disciplines take, namely, research. Although Nightingale may have provided the beginning impetus for research and theory, her impact was most keenly felt in nursing education. Education of nurses had predominantly occurred in diploma programs, but there was a beginning unrest regarding a different route for nurses' education.

This period was otherwise uneventful for nursing theory, except that the establishment of nursing research publications provided the framework for a questioning attitude that may have set the stage for inquiries into theoretical nursing.

1955–1960—The Birth of Nursing Theory: The Columbia University Teachers College Approach

Although Florence Nightingale's ideas about nursing, focusing on the relationship between health and environment, were developed in the early 1900s, it was not until the mid-1950s that nurses began to articulate a theoretical view of nursing. Questions about the nature of nursing, its mission and goals, and about nurses' roles drove nurse educators to capture the answers to these questions and present them in a more coherent whole. These questions grew out of an interest in changes in educational preparation of nurses from diploma to baccalaureate programs and out of concerns about what to include or exclude in curricula and about what nurses needed to learn to function as nurses.

Columbia University's Teachers College offered graduate programs that focused on education and administration to prepare graduates as expert educators and administrators. Although the focus was not on nursing science or nursing theory, participants in this program must have debated such questions. Significantly, most theorists who offered a conception of nursing during that decade were educated at Teachers College; these were Peplau, Henderson, Hall, Abdellah, King, Wiedenbach, and Rogers (Table 3-3).

Being prepared in the functional roles and experiencing a sense of competency in preparing syllabi, staffing patterns, and so on may have freed the creative abilities of these scholars for other aspects of the scholarly process, such as theory development or conceptual model development. Therefore, it may have been other experiences and

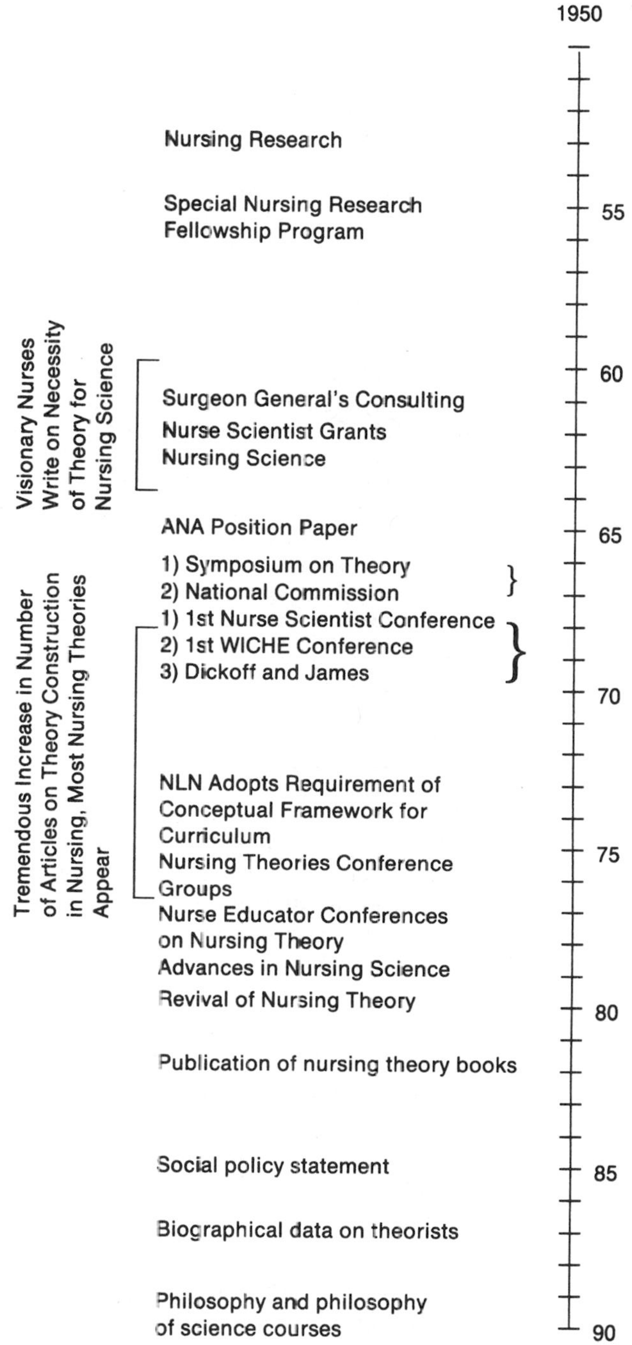

Figure 3–1 Chronology of the development of theoretical nursing.

Table 3-3 ***Nursing Theorists: 1950–1980***

1952	Hildegarde Peplau. *Interpersonal relations in nursing*. Also published 1962, 1963, 1969.
1955	Virginia Henderson. *Textbook of the principles and practice of nursing* (with B. Harmer). Also 1966, 1972, 1978.
1959	Dorothy Johnson. *A philosophy of nursing*. Also 1961, 1966, 1974.
1959	Lydia Hall. *A philosophy of nursing*. Also 1964 (and by others, 1975).
1960	Faye Abdellah. *Patient-centered approaches to nursing*. Also 1965, 1973.
1961	Ida Jean Orlando. *The dynamic nurse-patient relationship*.
1963	D. Howland and E. McDowell. A hospital system model.
1964	D. Howland and E. McDowell. The measurement of patient care: A conceptual framework.
1964	Joyce Travelbee. *Interpersonal aspects of nursing*. Also 1969, 1971, 1979.
1964	E. Wiedenbach. *Clinical nursing: A helping art*. Also 1967, 1969, 1970, 1977.
1966	Myra Levine. Adaptation and assessment.
1966	M. Harms and F. McDonald. A new curriculum design.
1967	Myra Levine. *Introduction to clinical nursing*. Also 1969, 1971, 1973.
1968	Imogene King. A conceptual framework of reference for nursing. Also 1971, 1975.
1969	Joyce Travelbee. *Interventions in psychiatric nursing*. Also 1971 (1979).
1970	Martha Rogers. *An introduction to the theoretical basis of nursing*. Also 1980.
1970	Sister Callista Roy. Adaptation: A conceptual framework for nursing. Also 1974, 1976, 1980, 1984.
1971	Imogene King. *Toward a theory for nursing: General concepts of human behavior.*
1971	Dorothea Orem. *Nursing: Concepts of practice*. Also 1981, 1982, 1985, 1991.
1972	Betty Neuman. The Betty Neuman health-care systems model. Also 1989.
1976	Josephine Patterson and L. Zderad. *Humanistic nursing*. Also 1988.

For complete citations, use Chapter 21 under appropriate authors.

programs that directly influenced these scholars in their theoretical pursuits (eg, Rogers' doctoral preparation at Johns Hopkins). However, whatever the other experiences were, it appears that the philosophy of Teachers College indirectly left an impact, not only on psychiatric theory and research, but also on theoretical thinking in all of nursing (Sills, 1977). Asking and answering questions about the influence of scholarly environments on preparing productive scholars may have stimulated the search for the nature of scholarship, which may have led to questions related to the nature of nursing identity.

Peplau (1952), using Harry Stack Sullivan's theory title and concepts to develop her own, produced the first articulated concept of nursing as an interpersonal relationship with components of interpersonal processes central to nursing needing to be elucidated and analyzed. The field of psychiatric nursing subsequently was substantially developed using Peplau's ideas. Other theories that evolved in the 1960s were based on those early conceptions of nursing. For example, Virginia Henderson, with Bershan Harmer, developed the early seeds of a nursing theory that was published in the mid-1950s in a textbook on the principles and practice of nursing.

The request from the International Council of Nursing (ICN) to define nursing and its mission led to the subsequent ICN statement in 1958 that appeared in a publication with wide distribution and that was adapted internationally (Henderson, 1966, p. 15).

The message given by both Peplau and Henderson was that nursing has a specific and unique mission and that this mission has some order and organization that can be communicated. These articulated wholes represented the beginnings of theories in nursing.

Abdellah's nursing theory, evolving from her work at Columbia University, is another example of the influence of that school on theoretical nursing (Abdellah, Beland, Martin, and Matheney, 1961). Abdellah's doctoral dissertation in 1953 at Teachers College, under the leadership of Hildegard Peplau, focused on determining covert aspects of nursing problems. The results of her research were subsequently published in *Nursing Research*, marking the beginning of her attempts at theorizing the nursing care process. Her conceptualization of nursing care evolved from the dissertation research and from another study completed in 1955 on the needs of patients for nursing care. The latter was based on data collected from patients, nurses, and doctors. Abdellah developed her conception of what nursing is by focusing attention on patients rather than on techniques (Abdellah, Beland, Martin, and Matheney, 1961).

Other theorists' ideas were formulated around the need for a binding framework to guide curricula, but their writing and publications did not have the instant impact that Peplau's, Henderson's, and Abdellah's had on theoretical nursing. Their conceptions were slow to have an impact on nursing. Orem's ideas were first published in a guide for developing a curriculum for practical nursing in 1959. Patient needs were also the focus. Hall developed, in 1959, and implemented, in 1963, a concept of nursing based on needs and interpersonal relations at the Loeb Center for Nursing and Rehabilitation. One can see the influence of both Peplau and Henderson in her writing (Hall, 1963).

Independent of the Teachers College group of theorists, Johnson was beginning to play a central role in conceptualizing nursing. Johnson's (1959) analysis of the nature of science in nursing was undoubtedly a milestone in drawing attention to the potential of nursing as a scientific discipline and in advocating the development of its unique knowledge base. At that time Johnson tentatively suggested that nursing knowledge is based on a theory of nursing diagnosis that is distinct and different from medical diagnosis. The substantive matter for such diagnosis, the beginning of Johnson's theory, was starting to be formulated at this time. (See Chap. 21 for appropriate citations for each theorist.)

Another milestone in nursing progress was the establishment of the special nursing research fellowship program to facilitate, support, and encourage nurses' education for research careers.

1961–1965—Theory: A National Goal for Nursing

From a reduced conception of a human being as "an illness" or "a surgery," with signs and symptoms, nursing theory, in the late 1950s, refocused nursing attention on the individual as a set of needs and nursing as a set of unique functions. Still, a reductionist approach to nursing existed. The 1960s, with its turbulent society, the Camelot goals of harmony and coexistence, and the influence of Peplau may have prompted the refocusing of nursing from its stated mission of meeting patients' needs to the goal of establishing a relationship between the nurse and client. If relationships are effectively established through interpersonal relationships (as previously articulated by Peplau, 1952, and as advocated by a new group of theorists), then nursing care can meet the needs of the patient—not as defined by nurses but as perceived by the patient.

During this period, the Yale School of Nursing's position, influenced by the Columbia Teachers College graduates who became faculty members at Yale, was beginning to be formulated. To them, nursing was considered a process rather than an end, an interaction rather than content, and a relationship between two human beings rather than an interaction between unrelated nurse and patient. Social forces that helped the Yale group to develop their ideas into concepts of nursing were multifold. Federal grant money was available for preparation ranging from psychiatric nursing to teaching positions, for identifying psychiatric concepts in nursing, and for developing an integrated curriculum. The availability of time and resources, therefore, was significant in providing the necessary push as well as the appropriate environment in which to reflect on nursing's mission and goals.

Although the work of the faculty of the Yale School of Nursing may have profoundly influenced nursing research in the United States in the 1960s, its influence on theory was not as marked at the time. There was a revival of that impact in the 1980s as nurses acknowledged Yale's strategies for theory development; this is evidenced by the reconsideration of Orlando's work (Schmieding, 1983, 1987, 1988) and by the paradigmatic shift in nursing research to phenomenology (Oiler, 1982; Omery, 1983; Silva and Rothbart, 1984). These writers' conceptualization of nursing therefore was not the milestone that prompted the evolution of the next stage of theory. Rather, it was the American Nurses' Association's (ANA) position paper in which nursing was defined as care, cure, and coordination and in which theory development was identified as a most significant goal for the profession of nursing that may have been influential in the further development of theoretical nursing (ANA, 1965).

Two other significant developments occurred during this period. Federal support was provided to nurses wishing to pursue doctoral education in one of the basic sciences. The graduates of these programs are those who, in the mid-1970s, further developed metatheoretical ideas. The second development was inauguration of the journal, *Nursing Science.* Although short-lived, it was a medium for exchange of ideas on theory and science in nursing and a confirmation that nursing is an evolving science with theoretical principles and underpinnings.

1966–1970—Theory Development: A Tangible Goal for Academics

With the ANA's recommendation that theory development was of highest priority in the profession, and with the availability of federal support, a symposium sponsored by Case Western Reserve University was held as part of the nursing science program. This symposium was divided into three parts. The part focusing on theory was held on October 7, 1967 and was considered a milestone during this period (Table 3-4). The papers were published in *Nursing Research* a year later. These publications supported what were previously considered simply perceptions and conceptions of theoretical nursing from an isolated number of theorists. Not only did a group of significant people in nursing

Table 3-4 ***Theory Development in Nursing: A Historical Perspective***

1860	Florence Nightingale addresses the need for research and the educational preparation of nurses.
1900–1950	Diploma schools served as major source of nurses—the Flexner Report for Medicine.
1952	*Nursing Research* first published.
1955	Establishment of the Special Nurse Research Fellowship Program in the National Institute of Health, Division of Nursing
1959	D.E. Johnson. The nature of a science of nursing. *Nursing Outlook, 7,* 292–294.
1960	R.N. Schlotfeldt. Reflections on nursing research. *American Journal of Nursing.* 60(4), 492–494. (The primary task of nursing research is to develop theories that serve as a guide to practice.)
1961	Surgeon General's Consultant Group on Nursing appointed to advise the Surgeon General on nursing needs and to identify the appropriate role of the federal government in assuring adequate nursing services in the nation. This group strongly supported nursing research and recommended a substantial increase in funds.
1961	D.E. Johnson. Patterns in professional nursing education. *Nursing Outlook,* 9, 608. (Nursing science may evolve more easily through the identification of common but major problems of patients that are of direct concern to nursing.)
1962	Nurse Scientist Graduate Training Grants Program
1963	*Nursing Science* first published
1963	M.E. Rogers. Some comments on the theoretical basis of nursing practice. *Nursing Science,* 1, 11–13. (The theoretical base of nursing practice is nursing science . . . a body of scientific knowledge characterized by descriptive, explanatory, and predictive principles . . . developed through synthesis and resynthesis of selected knowledges from the humanities and the biological, physical, and social sciences. . . It assumes its own "unique scientific" mix through selection and patterning of these knowledges.)
1963	M.E. Rogers. Building a strong educational foundation. *American Journal of Nursing,* 63(6), 941. (The explanatory and predictive principles of nursing make possible nursing diagnosis and knowledgeable intervention toward predictable goals . . . nursing science is not additive, but creative.)
1964	D.E. Johnson. Nursing and health education. *International Journal of Nursing Studies,*1, 219. (Nurses must be socialized as scholars and must develop commitment to inquiry and skill in the use of scientific knowledge.)
	J.S. Berthold. Theoretical and empirical clarification of concepts. *Nursing Science,* 406–422.
	M.I. Brown. (Spring). Research in the development of nursing theory. *Nursing Research,* 13, 109–112. (Assess progress of theory development in nursing and emphasizes need for explicit relationship of research to theory.)
	F.S. Wald and R. C. Leonard. (1964). Toward development of nursing practice theory. *Nursing Research,* 13(4), 309–313.
1965	American Nurses' Association. Educational preparation for nurse practitioners and assistants to nurses: A position paper.
	P. Putnam. A conceptual approach to nursing theory. *Nursing Science,* 430–442.
1967	V.S. Cleland. The use of existing theories. *Nursing Research,* 16(2), 118–121.
1967	L.H. Conant. (Spring). A search for resolution of existing problems in nursing. *Nursing Research,* 16, 115.
	Symposium on Theory Development in Nursing. (Reported in *Nursing Research,* 1968, 17(3).)
1967–1970	National Commission for the Study of Nursing and Nursing Education, Jerome F. Lysaught, director.

(continued)

Table 3-4 ***Theory Development in Nursing: A Historical Perspective*** *(Continued)*

1968	First Nurse Scientist Conference on The Nature of Science in Nursing. Sponsored by University of Colorado School of Nursing, Dr. Madeleine Leininger, chair. (Reported in *Nursing Research,* 1969, 18(5).)
	First Annual WCHEN Communicating Research Conference
1968	J. Dickoff and P. James. A theory of theories: A position paper. *Nursing Research,* 17(3), 197–206. (Professional disciplines are obligated to go a step further than explanation and prediction in theory construction, to the development of prescriptive theory.)
	J. Dickoff, P. James, and E. Wiedenbach. Theory in a practice discipline: Part I. Practice oriented theory. *Nursing Research,* 17(5), 415–435.
	Idem. theory in a practice discipline: Part II. Practice oriented theory. *Nursing Research,* 17(6), 545–554.
	R. Ellis. (1968). Characteristics of significant theories. *Nursing Research,* 17(3), 217–222.
	D.E. Johnson. Theory in nursing: Borrowed and unique. *Nursing Research,* 17(3), 206–209.
	M. Moore. Nursing: A scientific discipline. Forum, 7(4), 340–347.
	J.L. Sasmor. Toward developing theory in nursing. *Nursing Forum,* 7(2), 191–200.
1969	G. Mathwig. Nursing science: The theoretical core of nursing knowledge. *Image,* 3, 9–14, 20–23.
	R. McKay. Theories, models, and systems for nursing. *Nursing Research,* 18(5), 393–399.
	C.M. Norris (Ed.). Proceedings: First, second, and third nursing theory conference. University of Kansas, 1969 and 1970.
1971	F. Cleary. A theoretical model: Its potential for adaptation to nursing. *Image,* 4(1), 14–20.
	I.M. Harris. Theory building in nursing: A review of the literature. *Image,* 4(1), 6–10.
	M. Jacobson. Qualitative data as a potential source of theory in nursing. *Image,* 4(1), 10–14.
	J.F. Murphy (Ed.). *Theoretical issues in professional nursing.* New York: Appleton-Century-Crofts.
	I. Walker. Toward a clearer understanding of the concept of nursing theory. *Nursing Research,* 20(5), 428–435.
1972	M. Newman. Nursing's theoretical evolution. *Nursing Outlook,* 20(7), 449–453.
	NLN Council of Baccalaureate and Higher Degree Programs approved its "Criteria for the Appraisal of Baccalaureate and Higher Degree Programs in Nursing," including criterion stating that curricula should be based on a conceptual framework.
1973	M.E. Hardy. The nature of theories. In M. Hardy (Ed.), *Theoretical foundations for nursing.* New York: MSS Information Corporation.
	The Nursing Development Conference Group. (1973). *Concept formulation in nursing: Process and product.* Boston: Little, Brown & Co.
1974	M.E. Hardy. Theories: Components, development, evaluation. *Nursing Research,* 18, 100–107.
	A. Jacox. Theory construction in nursing: An overview. *Nursing Research,* 23, 4–13.
	D.E. Johnson. Development of theory: Requisite for nursing as a primary health profession. *Nursing Research,* 18, 372–377.
1975	Nursing Theories Conference Group. (Formed out of a concern for the need for materials to help students of nursing understand and use nursing theories in nursing practice.)

(continued)

Table 3-4 Theory Development in Nursing: A Historical Perspective (Continued)

1978	Advances in Nursing Science. S.K. Donaldson and D. Crowley. The Discipline of Nursing. *Nursing Outlook* 26(2), 113–120.
1979	M.A. Newman. *Theory Development in Nursing*. Philadelphia: F. A. Davis.
1982	M.J. Kim and D.A. Moritz. *Classifications of Nursing Diagnosis*. New York: McGraw-Hill.
1983	L.O. Walker and K.C. Avant. *Strategies for Theory Construction in Nursing*. New York: Appleton-Century-Crofts.
	J. Fitzpatrick and A. Whall. *Conceptual Models of Nursing: Analysis and Application*. R.J. Brady Co.
	P.L. Chinn and M.K. Jacobs. *Theory and Nursing: A Systematic Approach*. St. Louis: C.V. Mosby.
	H.S. Kim. *The Nature of Theoretical Thinking in Nursing*. New York: Appleton-Century-Crofts.
	I.W. Clements and F.B. Roberts. *Family Health: A Theoretical Approach to Nursing Care*. New York: John Wiley & Sons.
	P.L. Chinn. *Advances in Nursing Theory Development*. Rockville: Aspen Systems.
1984	J. Fawcett. *Analysis and Evaluation of Conceptual Models*. Philadelphia: F.A. Davis.

See Chapter 21 for evidence of increasing publications related to each of the theorists.

get together to discuss theory in nursing, but the official scientific journal of the field recognized the significance of these proceedings by publishing them.

Nurses also received confirmation from two philosophers and a nurse theorist who had been involved in teaching nurses at Yale for 5 years that theories are significant for the practice of nursing, that the practice of nursing is amenable to theoretical development, and that nurses are capable of developing theories (Dickoff, James, and Wiedenbach, 1968). The presentations and the subsequent publications influenced the discipline of nursing profoundly, as evidenced by the classic nature of those publications and by the acceleration in publications related to theory. Nursing theory was defined, goals for theory development were set, and the confirmation of outsiders (people outside the field of nursing, nonnursing philosophers) was productive.

Although the insiders (the nurse theorists) may have charted the course of action for theory development, the doubts and skepticism about theory (from the critics who viewed theory as scientific and as evolving from an empirical, positivistic model) that dominated nursing until then were somewhat squelched by the presentations and discussions that went on during that significant meeting in which Dickoff and colleagues presented their metatheory of nursing. (The evidence for skepticism is derived from omission rather than commission. When theories were used during this period, they were used in conjunction with education and not in practice or, except for the New York and Yale students, in research. Refer to the theory literature in Chap. 21 for documentation of the omission.)

The metatheorists in nursing started their questioning during this period. Questions of this era were related to what types of theories nurses should develop rather than to the nature of the substantive content of those theories. The first metatheorists were Ellis (1968) and Wiedenbach (Dickoff, James, and Wiedenbach, 1968). Dickoff and James (1968), philosophers by training, addressed metatheoretical concerns that focused on types of theories and content of theories. Debates occurred about whether the theories should be basic or borrowed, pure or applied, descriptive or prescriptive.

Accomplishments at this stage can be summarized as:

- Nursing is a field amenable to theorizing.
- Nurses can develop theories.
- Practice is a rich area for theory.
- Practice theory should be the goal for theory development in nursing.
- Nurses' highest theory goal should be prescriptive theory, but it is acceptable to develop descriptive and explanatory theories.

1971–1975—Theory Syntax

There was a period, just before the research enterprise in nursing focused on answering significant questions in the field, when nurse researchers focused on discussing and writing about research methodology. A parallel exists in the area of theory. The period from 1966 to 1970 resulted in a beginning focus on theory development, which was followed by attempts at identifying the structural components of theory (see Table 3-4). Metatheorists dominated this period. The emphasis was on articulating, defining, and explicating theory components and on the processes inherent in theory analysis and critique. Nurse theorists were no longer questioning whether nursing needed a theory or whether or not theory could be developed in nursing; questions of this period focused on what is meant by theory (Ellis, 1968, 1971; Walker, 1971), on what are the major components of theory (Hardy, 1974; Jacox, 1974), and on ways to analyze and critique theories (Duffey and Muhlenkamp, 1974). Education of nurses in basic, natural, and social sciences through the federally supported nurse–scientist programs produced a cadre of nurses who shared a common goal: the establishment of the unique knowledge base of nursing. Discussions of what constituted theory and the identification of theory syntax seemed to be the means to achieve that goal.

Just before the close of this period, a milestone was achieved. Just as the ANA acknowledged the significance of theory development during the previous period, the National League for Nursing not only acknowledged theory but also made theory-based curriculum a requirement for accreditation. Schools of nursing were expected to select, develop, and implement a conceptual framework for their curricula. This requirement for accreditation was both a moving force and a major barrier to theory development. To use theory for curriculum development further heightened awareness of academic nursing to the significance of theory and to the available nursing theories. However, this requirement diverted the goal of developing theories for practice (those theories that would answer significant questions related to practice) to the goal of using theory for education. Nevertheless, this milestone increased the use of theory and discussions about theory and prompted more writing about the syntax of theory to help academicians and students understand and use theories in curriculum and teaching. The limited number of journals that acknowledge and promote theoretical nursing, the focus on promoting the publication of empirical research findings, and the growing financial difficulties of some journals were barriers to written exchanges on theory and theorizing.

1976–1980—A Time to Reflect

Nurse theorists were invited to participate in presentations, discussions, and debates in conferences sponsored by nurse educators, marking a significant milestone in the progress of theoretical nursing. A national conference devoted to nursing theory and the formation of the Nursing Theory Think Tank in 1978 further supported the direction of the profession toward the utilization of existing theory and the development of further theory to describe and explain nursing phenomena, to predict relationships, and to guide nursing care (Preview, 1978). This was the time for nurse academicians, who had used nursing theories as guiding frameworks for curricula, to consider putting theory to other uses, particularly in practice.

The inauguration of the journal, *Advances in Nursing Science*, with its focus on "the full range of activities involved in the development of science," including "theory construction, concept, and analysis" and the application of theory, was another significant milestone during this period (Chinn, 1978) (see Table 3-4). The focus of the journal on theory and theory development added more support to the significance of theoretical nursing and simultaneously gave nurses who were interested in theory the necessary medium in which to present and discuss their ideas. It allowed for the questioning and debate that is necessary for the development of theoretical bases in any discipline.

This period is characterized by questioning if nursing's progress would benefit from the adoption of a single paradigm and a single theory of truth (Carper, 1978; Silva, 1977). More sophisticated debates about what types of theory nursing needs (Beckstrand, 1978a, 1978b, 1980) and about issues in theory (Crawford, Dufault, and Rudy, 1979) appeared in nursing literature. A more solid commitment to the development of theory emerged, combined with a specific direction to nurses' efforts in theory development (Donaldson and Crowley, 1978; Hardy, 1978). The links between theory and research were considered and discussed (Batey, 1977; Fawcett and Downs, 1986), the path was charted for bridging the theory–research gaps between theory and practice (Barnum, 1990), theory and philosophy were examined (Silva, 1977), and the role of each in the development of nursing knowledge was clarified (see Fig. 2-1). Domain concepts were beginning to be identified, and their acceptance was demonstrated in the next period.

1981–1985—Nursing Theories' Revival: Emergence of the Domain Concepts

In this period, theory began to be questioned less and pluralism debated less. This period was characterized by an acceptance of the significance of theory for nursing and, furthermore, by the inevitability of the need for the development of nursing theory. Doctoral programs in nursing incorporated theory into their curricula and considered it a core content area, ranking it at the top of all other core content (Beare, Gray, and Ptak, 1981).

A review of theory literature during this period reveals the lack of debate on whether or not to use theory–practice versus basic theory or borrowed versus nursing theory. Instead, there appeared to be more writing on the examination of nursing theories in relation to different research and practice problems and on comparisons between the different conceptualizations (Jacobson, 1984; Spangler and Spangler, 1983). Questions of this period included:

- What have we learned from theory?
- How can we use theory?

The second question was one that clinicians began to ask and for which there have been many useful dialogues.

Knowledge of the syntax emerging as a previous milestone was used to analyze existing theories (Fawcett, 1984; Fitzpatrick and Whall, 1983). In addition, existing theories came to be thought of as the means to develop unique nursing knowledge. Concepts central to nursing were identified, and existing theory, the source of the identified concepts, was in turn re-examined in terms of further development and refinement (Crawford, 1982; Reeder, 1984).

This period was characterized by the nursing *theory advocates* who pleaded for the use of a nursing perspective in general or for the specific utilization of nursing theory (Adam, 1983; Dickson and Lee-Villasenor, 1982). (See *Advances in Nursing Science, Journal of Nursing Administration*, and *American Journal of Nursing* for examples of the American advocates and *Journal of Advanced Nursing* for examples of international advocates.) Another group also emerged during this period: the *theory synthesizers.* The difference between the advocates and the synthesizers was in the level of the scope of analysis. The advocates promoted nursing theory and demonstrated its use in research projects or in a limited practice arena. The synthesizers went beyond that limited use to describe and analyze how nursing theory had influenced nursing practice, education, research, and administration. The synthesizers are exemplified by, but not limited to, Fitzpatrick and Whall (1983, 1996) and Fawcett (1984, 1995). The Rogerian First National Conference (1983) and subsequent ones, in which theoreticians, practitioners, and researchers discussed the utility of Rogers' theory from different perspectives, is a different example of an effective synthesis of different uses of a theory. The planners of this conference belong to the group of theory synthesizers.

A few of the synthesizers graduated from New York University in the mid-1970s. It is too early to determine a pattern among the synthesizers as a school of thought. One thing that cannot be ignored is made evident by a review of the titles of doctoral dissertations in nursing from New York University from 1941 to 1983, which affirm the significance of that school in nursing research and nursing theory. Most of the titles indicate a nursing perspective, and there appears to have been an attempt at cumulative knowledge development. How and in what ways such a pattern may have influenced and may continue to influence theory development is an area worth further investigation and analysis.

This period was characterized by an acceptance of theory as a tool that emanates from significant practice problems and can be used for practice and research. This period was also characterized by a greater clarity in the relationship between theory and research than between theory and practice.

One remaining confusion during this period was related to semantics. Conceptual models were referred to as conceptual frameworks, theories, metatheories, paradigms, and metaparadigms and, when differentiated, boundaries were not totally clear and properties not entirely distinct.

1986–1990—From Metatheory to Concept Development

Three characteristics of this milestone were epistemological debates, ontological analyses, and an increase in concept development and analyses. The epistemological debates included questions related to describing alternative approaches to knowledge development, such as the use of phenomenology, critical theory, and feminist or empiricist methodologies (eg, Allen, 1985; Allen, Benner, and Diekelman, 1986; Hagell, 1989; Leonard, 1989). Although the debates were focused on knowledge development in general rather than on theoretical development of the discipline, these debates were related as well to the development of theoretical nursing.

Effective analyses were those that focused on ontological beliefs related to central nursing concepts, for example, environment (Chopoorian, 1986; Stevens, 1989), and health (Allen, 1985, 1986; Benner, 1984). These analyses added substantially to a more contextual approach to understanding each concept. These analyses also raised the awareness and the consciousness of nurses to the necessity of using frameworks that allow for an integrative, holistic, and contextual description of nursing phenomena, phenomena that go beyond the individual clients. Such frameworks, these authors demonstrated, maintained the integrity of the basic ontological beliefs that have historically guided nursing practice, for example, holism, integrated responses, and relationship with environment.

The third property of this milestone was an increase in writings related to concept development. These developments were different from earlier theory developments that included answers to such general questions as "What is nursing?" These analyses were more practice oriented, were integrative, and represented early attempts in the development of single domain theories. This was also the period in which a plea for substance was made (Chinn, 1987; Downs, 1988; Meleis, 1987; Woods, 1987). These authors echoed the sentiment of other discipline members by urging discourse that was more focused on substantive issues that were confronting health care recipients.

Process debates became more a potential force for theory development when and if they were grounded in substantive disciplinary content. Therefore, instead of debating whether critical theory or feminist theories were more appropriate as a philosophical base for the discipline, one may argue whether it was more effective to view environment or comfort from either or both perspectives. Such substantive debates then would add to or revise parameters and dimensions of that area of knowledge.

1991–1995 Mid-Range and Situation Specific

One significant milestone that marks the considerable progress in knowledge development in nursing is manifested in the numerous mid-range theories that evolved during this period. Some of these were labeled as theories (eg, Younger's Theory of Mastery

[1991] or Mishel's Theory of Uncertainty [1990]). Others were considered in the process of becoming theories. (See Funk, Tornquist, Champage, Copp, and Wiese [1990] for discussions about key aspects of recovery and Hagerty, Lynch-Sauer, Patusky, and Bouwsema [1993] for their emerging theory of human relatedness.) Mid-range theories focus on specific nursing phenomena that reflect and emerge from nursing practice and focus on clinical process (Meleis, 1987). They provide a conceptual focus and a mental image that reflect the discipline's values, but they do not provide prescriptions for practice or specific practice guidelines (Chinn, 1994).

Situation-specific theories may be emerging as another milestone. They are theories that are more clinically specific, theories that reflect a particular context, and may include blueprints for action. They are less abstract than mid-range theories but far more abstract than individual nurses' frameworks for practice designed for a specific situation. These situation-specific theories may emerge from synthesizing and integrating research findings and clinical exemplars about a specific situation or population with the intent of giving a framework or blueprint to understand the particular situation of a group of clients. They are theories that are developed to answer a set of coherent questions about situations that are limited in scope and in focus. For example, a conceptualization of patterns of responses to health–illness transitions of Middle Eastern immigrants could be developed from the results of research studies, the clinical exemplars, and the experience of nurses in their care of this population (Meleis, Isenberg, Koerner, Lacey, and Stern, 1995). An example is work that has focused on Middle Eastern immigrants (Afghans, Iranians, Egyptians, and Arabs), supported by similar work on these populations in their native countries, which helps illuminate patterns of behavior and responses before immigration and helps in providing an historical and sociocultural context for the responses of immigrants in their new country.

Conclusion

This chapter presented significant historical themes that are related to an interest in theoretical nursing. Progress and development in theoretical nursing was defined in terms of stages and milestones. A view of historical development offers a significant perspective on which current and future theoretical thinking can be built. Analysis of present development is deficient without tracing these historical themes.

Acknowledgments

The first part of this chapter is based on: A.I. Meleis (1983). The evolving nursing scholarliness. In P.L. Chinn (Ed.), *Advances in nursing theory development*, pp. 19–34. Reprinted with permission of Aspen Publishers, Inc., 1983.

REFERENCES

Abdellah, F.G., Beland, I.L., Martin, A., and Matheney, R.V. (1961). *Patient-centered approaches to nursing.* New York: Macmillan.

Adam, E. (1983). Frontiers of nursing in the 21st century: Development of models and theories on the concept of nursing. *Journal of Advanced Nursing*, 8, 41–45.

Allen, D. (1985). Nursing research and social control: Alternative models of science that emphasize understanding and emancipation. *Image: The Journal of Nursing Scholarship*, XVII(2), 58–64.

Allen, D.G. (1986). Using philosophical and historical methodologies to understand the concept of health. In P.L. Chinn (Ed.), *Nursing research methodology: Issues and implementation*. Rockville, MD: Aspen Systems.

Allen, D.G. (1987). The social policy statement: A reappraisal. *Advances in Nursing Science*, 10(1), 39–48.

Allen, D.G., Benner, P., and Diekelman, N.K. (1986). Three paradigms for nursing research: Methodological implications. In P.C. Chinn (Ed.), *Nursing research methodology: Issues and implementations*. Rockville, MD: Aspen Systems.

American Nurses' Association. (1965). Educational preparation for nurse practitioners and assistants of nurses. *American Journal of Nursing*, 65(12), 106–111.

Barnum, B.S. (1990). *Nursing theory: Analysis, application and evaluation* (3rd ed.). Boston: Little, Brown.

Batey, M.V. (1977). Conceptualization: Knowledge and logic guiding empirical research. *Nursing Research*, 26(5), 324–329.

Beare, P.G., Gray, C.J., and Ptak, H.F. (1981). Doctoral curricula in nursing. *Nursing Outlook*, May, 311–316.

Beckstrand, J. (1978a). The notion of a practice theory and the relationship of scientific and ethical knowledge to practice. *Research in Nursing and Health*, 1(3), 131–136.

Beckstrand, J. (1978b). The need for a practice theory as indicated by the knowledge used in conduct of practice. *Research in Nursing and Health*, 1(4), 175–179.

Beckstrand, J. (1980). A critique of several conceptions of practice theory in nursing. *Research in Nursing and Health*, 3(2) 69–80.

Benner, P. (1984). *From novice to expert: Excellence and power in clinical nursing practice*. Menlo Park, CA: Addison-Wesley.

Benner, P. (Ed.). (1994). *Interpretive phenomenology: Embodiment, caring, and ethics in health and illness*. Thousand Oaks, CA: Sage.

Bradshaw, A. (1995). What are nurses doing to patients? A review of theories or nursing past and present. *Journal of Clinical Nursing*, 4, 81–92.

Carper, B.A. (1978). Practice oriented theory: Part 1. Fundamental patterns of knowing in nursing. *Advances in Nursing Science*, 1(1), 13–23.

Chinn, P.L. (1978). A model for theory development in nursing. *Advances in Nursing Science*, 1(1), 1–11.

Chinn, P.L. (1987). Response: Revision and passion. *Scholarly Inquiry for Nursing Practice: An International Journal*, 1(1), 21–24.

Chinn, P.L. (1994). *Developing substance: Mid-range theory in nursing* [preface]. Gaithersburg, MD: Aspen.

Chopoorian, T.J. (1986). Reconceptualizing the environment. In P. Moccia (Ed.), *New approaches to theory development*. New York: National League for Nursing.

Crawford, G. (1982). The concept of pattern in nursing: Conceptual development and measurement. *Advances in Nursing Science*, 5(1), 1–6.

Crawford, G., Dufault, K., and Rudy, E. (1979). Evolving issues in theory development. *Nursing Outlook*, 27(5), 346–351.

Dickoff, J. and James, P. (1968). A theory of theories: A position paper. *Nursing Research*, 17(3), 197–203.

Dickoff, J., James, P., and Wiedenbach, E. (1968). Theory in practice discipline: Part 1. Practice oriented theory. *Nursing Research*, 17(5), 415–435.

Dickson, G., and Lee-Villasenor, H. (1982). Nursing theory and practice: A self-care approach. *Advances in Nursing Science*, 5(1), 29–40.

Donaldson, S.K., and Crowley, D. (1978). The discipline of nursing. *Nursing Outlook*, 26(2), 113–120.

Downs, F. (1988). Doctoral education: Our claim to the future. *Nursing Outlook*, 36(1), 18–20.

Duffey, M., and Muhlenkamp, A.F. (1974). A framework for theory analysis. *Nursing Outlook*, 22(9), 570–574.

Ellis, R. (1968). Characteristics of significant theories. *Nursing Research*, 17(3), 217–222.

Ellis, R. (1971). Commentary on Walker's "Toward a clearer understanding of the concept of nursing theory." *Nursing Research*, 20(6), 493–494.

Ellis, R. (1983). Philosophic inquiry. In H. Werley and J. Fitzpatrick (Eds.), *Annual review of nursing research*. New York: Springer.

Fangary, A.S. (1980). *Rofaida: First nurse in Islam*. Kuwait: Dar el Kalaam.

Fawcett, J. (1984). *Analysis and evaluation of conceptual models of nursing*. Philadelphia: F.A. Davis.

Fawcett, J. (1995). *Analysis and evaluation of conceptual models of nursing* (3rd ed.). Philadelphia: F.A. Davis.

Fawcett, J., and Downs, F.S. (1986). *The relationship of theory and research*. East Norwalk, CT: Appleton-Century-Crofts.

Fitzpatrick, J., and Whall, A. (1983). *Conceptual models of nursing: Analysis and application*. Bowie, MD: Robert J. Brady Company.

Fitzpatrick, J., and Whall, A. (Eds.). (1996). *Conceptual models of nursing: Analysis and application*. Stamford, CT Appleton & Lange.

Fry, S.T. (1989). Toward a theory of nursing ethics. *Advances in Nursing Science*, 11, 9–22.

Funk S.G.,Tornquist, E.M., Champage, M.T., Copp, L.A., and Wiese, R.A. (Eds.). (1990). *Key aspects of recovery: Improving nutrition, rest, and mobility*. New York: Springer.

Gortner, S.R. (1980). Nursing science in transition. *Nursing Research*, 29(3), 180–183.

Gortner, S.R., and Nahm, H. (1977). An overview of nursing research in the United States. *Nursing Research*, 26(1), 10–33.

Hagell, R.I. (1989). Nursing knowledge: Women's knowledge. A sociological perspective. *Journal of Advanced Nursing*, 14, 226–233.

Hagerty, B.M.K., Lynch-Sauer, J., Patusky, K.L., and Bouwsema, M. (1993). An emerging theory of human relatedness. *Image: The Journal of Nursing Scholarship*, 25(4), 291–296.

Hall, L.E. (1963). Center for nursing. *Nursing Outlook*, 11, 805–806

Hardy, M.E. (1974). The nature of theories. In M.E. Hardy (Ed.), *Theoretical foundations for nursing*. New York: MSS Information Corporation.

Hardy, M.E. (1978). Practice oriented theory: Part 1. Perspectives on nursing theory. *Advances in Nursing Science*, 1(1), 37–48.

Henderson, V. (1966). *Nature of nursing.* New York: Macmillan.

Jacobson, S.F. (1984). A semantic differential for external comparison of conceptual nursing models. *Advances in Nursing Science*, 6(2), 58–70.

Jacox, A. (1974). Theory construction in nursing: An overview. *Nursing Research*, 23(1), 4–13.

Johnson, D.E. (1959). A philosophy of nursing. *Nursing Outlook*, 7(4), 198–200.

Johnson, D.E. (1980). The behavioral system model for nursing. In J.P. Riehl and C. Roy (Eds.), *Conceptual models for nursing practice* (2nd ed.). New York: Appleton-Century-Crofts.

Kuhn, T.S. (1970). The structure of scientific revolutions. In Neurath, O. (Ed.), *International encyclopedia of unified science* (2nd ed., Vol. 2). Chicago: University of Chicago Press.

Leininger, M. (1968). The research critique: Nature, function, and art. *Nursing Research*, 17, 444–449.

Leonard, V.W. (1989). A Heideggerian phenomenologic perspective on the concept of the person. *Advances in Nursing Science*, 11(4), 40–55.

Levine, M.E. (1967). The four conservation principles of nursing. *Nursing Forum*, 6(1), 45–59.

Meleis, A.I. (1987). Revisions in knowledge development: Being vs. becoming or being and becoming. *Health Care for Women International*, 8, 199–217.

Meleis, A.I., Isenberg, M., Koerner, J.E., Lacey, B., and Stern, P. (1995). Diversity, marginalization, and culturally competent health care issues in knowledge development. Washington, DC: American Academy of Nursing.

Merton, R.K. (1973). *The sociology of science: Theoretical and empirical investigations.* Chicago: University of Chicago Press.

Mishel, M.H. (1990). Reconceptualizing of the uncertainty in illness theory. *Image: The Journal of Nursing Scholarship*, 22, 256–262.

Newman, M.A. (1995). Theory for nursing practice. *Nursing Science Quarterly*, 7(4), 79–85.

Nightingale, F. (1946). *Notes on nursing: What it is and what it is not.* Philadelphia: J.B. Lippincott.

Nursing Theory Think Tank. (1979). *Advances in Nursing Science*, 1(3), 105.

Oiler, C. (1982). The phenomenological approach in nursing research. *Nursing Research*, 31(3), 178–181.

Omery, A. (1983). Phenomenology: A method for nursing research. *Advances in Nursing Science*, 5, 49–63.

Orem, D.E. (1971). *Nursing: Concepts of practice.* New York: McGraw-Hill.

Orem, D.E. (1985). *Nursing: Concepts of practice* (3rd ed.). New York: McGraw-Hill.

Peplau, H.E. (1952). *Interpersonal relations in nursing.* New York: G.P. Putnam's Sons.

Preview: The Second Annual Nurse Educator Conference. (1978). *Nurse Educator*, 3(6), 37–39.

Reeder, F. (1984). Philosophical issues in the Rogerian science of unitary human beings. *Advances in Nursing Science*, 6(2), 14–23.

Rogerian First National Conference. (1983, June). New York University, New York.

Rogers, M. (1970). *An introduction to the theoretical basis of nursing.* Philadelphia: F.A. Davis.

Roy, C.L. (1995). Developing nursing knowledge: Practice issues raised from four philosophical perspectives. *Nursing Science Quarterly*, 8(2), 79–85.

Sarter, B. (1987). Evolutionary idealism: A philosophical foundation for holistic nursing theory. *Advances in Nursing Science*, 9(2), 1–9.

Schlotfeldt, R.M. (1988). Structuring nursing knowledge: A priority for creating nursing's future. *Nursing Science Quarterly*, 1(1), 35–38.

Schmieding, N.J. (1983). An analysis of Orlando's nursing theory based on Kuhn's theory of science. In P.L. Chinn (Ed.), *Advances in nursing theory development.* Rockville, MD: Aspen Systems.

Schmieding, N.J. (1987). Problematic situations in nursing: Analysis of Orlando's theory based on Dewey's theory of inquiry. *Journal of Advanced Nursing*, 12, 431–440.

Schmieding, N.J. (1988). Action process of nurse administrators to problematic situations based on Orlando's theory. *Journal of Advanced Nursing*, 13, 99–107.

Sills, G.M. (1977). Research in the field of psychiatric nursing 1952–1977. *Nursing Research*, 26(3), 281–287.

Silva, M.C. (1977). Philosophy, science, theory: Interrelationships and implications for nursing research. *Image: The Journal of Nursing Scholarship*, 9(3), 59–63.

Silva, M.C. and Rothbart, D. (1984). An analysis of changing trends in philosophies of science on nursing theory development and testing. *Advances in Nursing Science*, 6(2), 1–13.

Silva, M.C., Sorrell, J.M., and Sorrell, D.S. (1995). From Carper's patterns of knowing to ways of being: An ontological philosophical shift in nursing. *Advances in Nursing Science*, 18(1), 1–13.

Spangler, Z.S., and Spangler, W.D. (1983). Self-care: A testable model. In P.L. Chinn (Ed.), *Advances in nursing theory development.* Rockville, MD: Aspen Systems.

Stevens, P. (1989). A critical social reconceptualization of environment in nursing: Implications for methodology. *Advances in Nursing Science*, 11(4), 56–68.

Stevenson, J.S., and Woods, N.F. (1986). Nursing science and contemporary science: Emerging paradigms. In G.E. Sorensen (Ed.), *Setting the agenda for the year 2000: Knowledge development in nursing.* (Publication No. G-a170, 3M, 5/86). Kansas City, MO: American Nurses Association.

Toulmin, S. (1977). *Human understanding: The collective use and evolution of concepts.* Princeton, NJ: Princeton University Press.

Walker, L.O. (1971). Toward a clearer understanding of the concept of nursing theory. *Nursing Research*, 20(5), 428–435.

Woods, N.F. (1987). Response: Early morning musings on the passion for substance. *Scholarly Inquiry for Nursing Practice: An International Journal*, 1(1), 25–28.

Younger, J.B. (1991). A theory of mastery. *Advances in Nursing Science*, 14(1), 76–89.

CHAPTER 4

From Can't to Kant: The Fantastic Voyage

The journey from the days of Florence Nightingale to modern nursing has been long, hard, and bumpy. Nightingale's attempts to establish professional nursing based on nursing's unique concern with the environment for promotion of health were preempted by an illness-oriented training that depended on other professions for existence and on hospitals for training and sustenance. Nursing has traveled from apprenticeship to education, from hospital service and training to the university, from mere implementation of doctors' orders to accountability and autonomy, from practical to theoretical applications.

The journey has included a major detour through the land of "Can't": a land of perceived inability to conceptualize or generalize; a land that espoused practice, concreteness, and practical relevance as antithetical to some generalizations, common propositions, and theoretical statements. The decades of the 1970s, 1980s, and 1990s mark our emergence from this land and our going back on course, back to where Nightingale began. On our return, however, we are more experienced, more assured, and more trusting in our perceptions. We are more accepting of the significance of patients' experiences and of the varied meanings of experience in the development of nursing knowledge.

We are reminded in this journey of Immanuel Kant, a dominant 19th century philosopher, who maintained that reality is not only a thing in and of itself but is also constructed by those who experience it. Reality in nursing history has been a synthesis of conditions that predisposed nurses to a nontheoretical existence and an *a priori* perception that helped to promote a lack of acceptance of theoretical themes.

Kant aptly distinguished between perception of experience and sensation of experience. Sensation of experience is confounded by temporal and spatial limitations. Experience, the basis of knowledge, has, in nursing, depended on this or that procedure as performed at a certain moment, or on the knowledge of this or that patient occupying a certain space and existing at a certain moment. Although knowledge begins with experience, Kant maintained that this does not mean that all knowledge evolves from experience. To him, our experiences have two components: an *a priori* impression of what may be experienced and impressions as they are actually received. Understanding is a synthesis of both. Therefore, a human being—a knowing, active, and experiencing subject, not a passive recipient—interprets and analyzes impression data in a certain way. That certain way—the *a priori* form by which experiences are shaped—is a synthesis of something that is out there and something that is constructed by the person experiencing it (Copleston, 1964).

During the journey of nurses from early to modern times, experience assumed different meanings with more profound explanations. Experience provided the impetus for describing and explaining phenomena central to nursing and perhaps was responsible for the development of new therapeutics to promote health, to change environments, or to control unwanted events related to health care. During this journey, some nurses were more accepting of the role of clinical experience in the development of clinical knowledge, others were reluctant to acknowledge that experience had any role in theoretical nursing, and still others preferred to rely on the experiences of scientists in other fields to shape their clinical knowledge. Some pioneering thinkers in nursing assumed that nurses can conceptualize and allowed themselves the luxury to consider patients' responses and experiences to help them, and others, better understand clients and their health care experiences. These thinkers helped the theoretical journey move forward. The journey is still in progress and will continue to be in progress in a human and dynamic discipline such as nursing. Within the discipline of nursing, evidence suggests a long journey to a more effective and useful theorizing; support is available for a more systematic development of nursing knowledge.

To enhance the development of theoretical knowledge, we must pause and ask why the journey was long and complex. Why did nursing go through such detours of seemingly nontheoretical periods and, more importantly, why did nurses appear to reject theory and theorizing during the journey, practically forcing the detour into a nontheoretical existence? Even when a small handful of nurses attempted to return, to put nursing on course by providing a theoretical view of what nursing is, it was almost two decades after the development of these conceptions that their notions and their stance began to be accepted. Why is it that some skeptics in nursing were still saying, at the end of the 20th century, that theory or theorizing in nursing is antithetical to the practice of nursing, that nursing practice is either a practically or theoretically oriented situation and therefore choosing one standpoint leaves no room and no need for the other? What conditions have prompted the beginning acceptance of theoretical nursing?

This chapter considers the forces that have hindered and fostered the development of nursing theory. Kant's writing on the synthesis between reality as a separate entity and reality as constructed by the subject who is experiencing it helps us understand the two meanings of these forces. Human and knowledge barriers and human and knowledge forces are two sides of the same coin. We can analyze these forces as both negative and positive in the development of nursing theory. The content may be the same (the sensation in Kant's analysis), but the form distinguishes between forces as barriers and forces as resources. Together, content and form (provided by sensation and mind) enhance knowledge and understanding of the dynamics of the journey from no theory to theory. As we begin to perceive constraints in a new light and through a new lens, we can shift the negative power of constraint to a positive force, and we can reconstruct new realities and develop new blueprints that are more congruent with the mission of nursing and health care needs nationally and internationally.

Barriers to Theory Development

Human Barriers: Nurses as Nurses

The type of student who is selecting nursing, the kind of education nursing students receive, and the nature of nursing may all have been related to the paucity of developments in nursing theory or to the rejection of the theoretical nature of nursing, particularly when nursing education was confined to hospitals and before baccalaureate programs became the norm. Evidence of these relationships varies from speculative to more empirical and verified. Before the 1970s, women who entered nursing may have done so because of its service orientation rather than its professional potential. Nursing may have attracted non–career-oriented individuals who were looking for an occupation that allowed them to get in and out conveniently as their families demanded. A decision to become a nurse may have depended on an image of nursing that was glamorized in the media but that was also paradoxically servile.

Whether nursing still attracts a unique group of individuals who are substantially different from students entering other fields is becoming increasingly debatable. Students are becoming attracted to nursing for its financial potential, its career possibilities, and its potential impact on society. No reported data substantiate that shift; however, it is apparent to educators that attitudes of nursing students are changing drastically as changes occur in other spheres of life, in other professions, and in economic status. Several nursing programs now attract graduates from other disciplines, more nurses are seeking graduate degrees, and fewer nurses are enrolling in diploma programs.

One example of this shift in attitude is the influx of graduate students (graduates from other fields) into community college nursing or baccalaureate nursing programs. These students are often women who are older and therefore more developmentally mature and more intellectually sophisticated. They have already experienced academic life, they have experienced different occupations based on their first degree, and they knowingly and deliberately selected a different educational path that has the potential for leading to financial independence and a new career. More men are also changing careers and choosing nursing. These differences between nursing students of the past and present may suggest a difference in attitudes toward nursing and its professional status as well as its theoretical underpinnings.

Although differences between students who select nursing and those who select other professions are inconclusive because of the sparseness of research, indications are that nursing education itself has created differences between nursing students and other students. Education plays a major role in training the mind to think beyond immediate action, to question situations, to link events, to generalize and, in short, to conceptualize.

Nursing education has a long history of squelching curiosity and replacing it with conformity and a nonquestioning attitude. Nursing education in the past prepared nurses to think of themselves as the handmaidens of physicians, the executors of doctors orders, and the implementers of hospital policy. It socialized students to roles that are not congruent with scholarship and discovery. Any independent thinking or critical attitude was the antithesis of what was expected of a nurse. Because nursing education was based more on apprenticeship, training, and experience than on ideas, knowledge, and learning, the nurse graduated only to find herself far more dependent on the medical and hospital systems than on her own problem-solving abilities. The educational system in nursing did not help nurses see themselves as sources of knowledge.

Theory creation is an active process, but early research characterized nurses as passive (Cleland, 1971; Edwards, 1969). The social climate in which nurses practiced did not encourage debate or freedom to experiment.

> [T]he subculture of nursing has encouraged the perpetuation of a feminine world that has been perveived to emphasize emphasizes routine and repetition, intuition and magical thinking, respectful obedience for authority, and covert rather than overt methods of control. Such a subculture does not provide a fertile field for the growth and development of curiosity and challenge of the status quo, both so necessary to scientific inquiry and scholarship. As a result, a number of nurses . . . have chosen to move to other disciplines for the substantive background and the mental stimulation so necessary to scholarly development (Benoliel, 1975, p. 25).

Functional orientation—the act of performing procedures rather than thinking, reflecting, and solving problems—is a theme apparent in the discipline of nursing (Loomis, 1974). The concept originated in the early inclusion of nursing training programs in hospital settings that socialized nurses to become intellectually subordinate.

The hospital's role was to provide service within its means; its role in education was minimal. Therefore, when hospitals agreed to take on the education of nurses, they did so to improve patient care and to save money. It was acceptable to have nurses work long hours and to allow them to attend lectures only when education did not interfere with the service they were providing. Nursing students were the lowest on the totem pole; they were taught how to respect physicians, how to believe in physicians, and how to totally submit to the hospital routine. Essentially, nurses were taught "intellectual subordination" (Bullough, 1975, p. 229).

Nursing students worked 12-hour shifts and were even further exhausted by being sent on home visits to bring in more revenue that was direly needed by the hospital. Decisions about home care were not predicated on goals of nursing nor on the outcome of nursing care but rather on the need for an economic boost through the use of students as cheap labor. As a result, nurses developed an attitude of task orientation and, for the most part, did not take time to think or reflect, which maintained nursing at a practical rather than a theoretical level. Doing and thinking are not mutually exclusive. Unfortunately, however, the education nurses received fostered an unquestioning acceptance of authority and a subservient attitude.

> The weight of past tradition, the subordination of nurses, the sex segregation, and the apprenticeship model in nursing education have left a mark on the attitudes of present-day nurses (Bullough, 1975, pp. 229–230).

The qualities necessary for theory development are thinking, reflecting, questioning, and perceiving the self as being capable of developing knowledge. The education nurses received may not have nurtured the development of these qualities, nor did it reinforce critical thinking in those who came to nursing with critical thinking abilities.

Nursing has also suffered from the paternalism of hospital administration and medical staff (Ashley, 1977). This paternalism has been internalized as the rules and regulations created by others have been replaced in recent years with rules and regulations created by nurses for nurses. Nurses may be following the rules unquestioningly or they may only be controlling their own questioning of the rules because as Street (1992) discovered in a critical ethnography of nursing practice, nurses are aware of the negative consequences of thinking or speaking critically. Therefore, questioning is still discouraged, rebelliousness is unthinkable, and disobedience is punished, but attrition is a personal option and many, indeed, resort to it.

Early on, the nurse's role was equated with a woman's or mother's role in the family, and the physician's role was equated with that of the father, the head of the family. Therefore, just as wives and mothers were relegated certain prescribed roles, the nurse was also plagued by the image of the sacrificing, altruistic, submissive placater, the fixer of all—a role detrimental to the creativity essential for theoretical thinking. Thinking, creating, and questioning were reserved for the head of the family. It is perhaps that same image that has helped perpetuate the duality of science and practice. Compassion (a characteristic of nurses in practice) cannot be replaced by the rigor, calculation, objectivity, and coolness of the scientist or the theoretician, although perhaps it could be complemented by such characteristics.

Academic nurses suffered from this concept of nursing just as greatly but in a different way. Because they were far removed from patient care, they were more interested in theorizing about student learning or curricula than about patient environment. Being new themselves to the halls of academia, they dissipated their energies in the struggle to prove they belonged there. They competed with others in more established disciplines and shied away from those in practice who pointed their finger at these "ivory tower" colleagues and said, "Your theories are too theoretical and your research is too esoteric; what do you know about practice anyhow?" or "Stick to teaching and leave practice to us."

The attitude of nurses toward theory development, shaped by personal attributes on entry into nursing or by educational and practice environments that are antithetical to theorizing and scientific endeavors, was also greatly influenced by the reward structure in the profession. Recognition of nurses was based on immediate actions, and rewards were based on expedient doing. Rewards were more easily bestowed on nurses in clinical roles or nurses in teaching roles than on those engaged in research or theory development. Rewards for scholarliness were not as tangible as rewards for these other roles, they were slow to come by, and the rationale for the rewards was not as well defined, especially as the discipline was still developing and had no agreed-on standards for reward (Gaston, 1975). In addition, the subculture of nursing had not promoted constructive debates and competition, which could have been helpful in discussing and developing theoretical ideals. What Benoliel said about competition in research applies to theory development:

> If scientific inquiry and production of knowledge are dependent on individuals who thrive on open competition, then perhaps the slow development of research in nursing is tied to a lack of competitive spirit among nurses in idea development. Reflecting on nursing's origins as a form of women's work, I find this slow development

> not too surprising. Compliance with the rules rather than challenge of authority has been an organizing theme in much of nursing's history, and a subculture that places high value on conforming behavior is not fertile soil for the development of practitioners who are comfortable with the aggressive rivalry of scientific endeavors.
>
> The subservient and self-effacing posture that nurses have traditionally held in their working relationships with physicians is not an effective stance for nurses engaged in scientific study. Rather, those who seek to be purveyors of new nursing knowledge can only do so when they carry a sense of self-confidence that permits them to see and experience the positive values of open competition in the world of ideas (Benoliel, 1973, p. 8).

Finally, collaboration, a hallmark of success in nursing practice and an activity about which nurses are most familiar, has not been attached to the scholarly development of disciplines. So, even this, which nurses can do well, was not acknowledged as a significant characteristic of development and progress in scientific disciplines until the late 1980s when Gilligan (1984) and others described and explained the differences in development between men and women. Women's development was described in terms of connection and collaboration. A tolerance for these differences was beginning to appear in the late 1980s and with it came a slow acceptance of alternate indicators to progress and development.

Human Barriers: Nurses as Women

Slowness in the development or acceptance of nursing theory can also be attributed to sex-role stereotyping. Theory development is a laborious process that requires flexibility in time, access to leisure time, access to resources, and freedom from apprehensions, none of which women possessed or obtained as readily as men did in the past (Keller, 1979). The Western view pictures a woman as a hard-working, home-bound person whose energies should be confined to rearing children and caring for a family. Many women have internalized this role ascribed to them by society. Even when women tried to break away from societal stereotypes, they were beset by the need to both fulfill the new employment roles and maintain their function in the old roles. The result has been overload—hardly conducive to reflecting, questioning, and cumulatively developing theory. As Cole (1981) noted, "It is in the domain of informal activities in science that the biggest gaps between men and women remain" (p. 388).

About 95% of nurses are women; therefore, the sex-role identity of nurses cannot be ignored when we discuss theory development and the potential for theoretical thinking. Nursing has always been an occupation with predominantly feminine characteristics, and it is still stereotyped with nurturing roles such as those of wife and mother. Whether the image of nursing as a feminine role evolved from recruitment of women into nursing or whether women were recruited into nursing because of its feminine image is a moot question. Ever since Nightingale recruited only women to accompany her to the Crimean War area to care for the wounded, the image of nurse was fused with the ministering, sacrificing, and altruistic image of women. The same pattern also was demonstrated in the Eastern image of a nurse, Rofaida Al-Islamiah, who is considered the mother of nursing in the Middle East. There is little doubt that many of the issues facing nursing emanated from the feminine image of nursing and the idea of nursing as a profession for women, particularly in societies in which women are relegated to secondary status (Dachelet, 1978; Heide, 1973; Wren, 1971).

Many characteristics of women have been considered antithetical to creativity and scientific productivity. Ample evidence indicates that women are reared and socialized differently than men from the minute they utter their first cry of life, which may lead to some differences in their cognitive structures. Women are considered more affective, more subordinate, more emotional, less aggressive, and less achievement oriented, and they are generally expected to apply rather than to create. Because ours is a patriarchal society, these differences, which could have been considered simply as differences without any value judgments, have been judged as negative toward women. In addition to this attitude, which has been more than devastating to women, women are also beset with many roles to juggle and many struggles to survive in career-oriented jobs (May, Meleis, and Winstead-Fry, 1982). Generally, women are conditioned to consider a professional career as secondary to family and home, which has not allowed them to reserve their energies for more creative endeavors such as theory development and theory testing.

Creativity and scholarly productivity embody curiosity, intellectual objectivity, the ability to be engaged in decision making, and independent judgment. These are socially desirable attributes so long as they are not adopted by women. Because nursing did not insist on independence or active striving for success, it has generally been perceived as a profession congruent with what is expected of women. Furthermore, nursing embodies subjectivity in caregiving, dependence on others for decision making, and expressiveness in relationships—all considered female traits. Street (1992), in a critical ethnography of nursing practice, describes how nurses are aware of the potential negative consequences of thinking and speaking critically. Therefore, nurses may have been socialized against thinking critically.

Even when women broke away from the mold, they suffered ambivalences. Horner (1972) demonstrated that anxiety in many women is created by achievement-related conflicts. Those qualities that are essential for "intellectual mastery," such as independence and active striving, are not female qualities. Therefore, women who defy the conventions of sex-appropriate behavior usually pay the price in anxiety.

Until recently, the message was, because women are biologically different, they are less than men. Nursing is a profession for women, and the attributes that women should strive for and maintain are epitomized in nursing. Therefore, women believed the congruence between societal expectations of women and nurses. The self-fulfilling prophecy of what education women should have and how they should act as women and nurses lingered. As a result, women who entered nursing, at least until the 1970s, had identified strongly with the roles of wife and mother and either believed that nursing would prepare them for the natural roles of women or that the nursing role was a way to earn a living until a knight came along and rescued them from the drudgery of full-time work. For most women, a career was not supposed to coexist with marriage and motherhood, so a woman had to choose between the two. Men, however, could easily combine career, fatherhood, and being a husband.

The self-identity of nursing students lay in their womanhood rather than in their profession or in their discipline. Women in nursing were different from women studying other professions in other ways as well. The self-concept of women who selected nursing, teaching, and dental hygiene included a perception of low autonomy, less chance for advancement, and less need for intellectual stimulus. They also asserted, by selecting nursing, that they had more favorable attitudes toward marriage and family. Students in nursing in the late 1960s and early 1970s ranked home and family roles as number one and career roles as number two, with their own identity being attached more to the former and less to the latter roles (Cleland, 1971; Olesen and Davis, 1966).

On the job, nurses' productivity was measured by their constantly doing, by their sense of urgency, and by their appearing busy. However, their identity remained first and foremost ascribed to simply being women. Their type of productivity was devalued because women were socialized to believe that what they do is of less worth then what men do. Their identity also suffered because they were allowed to receive validation mainly through the capacity to attract a marital partner, to bear and rear children, not through intellectual achievement, career advancement, or financial gain. Male productivity was valued, and a man's identity was measured by his job, career, achievements, and financial gains. The male identity, therefore, was measured by what men did in society and female identity by what women did for the family.

Other perceived differences between men and women might have constrained the development of nursing theory. For one thing, women in science were, in general, engaged in less scholarly production than men (Cole, 1981). Also, because nursing was fairly new to the scholarly arena, it was apparent that

> New scholars in the field have more obstacles and ambivalences to overcome in their attempt to integrate the scholarly role with the repertoire of other roles that constitute the self-concept (May, Meleis, and Winstead-Fry, 1982, p. 23).

Sex-role stereotyping has also impeded theoretical development of nursing in one more way. Many women have come to believe the stereotypes that they are unintellectual, subjective, and emotional (Keller, 1979, 1985). Women have become prejudiced against each other, have reinforced the myths against each other, and have perpetuated the myth about their inability to think theoretically and to develop theories (Goldberg, 1968).

Three patterns that have existed in nursing for some time may thus be questioned:

- Slow acceptance of the acts of theorizing in nursing
- Devaluation of the work of nurse theorists
- Uncritical acceptance of theories developed by nonnurses

These theories were mostly developed by male scholars in other disciplines who may not have reflected nursing concerns or women's perspectives. Is it possible that the slow adaptation and utilization of nursing theories may have occurred because they were theories developed by women and nurses as compared with other theories that were developed by men who were not nurses? These are questions worthy of further exploration by those interested in sex-role identity and perceptions and knowledge development in nursing.

Human Barriers: Nurses as Theorists

Nurse theorists have sometimes acted unwittingly as barriers to the further development of theory. In the minds of practitioners, theorists who were associated with educational institutions were castigated for being far removed from practice. The language that theorists used separated them from their colleagues in practice and other nursing arenas. The language of theories appeared to be esoteric to the rest of the nursing world, to say nothing of the outside world. A nursing client as an energy field, a system of behavior, or a self-care agent were all new and poorly defined concepts. To complicate matters, educators translated nursing theory to curricula rather than to propositions for testing. This intensified the schism between theory and practice and supported the perceived lack of relationship between theory and practice.

Nurse theorists, easily accessible to their immediate colleagues, appeared to practitioners to be remote and inaccessible. Academics in general are perceived to represent the "ivory tower" and are perceived far less to represent the real world. The lack of intertheory discussions and debates added a new dimension to the many intradisciplinary schisms. Schisms also appeared between disciples of the various theorists.

All theorists agree that the discipline of nursing needs to concur on the phenomena, perspectives, and problems central to the field and to the mission of nursing. But to select caring, adaptation, homeostasis, self-care, need fulfillment, or effective nurse–patient interactions as the mission of nursing may mean concentrating exclusively on one mission to the exclusion of others. Defining a nursing mission, advocated by the early nurse theorists, may have been interpreted to mean an exclusive mission. Therefore, the perception was that those who theorize tend to preach for one binding philosophy, one theory, or one conceptual model to guide nursing's research and practice. To accept one theory (argued the practitioners, educators, and researchers) that has not evolved from practice, or has been subjected to practice application, research validation, or the test of time (to the exclusion of others) was unacceptable. Misconceptions, such as believing it was necessary to have only one theory, drew the few believers further away from theoretical nursing.

Although there is no published documentation for this analytical posture, the lack of debate about and among nursing theories in the 1960s and 1970s may be an indication of such a misconception. There were numerous debates, though, among and between faculty members and clinicians regarding which theory to use and the inadvisability of such a choice. These debates were more ideological than substantive. Therefore, we can propose that nurses have been harsh in critiquing nursing theories, perhaps because (1) the theories did not appear to evolve from an empirical base; (2) these theories were developed by women; (3) each theory in itself was not able to describe, explain, and predict all nursing phenomena; and (4) the theories were not perceived to reflect the complexities of nursing practice. Harshness was also apparent in criticism of the nurse theorists for taking risks, which is another manifestation of what Ryan (1971) called "blaming the victim."

> Nurses have been admonished for contributing to their own oppression and inhibiting nursing from achieving the status of a profession (Stein, 1972). Much energy and

> time has been wasted, through intradisciplinary battles between nursing service and nursing education and over types of educational programs and levels of entry into practice. Nurses invalidate other nurses by bringing in "experts" from other disciplines to tell nurses how to do things that are already being done by nursing "experts." This blaming, self-flagellation, and infighting must be recognized by nurses as deriving from the more general social problems of women. And, like women generally, nurses must understand that they alone are not to blame for these problems (Yeaworth, 1978, p. 75).

Knowledge Barriers

Knowledge barriers also inhibit development in theoretical nursing. Knowledge barriers are manifested in the use of knowledge developed by other disciplines, the reluctance to use nursing theory developed within the discipline by members of the discipline, and the further development of knowledge that is more pertinent to the fields of preparation of nurses (ie, disciplines from which nurses received their doctorates before the development of doctoral programs in nursing).

An interesting phenomenon persisted for decades in nursing—the *what is imported is superior* phenomenon—in which imported knowledge was far more meaningful than that which is domestic and developed by nurses. By "imported" we mean theories developed by individuals other than nurses and those developed in a field other than nursing. Sometimes this importing of theories was done for legitimate reasons, but many times it was done with no rationale other than the obvious: someone who was not a nurse developed it, and it emerged from a nonnursing paradigm, therefore, it must be accepted and its effectiveness must not be questioned. Other forms of "conceptual imperialism" have been described that perpetuate the institutional world view (Smith, 1990). This is apparent in the unquestioning use of theories from other disciplines, the lack of reluctance to attribute the label of theory to conceptualizations that evolve from a nonnursing discipline (eg, role theory, when sociologists are still debating whether role is a concept, a construct, or a theory), and the concomitant reluctance to attribute the label of theory to nursing conceptual schemes.

Nursing has been shadowed first by the biomedical model and then by numerous other models, theories, and paradigms; therefore, theory development was left up to those in the different fields that are related to nursing. Few in those related fields saw fit to support nurses' efforts to look for their own individualized umbrella, their own perspective, their own paradigm. As expected, disciplines prefer to prepare their own students for research careers that include research in nursing rather than to prepare nurses for such careers.

> Sociologists, psychologists, and physiologists are much more comfortable with the idea of providing members of their discipline to do the research for nursing than with the idea of providing doctoral preparation for nurses who then return to nursing to apply their knowledge (Yeaworth, 1978, p. 75).

Because nurses had few role models who combined nursing and another field in their graduate programs and because nurses were away from nursing practice while studying theory and research, those with doctorates in nonnursing fields tended to explore phenomena using their new field's binoculars and neglected to synthesize the findings into theoretical nursing. The result has been to explore propositions from sociology, psychology, education, or physiology. These explorations often have implications for nursing practice but not for nursing theory. Many of these nurses educated in other disciplines may have believed that nursing had nothing unique to offer and therefore maintained that the quest for a unique domain is a quest for separation and noncollaboration. To some, to condone nursing theories and nursing's need to develop theories was to support a separationist notion. This view continues to persist among some members of the discipline.

Theory itself was a barrier. First, nurses said they needed theories to prove that nursing is a profession, not simply an occupation. They argued that what nursing lacked in its quest for professionalism was a systematic, coherent body of knowledge with boundaries. Theories fulfilled this requirement. As a result, theorists were suspected of developing theories for professionally selfish reasons. This turned off the practitioners, and theorists found themselves spending a great deal of energy trying to justify their theories rather than revising, further developing, or making them more clinically useful.

Another misguided goal evolved. Educators began to believe that theory—which was then called "conceptual framework"—was needed to develop conceptually based curricula. In fact, the National League for Nursing required that a curriculum should have a well articulated conceptual framework as a requirement for accreditation. The rationale was that if students were prepared in these programs, they would emerge and be agents of change in practice. Thus, from 1965 to 1975 faculty members of nursing schools began to try to fit square pegs into round holes. The result was curricula that overwhelmed students with esoteric content that was rarely used in practice after graduation. In fact, the schism that existed between the languages of clinicians and educators had convinced students of the uselessness of the esoteric content even before their own graduation and initiation into the work force.

Many graduate students have commented on trying to revive the knowledge of nursing theory they gained in their baccalaureate years, knowledge that to them had not been useful in practice. Many of them believe that a theoretically based curriculum both confined and liberated their thinking. It confined it to one approach and it liberated them to experiment with theory utilization. The decrease in the number of nursing theory-based programs may be a sign of progress. Curricula have become more coherent, systematic, and theoretical, and therefore do not need to be limited to one framework. The academic need for theory may have been already established. However, when theory-based curricula were first introduced, faculty focus on curricula may have caused them to lose sight of the reason for theory, which is quality nursing practice and patient care.

Another goal was for nursing to have a disciplinary status based on scientific foundations; this required the existence of theories. Theories, then, appeared to be a means to establish nursing as an academic discipline, one that is distinct from medicine and deserving of professional status. All these are worthy goals for nursing. They will not be achieved, however, by developing theories to guide curricula; theories must be developed through asking and answering the significant questions of the field. The central goal is the provision of effective nursing care of clients in any society. Significant questions arise from this goal, and theories help us understand, explain, predict, and prescribe the care. Secondary gains, then, comprise a professional and disciplinary status for nursing. During the 1980s and 1990s, nurses have realized the primacy of the goal of providing care to clients and have restructured their goals.

Conceptual Barriers

All these barriers—history, culture, and environment—contribute to the lack of conscious use of nursing theories, inhibit the potential for developing theories, and may have created conceptual barriers for nurses. Conceptual blocks are those closed gates that prevent nurses from perceiving or developing nursing phenomena beyond the immediate problem-solving need. According to Adams (1974), conceptual blocks are caused by perceptual, cultural, and environmental obstacles. Cultural and environmental blocks were discussed previously; the following section discusses perceptual blocks.

> Perceptual blocks are obstacles that prevent the problem solver from clearly perceiving either the problem itself or the information that is necessary to solve the problem (Adams, 1974, p. 13).

When used as a framework to describe the nursing situation, perceptual blocks may appear in the following six forms, as described by Adams (1974). First, a nurse may have difficulty delineating a phenomenon that is worthy of pursuance theoretically. She may be unable to perceive meaningful clues; she may focus on tangential issues, use *a priori* paradigms that do not permit a nursing perspective, or fail to see a phenomenon because of the lack of a defining framework.

Second, some nurses may put closer boundaries on a phenomenon—more acceptable boundaries in terms of societal expectations—to the detriment of understanding the phenomenon. For example, suppose an immigrant was admitted to the emergency room three times in the 6 weeks after his successful triple bypass surgery. Each time there was a question of another myocardial infarction, and each time the infarction was unsubstantiated. The causes of the unwarranted emergency room appearances were recorded as noncompliance, or diagnostic problems in the emergency room, or inability to communicate signs and symptoms. In this case, a premature closure on the phenomenon of repeated appearance prevented a careful exploration of the phenomenon within the context of the immigrant's experience and the cultural meanings attached to heart problems.

Similarly, a third perceptual block is lack of experience in considering a phenomenon from different perspectives.

Nurses also fall prey to a fourth type of perceptual block that is related to paradigms that have guided us for many generations and make us see what we expect to see. If we see the world through the biomedical model, we tend to see signs, symptoms, and biomedical antecedents. Our stereotypes of cultures and social classes and our likes and dislikes in values limit our perceptions and create blocks.

Immersion and experience are two-edged swords in theoretical development. Although both are essential in describing theoretically clinical practice, they also tend to prevent us from seeing a phenomenon from a fresh perspective. Anthropologists and sociologists have discussed this fifth perceptual block and advise distancing to allow a return to a fresh start. Another strategy is to consciously keep a journal of events related to the phenomenon. Putting the journal aside and picking it up again later permits the distancing and diffuses what Adams calls the problems of "saturation" (1974, p. 25).

The final perceptual block to be aware of is the nurse's potential inability to permit and accept all senses and intuitive inputs in delineating and developing a phenomenon theoretically.

Forces as Resources

Human Resources: Nurses as Nurses

Theory is a mental image and conception of reality. Tools for theory development are similar to tools that nurses use in their clinical practice and with which they are most experienced. One of the most significant tools for theorizing is the ability to observe. Nurses have ample opportunity to learn how to observe, to sharpen their observations, and to use all their senses in collecting data Observation is central to nursing practice; observation comes easily to the experienced clinician.

Another significant tool for theorizing is the ability to record what actually is happening in a nursing care situation. Nursing records offer a wealth of information and are patient specific, temporally limited, and have space boundaries that do not allow for generalization. With other tools—thinking and reflecting—providing legitimation for developing theories, the observation and recording of data could become the impetus for more general descriptions. Each one of these nursing care situations could become an exemplar for further generalization.

Examples from our theoretical history substantiate these abilities and their relationship to theory development. Nightingale reflected on the many functions and activities that nurses performed during the Crimean War. While in bed (Nightingale spent the last 30 years of her life in bed), she had uninterrupted time and resources to collate observations, critique actions, analyze perceptions of nursing, and arrive at the first systematic, comprehensive concept of nursing.

The field of nursing itself, a source for theory development, is a gold mine for those who wish to articulate its many components and incorporate them into theory. Nurses are dealing with many phenomena that need describing and explaining, and they are responsible for helping clients achieve their health goals through a wide range of activities, ranging from assessing to evaluating, from the technical to the highly abstract. A world of information exists in nursing, which needs to be described and put into order. Clinical stories from nurses' daily practice provide rich accounts of what nursing is about. These stories could provide the necessary data for developing exemplars and models for practice.

Unlike other disciplines that have doubtful social significance, nursing is needed as a human service and is sanctioned for its significance to health care. Nurses in practice settings spend a good deal of time with patients, and because practice is one of the most significant sources of theory, the central ingredient for theory development is therefore available.

In the 1960s, in the wake of nursing education and its attempt at integration, the Yale school of thought evolved to represent developing theories by observing patients, cajoling nurses to articulate what they had accomplished in patient care, and composing a view of nursing—its mission, its goals, and its prescription. These nurse educators used observation and recording skills they had mastered as nurses, and they used nursing clinicians' abilities to do the same. The result was an early conceptualization of nursing as an interpersonal process, which is useful to this day. One must consider, however, that federal funding at the time allowed those nurses the free time and flexible schedules to think, reflect, and develop theories.

Whereas earlier nursing education had been a deterrent to theory development, nursing education since the beginning of the 1980s has been a force headed toward its enhancement. When faculty of doctoral nursing programs in the United States were asked what they considered the core content in their respective programs, highest in rank order were nursing theory, theory development, and conceptual formulation (Beare, Gray, and Ptak, 1981). Students and recent graduates from doctoral programs in nursing, beginning in the 1980s, were practically the first purebreds in the science of nursing. The generation immediately preceding them had experienced a true hybrid of a multitude of programs. Therefore, it is natural that these purebred individuals address the central questions in the field by engaging in the much needed processes of theory development and organization of nursing knowledge. Many master's programs in the United States also offer nursing theory, and a few undergraduate programs are beginning to orient their students to the need for theorizing and for using nursing theory in practice.

Other quests make the nature of nursing a moving force in theory development. Theoretical knowledge is viewed as a "basis for power" (Chinn and Jacobs, 1987). Therefore, as nurses attempt to achieve their professional autonomy, theory becomes a most significant mechanism. As the novices recognize that they can defend ideas better when they approach the argument or debate from a theoretical basis, they will tend to use theory more. As the experienced push to have their services acknowledge nursing care outcomes as distinguishable from outcomes of other kinds of care, they will use theory to articulate their mission, their goals, and their focus. A move toward autonomy is indeed a moving force toward theory development and utilization.

Autonomy is linked to communication about patient care among nurses and between nursing and other health care professions. Communication is enhanced when it is in an understandable language that is common, if not to all health care professionals, then at least among nurses themselves. Communication is enhanced when it evolves from some guiding framework. As nurses value and respect each other's observations and diagnoses, and as they search for a common language with which to communicate, a language that represents nursing's goals and missions more than immediate patient care, then theory becomes a means to achieve better communication. Therefore, the quest for better communication about patient care and about patient care outcomes is a quest for theory development. Nursing practice and nursing education are present-day forces toward theorizing in nursing.

Finally, experiences of nurses as experts in nursing practice were formally acknowledged in the 1980s as a most significant source for nursing knowledge (Benner, 1984). Describing expert nursing practice as seen and practiced by nurses was considered a valued source if not the most significant source for articulating in a meaningful and coherent whole the fundamental and practice aspects of nursing.

Human Resources: Nurses as Women

Theorists and researchers are beginning to produce evidence to refute some of the myths surrounding female identity. Recent empirical investigations and theories do not show sex-role differentiation in sensitivity to social cues, in affiliative behavior, or in nurturing behavior. Women are neither more empathic nor more altruistic than men. Although the myth surrounding these differences still lingers, data are increasingly refuting them (Meeker and Weitzel-O'Neill, 1977). Therefore, some of the attributes of women that have been linked to lower productivity and paucity in theoretical thinking are questioned by more contemporary researchers (Bleier, 1990). These new findings, though, are still limited in distribution and in their power to refute earlier findings presented in this chapter. More research and more widespread distribution of knowledge about productivity-oriented female attributes that is occurring in the current decade will in the future drastically alter socialization practices that have perpetuated the myths.

In the meantime, the feminist movement has done a great deal of consciousness raising of women in general and nurses in particular. It has attempted to dissipate some of the myths that have been true barriers to the development of women for a long time. As early as the 1970s, nurses began to identify more with feminist movement ideals and with a view of nursing as a career rather than merely as a stepping stone toward motherhood (Moore, Decker, and Dowd, 1978; Stein, 1972). Research supports the presence of that shift. Graduate, baccalaureate, and associate degree program students had self-images more in harmony with the image of professional nursing (Stromborg, 1976). The shift is toward an image of independence, competence, and intellectual achievement, characteristics more congruent with a person who engages in idea development.

Research findings demonstrated that nursing students are not qualitatively different from other female college students in their sex-role identity and personality constructs (Meleis and Dagenais, 1981). These studies either dispelled the earlier myths that nursing students manifest more feminine characteristics than other women in college or demonstrated that drastic changes have occurred for women, and particularly for nurses.

When feminine characteristics of nursing students in programs at the three educational levels (diploma, associate, and baccalaureate) were compared with normative data of women in general, results demonstrated that nurses are generally similar to female college and university students in a number of personality constructs. When there were differences, they were congruent with what is expected in practice professions; that is, they did not differ in autonomy but rather in practical aspects (Meleis and Dagenais, 1981). Education plays a more significant role in perception of self than in sex-role identity. Changing sex-role identities through dispelling some of the myths surrounding women's abilities makes the environment more receptive to women's creativity in knowledge development.

Changing society's expectations of women and science are other forces in theory development in nursing. Women possess some attributes that may have been perceived in the past as inappropriate and incongruent with creativity but that are becoming more accepted in today's society (Weedon, 1991). Women have been described as intuitive. Increasingly, as Eastern and Western modes of knowledge development merge, intuition is seen in a more positive light and, indeed, as essential in idea development, as a component in different patterns of understanding reality, and as an accepted method for scientific inquiry (Carper, 1978; Silva, 1977). Intuition is part of the philosophical process, the mental labor that is central to the process of developing theories. Intuition played a significant role in Einstein's discovery and in Darwin's articulation of the evolutionary theory. Intuition, the "curse" of women's abilities, is a force in the 1990s for women's potential. Intuitive awareness of personal and social phenomena is a resource for women in nursing (Adams, 1972).

Although women may have been caught in a "compassion trap" of always being available as helpers in the past, Adams (1972) suggests that, as a result, women possess an attribute that is significant in today's world: flexibility. Women, as an oppressed minority, learned to deal with difficult situations when others controlled access to resources. In the process, they learned how to be flexible and how to be innovative in finding alternative resources essential for their development and for accomplishing their goals.

> Persons with these sensitive capacities undoubtedly perceive reality differently from those who occupy positions of social power and dominance, yet their perceptions have much to contribute to knowledge about nurturing and the care-taking process (Benoliel, 1975, p. 26).

Women's contextual cognitive style has been learned in a life of socialization. Juggling roles is more congruent with the contemporary need to consider sociocultural variables in scientific questions. Changes in sex-role identity, changes in the image of women, and a growing respect for intuition as a pattern of knowing, flexibility, and resourcefulness are all significant forces in theory development.

Women in nursing have an added advantage over women in other disciplines. Women scientists—in physics, chemistry, and social and behavioral sciences, among others—are a minority in their own fields. They have experienced prejudices, less support, and outright discrimination in resource allocation, among other social ills that result from the competition with a dominant group by an oppressed group. In such unfair competition, men tend to win to the detriment of women's progress in these disciplines (Cole, 1981; Keller, 1985).

The overwhelming majority of nurses are women; therefore, conflicts resulting from intradisciplinary sex-role competition are nonexistent. Female nurses have full citizenship within their own discipline. Moreover, we hope that the lessons we have learned from other disciplines will not permit prejudices against male nurses. Creative energy can be freed from the sex-role struggle for the benefit of theory development.

Women and nurses have exhibited a sense of humility as a corollary to humanity, which may have previously prevented them from generalizing beyond the immediate situation (Dickoff, James, and Wiedenbach, 1968). This sense of humility is now being replaced by self-assurance as nurses articulate their own conceptualizations of the different clinical realities they encounter (Parker and MacFarlane, 1991).

Knowledge as a Force and a Resource

Knowledge breeds knowledge; the more knowledge we need, the more we are stimulated and challenged to further develop an understanding of phenomena. Theory development in nursing is enhanced by the wealth of theoretical knowledge we already have. The theories developed by nurse scholars provide an impetus for further refinement and development. They lead to an agreed-on set of concepts that are central to nursing and point to phenomena of interest to nursing. They have set the stage for the next steps.

Debates surrounding which theories to develop, how to develop them, and whether or not to develop them have helped to clarify the mission of nursing. With a preliminary identification of content and a beginning articulation of methodology, the course is now clear for smoother sailing. All this has set the stage for shaping skills in analytical and critical thinking and has stimulated more nurse scholars to pursue development in theoretical nursing. Nursing has the potential for developing a feminist approach to science, or even a nonsexist science, by converting "value-free technology" to a "humane technology" that incorporates self-care (Ardetti, 1980).

Old paradigms of knowledge are being challenged by new paradigms, prompted by two significant social movements: the feminist movement and the women's health movement (McPherson, 1983). Essential components of the new paradigm represent a shift to include humanitarianism, holism, the incorporation of sociocultural content, perceptions of subjects of research, subjects and researchers collaborating in the research process, and a qualitative approach. The "new paradigm" is not new to nursing. Its newness stems more from social acceptance as the public is becoming more aware of ways to develop knowledge and demanding participation in the process. The newness is in the congruence rather than in a shift in thinking. There is wider acceptance of components of the "new paradigm" by consumers who care. That is a force that will help nurses further develop knowledge. The energy that used to be expended by those defending components of a paradigm that was incongruent with a prevailing scientific perspective can now be channeled from the creativity of reaction to the creativity of action.

A new world view emerged, a view that had even changed physics from the mechanistic conceptions advanced by Descartes and Newton to a more holistic and ecological view (Capra, 1983). The new world view is congruent with women's views of science and nurses' views of health. It is a view that has shifted focus from a causative view to a more interpretive view. It is heightened by phenomenology and qualitative research.

Conceptual Resources

To use all senses, experiences, and intuition requires involvement and immersion in situations as a whole, and to describe patterns of responses theoretically requires longer periods of engagement in situations where nursing phenomena occur. The nature of nursing, the process of nursing care, the history of the profession, and the predominant gender orientation of the profession enhance the conceptual resources for nurses.

Nurses are trained to observe, to record, to analyze, and to solve problems. Whether we admit it or not, we tend to use our own and others' experiences in providing care, and in doing so we rely on all our senses and intuitions, just as we rely on science principles to guide our action.

Nurses spend long hours with patients, families, and communities; this time allows an understanding of patterns of behaviors rather than isolated incidents. Diversity in nurses and in their cultural, educational, and socioeconomic backgrounds can be a resource to allow for diverse views, a safeguard against premature closure on a phenomenon and against narrow perspectives. Diversity in caregivers, in some instances considered problematic, could become a useful resource for theoretical development. This resource could help remove perceptual blocks.

Nurses have effective interviewing skills for which they have been meticulously trained. They have mastered questioning, they know how to prioritize, and they know how to participate in dialogue. They have opportunities to confirm observations and hunches during clinical rounds at the end or beginning of shift reports, during impromptu meetings at the nurses' stations, in meetings with other members of the family, and during their many regular daily roles and activities that involve talking, listening, questioning, answering, and writing. Each one of these tasks enhances perception, and each is a resource and an asset for conceptualization.

Other Forces for Theory Use and Development

The journey to theoretical thinking has been a progression through self-effacing stops, self-doubt detours, humility delays, collisions with opposing and dominating paradigms, and near misses due to embarking on unfamiliar territory or unpaved terrain. Nursing and nurses are emerging theoretically stronger and far better prepared to embark on a task of theoretical clarification. The quality of the journey could be enhanced by coaching, mentorship, and sponsorship toward the development of the scholarly role.

Nurses are no longer resistant to the use of nursing theory in their practice or to their potential involvement in theory development. Rather, they are asking how they can use theory and looking for those they can emulate in the process. One example of nurses' interest in theory was a national conference held in 1983 by clinical specialists, in which the topic of theory development and utilization dominated a full half day of the 2-day conference (Clinical Nurse Specialists, 1983).

Planners of the conference were concerned about the responses of the attendants to what might appear as highly abstract ideas not directly related to everyday care issues. The results were astonishing, the evaluations were heartening, and the request came for another session the following year, focusing on how to bring acceptance to theory utilization and development in clinical areas (Clinical Nurse Specialists, 1984). In short, nurses were asking for role modeling, role clarification, and role rehearsal—all properties of mentorship (May, Meleis, and Winstead-Fry, 1982).

> Mentorship is an intense relationship calling for a high degree of involvement between a novice in a discipline and a person who is knowledgeable and wise in that area. ...In the process of helping the beginning scholar to fit resources to her needs and capabilities, the mentor provides options, opens up new opportunities,

> and helps to make corrections. This means that, on cognitive and affective levels, the mentor is involved with the novice as a whole person and feels a sense of responsibility for her (May, Meleis, and Winstead-Fry, 1982, p. 23).

Role modeling, which is teaching by example and emulation, then fosters the learning of these behaviors (Bandura, 1962; Meleis, 1975). Role clarification provides an opportunity to understand the subtle intricacies of the role to be emulated. What does it mean to have a role in the theoretical development of nursing? What cues are needed to perform that role? Role clarification in theory use and development may include spelling out the differences between the various theories, the different strategies in theory development, the different barriers to use of theory, and some strategies for handling all of these. Mentorship also includes opportunities for role rehearsal. Use of theory in theoretical patient care studies and use of different strategies in theory development are examples of staged situations to practice behaviors central to the use and development of theory (May, Meleis, and Winstead-Fry, 1982; Meleis and May, 1981).

Time and sociocultural conditions are right for the development of theoretical nursing, which in turn is significant for patient care, and nurses are "going for it." If, indeed, there is a woman's way to understand the world, and if there are areas of knowledge that are better understood when seen through the eyes of women and through the use of feminine logic, then nursing is ready on all of these accounts, and nurses are prepared to pursue that knowledge.

Nursing education can provide supportive conditions through programs that focus on scholarly productivity (Meleis and May, 1981; Meleis, Wilson, and Chater, 1980). Theory and theory development should not be limited to graduate programs. Theoretical thinking should be the *modus operandi* for conscientious patient care from day one in nursing education. Nursing practice has an equal commitment to provide avenues by which nurses can communicate their findings in theoretical terms and can have the opportunity to translate their hunches into theoretical terms. Nurses in the appropriate atmosphere should be able to try using different theories in practice for the purpose of refining and extending them.

Similar supportive environments could be provided by nurse administrators to help in the development of a theoretical culture that allows dialogues, debates, and discussions that go beyond the immediate day-by-day problem solving and decision making. Strategies to be used by nurse administrators and educators for the enhancement of theory development include creating a theoretical culture, supporting critical thinking, refocusing dialogues and discussions on concepts, defining nursing territory, exploring ambiguous ideas, allowing uncertainty about phenomena to linger, avoiding premature closure on ideas, facing views of phenomena from different perspectives, and providing such resources as library time, observation time, and writing time (Jennings and Meleis, 1988; Meleis and Jennings, 1989; Meleis and Price, 1988).

Conclusion

Nurses are now in the land of Kant rather than the land of "Can't." Kant maintained that knowledge depends on experience and experience on observation, but observations by themselves do not form experience nor give meaning to experience. Observations have to be organized *a priori* by the mind to develop into knowledge. In so organizing our observations, we tend to reconstruct reality.

Nurses may have reconstructed the meaning of theoretical constraints into forces that foster the further development of theoretical nurses. They can use the tools of practice for theory development, relying on the same abilities they have used for practice, research, teaching, administering, and translating these skills to theorize and to use theory, perhaps thereby becoming convinced that their experiences comprise the appropriate impetus for theory development.

The synthesis between continental rationalism and British empiricism espoused by Kant may be helpful in increasing our knowledge of nursing realities.

REFERENCES

Adams, M. (1972). The compassion trap. In V. Goernick and B.K. Moran (Eds.), *Women in sexist society.* New York: Signet Books.

Adams, J. (1974). *Conceptual block busting: A guide to better ideas.* San Francisco: W.H. Freeman.

Ardetti, R. (1980). Feminism and science. In R. Ardetti, P. Brennan, and S. Cavrak (Eds.), *Science and liberation.* Boston: South End Press.

Ashley, J.A. (1977). *Hospitals, paternalism, and the role of the nurse.* New York: Teachers College, Columbia University.

Bandura, A. (1962). Social learning through imitation. In M.R. Jones (Ed.), *Nebraska symposium on motivation.* Lincoln: University of Nebraska Press.

Beare, P.G., Gray, C.J., and Ptak, H.F. (1981). Doctoral curricula in nursing. *Nursing Outlook,* 29(5), 311–316.

Benner, P. (1984). *From novice to expert: Excellence and power in clinical nursing practice.* Menlo Park, CA: Addison-Wesley.

Benoliel, J.Q. (1973). Collaboration and competition in nursing research. In *Communicating nursing research: Collaboration and competition.* Boulder, CO: Western Interstate Commission for Higher Education.

Benoliel, J.Q. (1975). Scholarship: A woman's perspective. *Image,* 7(2), 22–27.

Bleier, R. (1990). Sex differences research: Science or belief. In R. Bleier, (Ed.), *Feminist approaches to science* (pp. 147–164). New York: Pergamon Press.

Bullough, B. (1975). Barriers to the nurse practitioner movement: Problems of women in a woman's field. *International Journal of Health Services,* 5(2), 225–233.

Capra, F. (1983). *The turning point: Science, society, and the rising culture.* New York: Bantam.

Carper, B.A. (1978). Practice oriented theory: Part 1. Fundamental patterns of knowing in nursing. *Advances in Nursing Science,* 1(1), 13–23.

Chinn, P.L. and Jacobs, M.K. (1987). *Theory and nursing: A systematic approach* (2nd ed.). St. Louis: C.V. Mosby.

Cleland, V. (1971). Sex discrimination: Nursing's most pervasive problem. *American Journal of Nursing,* 71(8), 1542–1547.

Clinical Nurse Specialists Annual Conference (1983, February 17–18). San Francisco.

Clinical Nurse Specialists Annual Conference (1984, February 16–17). San Francisco.

Cole, J.R. (1981, July/August). Women in science. *American Scientist,* 69, 385–391.

Copleston, F. (1964). *A history of philosophy. Modern philosophy: Kant* (Vol. 6, Part II). Garden City: Image Books.

Dachelet, C.Z. (1978). Nursing's bid for increased status. *Nursing Forum,* 17(1), 18–45.

Dickoff, J., James, P., and Wiedenbach, E. (1968). Theory in practice discipline: Part 1. Practice oriented theory. *Nursing Research,* 17(5), 415–435.

Edwards, C.N. (1969). The student nurse: A study in sex-role transition. *Psychology Report,* 25(3), 975–990.

Gaston, J. (1975). Social organization, codification of knowledge, and the reward structure in science. *Journal of Social Psychology,* 18, 285–303. (Koln, Germany)

Gilligan, C. (1984). *In a different voice: Psychological theory and women's development.* Cambridge, MA: Harvard University Press.

Goldberg, P. (1968, April). Are women prejudiced against women? *Trans-Action,* 5, 28–30.

Heide, W.S. (1973). Nursing and women's liberation—A parallel. *American Journal of Nursing,* 73(5), 824–827.

Horner, M. (1972). Toward an understanding of achievement-related conflicts in women. *Journal of Social Issues,* 28(2), 157–175.

Jennings, B. and Meleis, A.I. (1988). Nursing theory and administrative practice: Agenda for the 1990s. *Advances in Nursing Science,* 10(3), 56–69.

Keller, E. (1979). The effect of sexual stereotyping on the development of nursing theory. *American Journal of Nursing,* 79(9), 1585–1586.

Keller, E. (1985). *Reflections on gender and science.* New Haven, CT: Yale University Press.

Loomis, M.E. (1974). Collegiate nursing education: An ambivalent professionalism. *The Journal of Nursing Education,* November, 39–48.

May, K.M., Meleis, A.I., and Winstead-Fry, P. (1982). Mentorship for scholarliness: Opportunities and dilemmas. *Nursing Outlook,* 30(11), 22–28.

McPherson, K.I. (1983). Feminist methods: A new paradigm for nursing research. *Advances in Nursing Science,* 5(2), 17–36.

Meeker, B.F. and Weitzel-O'Neill. (1977, February). Sex roles and interpersonal behavior in task-oriented groups. *American Sociological Review*, 42, 91–5.

Meleis, A.I. (1975). Role insufficiency and role supplementation: A conceptual framework. *Nursing Research*, 24(4), 264–271.

Meleis, A.I. and Dagenais, F. (1981). Sex-role identity and perception of professional self in graduates of three nursing programs. *Nursing Research*, 30(3), 162–167.

Meleis, A.I. and Jennings, B. (1989). Theoretical nursing administration: Today's challenges, tomorrow's bridges. In B. Henry, C. Arndt, M. DiVincenti, and A. Marriner (Eds.), *Dimensions and issues in nursing administration.* Boston: Blackwell Scientific Publications.

Meleis, A.I. and May, K.M. (1981). Nursing theory and scholarliness in the doctoral program. *Advances in Nursing Science*, 4(1), 31–41.

Meleis, A.I. and Price, M. (1988). Strategies and conditions for nursing: An international perspective. *Journal of Advanced Nursing*, 13, 592–604.

Meleis, A.I., Wilson, H.S., and Chater, S. (1980). Toward scholarliness in doctoral dissertations: An analytical model. *Journal of Research in Nursing and Health*, 3, 115–124.

Moore, D.S., Decker, S.D., and Dowd, M.W. (1978). Baccalaureate nursing students' identification with the women's movement. *Nursing Research*, 27(5), 291–295.

Olesen, V.L. and Davis, F. (1966). Baccalaureate students' images of nursing: A follow-up report. *Nursing Research*, 15(2), 151–158.

Parker, B., and McFarlane, J. (1991). Feminist theory and nursing: An empowerment model for research. *Advances in Nursing Science*, 13(3), 59–67.

Ryan, W. (1971). *Blaming the victim.* New York: Random House.

Silva, M.C. (1977). Philosophy, science, theory: Interrelationships and implications for nursing research. *Image*, 9(3), 59–63.

Smith, D. (1990). *The conceptual practices of power: A feminist sociology of knowledge.* Toronto: University of Toronto Press

Stein, L.I. (1972). Liberation movement: Impact on nursing. *AORN Journal*, 15(4), 67–85.

Street, A.F. (1992). *Inside nursing: A critical ethnography of clinical nursing practice.* Albany: State University of New York Press.

Stromborg, M.F. (1976). Relationship of sex-role identity to occupational image of female nursing students. *Nursing Research*, 25(5), 363–369.

Weedon, C. (1991). *Feminist practice and post-structuralist theory* Cambridge, MA: Basil Blackwell.

Wren, G.R. (1971) Some characteristics of freshman students in baccalaureate, diploma, and associate degree nursing programs. *Nursing Research*, 20(2), 167–172.

Yeaworth, R. (1978). Feminism and the nursing profession. In N. Chaska (Ed.), *The nursing profession: Views through the mist.* New York: McGraw-Hill.

CHAPTER 5

Toward the Development of the Discipline of Nursing: Epistemological Issues

Epistemology is the branch of philosophy that considers the history of knowledge. It raises and answers questions related to the kinds, the origin, the nature, the structure, the scope, the trustworthiness, the methods, and the limitations in knowledge development and outlines the various criteria by which knowledge is accepted. This chapter discusses several issues that have preoccupied the discipline of nursing in the past. These are:

- Theoretical growth: Revolution, evolution, or integration
- From the received view to the perceived view
- From correspondence to Weltanschauung

Understanding how knowledge evolves, how science is accumulated, and how knowledge is accepted is essential for development and progress in any field. Such understanding helps to further define goals to be pursued, either for the individual scientist or for the discipline as a whole (Andreoli and Thompson, 1977; Baer, 1979; Carper, 1978; Silva, 1977). Therefore, a study of epistemological issues helps us to accomplish the following:

- Increase our awareness of the complexity and diversity of perspectives, views, and theories (sometimes conflicting) of scientific progress, truth, and the methodology of truth
- Distinguish between different kinds of problems in knowledge and development and therefore deliberately pursue those that seem most germane to the theoretical progress of the nursing discipline
- Deal with potential epistemological constraints, however inappropriate, that evolve from *de facto* acceptance of one view, one theory, or one perspective without careful study of alternatives

During the past few decades, we have accumulated a good deal of nursing knowledge about caring, interacting, promoting healthy environments, supplementing roles, enhancing recovery, and supporting healing. If we allow our knowledge to continue to develop haphazardly, disconnectedly, or aimlessly, it may not progress as expediently as we wish, or in the direction we choose. A period of reflection on the course of the development of nursing's knowledge base, particularly its theoretical progress, allows us to appreciate our progress and, at the same time, gives us the pause necessary for a more organized future development.

The concern in this book is the role of theory in the development of nursing knowledge, although it is understood that knowledge encompasses far more than theory—it includes research, common sense, and philosophy as well as extant and ought-to-be nursing practice. The following discussion is about, but not limited to, the evolution of theory in nursing.

Theoretical Growth: Revolution, Evolution, or Integration

Scientific growth has been studied by many philosophers and scientists. Several theories have been advanced to describe patterns of scientific progress based on retrospective analysis of physical and social science progress. The question of how sciences develop, which has occupied philosophers of science, has also become one of nursing's significant questions. What processes did nursing go through leading to its current stage of development? To answer these questions, nurses have resorted to patterns that have been previously identified. Using patterns that are more congruent with scientific progress in the physical sciences may have impeded the theoretical growth of the discipline of nursing.

A Theory of Revolution

Kuhn (1970, 1977), a physicist by training, is credited with developing the revolutionary theory of scientific development. *Revolution* is defined by *Webster's Third New International Dictionary* as "a sudden, radical, or complete change" characterized by "overthrowing" fundamental changes.* Kuhn's theory is based on this definition and is congruent with its sentiment. Sciences, to Kuhn, develop by leaps and bounds only through periods of crisis in which theories compete, anomalies are identified, and inadequacies are highlighted—leading to predominance of one theory over all others.

This period of scientific unrest is followed by a tranquil period that Kuhn calls normal science. This period marks the acceptability of one theory over all others. Normal science is a period when members of the field accept in a unified way a common paradigm. The transition from a crisis to normal science marks a scientific revolution. Kuhn asserts that scientific revolutions are inevitable for the development of a science and that scientific development is noncumulative, meaning an aspect of one theory that is useful is not added to another competing theory to render it more useful. The competition between paradigms does not evolve into collaborative paradigms; rather, only one

*By permission. From *Webster's Third New International Dictionary 1986* by Merriam-Webster Inc., publisher of the Merriam-Webster dictionaries.

prevails to the destruction of others. In other words, older paradigms, whether or not useful on the whole or in part, are incompatible with newly conceived paradigms (Kuhn, 1970).

Kuhn was a prolific writer and speaker who should be amply credited for giving credence to the philosophy of science as a field worthy of exploration and investigation. His central ideas are:

1. A *paradigm* is defined as an entire repertoire of beliefs, values, laws, principles, theory methodologies, ways of application, and instrumentation.
2. A paradigm encompasses substantive theoretical assumptions about the subject matter of the discipline and methodological strategies as well as a degree of consensus about theory methods and techniques.
3. A paradigm includes the questionable areas in the field and some puzzle solutions that could act as examples to help members of that scientific community solve the remainder of the normal science problems in the discipline.
4. A discipline matures when it has such a paradigm. Before its paradigmatic stage, however, there is haphazard and variable fact finding in the processes used to answer the discipline questions. This period is characterized as a preparadigmatic stage of the discipline. The movement toward a paradigmatic stage occurs only when one of the paradigms becomes dominant and is accepted by the community of scholars. It is then and only then that the period of normal science is achieved.

The process is a revolutionary one characterized by sudden changes, and its cornerstone is competition. Development is not possible without competition, the result of which is the predominance of one paradigm over all others. The revolution occurs because none of the earlier paradigms work any more. A paradigm may be discarded and replaced by another competing paradigm because the exemplar attached to it is more successful and others in the field are in agreement with it. Rejection of all other paradigms occurs at this time.

Once a paradigm dominates, competition is halted because one paradigm clearly prevails. This is the period of normal science. Collaboration, then, replaces competition, and the scientific community prevents any alternative paradigms from emerging during this period. Even when theoretical or methodological issues evolve, the scientific community avoids and ignores them, permitting the continuing dominance of the prevailing paradigm.

Kuhn's ideas led to a belief that disciplines develop by convergence. Converging on one paradigm is then accepted as the goal of disciplines to lead them to progress. A *convergent process* is a closed rather than an open process—a process that is antithetical to the nature of science, which is characterized as being open to new development and tolerant of competition.

The term *paradigm* was substituted in Kuhn's later writing with *disciplinary matrix*, denoting the same definition of paradigm but with the addition of *shared exemplars* (Kuhn, 1970, pp. 181–210). Because content boundaries of paradigms are not entirely explicit but rather implicit, exemplars are provided to identify the problems and the solutions in the discipline. They are models for problems and solutions that are accepted by scientists during the period of normal science.

Kuhn's ideas have been both revered and criticized. Many writers have taken issue with his admonitions and questioned the capability of his theory to describe and predict the developmental process in the progress of science. More specifically, Kuhn's notion of the development of scientific disciplines through crises and through scientific revolutions has fostered numerous debates in the field of philosophy of science. Some have pointed to historical inconsistencies between Kuhn's analysis of several of the established scientific disciplines and his generalization about such developments; these inconsistencies point to the harmonious coexistence between numerous competing paradigms.

In the view of those who have pointed out such inconsistencies, coexistence between competing paradigms leads to appropriate debates within a given field. Critics pointed out disciplines that were established despite having no single guiding framework. Why, Dudley Shapere (1981, p. 58) asks, should we only have the extremes, the absolute differences in competing paradigms (thus a crisis) or the absolute identity within one paradigm (thus a revolution) followed by normal science? Is it not possible to have, at any one point in time, both similarities and differences, both competition and collaboration?

Laudan also challenged Kuhn's assertion and proposed that competition is continuous and that scientific disciplines include a variety of coexisting research traditions (Laudan, 1981, p. 153). Laudan identified five major flaws in Kuhn's philosophical view of the development of scientific discipline (Kuhn, 1977, pp. 74–76). These have implications for nursing.

1. "Kuhn's failure to see the role of conceptual problems in scientific debates and in paradigm evaluation." Kuhn appears to be using only a positivistic view of science by comparing the number of facts a theory is able to address and the congruence between these facts in theory and in real life. An empirical view addresses elements in verification and falsification of theories; but no conceptual coherence, logic, social congruence, or other significant components of usefulness.
2. "Kuhn never really resolves the crucial question of the relationship between a paradigm and its constituent theories." Does a paradigm encompass all theories? Do theories explain and describe the paradigm or vice versa? Which gives evidence to the other?
3. The notion of a prevailing paradigm does not allow for the changes and discoveries that characterize our present science, where misconceptions are corrected, parts of theories are justified, and others are changed. Scientific discovery is a continuous process; present tools allow for a fast pace. Kuhn's theory of scientific development appears to provide a rigid structure that limits the continuous development of theories and the continuous correction of the paradigm's weaknesses, which may become apparent over time.
4. Kuhn does not advocate explicit articulation of paradigms or disciplinary matrices. Therefore, such implicitness does not account for nursing's attempt to make the boundaries of the discipline explicit or the assumptions debatable, nor does such implicitness promote the many controversies that Kuhn considers essential to the development of science. Scientists can debate explicit matrices but can avoid implicit ones.

5. "Because paradigms are so implicit and can only be identified by pointing to their *exemplars* (basically an archetypal application of a mathematical formulation to an experimental problem), it follows that whenever two scientists use the same exemplars they are, for Kuhn, *ipso facto* committed to the same paradigm" (Laudan, 1981, p. 85). If more scientists work in this way, we come closer to a revolution. Some exemplars have been used in nursing by nurses who hold divergent views about the most basic conceptual and methodological questions. Helping people cope with transitions is an area providing exemplars in health/illness transitions, developmental transitions, or situational transitions. These exemplars have been treated effectively by those who adhere to psychoanalytical views and just as effectively by those adhering to sociocultural views in nursing. Therefore, the exemplars themselves would not mean commitment to some paradigm. Commitment to one paradigm over another is apparent only by making paradigms explicit and not by maintaining implicitness.

Finally, a sixth flaw apparent in Kuhn's philosophy has been identified by Toulmin (1972):

6. How the transitions from competing paradigms, to revolution, to normal science occur is not clear in Kuhn's writing. Does a community of scholars hold a mass meeting to denounce one competing paradigm and adopt another? Considering that, according to Kuhn, followers of each paradigm are supposedly entrenched in the paradigm they use and do not always seem to communicate, nor do they always share a common language or world view, how could they agree on one rather than another paradigm? Contrary to Kuhn's ideas regarding the lack of communication during the crisis period, Toulmin offers many historical examples of careful communication, debate, discussion, or proposed modification in physics before any minute change was made or any modification was incorporated into the established body of the discipline (Toulmin, 1972, p. 10).

Some nursing scholars seem to have accepted Kuhn's theory of progress and have adhered to the position that nursing is following the same patterns of revolutionary development as the other physical sciences analyzed by Kuhn. Nursing progress has thus been measured against the canons proposed by him (Hardy, 1978). The result has been a negatively critical assessment of nursing progress and anticipation of a nursing scientific revolution in which one paradigm prevails and is accepted by the nursing community. According to these scholars, nursing is in its preparadigmatic stage. It is possible that the nursing scientific revolution may never come, not because nursing is not progressing but because there may never be periods of normal science. Other natural and behavioral science disciplines continue to progress and have competing paradigms to describe and predict the phenomena of their disciplines. In addition, the notion of one paradigm is not acceptable to sciences, particularly to nursing, which deals with human beings and complex health/illness situations.

Some nurses have presented a view of nursing as something that has arrived at the beginnings of a paradigm (Munhall, 1982; Newman, 1983) or is undergoing a paradigm shift. However, the processes depicted do not demonstrate competition, rejection, and dominance as much as an evolutionary process. Therefore, the appropriateness of using the revolutionary theory to describe progress and development of nursing knowledge should continue to be debated, other theories should be discussed, and analyses of consequences should be carefully considered.

A Theory of Evolution

A second approach to critically assessing progress in knowledge development is by using an evolutionary lens. Evolution denotes change in a certain direction, unfolding from lower to higher and from simpler to more complex and headed in the direction of greater coherence. Evolution denotes a sense of continuity and gives the impression of long-term cumulative changes. An evolutionary view of a scientific discipline combines instances of intellectual innovation that are complemented by a continuing process of critical assessment and selection An evolutionary stand acknowledges competition but accepts the inevitability of cumulation in knowledge development. An evolutionary stand also acknowledges the significance of the genealogy of ideas in the progress of knowledge.

Toulmin (1972) used the evolutionary theory of Darwin as the basis on which he formulated the evolution framework to explain the process of knowledge development. He identified four basic principles for Darwinian theory. These four principles have their counterparts in the evolution of scientific disciplines. *First*, each discipline contains its own body of concepts, areas of concern, methodologies, and goals, all of which can change drastically but slowly through a mutable process. Nevertheless, there is a definite continuity that can be detected in the major ideas of the discipline. Conceptual thoughts in each of the disciplines, while having coherence and continuity, also manifest slow, long-term changes, with each new conceptual thought based on previous ideas, and with the more developed concepts superseding older ones.

Second, all ideas, concepts, and methodologies are given a chance to compete, to be discussed, to be weeded out. Only the discoveries and innovations that fit will flourish and survive from one generation to the next. This process of retention of some conceptual thoughts, mutation of others, and rejection of still others explains the stability of intellectual thought in disciplines and accounts for transformations into new theories.

Third, marked substantive changes in the field are possible when a number of conditions exist. One important condition is the existence of qualified people in the discipline who are capable of inventing new ideas, exploring new problems, and developing new theories. An evolutionary position presupposes the presence of an arena for debate, critique, and competition of ideas and concepts. Another necessary condition is that there be enough openness in the discipline to allow for new ideas to develop and survive long enough to prove their suitability or to be refuted.

Fourth, the selection of the more useful ideas, concepts, and theories is based on which of them helps to meet the demands of the local intellectual environment within the discipline. The selection process is also based on the congruence between the demands, the issues, the current problem areas, and the innovative ideas that are being offered (Toulmin, 1972, pp. 139–143). Other competing ideas continue to be adhered to, refined, and further developed.

An evolutionary process of knowledge development contains such units of analysis as merits, competitions, demands, and successes. When contrasting the Darwinian zoological evolutionary process of the species with the Toulmin intellectual evolutionary process of disciplines, one finds a pattern of development based on innovation, comparison of ideas, survival of the fittest, and a systematic patterns of selection of the best among the competing paradigms. One theory, one set of ideas that may have more explanatory power to resolve some significant conceptual problem, is generally selected over another theory, however well established it may have been. It may incorporate parts of the previous theory and reject other parts. Progress in the physical sciences is not revolutionary, according to Toulmin, but evolutionary. It has taken a cumulative pattern.

The evolutionary theory of knowledge presupposes that the problem areas of the field and the criteria for truth and explanation are agreed on. In addition, certain conditions should exist as indicators that a discipline has developed cumulatively. These conditions, the first four of which have been identified by Freese (1972), are:

1. Modification of truth value: generalizations are cumulative when one generalization modifies a previous generalization; that is, one generalization causes change to or from truth, falsity, or indetermination. An empirical confirmation of the second generalization modifies the truth inherent in the first.
2. Modification of antecedent value: generalizations are cumulative if the empirical verification or falsification of a second subsequent generalization modifies the antecedent in the first generalization. Change of one to the other of the following would fulfill this condition: necessary but not sufficient, sufficient but not necessary, necessary and sufficient, sufficient with necessity indeterminate, and necessary with sufficiency indeterminate.
3. Premise or derivation in a deductive chain: this applies to cases in which a confirmed proposition in one theory becomes a premise preceding another proposition in another theory. Theory is cumulative when the propositions of one theory are based on or help modify the premises of another theory.
4. Space–time independence: theories are cumulative when their propositions transcend geography and time.
5. Practice–research–practice-dependent link: this link presupposes modification of practice based on theory or research, or vice versa. Cumulation occurs when a direct ripple effect occurs between practice and research.

If we accept these premises for cumulative knowledge, then physical sciences (using revolutionary criteria) are based on paradigms and (using the evolutionary process) are established disciplines. Social and behavioral sciences, on the other hand, are classified as being in a preparadigmatic stage or are, in Toulmin's terms, "would-be disciplines." One can readily detect conditions of cumulation in the physical sciences, very little of which exists in the social and behavioral sciences or, indeed, in nursing.

Propositions emanating from theoretical nursing do not fit in a deductively tight, logically interrelated cumulative model. Systematic cumulative development that begins from a common point and expands upward to become another canon cannot be detected in nursing knowledge. If cumulation is the unit of analysis for the evolution of disciplines, then nursing scientific development is not closely congruent with either a revolutionary or an evolutionary concept. Rather, it has followed a course that may be considered unsystematic, haphazard, and lacking direction—if we impose on it the two theories discussed previously.

A Theory of Integration

It is possible that the development of the discipline of nursing did not follow a strictly revolutionary or evolutionary path. The revolutionary one would deny nursing's scientific status and the evolutionary one presumes systematic development with research based on theory and theory evolving out of research. The discipline of nursing evolved through peaks, valleys, detours, circular paths, retracing of steps, and series of crises as well as through an evolutionary process. These are features and patterns in nursing that are unique to the discipline that may support a more integrative approach to describe its development. One unique feature is its *theory development*. The development of nursing theory was not based on the research of the discipline, nor did every research project make a contribution to the development of theory (Batey, 1977; Fawcett, 1978). Another unique feature of the discipline is that its competing ideas exist simultaneously and have existed for decades (different research methodologies, conceptual approaches to care, comfort, and pain), and in fact, competing theories are being used even within the same institution. To be sure, there are areas of agreement: significance of environment, focus on health and coping, interest in transitions, fascination with human responses to health and illness. Although each of these concepts may be viewed from a different theoretical background, there is more and more growing agreement that these concepts are central to the discipline. Even with more agreement on major concepts that are central to the discipline of nursing, different theories continue to explain, describe, and predict the different concepts. In some instances different theories best explain different situations related to the same concept. Human conditions dictate the appropriateness of different uses of theories.

One may argue that the discipline has been in continuous crisis over the origins of its knowledge base for many years (practice, teaching, or administration) and that the agreement now is that knowledge develops, for the most part, from clinical practice. However, there is agreement that the discipline of nursing incorporates professional practice, research, education, and teaching. There are also areas of disagreement, such as on the nature of the nursing client and on methodologies that are most congruent with the subject matter of nursing and its philosophical stand.

In a discipline that deals with human beings, it is perhaps not feasible that only one theory should explain, describe, predict, and change all the discipline's phenomena. For example, medicine uses the biomedical model based on the structure and function of biologic systems; however, it also uses a variety of means for auscultation, palpitation, and laboratory tests by computer or mechanical means, all of which are accompanied by different theories that compete but coexist (Frank, 1957, pp. 356–358).

A case for paradigmatic pluralism has to be made in nursing because there is a need for theories about people, interactions, illness, health, and nursing interventions.

In fact, currently there are many different theories that, although seen by some as competing with each other, address different relationships and focus on different phenomena, thereby actually complementing each other. These theories evolved from a variety of paradigms (adaptation, system, and interactionist, among others). Nursing deals with human behavior, and human behavior could not be explained through

> a single, completely general and comprehensive theory; instead, the desire for a single, all-embracing "scientific psychology" may itself prove to be a will-o'-the-wisp. Certainly, a similar will-o'-the-wisp had to be disregarded before modern physics could become the discipline it now is; and the reasons why this was so throw some light on the contemporary state of behavioral science (Toulmin, 1972, p. 386).

Another feature of nursing that supports its uniqueness is that as a profession it exists in an open system and has to be influenced by and be responsive to society's needs at all times. Therefore, nursing cannot afford to converge on one paradigm to the exclusion of others. Nurses' and clients' actions continue to be shaped by each other and by their social environment. This is where the analogy between nursing and sociology appears (Urry, 1973); both disciplines must be dynamic and changing, and both develop through integration and not through evolutions or revolutions. There are many communities in nursing, but there is not one community that could act as a unit to support one competing theory over another, nor are there unified communities in any of the other disciplines. If we decide to wait for that total agreement, perhaps we will not be able to work diligently on the much needed conceptual clarity and the further development of existing competing thoughts.

Another pattern of knowledge development in nursing is the compromise between the old and the new concepts. Researchers focus on the family and on the individual, on parts of individuals and on individuals as wholes; they use quantitative and qualitative techniques, and they explore administrative and clinical questions. In instances in which there are changes, old paradigms are redefined rather than totally rejected. For example, even as there is a revival of Nightingale's concept of environment, new paradigms, such as Rogers', are redefining her ideas.

It is the presence of competing theories, competing schools of thought, and debatable ideas that makes a discipline scholarly. The right to question, critique, and challenge has characterized all advanced disciplines (Toulmin, 1972, p. 110). If nursing were to adopt a revolutionary philosophy for its growth, it could put an end to this significant property of scholarliness (Laudan, 1977, pp. 73–76). Competition, creativity, and innovation are the hallmarks of scientific growth.

The discussion thus far has attempted to address the unique features of nursing that may make an evolutionary or revolutionary development unsuitable for describing nursing development (at best) and that may distort such developments (at worst) (Table 5-1). The thesis of this discussion is that *nursing progress seems to have charted its own path;* ideas that were rejected in one stage of development have been accepted at a different stage. Examples of this are the early rejection of nursing theories, the revival of Nightingale's focus on health and environment, and on spirituality (MacRae, 1995), the preoccupation with quantitative research methodology in the 1960s, the more recent revival of meaning of experience, the greater acceptance of alternate designs for research such as phenomenology, and the arguments for reclaiming our traditions

Table 5-1 Comparison Among Three Processes of Progress in the Discipline: Revolution, Evolution, and Integration

Analytical Unit	Revolution	Evolution	Integration
Sentiment	Aggression: crises	Adaptation	Change
Interaction	Competition	Cumulation	Collaboration
Goals	Conquering Overthrowing	Building Developing	Progressing Understanding
Process	Substitution Elimination Discontinuity	Lower to higher Selection Simple to complex Continuity	Openness Flexibility Contemporary and traditional Innovation
Pattern of development	Convergence	Mutation Slow, long range	Diversion
Reasoning	Adversarial	Logical	Dialectical
Mode	Rejection	Acceptance	Understanding
Evaluation	Criticize to destroy	Analyze to construct	Dialogue to develop
Environment	Critical Challenge	Restrictive	Supportive
Options	No option during normal science	Limited options	Open/unlimited options
Units of analysis	Paradigms Changes	Merits Competitions Demands Successes	History Patterns Development of members Number of unique phenomena identified Quality of questions answered Actualizing relationships between research, theory, and practice
Nursing	Preparadigmatic	Would-be discipline	Discipline

(Bradshaw, 1995). Ideas have been cumulative at times and unrelated to previous stages at others. Toulmin (1972), despite his interest in cumulation, observed that:

> [t]he leading ideas current at any stage in the development of 20th-century social science have tended to resemble those current two or three generations before, more than they have resembled those of the immediately previous generation (p. 385).

Popular theories of knowledge development call for a pattern of progress that is not manifested in its entirety in nursing. Therefore, nursing progress has been minimized, and its delays and limitations have been highlighted. An integrative process of development allows for an explanation of competitions and collaborations, acceptances and rejections, cumulations and innovations, peaks and valleys, reconsideration, development, evolution, and convolution. *Webster's Third New International Dictionary* defines a *convolution* as a complex, twisting, winding form or design.*

Integration is neither a nonpattern nor a negative pattern; rather it allows for pendulum swings and is explained as a pattern in progress. It is not a pattern toward the conventional idea of progress, toward a paradigm; it is a pattern of progress depicting

---

*By permission. From *Webster's Third New International Dictionary 1986* by Merriam-Webster Inc., publisher of the Merriam-Webster dictionaries.

nursing's accomplishments and its solid theoretical present through accommodation, refinement, and collaboration between thoughts, ideas, and individuals. This pattern of progress does not underestimate the further need for progress that is inherent in all scientific disciplines. It allows for careful critique of what has been accomplished and what is yet to be accomplished.

Table 5-1 illustrates the differences and similarities between the three processes of knowledge progress discussed here. When the progress of nursing is analyzed through each of the three philosophical views, different conclusions can be drawn. To a revolutionist, nursing is in a preparadigmatic stage; to an evolutionist, nursing is a would-be discipline; to an integrationist, nursing has achieved a disciplinary status. A careful assessment of patterns of growth and development in nursing, milestones, stages, and phenomena identified demonstrate the quality and significance of questions asked and answers provided. These units of analyses represent a synthesis between research, theory, and practice. When nursing is analyzed in terms of these, then it has achieved a disciplinary status.

From the Received View to the Perceived View

A number of philosophers in nursing have been concerned in the past that nurses may have adopted a limited view of science that is in direct contradiction to nursing's philosophy, its heritage, and its goals. The view perceived by these writers could be summarized under the rubric of "the received view," which others may call the scientific method (Suppe, 1977). The received view is philosophically old and outdated, but its effects lingered longer in nursing than in the field of philosophy of science (Suppe and Jacox, 1985).

The *received view* in any discipline usually denotes a set of ideas that are not to be challenged, the philosophical equivalent of being engraved in stone. It is the same premise that declares that holy books were received and therefore should not be challenged. Received view is also a label given to the "empirical positivism" movement or to "logical positivism," a 19th century philosophical movement closely aligned with Rudolf Carnap and rooted in the celebrated Vienna circle of philosophers. This circle, which met regularly during the 1880s in a seminar led by Moritz Schlick, a professor of philosophy at the University of Vienna, advocated an amalgamation of logic with the goals of empiricism in the development of scientific theories (Runggaldier, 1984). Eventually, the concept of "positivism" was dropped and replaced with "empiricism" to avoid the connection with Auguste Comte, whose ideas were coming into disfavor at that time. When Carnap joined the University of Chicago in 1936, logical empiricism was introduced to the United States (White, 1955, pp. 203–225).

The following are the tenets of logical empiricism:

1. Statements that cannot be confirmed by sensory data and through sensory experiences are not considered theoretical statements worthy of pursuing. As a result, they are disqualified as common sense statements and are therefore nonsense. Predictive statements that have no sensory data corroboration are not scientific. A direct relationship has to exist between experience and a meaningful theory.

2. True statements are only considered to be those that are *a posteriori.* That is, they are based on experience and known from experience.
3. Positivists regard most traditional metaphysics and ethical considerations as meaningless. Positivists regard such questions as possessing "emotive" meaning and as being "cognitively meaningless" (White, 1955).
4. Analyses of theories are based on analyses of completed theories, and completed theories are based on empirical data (Suppe, 1977, p. 125). The context of justification—that is, the verification and falsification of completed theory propositions—is the only significant context for consideration by scientists and philosophers alike. On the other hand, the contexts of discovery, such as conceptual issues, contexts within which theories are developed, logic in theory development, and usefulness, should be within the province of the sociologists of knowledge: the psychologist and historian (Reichenback, 1968).
5. Because the received view considers theories to reflect *a posteriori* depictions of reality, documented by sensory experiences, it therefore follows that propositions of theories are presented in a symbolic, formal, and axiomatic manner. There is room for *a priori* analysis, although it is only mathematical in nature.
6. Science is value free, and there is only one method for science, which is the scientific method.

The "ghost of the received view" loomed over nursing in its quest for a scientific base, according to Webster, Jacox, and Baldwin (1981). Others, such as Watson (1981) and Winstead-Fry (1980), also joined in blaming nursing's slow scientific progress on the insistence of its leaders to use the outdated scientific method as its model and to strive for one scientific method. The scientific method that they were speaking of is one based on the received view, one that espouses "reductionism, quantifiability, objectivity, and operationalization" (Watson, 1981, p. 414).

As a result, significant holistic problems in nursing have been ignored because they are neither reducible, quantifiable, nor objective. The scientific method adapted by nursing reduced a problem to its smallest unit or its most insignificant form and stripped it of the rich context from whence it emanated (Newman, 1981). The scientific method, oriented toward quantitative methods and highly accepted and respected, could not address theory and developing theory; therefore, it has not helped nursing to develop meaningful theories or advanced nursing to its projected goal of a scientific discipline.

There is some justification in blaming the received view for the slow progress and development of nursing. Many examples exist that support the view that nurses have been somewhat disillusioned by a philosophical view of science that is outmoded and ineffective (Newman, 1994). One example is the many theoretically disconnected but methodologically immaculate research projects that nurses have produced, a view that is shared by Batey (1977). However, there is more evidence than we have been led to believe supporting the view that nursing has, in fact, considered and followed a scientific path that is broader in scope and more integrative in approach than the received view.

Nursing theorists who have worked diligently to give us their conception of the discipline of nursing have not followed a received view approach. They have offered a number of conceptualizations that encompass the whole of nursing—a perceived view—based on their experiences and incorporating ideas that are subjective, intuitive, humanistic, integrative and, in many instances, not based on sense-oriented data. (See Chap. 21 for citations reflecting this statement.)

Discovery of field concepts, theory development, and processes of theorizing in nursing has not been based on the received view or on a structured and strict scientific approach. The context of discovery of these ideas has been traditional: case studies, personal anecdotes, and group insights. Acceptance of those visions that emanated from our nurse theorists has been slow because the theories have been branded by some as unscientific. Therein lies the problem.

To generalize, saying that nursing has followed a positivistic path is akin to saying that physics has followed an intuitive one. The theoreticians in nursing, those who have developed conceptualizations encompassing the field as a whole, have used the *perceived view*, which is a combination of phenomenological and philosophical approaches, as alternate methods of theory development. (See Chap. 11–for support of this view.) Perhaps the scholars in the field who believe that knowledge emanates from the context of justification have helped to orient nursing toward considering concepts such as sensory data, verification, and falsification as ways to accept or reject nursing conceptualizations. These scholars have therefore precipitated the early mass rejection of nursing theory as well as the continuous rejection by many in the field who are skeptical about the use or the effectiveness of nursing theories.

What we see in nursing today is a shift from the insistence of a few to adhere to the scientific method. Instead of ignoring nursing theoretical perspective until all propositions are tested and verified, the move is toward analysis of theories that are in process, as evidenced by the outpouring of books and articles that focus on and encourage the further development of nursing theory. There is a belief that analysis of these theories does not begin when theories are accomplished facts or when they are accepted or rejected. Rather, proposed analyses consider other epistemic factors related to the context of discovery. This context calls for explorations to discover which questions are more significant and which answers will be more acceptable. It is a view of science that accepts values, subjectivity, intuition, history, tradition, and multiple realities—a view that is more congruent with nursing and its commitment to human beings (Munhall, 1982; Oiler, 1982; Winstead-Fry, 1979).

To summarize, perhaps the dominant evaluative criteria for nursing research by our funding agencies has been a received view approach. In the meantime, the guiding paradigm for nursing practice, nursing theory, and, for that matter, nursing education has been more open, more variable, more relativistic, and more subject to experiences and personal interpretations. It has used a holistic approach, a view based on perceptions of both the clients and the theoreticians of their experiences; therefore, a perceived view.

It was perhaps the incongruence between the perceptions of the few (who evaluated research for publishing and for funding) and the perceptions of the majority of nurses (scientists, theoreticians, and clinicians) regarding knowledge development that delayed the acceptance of the perceived view. The research evaluators were slow in accepting the perceptions of the nursing majority. The views of the former, although leaders in nursing, did not seem to reflect the viewpoint of the majority in nursing. Table 5-2 demonstrates some of the similarities and differences between the received and perceived views.

Table 5-2 ***Comparison of the Received and Perceived Views of Science****

Received View	Perceived View
Objectivity	Subjectivity
Deduction	Induction
One truth	Multiple truths
Validation and replication	Trends and patterns
Justification	Discovery
Prediction and control	Description and understanding
Particulars	Patterns
Reductionism	Holism
Generalization	Individuation
Empirical positivism	Historicism

* *Based on Meleis, A.I. (1985). Theoretical nursing, Philadelphia: Lippincott; and Stevenson, J.S. and Woods, N.F. (1985). Nursing science and contemporary science: Emerging paradigms. In G. Sorenson (Ed.), Setting the agenda for the year 2000: Knowledge development in nursing. Kansas City, MO: American Academy of Nursing.*

Truth: From Correspondence to Weltanschauung

There is another subject of concern to those who are inquisitive about nursing's progress toward the development of its knowledge. What criteria have been used by nursing to accept or reject its theoretical notions? What concepts of truth should be used in the future? When do experiences become knowledge, and when does knowledge become truth? Does reality exist or appear?

Philosophers since Plato have addressed these epistemological questions. Over the centuries, three views have emerged: correspondence, coherence, and pragmatism (Armour, 1969; Kaplan, 1964).

The first view is that of *correspondence*, which, with its careful rules, calls for sensory data, very small variables, and operational definitions. For generations, this view has dominated science, research, and theory construction in the physical and natural sciences. It is the method of truth on which the received or scientific view is based. Indeed, many philosophers of science consider truth by correspondence and the received view one and the same. However, the received view and truth represent two different processes. The former addresses the process of research, the methodology by which data are collected and theories are developed; the latter attends to examining realities, the results of the findings. Whereas the former asks what to do to know, the latter asks how to know.

The empiricists, such as Bertrand Russell, and rationalists, such as J.E. McTaggart, preferring to view truth through correspondence, have designed a set of rules and norms against which theory development and research are expected to be analyzed. The most significant norm is that of truism of facts and their correspondence with the theories that encompass them. One of the most significant correspondence norms is total objectivity, a separation of the observer from the observed world. Validation is based on congruence between propositions and reality; that reality being one reality, an existing reality, and not reality as it may appear to different viewers. The theorist's role is to match the world with assertions and match the facts with concepts.

The positivists assert that correspondence truth is achieved through corroboration by verification. Popper (1959) modified the positivist view and developed the argument for falsification. He asserted that the central concept in scientific discovery is "marcation.' *Demarcation criteria* require that we consider a proposition scientific only if it has the potential for being falsified. Verification of the opposite statement occurs with multiple incidents of falsification of the statement through experience. Once a proposition is countered by a single falsifying instance, it should be rejected. On the other hand, it is not scientific if it does not have the potential for falsification. Continuous attempts to falsify statements make the scientific process rigorous. Truth is achieved when we have exhausted all attempts at falsifying propositions.

Although Popper warns against the potential for any entirely conclusive statement due to problems of reliability in testing, we nevertheless come closer to the truth by testing and retesting with the objective of attempting to nullify and to falsify the proposition under exploration. To the correspondence theorists, whether verification or falsification is the focus, truth is achieved through sensory data and controlled experiments. The correspondence of existing reality, of facts and propositions, is the goal. No room exists for metaphysics, for conceptual truths, for multiple realities, or for perceptions of reality. There are other problems when viewing truth in mainly correspondence terms. If facts exist, are not facts already affected by the concepts introduced to explain the facts?

Truth through *coherence* differs considerably from truth through correspondence. The truth through coherence is manifested in the logical way in which relationships and judgments relate. Whereas the norms for correspondence are verification and falsification with sensory data, the norms for coherence are an integration of relationships, simplicity of presentation, and a certain beauty of propositions. When separate components of a phenomenon "suddenly fall into a pattern of relatedness, when they click into position," then truth has been achieved (Kaplan, 1964 p. 314). Truth according to this theory endures, but perhaps in a more transitory fashion, in ways that may not be reproducible but are no less recognizable. If the proposition is sufficient for today, then there is truth in it.

The coherence norms of logic, simplicity, and aesthetic presentation appear to be norms to be used for both the context of discovery and the context of justification. They are most suitable, however, for the discovery of apparent realities. They lend themselves more to the evaluation of concepts that are in the process of development than those in the process of testing. Although norms of correspondence and coherence may appear to contradict each other, it is nonetheless possible to consider them as complementary. While using the coherence norms to judge and evaluate theories, we can also use correspondence norms to judge propositions that evolve out of research.

In the 1930s, a third type of theory about truth was advanced by a group of American philosophers called pragmatists. In fact, according to Leslie Armour (1969), there are two types of *pragmatic* theories of truth. *First*, an assertion is true if it produces the right type of influence on its followers. In other words, a proposition is declared to be true when its usefulness is determined by its users. Experience and the ability to solve problems are two of the norms considered in this view of truth. *Second,* a proposition or any theorized relationship is true if it receives confirmation from a person or persons who may have conducted the right investigations or who are designated as significant by the community of scholars. Pierce (cited in Kaplan, 1964) suggests that, according to this theory, a consensus between significant theoreticians or investigators is what constitutes truth.

Pragmatic truth is not as dependent on evidence as it is on observation—on a declaration of effectiveness by whatever methods the significant members of a community of scholars use. These measures of effectiveness may be subjective, political, social, or objective. To the proponents of this view, "a theory is validated, not by showing it to be invulnerable to criticism, but by putting it to good use, in one's own problems or in those problems of co-workers" (Kaplan, 1964).

A pragmatic theory of truth allows for validation of theories through restructuring, use of new techniques, or even better awareness and realizations of the meaning of old relationships. The value of these new relationships lies not in the answers they may provide as much as in the new questions they may ask and the consequences that result from their use (Kaplan, 1964). Humanity tentativeness, subjectivity, collectivity, and usefulness are all qualities attached to this concept of pragmatic truth, which evolved out of the Chicago school of thought (Table 5-3.)

Some conceptual problems are not as well addressed by any one of the theories of truth in isolation. Laudan (1977, p. 54) identified three. The first of these problems is an intrascientific problem, which results from two theories representing two domains that are inconsistent. An example may be Rogers' (1970) view of a unitary human being as an energy field and behavior as the manifestation of the pattern and organization of the energy field, which presupposes a methodological approach to the study of a human being and his energy field as a whole. Johnson (1974), on the other hand, views a social behavioral system with seven subsystems revolving around subsystem goals and manifested in observable behavior. Johnson presupposes a study of man by reducing man to behaviors.

Table 5-3 Comparison of Different Theories of Truth

Analytical Unit	Correspondence	Coherence	Pragmatism
Norms	Corroboration	Logic	Experience
Contexts	Context of justification	Context of experience	Context of discovery and justification
Goals	Acceptance/rejection	Support	Understanding
Reality	One		Multiple
Role of theorist	Match world with assertions Distance	Match with assertions Involvement	Match with users Humanness
Evaluation	Verification Falsification	Simplicity Beauty	Utility Problem solving
Process	End	Process	Process
Validation	Congruence between propositions and reality	Endurance of ideas	Consensus of users

Because of the theoretical incompatibility between the two fundamental views of the nursing client, the nursing community may attempt (perhaps prematurely) to accept one in favor of the other. The theorist's commitment to adequacy and effectiveness may also prompt one to concede to the other. Either of those alternatives to resolving the problem may not do so because of the level of conceptual and methodological knowledge. To reject Rogers' conception of a unitary human being as an energy field and behavior as a manifestation of pattern and organization of the energy field will either create a reductionist scientific school of thought in nursing or will prompt Rogers, a committed theorist, to continue to work on developing a more adequate theory of the unitary human being. The latter is an acceptable option for scientific development, but the former may impede development because of its prematurity.

It is also possible that the newness of nursing as a discipline makes it easier to reject both competing views in favor of another, more established view of a human being (such as a person as a biologic system) to the detriment of solving the central problem. Neither correspondence nor coherence criteria could solve this issue; it is best addressed through a pragmatic approach to truth.

Nursing has also been beset by other philosophical inconsistencies (Munhall, 1982). Existential and pragmatic philosophies have dominated clinical nursing, and positivistic, empirical philosophies have attempted to dominate the academic discipline. This theoretical confusion has only managed to impede nursing's theoretical development. Laudan refers to such conflict between emerging conflicting theoretical and methodological paradigms as normative difficulties. Those who believe that nursing has been dominated by the correspondence norm would attribute the early rejection of nursing theories to this paradox.

There was a belief that the only credible theories in nursing were those that were inferred from observable data. Others asserted that a nursing philosophy that espoused holism, integration, and health was in direct conflict with its methodology of reductionism, objectivity, logic, measurement, verification, and falsification. Where does the truth lie? Which of the two options should nursing follow—the methodological view or the philosophical premise? Who determines the truth—the methodologists or the theoreticians? None of the norms in isolation would provide us with the truth. A combination of all may bring us closer.

The third difficulty that confronts theorists and cannot be resolved by any one of the theories, Laudan calls "prevalent world view difficulties" (Laudan, 1977, p. 61). This phenomenon is observed when the myths, the beliefs, the history, and the practice are in opposition with the developing theories. The prevalent nursing view ascribed to by clinicians is that nursing is practical and skill oriented and that its principles as well as its skills are derived from other disciplines. Nursing is not theoretical, says this world view, or academic.

Tension also exists between the researchers, who hold the world belief that theories develop only from research, and the theoreticians, who believe that theories are culminations of experience, history, and intuition as well as research findings. There have been many "world views" in nursing, with very few ascribing to a theoretical world view. Weltanschauung attempts to address the many problems that none of the truth theories are able to address in isolation.

Multiple Truths in Nursing

In offering alternatives to correspondence norms and to the received view, Suppe (1977) suggested that what is needed is a different way by which theories are analyzed; he called this new way Weltanschauung. He defined it as "a comprehensive world view, especially from a specified standpoint." According to Suppe, Weltanschauung is:

> [an] analysis of theories which concerns itself with the epistemic factors governing the discovery, development, and acceptance or rejecting of theories; such an analysis must give serious attention to the idea that science is done from within a conceptual perspective which determines in large part which questions are worth investigating and what sorts of answers are acceptable; the perspective provides a way of thinking about a class of phenomena which define[s] the class of legitimate problems and delimits the standards for their acceptable solution. Such a perspective is intimately tied to one's language which conceptually shapes the way one experiences the world (p. 126).

There is a Weltanschauung, or world view, of truth in theoretical nursing that includes an integration of norms emanating from different theories of truth. It combines rigor and intuition, sensory data as they exist and as they appear, perceptions of the subject and of the theoretician, and logic with observable clinical data. What have been advocated by different theorists and researchers merely as norms for acceptance of propositions are not contradictory norms because in some situations, events, and experiences, one set of norms is more appropriate than another. Some research in nursing has been guided by the positivists' views and by correspondence. Some theory development has been guided by these norms as well; for example, Orlando and Johnson focused on observable, verifiable behavior in developing theories (Johnson, 1974; Orlando, 1961). Rogers spoke of experiences beyond the five senses (1970).

Nursing theoreticians, however, would not have developed their theories if they adhered to correspondence norms. There are numerous examples that nursing has used a pragmatic theory of truth. Johnson, in 1974, spoke about criteria for acceptance of knowledge as based on social responsibility and about how knowledge and nursing action should make a valuable difference in the people's lives. Whether the model guiding nursing is right or wrong is a social decision and not a theorist's or researcher's decision exclusively.

Rogers (1970), in conceptualizing a unitary man as an energy field, spoke of experiences beyond the five senses and therefore could not use correspondence norms to verify her conceptualization, but instead used coherence norms. Many others supported the necessity of considering coherence norms in conceptualizing nursing and suggested that truth emanated from logic (Batey, 1977; Beckstrand, 1978a, 1978b; Dickoff, James, and Wiedenbach, 1968).

The Weltanschauung of truth in nursing theory uses validation, verification, simplicity, logic, consequences, clients, theorists, and actual or potential experiences as norms against which truth of the theory is compared. It accepts multiple realities and "a composite of realities" (Oiler, 1982). It accepts different expressions, different sources, and criteria such as a number of solved problems within a discipline (Laudan, 1977).

Conclusion

Three epistemological issues may have influenced the course of theory development in nursing and, indeed, all knowledge in nursing. The first addressed the course that nursing has taken to achieve a disciplinary status. Two prevailing theories of progress were discussed and analyzed: revolution and evolution. Neither could adequately describe the unique path that nursing has taken, and both cast a dark shadow on nursing progress because accomplishments in nursing could not be entirely credited under either of them. A third approach of integration was proposed as being more congruent with nursing progress. It considers the nature of nursing and its detours.

The second issue is related to the pull between the received view of science and the perceived view. The former provided the canons for acceptance and rejection of the road that nurses have taken in theory development, but perhaps is a more acceptable approach to analysis and evaluation of work within the context of justification. The perceived view, the guiding paradigm for nursing practice, nursing theory, and, for that matter, nursing education, has been more open, more variable, relativistic, and subject to experience and personal interpretations. It is a view that is holistic in approach, a view that is based on the perceptions of both the client and the theoretician. The perceived view is more appropriate for the context of discovery.

The third subject that has created issues of acceptance and rejection of nursing knowledge comprises questions such as: What counts as truth? How do we go about finding it? What criteria do we have for acceptance of nursing's major questions, assumptions, and answers? Three theories of truth were discussed and related to the view of truth that has emerged in nursing.

Progress in nursing has been unique and phenomenal in acceleration in the past decade. In the late 1980s, theorists and researchers in nursing began to accept the differences between nursing and other sciences, the uniqueness of nursing, and the capabilities of its scholars to develop knowledge. Nursing deals with wholeness, perceptions, experiences, multiple realities, appearances of phenomena, and the existence of phenomena. Whether it needs to or should use any of the theories of truth discussed in this chapter is up to you and the future theoreticians in nursing. This chapter intended to bring you current discussions and to encourage you to go beyond this limited discussion to explore theories of probabilities and theories that espouse the use of the criteria of a number of solved problems within a discipline rather than truth theories.

REFERENCES

Andreoli, K.G. and Thompson, C.E. (1977). The nature of science in nursing. *Image*, 9(2), 32–37.

Armour, L. (1969). *The concept of truth*. Assen, Germany: Van Gorcum and Co.

Baer, E.D. (1979). Philosophy provides the rationale for nursing's multiple research directions. *Image*, 11(3), 72–74.

Batey, M.V. (1977). Conceptualization: Knowledge and logic guiding empirical research. *Nursing Research*, 26(5), 324–329.

Beckstrand, J. (1978a). The notion of practice theory and the relationship of scientific and ethical knowledge to practice. *Research in Nursing and Health*, 1(3), 131–136.

Beckstrand, J. (1978b). The need for a practice theory as indicated by the knowledge used in conduct of practice. *Research in Nursing and Health*, 1(4), 175–179.

Bradshaw, A. (1995). What are nurses doing to patients? A review of theories or nursing past and present. *Journal of Clinical Nursing*, 4, 81–92.

Carper, B.A. (1978). Practice oriented theory: Part 1. Fundamental patterns of knowing in nursing. *Advances in Nursing Science*, 1(1), 13–23.

Dickoff, J., James, P., and Wiedenbach, E. (1968). Theory in a practice discipline: Part 1. Practice oriented theory. *Nursing Research*, 17(5), 415–435.

Fawcett, J. (1978). The relationship between theory and research: A double helix. *Advances in Nursing Science*, 1(1), 49–62.

Frank, P. (1957). *Philosophy of science*. Englewood Cliffs, NJ: Prentice-Hall.

Freese, L. (1972). Cumulative sociological knowledge. *American Sociological Review*, 37(4), 472–482.

Hardy, M.E. (1978). Practice oriented theory: Part 1. Perspectives on nursing theory. *Advances in Nursing Science*, 1(1), 37–48.

Johnson, D.E. (1974). Development of theory: A requisite for nursing as a primary health profession. *Nursing Research*, 23(5), 372–377.

Kaplan, A. (1964). *The conduct of inquiry: Methodology of behavioral science*. San Francisco: Chandler Publishing Company.

Kuhn, T.S. (1970). The structure of scientific revolutions. In Neurath, O. (Ed.), *International encyclopedia of unified science* (2nd ed., Vol. 2). Chicago: University of Chicago Press.

Kuhn, T.S. (1977). *The essential tension: Selected studies in scientific tradition and change*. Chicago: University of Chicago Press.

Laudan, L. (1977). *Progress and its problems: Toward a theory of scientific growth*. Berkeley: University of California Press.

Laudan, L. (1981). A problem-solving approach to scientific progress. In I. Hacking (Ed.), *Scientific revolutions*. New York: Oxford University Press.

Macrae, J. (1995). Nightingale's spiritual philosophy and its significance for modern nursing. *Image: Journal of Nursing Scholarship*, 27(1), 8–10.

Munhall, P.L. (1982). In opposition or apposition. *Nursing Research*, 31(3), 175–177.

Newman, M. (1981, October). *Methodology of pattern*. Paper presented at the Nursing Theory Think Tank, Denver.

Newman, M.A. (1983). The continuing revolution: A history of nursing science. In N.L. Chaska (Ed.), *The nursing profession: A time to speak*. New York: McGraw-Hill.

Newman, M.A. (1994). Theory for nursing practice. *Nursing Science Quarterly*, 7(4), 153–157.

Oiler, C. (1982). The phenomenological approach in nursing research. *Nursing Research*, 31(3), 178–181.

Orlando I.J. (1961). *The dynamic nurse-patient relationship*. New York: G.P. Putman's Sons.

Popper, K. (1959). *The logic of scientific discovery*. London: Hutchinson.

Reichenback, H. (1968). *The rise of scientific philosophy*. Berkeley: University of California Press.

Rogers, M. (1970). *An introduction to the theoretical basis of nursing*. Philadelphia: F.A. Davis.

Runggaldier, E. (1984). *Carnap's early conventionalism: An inquiry into the historical background of the Vienna circle*. Amsterdam: Rodopi.

Shapere, D. (1981). Meaning and scientific change. In I. Hacking (Ed.), *Scientific revolutions*. New York: Oxford University Press.

Silva, M.C. (1977). Philosophy, science, theory: Interrelationships and implications for nursing research. *Image*, 9(3), 59–63.

Stevenson, J.S. and Woods, N.F. (1986). Nursing science and contemporary science: Emerging paradigms. In G. Sorenson (Ed.), *Setting the agenda for the year 2000: Knowledge development in nursing*. Kansas City, MO: American Academy of Nursing.

Suppe, F. (Ed.). (1977). *The structure of scientific theories* (2nd ed.). Champaign: University of Illinois Press.

Suppe, F. and Jacox, A.K. (1985). Philosophy of science and the development of nursing theory. In *Annual Review of Nursing Research*, 3, 241–267.

Toulmin, S. (1972). *Human understanding: The collective use and evolution of concepts*. Princeton, NJ: Princeton University Press.

Urry, J. (1973). Thomas S. Kuhn as sociologist of knowledge. *British Journal of Sociology*, 24(4), 462–473.

Watson, J. (1981). Nursing's scientific quest. *Nursing Outlook*, 29(7), 413–416.

Webster, G., Jacox, A., and Baldwin, B. (1981). Nursing theory and the ghost of the received view. In J.C. McClosky and H.K. Grace (Eds.), *Current issues in nursing*. Oxford: Blackwell Scientific Publications.

White, M. (1955). *The age of analysis: 20th century philosophers*. Boston: Houghton Mifflin.

Winstead-Fry, P. (1979, June). Defining clinical content of nursing. In *Proceedings of the 1979 Forum on Doctoral Education in Nursing*. San Francisco: University of California.

Winstead-Fry, P. (1980). The scientific method and its impact on holistic health. *Advances in Nursing Science*, 2(3), 1–7.

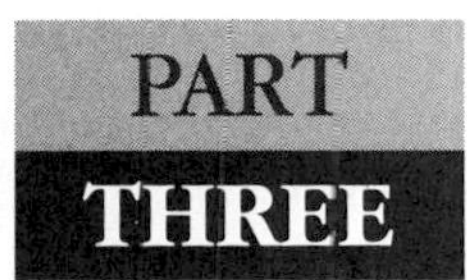

Our Discipline and Its Structure

A pause to reflect critically on a discipline's progress is significant to its continuous growth. This part of the journey focuses on analyses of the meaning of the discipline and the components that define our nursing discipline.

In this part there is a bridge between past and present in three distinct areas: the meaning and the structure of the evolved discilpline, sources and resources for theoretical nursing, and the paradoxes that may have contributed to paucity in the development of theoretical nursing. Two themes are apparent: an historical and a more contemporary view in the history of science and an historical and a more contemporary view in nursing theory. The tension between the opposite poles in these two themes is a healthy and effective tension, so long as work is not stunted while the tension is resolved. Perhaps the tensions, the inconsistencies, and the paradoxes could be considered as integral parts of nursing's theoretical progress, and the discipline of nursing and its scientific base could be considered as a process rather than an end result. If this is true, then we can view the effectiveness of an epistemology in its process and in the number of problems in nursing that it has been able to solve.

Understanding the structure of the discipline and defining the boundaries of a discipline, however flexible and open those boundaries are, is vital for focusing individual and group scholarly work and for the continuous growth and development of disciplines. Scholarship may be considered as the ability of a scholar to focus and connect her inquiries to the discipline's ultimate mission and focus. The question is: how could members of a discipline engage in cumulative knowledge development without giving attention to the focus and nature of inquiry in the discipline or to the primary mission of a discipline?

A *discipline* is defined as "a branch of knowledge or teaching," and as the "training expected to produce a specific character or pattern of behavior" (*American Heritage Dictionary*, 1992). A discipline includes "a branch of knowledge or teaching" and a regulatory "set of rules or methods" that govern practice (*American Heritage Dictionary*, 1992). It is also "a unique perspective, a distinct way of viewing all phenomena," and it provides the boundaries that define the nature of the questions investigated (Donaldson and Crowley, 1978, p. 113; Moore, 1990). The discipline of nursing includes the content and processes related to all the roles that nurses play, including administrator, teacher, politician, clinician, and consultant. A discipline also includes the theories developed to describe, explain, and prescribe, as well as the research findings related to the discipline's central phenomena and other related disciplines that are essential for the functioning of members of a discipline or for the continuous growth of the discipline.

Several components define the discipline of nursing. These are a perspective, a domain, existing and accepted definitions of nursing, and patterns of knowing in the discipline. In Chapter 6, the nursing perspective is defined. A perspective in nursing evolved from the nature of its defining characteristics. In Chapter 7, the domain of the discipline, its definitions, its components, and the unique characteristics of nursing are presented and discussed. The structure of a discipline could also be determined by the sources that drive its questions, the resources used to develop knowledge, and the nature and progress of a discipline, which is also influenced by the issues and paradoxes that its members encounter. A discussion about these is provided in Chapter 8. Chapter 8 also addresses conditions essential for theory development, such as nurses as resources of theory, and nursing practice as one of the sources for theory, among numerous others. Finally, the chapter focuses on two paradoxes that occupied the field of metatheory for some time: conceptual models versus theories and nursing theory versus borrowed theory. A discipline is also defined by the patterns that the discipline's members use to establish what is known in the discipline. In Chapter 9, the different patterns of knowing and the human processes involved are discussed. These human processes—of the theorist, the nurse, and the client—are an integral part of nursing and its theory. Aspects of empiricism are still significant and useful for nursing, added to other processes and aspects of knowing.

No attempt is made in this part to discredit one philosophy and promote another; an attempt is made, however, to display our options in the development and progress of theoretical nursing. An attempt is also made to highlight the tensions, to demonstrate what aspects of the different paradoxes are congruent with nursing and its mission and, finally, to emphasize human aspects of nursing in general and theoretical nursing in particular.

CHAPTER 6

Nursing Perspective

Each of us has a perspective of the world around us and each of us has a perspective through which we perceive, comprehend, and interpret situations and events in our lives. As nurses, we have developed some shared views that define the ways by which we come to assess our clients and their situations. Our individual and shared perspectives reflect our culture, education work experiences, and values, and these perspectives, in turn, influence our views of events and situations. Disciplines are characterized by perspectives shared by the discipline's members. Disciplines are characterized by a perspective that shapes the way members of a discipline tend to view the phenomena within the discipline, as well as those outside the discipline. A perspective is defined as the way members of a group view and characterize a situation. It is the sum total of the attitudes and the outlook that help members of a defined group to develop a position or a viewpoint. A perspective provides the panoramic view of situations, it provides the signposts that characterize the outlook on the world. A perspective is based on a set of values that help in characterizing the nature of the world for members of a group. It contains the preferences for certain views and for certain ways of observing and reacting to situations. A perspective, according to Rosemary Ellis, is the prevailing view held by members of a discipline or a profession (Algase and Whall, 1993). A nursing perspective is defined by its unique aspects, the history of the profession, the sociopolitical context in which nursing care is provided and the nature of the orientation of members of the nursing profession, as well as the discipline.

The perspective of clinicians and scholars in nursing reflects the academic and professional approaches to knowledge development, a history of second-class citizenship, a history of devaluation of its mission of caring, and a history of oppression of its members that reflects worldwide oppression of women and subordination of nurses to bureaucratic and professional structures. Therefore, nurses may be more experientially prepared to examine and analyze similar processes that may be encountered by nursing clients. By necessity, too, these experiences drive the kinds of analyses and interpretations of progress and development of the discipline. They shape the perspective that evolves and characterizes a discipline. A nursing perspective is shaped by many defining characteristics. Four important defining characteristics that determine our perspective are the:

- nature of nursing science as a human science
- practice aspects of nursing

- caring relationships that nurses and patients develop
- health and wellness perspective

Each aspect of the nursing perspective is presented and discussed below.

Nursing: A Human Science

The science underlying the discipline of nursing has been described as a human science. A human science has several properties, each of which is significant in shaping its perspective and in selecting appropriate strategies for knowledge development. Meleis (1992), McWhinney (1989), and Holmes (1990) identified some of these properties of human science.

1. A human science focuses on human beings as wholes and advocates understanding the particulars in terms of the whole.
2. A human science has at its core an understanding of experiences as lived by its members.
3. A human science deals with meanings as seen and perceived by its members. Meanings include those attached to responses, symbols, events, and situations.
4. To be able to understand meanings and experiences, a scientist needs to enter into a meaningful dialogue with participants. Interaction is the prime source of meanings and perceptions of experiences. Participants in the activities of knowledge development are those who are developing and structuring knowledge and those about whom knowledge is developed. All participants have to verify the meanings of these experiences.
5. "The scope for generalization for a human science is limited" (McWhinney, 1989, p. 298). A generalization has to be made within a context; therefore, generalization may be presented in terms of patterns.
6. Some conditions, situations, behaviors, and events are reducible for purposes of description.

Nursing as a human science is concerned with the experiences of human beings and with health and illness matters. Because these experiences are shaped by history, significant others, politics, social structures, gender, and culture, nurses also are concerned with how these perspectives shape actions and reactions of human beings. It is precisely that concern that makes nursing a practice discipline, which in turn helps to define its perspective.

Nursing: A Practice-Oriented Discipline

The practice aspects of nursing are a second defining characteristic that shape its perspective. Nursing exists to provide nursing care for clients who experience illness, as well as those who may experience potential health care problems. Nursing has been described as a clinical discipline, an applied field, or a practice-oriented discipline. What do we mean when we say that nursing is a practice-oriented discipline? It means that it has a primary mission related to practice. Therefore, its members seek knowledge of human beings' responses to health and illness to help in monitoring and promoting health, to help in caring for them, to help in assisting them to care for themselves, and to help in empowering them to develop and use resources (Bottorff, 1991). Nursing may use basic and applied knowledge to achieve its goals, but it is still a practice-oriented discipline.

Nurses need basic knowledge to understand the basic phenomena related to the goals and the mission of nursing, for example, how certain groups of people tend to seek help, how certain connections tend to maintain their balance and health, and how different patterns of responses to such events as pain, intrusive interventions, hospitalization, and discharge exert their influence. Basic understanding of such phenomena as comfort, touch, confusion, ambiguity, sleeplessness, and restlessness is essential for the subsequent development of applied knowledge. Applied knowledge is that which provides guidelines to maintain, ameliorate, develop, inhibit, support, change, advocate, clarify, or suppress some of these basic phenomena. Both basic and applied knowledge are the cornerstones of nursing as a practice-oriented discipline. Nurses also seek knowledge related to the practical care they provide. Practical aspects of nursing have been dichotomized with its theoretical aspects rather than integrating, incorporating, and using them as a springboard for further development of the discipline. The shift by nurse scholars away from practical aspects, and in particular from clinical skills, has been manifested in limited interest in research related to clinical concerns, in uncovering the daily work of nurses, in the conflicts between educators and administrators in defining educational end products, and in the decreasing emphasis on clinical skills among others (Bjørk, 1995; Clarke, 1986; Titler, Buckwalter, and Maas, 1993).

The goal of knowledge development, then, is to understand the nurisng care needs of people and to learn how to better care for them; therefore, the caring activities that nurses are involved in on a daily basis may be the focus for knowledge development and may be congruent with activities involved in knowledge structuring, particularly because the participants in both activities are human beings. Two types of knowledge development goals drive the activities and the progress in knowledge. There is "knowledge for the sake of knowledge" and knowledge to provide better nursing care to people through solving central problems of concern to the discipline (Laudan, 1977, 1981). Nursing as a discipline and nurses as scientists whose mission is to care for people and enhance their well-being cannot afford to participate only in developing knowledge for the sake of knowledge development.

Thus, the purposes of knowledge development in nursing are shaped by its practice orientation, which in turn shapes the nursing perspective. The nursing perspective reflects nurses' interest in:

- Empowering the discipline of nursing with knowledge related to patients and their care
- Empowering nurses to enhance well-being of clients and empower them with the necessary knowledge for their daily work
- Empowering clients to care for themselves by fully utiilizing available resources and creating new resources

If these are the main purposes for developing knowledge in nursing, then we have to consider approaches to knowledge development that make these purposes possible. To empower the discipline and its members, nurses look for and identify the same skills that made them effective and caring clinicians and build on these skills as well as other skills that could enhance knowledge development. These skills are related to nurses' daily work activities and its uniqueness.

A unique aspect of nursing as a practice discipline that further defines its perspective is around-the-clock care provided by nurses working in institutions. When nurses see patients around-the-clock, they tend to know more about their daily life processes and patterns and therefore are more likely to better understand their lived experiences and their health care needs. There is also more continuity to their knowledge of their patients. These provide a more textured context for the clients' needs and responses. Nurses who care for patients in primary health care settings, including home care, may have to structure their encounters in more creative ways to increase their understanding of the daily life processes and the integrated patterns of responses of their clients to health and illness within a context of limited time and a different space. Whether in a hospital, a clinic, or a home, nursing encounters are characterized by continuity, intensity, and involvement in ways that other health care professionals do not experience. Nurses also monitor and coordinate the care of their patients; this includes their own caregiving as well as the care offered by others in the health care team.

Nurses spend more time with clients (Masson, 1985); they conduct comprehensive assessments, including taking down family and medical histories to establish a better care context and gain a better understanding of the client's responses, perform daily activities such as bed baths, provide for daily hygienic needs, give medication, and carry out treatments. Therefore, experiences and responses of clients to health and illness tend to be viewed within a context of the client's life relationships, culture, goals, and daily experiences. The ongoing relationship with nurses prompts clients to share their experiences in more narrative dialogues allowing more details, meanings, and history that makes their health and illness experiences more understandable and allows for more congruent plans of action. If patients are given indications that these experiences are important for the caring processes, they tend to share more freely with nurses the effects of the complaint, the medical diagnoses, or the intervention on their daily life and on the significant others in their families. In other words, patients naturally are more interested in ways by which illness, altering conditions, or treatments affect their daily lives and daily routines. Nurses are in more opportune positions to get the benefit of hearing narratively about the experiences of their patients. Nurses tend to get to know the patient differently and more profoundly (Jenny and Logan, 1992).

Nursing: A Caring Discipline

The caring aspects of nursing also help define its perspective. Many questions have been raised about the concept of caring. Is caring the essence of nursing, is it the field's special knowledge area, is it equal to the discipline of nursing, is it a central concept in nursing, or is it the core of its domain? Is it the goal or the mission nursing, or is it a goal and a mission of nursing? Caring has been considered and discussed through each of these prisms, and there are enough writings in nursing to support each of these positions (Cohen, 1991).

Caring, which has been an integral part of the private domain of women, has been discussed recently as a component of both the public and private domains. Condon (1992) goes further by suggesting that caring may be the glue that will connect nurses' public and private domains and will decrease "the discrepancies between the demands of the private and public domains" (p. 19). She also proposes that caring and nursing are compatible, and caring and feminist ideals are compatible. Caring, for her, is the foundational moral value for nursing. It is detrimental to nursing if it continues to be viewed as a component of public domains and is relegated only to women in society. She further proposes that we explore how the philosophy of professionalism may conflict with the ethics of caring.

Condon (1992) calls for a new metaphor for nursing caring to substitute for the metaphors of duty and religious calling. There are numerous such metaphors in nursing. Watson (1988, 1990) describes caring more from an existential philosophy, and she reviews the spiritual bases of caring. To her, caring is the moral ideal of nursing. Leininger (1981) discusses caring from a cultural perspective. For Brody (1988), caring is the central virtue of nursing. Gendron (1988, 1994) provides innovative arguments, likening caring to the creativity that is woven on as a structure for the substance in nursing. The structure is based on the contextual knowledge of scientific facts as well as conceptual frameworks. The structure also includes skills, nursing interventions, and policies among other aspects of structure. All these are brought to the patient's bedside or home through creative patterns in an artistic way. To match nursing actions to people, a nurse needs to know how to synchronize with a person, and she must know when she is synchronized. The challenge is then not only in the development of the knowledge base required to provide these caring actions, but also in how to prepare clinicians who are able to develop a self-client relationship that is synchronized. A synchronized relationship is based on "sensing subjective tacit meaning" of experiences and situations and on attuning "one's self and others" to these experiences and their meanings. To develop and carry out these aspects of the caring processes, Gendron (1994) proposes using "reflective journals" and an "emphasis on dialogue in the sharing of students' experiences through narrative" (p. 29) story telling and analysis.

The art of nursing has also been used as a synonym for caring. An epistemological analysis by Johnson (1994) about the meaning of art in nursing identified five separate senses of art in nursing. Nursing art is exemplified when nurses are able to grasp the meaning that is inherent in their encounter with patients, when they are able to establish connections, when they are able to skillfully perform nursing activities, when they choose between alternatives, and when they morally conduct nursing practice. **Grasping meaning** is attributed to perceptions rather than intellect; it depends on observations, feelings, imagination, and understanding that go beyond description—it depends on inner experiences and is holistic in nature. **Connecting with patients** is more than establishing a relationship; rather, it consists of the experiences in everything the nurse does with patients, including nonverbal communication. There is an authenticity to this communication that occurs between human beings. **Skill in nursing activ-**

ities is a behavioral ability in which there is an understanding about the skills needed for providing care and in which there is embedded understanding of these skills. The skills in such nursing activities can be learned, and they are expressed through ease and fluidity of movements among other characteristics yet to be defined. **Determining a course of action** is expressed by the group of authors who contend that the nursing art is practical, and it is through assumptions derived from a disciplinary structure that nurses are making decisions, based on a thorough understanding of all options. The nursing process proponents build their case on the artistic aspects of nursing as described in this category of definitions. **To practice morally** is a definition of nursing art that includes the view that skills are important but not a substitute for other aspects of practice, nor are they enough for the care that patients need. If a nurse does not make moral choices or address the moral dilemmas in her practice, then she is not using the artistic aspects of the discipline.

Morse, Bottorff, Neander, and Solberg, (1991) and Morse, Solberg, Neander, Bottorff, and Johnson (1990) describe caring as human trait, moral imperative, affect, interpersonal relationships, and therapeutic intervention. Caring is further described in nursing literature in the following ways:

1. As a human trait, it should be considered from a personal, psychological, or cultural perspective.
2. As a moral imperative, Gadow (1985) and Watson (1988, 1990) view the fundamental essence of nursing as preserving the dignity of others. This meaning of caring provides the base for all nursing interventions, assessments, and activities.
3. As an affect this is manifested through emotional feelings or empathy, feelings of dedication. Demands on time may change this.
4. The nurse–patient relationship is the essence of caring.
5. Caring is also seen as a therapeutic intervention.

Caring for clients is a component of what defines a nursing perspective (Clifford, 1995). It is one of the traditions handed down over the decades (Olson, 1993). It is another lens by which nurses as clinicians view their clients. It is the core activity in nursing practice (Benner and Wrubel, 1989). It may also be the same lens that nurses as scholars need to see the subject matter for their research or theory development. If caring is an integral part of a nursing perspective, it could also be an integral component of the subject matter of the theories developed (Newman, Sime, and Corcoran-Perry, 1991) or the guiding force for the strategies by; which theories are developed and research is formatted (Feldman, 1993). A caring perspective has shaped the processes used for knowledge development. It is encouraging to observe that there is increasingly more openness in Western societies to acknowledge the caring aspects of relationships and to bring caring more into the public domain, a practice that has always been more prevalent in developing countries. The art of nursing and its caring aspects requires time, energy, and skills that are not well acknowledged or rewarded through appropriate policies. Therefore the question is: Are nurses rewarded for their caring activities? MacPherson (1989) contends that nurses are not rewarded for trying to care and for the time they spend in caring for their patient communities. Educators, clinicians, and administrators may have to hold and drive the notion that caring is not a negotiated commodity. Defining caring as a component of the nursing perspective may provide them with the rationale to support their quest for supportive and rewarding caring activities.

Nursing: A Health-Oriented Discipline

To say that a nursing perspective is shaped by its health orientation is not to deny the work and the caring that nurses provide for clients who are sick, who are experiencing traumas, or who are recovering from illness. Nurses' orientation to the health of individuals and populations is historical, beginning with Nightingale's writings (1859) in which she defined nurses' work in terms of maintaining health and bringing a state of health back to the individual. Health has been considered integral to nursing (Allen, 1986), a goal (Rogers, 1970), a construct (Tripp-Reimer, 1984), an idea in nursing (Smith, 1981), a metaparadigm concept (Fawcett, 1995), a theory (Newman, 1986), and a concept (Reynolds, 1988).

Health is also a perspective that defines what we consider in our assessments, in making plans for interventions, in evaluating our interventions, or in considering changes in our interventions (Meleis, 1990). It is the lens by which we view our clients during the course of their illness, as well as when we attempt to maintain or promote their health. Moch (1989) provided a compelling argument for the development of the concept of health within illness and demonstrated how such a perspective is receiving more support in health-related theory development. Examples are Moss (1985) who described the transformational aspects of illness. Such a view is supported by many personal accounts of patients particularly as discussed in the literature on patients with human immunodeficiency virus and acquired immunodeficiency syndrome. The notion of healthy dying (Fitzpatrick, 1983) might be another supportive argument for "health" as an important component of the discipline's perspective.

There is also support for a health perspective in the daily work of nurses. Patients are assessed in terms of their perception of their well-being throughout their experiences with health care professionals, how they could maintain their health despite a grave diagnosis or intrusive procedure. Many theorists speak of this perspective such as Travelbee (1966; 1971) who was a pioneer in encouraging nurses to help their clients find meaning in their illness experience. Paterson and Zderad (1976) described their nursing perspective in terms of health and connected interactions with clients. Although health for Newman (1986) may be the goal for caring, or as a process of expanding consciousness, and for Jones and Meleis (1993) as a process of empowerment, these analyses provide more support for a more prevailing view of nursing as understood from within a health perspective. Through the process of nursing care, nurses uncover health strengths, mobilize these strengths, and support the available resources so that the patient may take charge and fight the illness or the injury.

Community health nurses provide useful examples of a health perspective in their work. They speak of positive resources, of available support, of healthful habits, and how to empower clients using their healthy resources. Although nurses in the intensive care unit (ICU) may consider their approach more illness oriented, on careful analysis, we find that ICU nurses are concerned with patients' safety, well-being, promoting increasing health, maintaining healthful habits, and supporting as much of normality in daily life as possible. These activities and goals reflect a health perspective.

Conclusion

By identifying, acknowledging, and affirming the discipline's perspective, we could focus our knowledge development efforts on the phenomena that nurses deal with, using a perspective that best reflects nursing views and values. A nursing perspective is known by exploring nursing as a human science, with a practice orientation, caring tradition, and a health orientation.

REFERENCES

Algase, D. L. and Whall, A.F. (1993). Rosemary Ellis' views on the substantive structure of nursing. *Image: Journal of Nursing Scholarship*, 25, 69–72.

Allen, D. (1986). Using philosophical and historical methodologies to understand the concept of health. In P.L. Chinn (Ed.), *Nursing research methodology: Issues and implementation.* Rockville, MD: Aspen Systems.

American Heritage Dictionary (3rd ed.). (1992). Boston: Houghton-Mifflin.

Benner, P. and Wrubel, J. (1989). *The primacy of caring.* Menlo Park, CA: Addison-Wesley.

Bjørk, I.T. (1995). Neglected conflicts in the discipline of nursing: Perceptions of the importance and value of practical skill. *Journal of Advanced Nursing*, 22, 6–12.

Bottorff, J.L. (1991). Nursing: A practical science of caring. *Advances in Nursing Science*, 14(1), 26–39.

Brody, J.K. (1988). Virtue ethics, caring, and nursing. *Scholarly Inquiry for Nursing Practice: An International Journal*, 2(2), 87–96.

Clarke, M. (1986). Action and reflection: Practice and theory in nursing. *Journal of Advanced Nursing*, 11, 3–11.

Clifford, C. (1995). Caring: Fitting the concept to nursing practice. *Journal of Clinical Nursing*, 4, 37–41.

Cohen, J.A. (1991). Two portraits of caring: A comparison of the artists, Leininger and Watson. *Journal of Advanced Nursing*, 16(8), 899–909.

Condon, E.H. (1992). Nursing and the caring metaphor: Gender and political influences on an ethics of care. *Nursing Outlook, 40,* 14–19.

Donaldson, S.K. and Crowley, D. (1978). The discipline of nursing. *Nursing Outlook*, 26(2), 113–120.

Fawcett, J. (1995). *Analysis and evaluation of conceptual models of nursing* (3rd ed.). Philadelphia: F.A. Davis.

Feldman, M.E. (1993). Uncovering clinical knowledge and caring practices. *Journal of Post Anesthesia Nursing*, 8(3), 159–162.

Fitzpatrick, J.J. (1983). A life-perspective rhythm model. In J.J. Fitzpatrick and A. Whall (Eds.), *Conceptual models of nursing* (pp. 295–302). Bowie, MD: Robert J. Brady.

Gadow, S. (1985). Nurse and patient: The caring relationship. In A.A. Bishop and J.R. Scudder (Eds.), *Caring, curing, coping. Nurse-physician-patient relationships* (pp. 31–43). Birmingham: University of Alabama Press.

Gendron, D. (1988). *The expressive form of caring.* Toronto: University of Toronto.

Gendron, D. (1994). The tapestry of care. *Advances in Nursing Science*, 17(1), 25–30.

Holmes, C.A. (1990). Alternatives to natural science foundations for nursing. *International Journal of Nursing Studies*, 27(3), 187–198.

Jenny, J. and Logan, J. (1992). Knowing the patient: One aspect of clinical knowledge. *Image: Journal of Nursing Scholarship*, 24, 254–258.

Johnson, J. (1994). A dialectical examination of nursing art. *Advances in Nursing Science*, 17(1), 1–14.

Jones, P.S. and Meleis, A.I. (1993). Health is empowerment. *Advances in Nursing Science, 15*(3), 1–14.

Laudan, L. (1977). *Progress and its problems: Toward a theory of scientific growth.* Berkeley: University of California Press.

Laudan, L. (1981). A problem-solving approach to scientific progress. In I. Hacking (Ed.), *Scientific revolutions.* New York: Oxford University Press.

Leininger, M.M. (1981). The phenomenon of caring: Importance, research questions and theoretical considerations. In M.M. Leininger (Ed.)., *Caring: An essential human need* (pp. 3–16). Thorofare, NY: Charles B. Slack.

MacPherson, K.I. (1989). A new perspective on nursing and caring in a corporate context. *Advances in Nursing Science*, 11(4), 32–39.

Masson, V. (1985). Nurses and doctors as healers. *Nursing Outlook*, 33(2), 70–73.

McWhinney, I.R. (1989). "An acquaintance with particulars . . ." *Family Medicine*, 21(4), 296–298.

Meleis, A.I. (1990). Being and becoming healthy: The core of nursing knowledge. *Nursing Science Quarterly*, 3(3), 107–114.

Meleis, A.I. (1992). Nursing: A caring science with a distinct domain. *SAIRAANHOITAJA*, 6, 8–12.

Moch, S.D. (1989) Health within illness: Conceptual evolution and practice possibilities. *Advances in Nursing Science*, 11(4), 23–31.

Moore, S. (1990). Thoughts on the discipline of nursing as we approach the year 2000. *Journal of Advanced Nursing*, 15, 825–828.

Morse, J. M., Bottorff, J., Neander, W., and Solberg, S. (1991). Comparative analysis of conceptualizations and theories of caring. *Image: Journal of Nursing Scholarship*, 23, 119–126.

Morse, J.M., Solberg, S.M., Neander, W.L., Bottorff, J.L., and Johnson, J.L. (1990). Concepts of caring and caring as concept. *Advances in Nursing Science*, 13(1), 1–14.

Moss, R. (1985). *How shall I live: Transforming surgery or any health crisis into greater aliveness.* Berkeley, CA: Celestial Arts.

Newman, M.A. (1986). *Health as expanding consciousness.* St. Louis: C.V. Mosby.

Newman, M.A., Sime, A.M., and Corcoran-Perry, S.A. (1991). The focus of the discipline of nursing. *Advances in Nursing Science*, 14(1), 1–6.

Nightingale, F. (1859). *Notes on nursing: What is it and what it is not.* London: Harrison.

Olson, T.C. (1993). Laying claim to caring: Nursing and the language of training, 1915–1937. *Nursing Outlook*, 41(2), 68–72.

Paterson, J.G. and Zderad, L.T. (1976). *Humanistic nursing.* New York: John Wiley & Sons.

Reynolds, C (1988). The measurement of health in nursing research. *Advances in Nursing Science*, 10(4), 23–31.

Rogers, M.E. (1970). *An introduction to the theoretical basis of nursing.* Philadelphia: F.A. Davis.

Smith, J.A. (1981). The idea of health: A philosophical inquiry. *Advances in Nursing Science*, 3, 43–50.

Titler, M.C., Buckwalter, K.C., and Maas, M.L. (1993). Critical issues for the development of clinical nursing knowledge. *Advances in Clinical Nursing Research*, 28(2), 475–477.

Travelbee, J. (1966). *Interpersonal aspects of nursing.* Philadelphia: F.A. Davis.

Travelbee, J. (1971). *Interpersonal aspects of nursing* (2nd ed.). Philadelphia: F.A. Davis.

Tripp-Reimer, T. (1984). Reconceptualizing the construct of health: Integrating emic and etic perspectives. *Research in Nursing and Health*, 7, 101–109.

Watson, J. (1988). New dimensions of human caring theory. *Nursing Science Quarterly*, 1, 175–181.Watson, J. (1990). Caring knowledge and informed moral passion. *Advances in Nursing Science*, 13(1), 15–24.

CHAPTER 7

The Domain of Nursing Knowledge

Discipline-specific inquiry, explorations, and theory development are vital for the development of nursing knowledge. All disciplines are formed around a domain of knowledge. A domain of knowledge is the crux of a discipline (Fig. 7-1). A *domain* is a territory that has both theoretical and practical boundaries. The practical boundaries represent the current state of investigative interests that emerge from questions significant to members of the domain. The theoretical boundaries are formulated by the visionary questions proposed for exploration, as well as those that occupy the intellectual energies of members of disciplines. These visionary questions are not bound by, or limited to, current concerns of the members of the discipline. Certain aspects of a domain are the core and are less dynamic, such as the phenomenon of interest and of concern to the members. Other aspects of the domain are more dynamic and changeable, such as the way the phenomena are conceptualized, the nature of the questions asked about the phenomena, as well as those phenomena that reflect societal or policy changes, and during periods of transition, phenomena that result from these changes. For example, some current questions that determine the territory of nursing include what is involved in caring for people who are not able to care for themselves because of illness or anticipated illness; how best to help individuals and populations to maintain their health and well-being; what is involved in self-care and how to support the promotion of self-care activities; and what are the best strategies that nurses could use to maintain or promote health, support recovery, and manage illness. In the future, theoretical boundaries may extend to include questions about caring for individuals who are in hemispheric transition or who may reside in a space shuttle for an extended period of time. Some elements of the domain may be maintained, for example, a focus on human beings and their environment; others may require some modification, for example, the nature and the content of the environment may have to be changed considerably to reflect changing environments. Environment for clients living on earth may have similar as well as different characteristics from environment for individuals living in space stations, or in the future, on other planets. The language used, the concepts defined, and the questions explored and examined are shaped by the

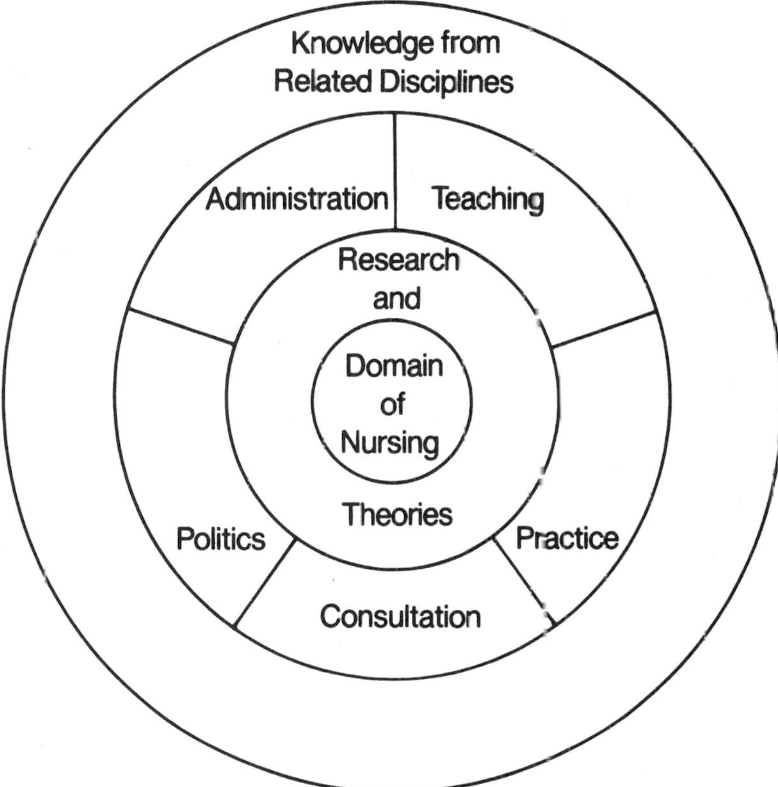

Figure 7–1 The discipline of nursing.

structure of the discipline. The structure, in turn, shapes the nature of questions asked about the phenomena (Mitchell, 1994).

Domains: A Definition

Domains are defined differently by different philosophers of science. The following definitions of a domain synthesize some aspects of Kuhn (1970), Merton (1973), Parsons (1968), and Toulmin (1972).

- A domain has some broad basic concepts.
- It contains the major problem areas of the field that make up the canons for significant statements.
- Some units of analysis used in its investigations are identified.
- There is evidence of beginning agreement and genealogy of ideas.
- Its members allow for a synthesis of a number of paradigms.

- Its members are knowledgeable about the different schools of thought, and they acknowledge and accept the use of different paradigms.
- There are accumulated experiences of its members. These experiences are respected, critically assessed, and accepted. The grounds for analysis and critique are clear and subject to debate.
- The norms and the tools for knowledge development are defined within the domain. These norms and tools emerge from the domain goals and are congruent with its shared assumptions.
- A domain informs and is informed by all outer circles of the discipline (see Fig. 7-1). That is, a domain is revised and developed through the wisdom and expertise of members of the discipline, through accumulated research and theory, and through knowledge developed in other disciplines. In sum, a domain has certain focal elements of stability, but the nature of its content is dynamic and responsive to changes occurring in other spheres.

A Nursing Domain

When we consider nursing analytically, we find numerous indications that nursing is indeed a discipline with a particular perspective and a defined domain (Fig. 7-2). The perspective of the discipline is defined in Chapter 6, and the nursing domain as it evolved is introduced and discussed in this chapter. As you reflect on what constitutes our disciplinary domain, keep in mind that the central problems of the domain of nursing may be examined by other sciences; however, the centrality of these problems to the domain is what determines primary domain affiliation. Comforting patients during intrusive procedures may be of concern to a number of health science disciplines, but comfort of clients during all life processes related to health and illness situations as well as ways by which comfort is enhanced are central concerns of nurses and nursing.

Some interests of some disciplines overlap others. An example of another discipline that may encounter such overlap is engineering. Premises on which the discipline

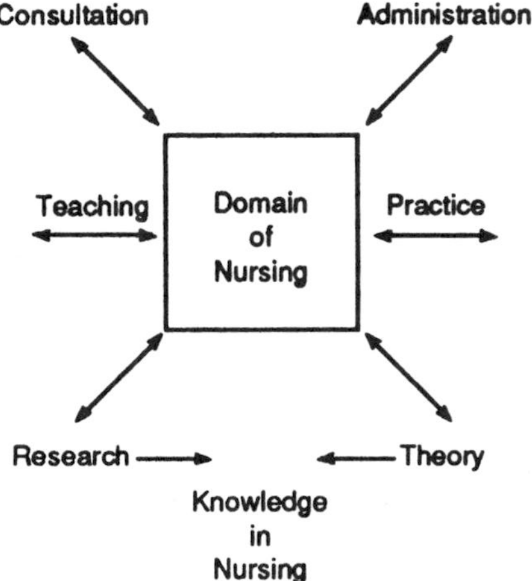

Figure 7–2 The domain of nursing.

of engineering is built may come from physics, chemistry, economics, and behavioral sciences, but the synthesis is uniquely engineering for the purpose of describing, explaining, and predicting phenomena central to engineering, for example, the shielding of nuclear power plants. The problem of shielding is central to the field of nuclear engineering but only peripheral to physics, chemistry, and other sciences.

The nursing domain does not simply encompass results of research (IE, nursing science), nursing theories, or nursing practice; rather it encompasses knowledge of nursing practice (Newman, 1983), which is based on philosophy, history, former practice, common sense, research findings, theory, and genealogy of ideas (see Fig. 7-2). The nursing domain encompasses units of analysis, congruent methodology, nursing processes, holistic approaches to assessment, and other practice and methodological procedures that are essential to knowledge development. Central components of the nursing domain are:

- Major concepts and problems of the field
- Processes for assessment, diagnosis, and intervention
- Tools to assess, diagnose, and intervene
- Research designs and methodologies that are most congruent with nursing knowledge

Theoretical boundaries of the nursing domain result from an explication of the first three components listed. Research designs and methodologies evolve from acceptable philosophical principles in nursing and complement knowledge development related to its central concepts, problems, and goals of the discipline. Research designs and methodologies also help identify and develop components of the domain of nursing. Nursing theories are a component of the domain of nursing, and they provide nurses with different perspectives on nursing and nursing phenomenon.

In 1975, Yura and Torres delineated and described the major concepts used in baccalaureate programs that were central to the different conceptual models and frameworks used for nursing curricula. Four focal concepts emerged: person, society, health, and nursing (Yura and Torres, 1975). The centrality of these concepts in the discipline of nursing continued to be supported through the 1980s. For example, Newman (1983) asserted that the "domain of nursing has always included the nurse, the patient, the situation in which they find themselves, and the purpose of their being together, or the health of the patient" (p. 388). Therefore, she agreed that the major components of concern to nursing are "nursing (as an action), client (human being), environment (of the client and of the nurse-client), and health" (p. 389). Others modified the list to exclude environment (Barnum, 1994), or they expanded the meaning of "person" to encompass both human being and patient (Barnum, 1994), or they redefined "client" to mean "pluralities of persons and internal units, such as families, groups, and communities" (Schultz, 1987, p. 71). Nursing theory, it was argued by some, could include one or more of these concepts (Fawcett, 1989), for example, client, society, health, or nursing, or, others argued, nursing theories should include the concept of nursing as an activity in addition to any one of the other concepts (Flaskerud and Halloran, 1980), such as any set of "commonplaces" (nursing act, patient, health, nurse–patient relationships, nursing acts and health, and patient and health), these "commonplaces" differentiate nursing from other disciplines (Barnum, 1994, pp. 14–15). Still others emphasized that nursing theories should include health and the direction for nursing actions to facilitate the processes of health (Newman, 1983, p. 390). None of the positions objected to inclusion of all domain concepts, if indeed a theory is able to address them all.

As indicated, there were variations in the recommendations of metatheorists in what, how many, and which central concepts should be included in nursing theories. The position adopted in this text has its own unique features also, but it falls within general patterns of agreement within the discipline. Concepts identified as central to the domain of nursing are nursing client, transitions, interaction, nursing process, environment, nursing therapeutics, and health. It is proposed that the nurse interacts (*interaction*) with a human being in a health/illness situation (*nursing client*) who is in an integral part of his sociocultural context (*environment*) and who is in some sort of transition or is anticipating a transition (*transition*); the nurse–patient interactions are organized around some purpose (*nursing process, problem solving, holistic assessment, or caring actions*), and the nurse uses some actions (*nursing therapeutics*) to enhance, bring about, or facilitate health (*health*).

It is argued here that theories developed related to any of the concepts listed above are nursing theories when the ultimate goal is related to the maintenance, promotion, or facilitation of health and well-being, even though the theory may not specify the nursing actions. It is also argued that nursing is an encompassing concept that includes all the concepts listed previously and is therefore defined by them. It would be an instance of tautological conceptualizing to define nursing by all the concepts and then include nursing as one of the concepts. Other disciplines may use nursing theories for different goals, and nursing theories therefore lose the original goal, become adapted, and become "shared" theories (Barnum, 1994).

A conceptual definition is provided for each of the central concepts in nursing. These definitions, evolving from contemporary shared knowledge in nursing and from a current world view, are provided as working definitions. The reader should use them as a springboard for further development and refinement.

The Nursing Client

The most central concept within the domain of nursing is the recipient of care or the potential recipient of care—the nursing client. Although a client is also central to a number of other disciplines, the perspective from which that client is considered is invariably different and evolves from the domain of the discipline. Nurses have claimed that individuals are the focus of their actions ever since nurses began caring for patients and ever since they attempted to describe the care they provide. For example, Nightingale described nursing as having to "put the patient in the best condition for nature to act upon him" (Nightingale, 1946, p. 74). Others spoke of nursing in terms of helping individuals develop their self-care activities (Orem, 1988) and doing what needs to be done to help individuals adapt to their illness or environment (Roy, 1984).

To illustrate, when a physician thinks of a person, the image is one of biologic systems with structure and function. That image may include a person's occupation, family, socioeconomic class, or other variable; however, the central image is of a biologic system. When a sociologist thinks of a person, she thinks of roles, status, interaction, and significant others, of individuals as part of a society. When a psychologist thinks of a human being, she thinks in terms of intrapsychic processes. A human being to a cell biologist is made up of groups of cells.

Nursing theories claim that nursing focuses on the person whose needs are not met because of illness or the person who needs help in maintaining or enhancing wellness. Nurse theorists provide us with several views of our clients. A nursing client probably is a composite of all of the conceptions provided by these nurses theorists, and perhaps the context determines which image is more central at the time. Some of these conceptions are complementary, whereas others are based on conflicting value systems. The following are some examples of nurse theorist's conceptions of the nursing client:

- The nursing client has a set of basic human needs (Abdellah [1969]—21 problems; Henderson [1966]—14 daily activities; Orem [1988]—the deficit between self-care capabilities and self-care demands). The focus of nursing is on assisting with activities to fulfill the client's needs.
- The nursing client is an open system, an adaptive being who changes to accommodate outside changes.
- A nursing client is conceptualized as a person in disequilibrium or at risk of disequilibrium due to insufficiency or incompatibility between one or more of the subsystems.
- A nursing client is a person who is unable, or is at risk of being unable, to be a self-care agent.

These theories provided us with varied conceptions described in the social policy statement (American Nurses Association [ANA], 1995). These conceptions should be used as guidelines for analyses to determine which conceptions are more congruent with the values and the mission of the discipline (Allen, 1987). A *nursing client* is defined here as a human being with needs who is in constant interaction with the environment and has an ability to adapt to that environment but, due to illness, risk, or vulnerability to potential illness, is experiencing disequilibrium or is at risk of experiencing disequilibrium. *Disequilibrium* is manifested in unmet needs, inability to take care of oneself, and nonadaptive responses.

Theoretical developments of phenomena related to nursing clients encompass but are not limited to six areas.

1. Research and theories to describe philosophical principles governing views of human beings in nursing, including analyses of values and norms related to human beings and their relationships
2. Research and theories that relate to the fundamental process of responses to human and environmental conditions that are considered within normal ranges
3. Research and theories to describe, explain, and predict responses of human beings to health and illness situations
4. Research and theories to describe human responses to nursing therapeutics
5. Research and theories to describe groups, communities, and organizational responses to health and illness and nursing therapeutics
6. Theoretical development of person models that are congruent with the disciplinary values

The nursing client is increasingly defined by his or her experiences (McIntyre, 1995). These experiences are expressed and related to others in continuous and discontinuous ways, in isolation or within a context, and are expressed through narration and various responses whether verbal, written, nonverbal, or through silences. Experiences can be uncovered and understood through involvement and participation in dialogues and discourses.

One of the discipline's immediate goals is to discover and develop techniques and methodologies to capture the holistic nature of human beings and the nature of integrated responses to the environment that are considered central to the domain of nursing. It is also to develop ways by which the nature of the lived experiences of human beings can be accessed, captured, and used as the basis for caring for people (McIntyre, 1995). Until this goal is realized, nurses may have to continue to resort to a more reductionist approach to the study of clients. Another goal is to focus knowledge development on populations that have been marginalized in the health care systems in particular and in society in general.

Examples of the types of theories that need to be developed are:

1. Descriptive theories (eg, patterns of normal responses)
2. Explanatory theories (eg, how and why different groups of clients respond in certain ways to noxious stimuli)
3. Prescriptive theories (eg, how and in what ways nurses enhance a sense of comfort or well-being in clients)

Transitions

Nurses deal with people who are experiencing transition, anticipating transition, or completing the act of transition (Meleis and Trangenstein, 1994). *Transition* denotes a change in health status, in role relationships, expectations, or abilities. It denotes changes in needs of all human systems. Transition requires the person to incorporate new knowledge, to alter behavior, and therefore to change the definition of self in social context. Transitions are developmental, situational, or health/illness events. Two significant developmental transitions may be associated with health problems (both psychosocial and biophysiologic): the transition from childhood to adolescence, which has the potential of being associated with ensuing problems such as substance abuse and teen pregnancies; and the transition from adulthood to mature adulthood, a period accompanied by gerontologic problems relating to identity, retirement, and chronic illness.

Another transition falling within the domain of nursing is the situational transition, which includes the addition or loss of a member of the family through birth or death. Each situation requires a definition or redefinition of the roles that the client (a person or a family) is involved in. The transition from a nonparental role to a parental one, the change from double parenting to single parenting, and the attempts of women to move from the battered role to the nonbattered role are three examples of situational transitions that affect a human being in totality, although we are concerned with them in terms of health. Nurses are also concerned with the transition from institutional care to community care.

The last, but not least important, transition category is the health/illness transition. This category includes such transitions as sudden role changes that result from moving from a well state to an acute illness, from wellness to chronic illness, or from chronicity to a new wellness that encompasses the chronicity (Tornberg, McGrath, and Benoliel, 1984). Transitions are therefore one component of the nursing domain.

The sociologist, the psychologist, the biologist, and the physiologist are all interested in transitions at the micro and macro levels, and the objective of their interest is to know. Because domains are not only identified by the types of objects with which they deal but also by the questions they ask, the different domain interests can be differentiated by considering types of questions that nurses ask. Only the nurse is interested in articulating transitions that are biopsychosociocultural—not only to know but ultimately to have knowledge of the utility of what we know and, in particular, to have ways to effectively use that knowledge. Unlike other academic disciplines, nursing is accountable to the public; it is expected to meet the public's needs.

An example of a multidimensional transitional interest is my own interest in the health care of immigrants, which arose from the needs of health care systems dealing with this population and the need for a broader knowledge base to support the provision of culturally competent care. It concerns immigrants in sociocultural transition and considers the effect of transition on clients' biologic, psychological, sociological, and cultural needs and the effect of transitions on health behavior, illness behavior, illness episodes, and coping styles of any group of immigrants to the United States. The interest evolved from a nursing perspective, uses a sociological model, and will add to the domain of nursing.

Nursing does not deal with transition of an individual, a family, or a community in isolation from an environment. How human beings cope with transition and how the environment affects that coping are fundamental questions for nursing. Nursing seeks to maximize clients' strengths, assets, and potentials or to contribute to restoration of the client to optimal levels of health, function, comfort, and self-fulfillment. Coping and adapting are multidisciplinary and interdisciplinary concepts. The menopausal experience, for example, is a developmental transition and a multidomain concept. Although research in nursing considers menopause from a biopsychosociocultural perspective, the sociologist looks at it in terms of societal expectations, with the roles and status normatively accorded the menopausal woman. The psychologist views menopause from an intrapsychic perspective; the physician views it in terms of changes in cells in the endocrine system. The nurse researcher considers the subjective meaning of the entire experience, what biopsychosociocultural variables influence that meaning, what the consequences are for the person as well as for that person's significant others, how the person is adapting to changes, and, finally, how the nurse can help the menopausal woman cope with the experience, if indeed there is a need to do so.

Clients in transition share some commonalities. These were defined by Chick and Meleis (1986) and Meleis (1986) as a perception of "disconnectedness from usual social network and social support systems," "temporary loss of familiar reference points or significant objects or subjects," "new needs that may arise," or "old needs that remain unmet," and "old sets of expectations no longer congruent with changing situations" (Meleis, 1986, p. 19). These characteristics were further refined through the review of

310 literature citations from 1986 to 1992. Universal properties of transitions that emerged were process, changes in identities, roles, relations, abilities, and patterns of behavior. Several conditions were identified that affect transition processes. These are meanings, expectations, levels of knowledge and skills, environment, levels of planning, and emotional and physical well-being (Schumacher and Meleis, 1994). The delineation of the concept of transitions has resulted in a continuing process of development of the concept and may have dialectically promoted some more focused research studies to answer fundamental questions related to recovery transitions.

Although each nurse researcher considers the nursing phenomenon according to the basic premises of the field and according to a total view of the human being, the goals of research will dictate the dominant model. For example, one nurse researcher conceptualizes phenomena predominantly from a physiologic model, whereas another may use a sociological model. Both explicate nursing phenomena and work toward the goals of enhancing healthful living, an adaptive stance, and a higher sense of well-being. Both are adding to the nursing conceptualization of an experience.

Theories are needed to describe the nature of transitions and normal patterns of responses to transitions, to explain relationships between transitions and health, and to provide guidelines for enhancing a perception of well-being.

Interaction

Some theorists focused on the process and tools of assessment and therefore viewed nursing as an interaction process. Together they provided us with the genesis of one or more interaction theories. They all spoke of properties of the nurse–patient dialogue, of therapeutic interaction, and of the components of interacting as being the sensing, perceiving, and validating of the patient's need for help and the sharing of information. They explicated properties of perception, thought, and feelings during health and illness situations. Together they provided us with a framework that contains major concepts central to nursing. Theories relating these concepts could come from inside or outside nursing. They could evolve from studying the work of the different theories in conjunction with patient care situations or in conjunction with other interaction theories, such as those of Sullivan (1953) and Mead (1937).

Interaction is one of the central concepts in nursing for the following reasons:

1. A nursing client is in constant interaction with the environment (Rogers, 1970; King, 1981; Nightingale, 1946). Therefore, nursing focuses not only on individuals but also on monitoring, regulating, maintaining, and changing environments.
2. Interaction is the major tool by which nurses assess client's needs and resources, and it is also a central tool in providing nursing therapeutics (Orlando (1961), Wiedenbach (1963), King (1981), Travelbee (1971), Paterson and Zderad (1976).

There is some agreement that interaction is a domain concept and that there are interactions as person–environment interactions (Flaskerud and Halloran, 1980;

Forchuk, 1995) and nurse–patient interactions (Barnum, 1994). Interaction is considered here in its broadest sense to incorporate both of these types of interactions.

Several kinds of theories related to interactions need to be developed, including the following:

1. Theories that describe normal patterns of interactions of human beings with significant aspects of their environments
2. Theories that describe normal patterns of interactions between clients and their environments within a context of health and illness, which should account for developmental, sociocultural, and cognitive variations
3. Theories that describe and explain interactions and consequences of interactions that are related to assessment, diagnosis, and interventions

Kim (1987) identified four sets of variables that are related to client–nurse contacts for providing nursing care: client and nurse, a social context for the contact, a process of interaction, and outcomes. The conceptual linkages between each of these sets of variables are then amenable to theory development (Kim, 1987, p. 105).

Nurses have claimed nurse–patient interactions as central to the nursing diagnosis; however, Kim (1987) reminded us:

> While there has been a great deal of theoretical emphasis on the importance of client–nurse interaction in the delivery of nursing care, very little has been done either in theory development or in empirical testing of these theories. More needs to be done on the meaning of therapeutic relationships and ways by which such relationships are established, nurtured, supported, discouraged, or avoided. There is a rich array of theoretical and empirical work accomplished in sociology and social psychology that is transferable to this nursing domain. There is a need to have an understanding of how the special nature of client–nurse interactions modifies sociological, social, psychological, and communication theories. Much work, therefore, needs to be done to revise and reformulate existing knowledge to explain and predict phenomena in the client–nurse domain (Kim, 1987, p. 107).

Nursing Process

Another concept that is central to the discipline of nursing as demonstrated in the many discourses in the literature as well as demonstrated in many of the nursing theories is that of the nursing process. The distinct properties of the nursing process as they differ from client–nurse or client–environment interactions have not been as clearly defined and distinguished. Despite some apparent overlap, it is proposed here that propositions about the nursing process, about approaches that are more effective in the process of assessing, diagnosing, or providing nursing therapeutics, and about the goals of the nursing process can be derived from the work of several theorists: Abdellah, Henderson, Orem, Orlando, Travelbee, and Wiedenbach. Together they provided nursing with a perspective on assessment, diagnosis, plan for intervention, and evaluation (Abdellah, 1969; Henderson, 1966; Orem, 1988), on the process of defining and attaining goals (King, 1981), and with emphasis on the patient's perception of his own condition (Wiedenbach,

1963). In proposing the nursing process as a concept with the potential for development of middle-range theory, Hall (1982) makes the following comments:*

> Nurses and teachers of nursing find it useful to organize their knowledge in a way that depicts nursing as orderly and sequential. It is also useful because it structures reality and acts as a focus for the nurse's attention. It limits the duration of the nurse's interaction and it spells out clearly the phases or the steps that should occur and in what order. It thus confines the nurse and the patient to a relationship with each other that has a specific function, is temporary, and has signposts that indicate progress.
>
> Therefore nursing needs a process theory because concern with patients inevitably involves a relationship that has temporal elements. Different knowledge and actions are called for as the relationship proceeds through stages from the beginning to the end. The theories, however, need to pay attention to the details of the model itself rather than focus on content. The significant process variables connected with the beginning, the middle, and the end cannot be given short shrift. One cannot find any theoretical approach in the literature that claims to teach us how to develop a process theory, or even what one is, specifically. There are some examples of this approach, though, and these will be cited in this paper so we can arrive at the elements of a process theory inductively.
>
> From the field of sociology there are no better examples of process theory than those developed by the symbolic interactionists, Becker, Strauss, and Glaser (Becker, 1963; Becker, Geer, Hughes, and Strauss, 1961; Glaser and Strauss, 1964, 1967). These process theories are called, variously, career sequence, commitment, and status passage. They all rest on the assumption that behavior occurs in an orderly sequence that can be observed, recorded, and then generalized as a process. Essentially, the process metaphor presents identity as a series of movements or steps in a sequence. Passage from one sequence to another is a study of the orderly steps or changes over time. Becker says that, when viewed as a process, the variables in this sequence model are a description of the steps in the process accompanied by an explanation of each step.
>
> Becker's (1963) conception of sequential models was developed from Hughes' (1956) work on occupational careers. Becker used Hughes' idea of career as a "moving perspective" to develop his own thoughts on career contingencies and career flow. Becker reasoned that at various stages of the career process, factors come into play such as recruitment, replacement, crucial contingencies, timing, sequencing, and sponsorship. These factors then become the dimensions of the process. Each one serves to further the career, socialize the recruit, foster identity with the occupation, and ensure that critical choices are made with appropriate help. From the point of view of the occupation, the process ensures that the members entering the occupation will have sufficient socialization to develop appropriate attitudes, values, and skills necessary to good functioning.
>
> Thus, instead of the simplistic stages depicted by the nursing process, we have a process comprised of stages that presents a moving picture of the significant career variables in each stage and culminates in the achievement of a new identity for the occupational recruit. Becker depicts occupational identity as career process because the two, from his perspective, are inseparable.
>
> Further study of Becker's work, though, reveals that Becker did not use the above theory to establish a middle-range substantive theory of occupational careers. Rather, he went on to develop from this process a formal theory of career process. The variables of recruitment, replacement, crucial contingencies, timing, and sponsorship are

---

*Reprinted with permission from Beverly A. Hall.

> the "form" of a career, whether the career is occupational or some other kind. Career is literally a moving perspective, to go back to Hughes, and we can use that "form" to study other processes such as dying and the study of social deviance.
>
> In the case of the deviant, the first step in a deviant career is the commission of a nonconforming act. This is a necessary condition but not a sufficient condition because acts are committed by persons who do not go on to a deviant career. Individuals who are to become deviant learn their careers in the same way people learn any career, by having crucial experiences along the career process that enforce a deviant identity, such as sponsorship, public labeling, and recruitment into the inner circle of a subgroup. Eventually, as the person goes through these stages of a career, the growing commitment strengthens identification as a deviant.
>
> Becker used this same sequence model to study professional careers, marijuana users, and dance musicians. The notion of career sequence was further developed by Glaser and Strauss in their study of status passage in which the sequence model was applied to the dying patient. This latter example is well known in nursing. Glaser and Strauss developed a "low level" theory of dying in hospitals. They then began to apply this to many areas. This step developed the theory of dying into a theory of status passage which has been applied to many areas of status and role change—retirement, career mobility, deviant behavior, and adjustment to the sick role. It is at this stage that Denzin (1970) says we have a multifocused formal theory, that is, one that describes a form that can be applied to a number of substantive areas.
>
> Although Becker, Strauss, and Glaser do not discuss patterns per se, I believe that if a process is developed and studied in its complex detail, it would take on the characteristics of a pattern. A pattern in process theory would appear to be simply a stage or a step in the process that is normative or at least modal, along with the clustered variables in each stage.
>
> Furthermore, these patterns could be developed along the lines of formal sociological theory. That is, we could discover formal patterns that would cut across substantive areas. These would include both process and content. In the so-called nursing process there is virtually no content, although it is implied by the process and could be developed. A good process would lead to the development of content that is inseparable from the form. Form and content can be isolated from each other, just as they are in grammar, so that the form can have life without the content. However, it would seem to me that the content cannot have life without the form. That is the purpose of form; it allows the content to be interpreted.
>
> In summary, nursing could probably benefit by attention to its process in which basic forms would be developed. Formal theory may begin in its development by focusing on a single process. It then becomes multifocused as it is extended to explain phenomena other than that for which it was originally developed.

The nursing process, a tool for nursing practice, was introduced to nursing first by Orlando (1961) and became central to many publications in nursing and has even been considered a framework for nursing practice and nursing education (Yura and Walsh, 1978a, 1978b). Most of the theorists described and discussed the nursing process. Although some components of the process of clinical judgments are an integral part of all professional–client relationships, the process in nursing differs in that the goals of each profession are different. It is proposed here that the nursing process is a central concept in the domain of nursing.

Many nurse metatheorists agree with this position (eg, Torres, 1986; Walker and Avant, 1995), as demonstrated by the extensive literature on and use of the nursing process, and by those who maintain that emerging theories and models in nursing must consider the nursing process (Thibodeau, 1983). Others question the compatibility of the holistic mission of nursing and the reductionist approach dictated by the use of the nursing process (Barnum, 1987). Barnum (1987) pointed out the potential for other processes in decision making to be more compatible with the holistic principles of nursing, such as the problematic method described by Dewey in 1966. These debates in the nursing literature demonstrate the need for further theoretical development of different processes for assessment and diagnoses and for providing nursing therapeutics.

One significant component of the nursing process that has received the attention of the discipline throughout the 1980s is a taxonomy of nursing diagnoses. The movement toward the development of the taxonomy began in the early 1970s by Kristine Gebbie (a graduate of University of California, Los Angeles, a faculty member at UCLA, and a collaborative author with Betty Neuman). The nursing diagnoses described by participants in annual nursing diagnoses conferences were without a binding theoretical framework to guide their development. Although these taxonomies appear to be a unifying diagnostic language for communication between nurses, they

> cannot contribute to the development of scientific solutions (IE, nursing therapeutics), [because] nursing diagnoses that are not developed within an explanatory framework have to be accepted only as descriptive "averages" to be used for the purpose of communication and documentation only (Kim, 1987, p. 102).

Several types of theories related to the nursing process need to be developed (Frisch, 1994). Examples of these are: theories to describe the actual processes that nurses use in assessing, diagnosing, and providing nursing therapeutics to different types and categories of clients; theories to describe nursing diagnoses and those that can "give order to the nomenclature" (Kim, 1987, p. 103); theories to explain diagnostic categories within the different contexts; and theories that explain nurse–patient contacts within the contexts of client variables and diagnostic categories. Processes for assessment, diagnosis, and intervention have emerged as central to nursing and its mission.

Finally, a dialogue about the congruency between a reductionist approach to viewing nursing phenomenon, as assumed through using the nursing process, and the assumptions of holism, needs to continue. This dialogue began with effective arguments supporting the incongruity between assumptions inherent in theories of nursing process and the nature of holism in nursing (Barnum, 1987). Similarly, questions arise about the role of nursing process in curricula and in nursing science that evolve from considering it as central to nursing. Duldt (1995) argued for better clarification of the properties inherent in the nursing process, as differentiated from the clinical inquiry process and the research processes, and proposed that such differentiation enhances the potential of using these differentiated processes to structure advanced nurse practitioner courses. Students may be better able to move easily between the different processes when they are aware of their similarities and differences in process and in goals.

Environment

Ever since Florence Nightingale (1946) identified nursing in relation to a focus on optimizing an environment to promote healing and optimal health, environment has been a concept central to the nursing domain. Nightingale considered both the discomfort and suffering that patients experience as results of inadequacies in the environment and nurses' actions as focusing on that environment. We lost track of this concept during the years when the biologic systems dominated nursing and when nursing focused on illness, medical treatment, and assistance with a medical regimen. As central as the concept may be, nursing theorists have not addressed it in the same depth and with the same conviction about its centrality as did Nightingale—nor as they did when considering the individual. Clinicians appear to pay lip service to it.

More contemporary theorists see the environment as central to nursing, particularly as it relates to human beings and their responses (eg, Rogers, 1970; Paterson and Zderad; 1976). To these theorists, environment encompasses energy fields, social systems, family, society, culture, the patient's room, the nurse, and all that surrounds the client. Rogers' theory focuses on a description of person and environment energy fields as inseparable and on the dynamics of human being–"environment" interactions. According to her, the process inherent in such interactions can only be understood through a careful consideration of the environment. This view assumes the person and the environment as being in constant interaction and recognizes changes in one as integral and simultaneous to changes in the other. Therefore, the aim of nursing intervention is to promote, maintain, regulate, or change the environmentand/or the life processes of people to affect changes in either or in both.

Chopoorian (1986) argued for considering the environment as the central focus for nursing interventions and warned us against continuing to develop knowledge based on the centrality of clients. She suggested her thesis by demonstrating the limited roles that nurses play in instituting policy changes when clients are considered the central focus for nursing. In reconceptualizing environment for the discipline of nursing, she suggested that, "nurses develop a consciousness of environment as social, economic, and political structures; . . . as human social relations, . . . as everyday life" (Chopoorian, 1986, p. 47). She further argued that this approach has the potential for opening up new opportunities for nurses to go beyond the acceptance of the status quo for patients' and for making contributions to resolving society's problems (p. 53). A focus on environment may prompt nurses to reconsider their goals and the mission of the discipline.

Environment, as a central domain concept, includes but is not limited to immediate client settings, family, significant others, health care professionals, and the socioeconomic and political contexts of the client's families and communities (Hedin, 1986). Stevens (1989) proposes the use of critical theory to illuminate oppressive environmental factors that influence health, hinder human potential and life possibilities, and "restrict their equal and fully conscious participation in society" (p. 63).

Several types of theories related to environment need to be developed. Theories centering on environment are expected to describe properties, components, and dimensions of environment that are healthy or that help in maintaining or in changing health care outcomes. They are also expected to describe the environment, which promotes the client's abilaities for self-care and adaptation. In addition, they are expected to guide the development of effective interventions that may change systems that constrain access and equality in giving and receiving health care. Examples of nursing theories are descriptive theories of healthy environments; theories to describe societal mechanisms in constraining the development, provision, and maintenance of healthy environments; theories that describe and explain policies for health care; and theories that guide actions for environmental changes (Salazar and Primomo, 1994).

Nursing Therapeutics

Nursing therapeutics is defined as all nursing activities and actions deliberately designed to care for nursing clients (Barnard, 1980; 1983). Although the nursing process addresses patterns in assessing, diagnosing, and intervening, nursing therapeutics considers the content of nursing interventions and the goals of intervention. The ultimate goal of theory development in nursing is to develop theories that guide the care nurses give to patients. The existing nursing theories, as categories, provide nursing with the beginnings of nursing therapeutics. For example, interaction theorists suggest that because we define nursing as a process and as an interaction, the nursing problems reflect process and interactional problems; therefore, to these theorists nursing therapeutics are related to making the interaction process more effective. These theorists recommend the development of empathy, the use of validation, and the use of deliberative nursing process as strategies to deal with communication and interaction problems.

Examples of nursing therapeutics that are being used in the nursing literature are:

- Touch (stimulation and repatterning of human fields) (Krieger, Johnson, Weiss, Rogers, Neuman)
- Care (Orem, Henderson, Leininger)
- Role supplementation (Meleis, Swendsen, Dracup)
- Protection (Johnson, Norris)
- Manipulation of focal, residual, and contextual stimuli (Roy)
- Comfort (Arruda, Larson, and Meleis; Morse)
- Use of self as a nursing therapeutic

Each of these concepts related to nursing therapeutics could become the nucleus of a middle range or a situation-specific theory in therapeutics (see also Chapters 8 and 19).

Health

Health, a goal shared by a number of health professions, emerged as a central goal in nursing in the writings of Florence Nightingale in the mid-1800s. Since then, theorists have considered health with different degrees of specificity, reductionism, and centrality. Health has been accepted as more than the absence of disease, and that concept is becoming more emphasized in nursing (Newman, 1983, 1986; Smith, 1983; Neuman, 1989).

Several different models of health were identified from the nursing literature (Meleis, 1990): health as an absence of disease (Smith, 1983), health as an internal homeostasis (Johnson, 1980), health as adaptation (Roy, 1984; Smith, 1982), health as performing roles and functions (Orem, 1988; Smith, 1982), and an existential view of health that focuses on symbolism and the place of the self in an intricate web of relations among objects and subjects (Paterson and Zderad, 1976; Travelbee, 1971). A sixth model relies on space/time/energy and consciousness expansion; health in this model is viewed in terms of awareness, personal control, personal empowerment, and mastery over body (Newman, 1986; Rogers, 1970). The last model considers the cultural/social/political aspects of health (Allen, 1986; Jones and Meleis, 1993; Meleis, 1990; Tripp-Reimer, 1984). For further theoretical development of health as a central concept, the unity and diversity among these models need to be addressed, compared, and contrasted. Several conditions were identified as needing to be included in further theoretical development of health. These are the need for focusing on an understanding of the health care needs of underserved populations, the potential advantage in using a feminist framework, the integration between a static conception of being healthy, and a process/dynamic/becoming conception of health (Meleis, 1990).

Nursing Defined

A domain is also shaped, and it reflects the definition attached to it by its members and by the society at large. Several definitions of nursing could drive the process and the goals of knowledge development and, in turn, help to further define the structure of the discipline. These definitions, in turn, were shaped by the progress made in theoretical nursing. One of the most influential definitions of nursing has been the one offered by Nightingale (1859, 1946) in which nursing was defined as "taking charge of the personal health" of individuals and to "put" the individual in the best possible state and "allow nature to act upon him." This definition though old, continues to be contemporary, and it set the stage for nursing to claim "personal health" as part of its domain.

A second influential definition is one that was commissioned by the International Council of Nurses (ICN) for international use. Henderson offered a definition that emphasized a unique role for nursing and brought in the notion that patients have a role in caring for themselves; when patients are not able to care for themselves due to health problems, nurses provide the care they need. Once the patient is again capable, self-care can resume and nurses are then not expected to do for patients what they are capable of doing for themselves (Henderson, 1966).

A third significant definition is that offered by the ANA (1980). Nursing is defined as "the diagnosis and treatment of human responses to actual or potential health problems" (p. 9). This earlier version (1980) of the definition has been discussed and critiqued for ignoring the environment, for its inconsistency with nursing values, for its limitation to individual care instead of community care, and for its problem orientation and lack of health orientation (Allen, 1987; Field, Kritek, Christman et al., 1983; Silva, 1983; White, 1984). However, the definition has helped in further identifying the domain of the discipline and in providing boundaries that have been reflected in theory development and in research priorities. An updated version of this definition included affirmation that nursing is committed to caring for ill and well people, as individuals, groups, or communities (ANA, 1995). The concept, "responses," is yet to be fully defined; nevertheless, it reflects a more integrated approach to viewing clients' behaviors and actions. The definition legitimized nurses' abilities to diagnose and treat or deal with these responses and acknowledge the significance of giving attention tothe daily lived human experiences. The taxonomy of responses provided as examples reflects the influence of theoretical nursing. Future definitions will need to reflect progress in other components of the domain such as the emphasis on environment and its relationship to nursing care.

I have selected two other definitions to illustrate the dialectic relationship between domain definitions and progress and development in disciplines. Based on earlier definitions of nursing, on the identification of central concepts, and on the authors' theoretical research and curricular explorations, Newman, Sime, and Corcoran-Perry (1991) defined the focus of the discipline of nursing as the "study of caring in the human health experience" (p. 3). Similarly, Meleis and Trangenstein (1994) defined nursing as being concerned with the process and the experiences of human beings undergoing transitions; therefore nursing is defined as "facilitating transitions to enhance a sense of well-being" (p. 257). Both definitions evolved from previous definitions of nursing, from identification of central concepts, from established research traditions, and from previous theoretical work by nurse scholars. Each of these definitions drives the development of different levels of investigation, one relating to caring acts and lived experiences in health and illness, and the other focusing on the nature of transitions, responses and consequences of transitions, and the different strategies by which nurses can enhance healthy transitions.

Conclusion

The domain of nursing deals with clients who are assumed to be in constant interaction with their environments, human beings who have unmet needs related to their health or illness status, who are not able to care for themselves or are not adapting to their environments due to interruptions or potential interruptions in health. The domain of nursing incorporates a central focus on environments that includes sociopolitical and economic contexts for nursing clients and their significant others. The domain of nursing includes a focus on nursing therapeutics to help in meeting the needs of human beings for health and health care, to enhance adaptation capability, to develop self-care abilities, and to maintain or promote health and well-being. Theory and research are the processes by which the domain concepts and problems are developed, validated, and communicated. Practice, education, and administration are the means by which the domain goals are implemented. Domains are redefined through theoretical and research processes and there is a dialectic relationship between domains, definitions, and theory and research traditions. All these are part of the structure of the discipline of nursing.

REFERENCES

Abdellah, F.G. (1969). The nature of nursing science. *Nursing Research*, 18, 390–393.

Allen, D.G. (1986). Using philosophical and historical methodologies to understand the concept of health. In P.L. Chinn (Ed.), *Nursing research methodology: Issues and implementation.* Rockville, MD: Aspen Systems.

Allen, D.G. (1987). The social policy statement: A reappraisal. *Advances in Nursing Science*, 10(1), 39–48.

American Nurses Association. (1980). *Nursing: A social policy statement.* Kansas City, MO: Author.

American Nurses Association. (1995). *Nursing's social policy statement* (Publication No. NP-107). Washington, DC: Author.

Barnard, K. (1980). Knowledge for practice: Directions for the future. *Nursing Research*, 29, 208–212.

Barnard, K. (1983). Social policy statement can move nursing ahead. *American Nurse*, 15(1), 4–14.

Barnum, B.J. (1987). Holistic nursing and nursing process. *Holistic Nursing Practice*, 1(3), 27–35.

Barnum, B.J.S. (1994). *Nursing theory: Analysis, application, and evaluation* (4th ed.). Philadelphia: J.B. Lippincott.

Becker, H.S. (1963). *Outsiders: Studies in the sociology of deviance.* New York: Free Press.

Becker, H.S., Geer, B., Hughes, E.C., and Strauss, A.L. (1961). *Boys in white.* Chicago: University of Chicago Press.

Chick, N. and Meleis, A.I. (1986). Transitions: A nursing concern. In P.L. Chinn (Ed.), *Nursing research methodology.* Boulder, CO: Aspen.

Chopoorian, T.J. (1986). Reconceptualizing the environment. In P. Moccia (Ed.), *New approaches to theory development.* New York: National League for Nursing.

Denzin, N.K. (1970). *The research act.* Chicago: Aldine.

Dewey, J. (1966). *Democracy and education.* New York: Macmillan.

Duldt, B.W. (1995) Nursing process: The science of nursing in the curriculum. *Nurse Educator,* 20(1), 24–29.

Fawcett, J. (1989). *Conceptual models of nursing* (2nd ed.). Philadelphia: F.A. Davis.

Field, L., Kritek, P., Christman, L., et al. (1983). Five nurse leaders discuss social policy statement. *American Nurse,* 15(2), 4, 6, 14.

Flaskerud, J.H. and Halloran, E.J. (1980). Areas of agreement in nursing theory development. *Advances in Nursing Science,* 3(1), 1–7.

Forchuk, C. (1995). Uniqueness within the nurse-client relationship. *Archives of Psychiatric Nursing,* 9(1), 34–39.

Frisch, N. (1994). The nursing process revisited [editorial]. *Nursing Diagnosis,* 5(2), 51.

Glaser, B.G. and Strauss, A.L. (1964). *Awareness of dying.* Chicago: Aldine

Glaser, B.G. and Strauss, A.L. (1967). *The discovery of grounded theory.* Chicago: Aldine.

Hall, B. (1982, September). *The nursing process as a middle-range theory.* Paper presented at Nursing Theory Think Tank, Dallas, Texas.

Hedin, B.A. (1986). Nursing, education, and emancipation: Applying the critical theoretical approach to nursing research. In P.L. Chinn (Ed.), *Nursing research methodology: Issues and implementation.* Rockville, MD: Aspen Systems.

Henderson, V. (1966). *The nature of nursing.* New York: Macmillan.

Hughes, E.C. (1955). *Men and their work.* Glencoe, IL: Free Press.

Johnson, D.E. (1980). The behavioral system model for nursing. In J.P. Riehl and C. Roy (Eds.), *Conceptual models for nursing practice* (2nd ed.). New York: Appleton-Century-Crofts.

Jones, P.S., and Meleis, A.I. (1993). Health is empowerment. *Advances in Nursing Science,* 15(3), 1–14.

Kim, H.S. (1987). Structuring the nursing knowledge system: A typology of four domains. *Scholarly Inquiry for Nursing Practice,* 1(2), 99–110.

King, I.M. (1981). *A theory for nursing: Systems, concepts, process.* New York: John Wiley & Sons.

Kuhn, T.S. (1970) The structure of scientific revolutions. In O. Neurath (Ed.), *International encyclopedia of unified science* (2nd ed., Vols. 1 and 2). Chicago: University of Chicago Press.

McIntyre, M. (1995). The focus of the discipline of nursing: A critique and extension. *Advances in Nursing Science,* 18(1), 27–35.

Mead, G.H. (1937). *Mind, self, and society.* Introduction by C.W. Morris. Chicago: University of Chicago Press.

Meleis, A.I. (1986). Theory development and domain concepts. In P. Moccia (Ed.), *New approaches to theory development.* New York: National League for Nursing.

Meleis, A.I. (1990). Being and becoming healthy: The core of nursing knowledge. *Nursing Science Quarterly,* 3(3), 107–114.

Meleis, A.I., and Trangenstein, P.A. (1994). Facilitating transitions: Redefinition of the nursing mission. *Nursing Outlook,* 42, 255–259.

Merton, R.K. (1973). *The sociology of science: Theoretical and empirical investigation.* Chicago: University of Chicago Press.

Mitchell, G.J. (1994). Discipline-specific inquiry: The hermeneutics of theory-guided nursing research. *Nursing Outlook,* 42, 224–248.

Newman, M. (1983). The continuing revolution: A history of nursing science. In N. Chaska (Ed.), *The nursing profession: A time to speak.* New York: McGraw-Hill.

Newman, M. (1986). *Health as expanding consciousness.* St. Louis: C.V. Mosby.

Neuman, B. (1989). *The Neuman systems model* (2nd ed.). East Norwalk, CT: Appleton & Lange.

Newman, M. A., Sime, A.M., and Corcoran-Perry, S.A. (1991). The focus of the discipline of nursing. *Advances in Nursing Science,* 14(1), 1–6.

Nightingale, F. (1946). *Notes on nursing.* Philadelphia: J.B. Lippincott. [originally published in 1859]

Orem, D.E. (1988). *Nursing: Concepts of practice* (3rd ed.). New York: McGraw-Hill.

Orlando, I.J. (1961). *The dynamic nurse–patient relationship.* New York: G.P. Putnam's Sons.

Parsons, T. (1968). *Sociological theory and modern society* (2nd ed.). New York: Free Press.

Paterson, J.G. and Zderad, L.T. (1976). *Humanistic nursing.* New York: John Wiley & Sons.

Rogers, M.E. (1970). *An introduction to the theoretical basis of nursing.* Philadelphia: F.A. Davis.

Roy, C. (1984). *Introduction to nursing: An adaptation model* (2nd ed.). Englewood Cliffs, NJ: Prentice-Hall.

Salazar, M.K. and Primomo, J. (1994). Taking the lead in environmental health. *AAOHN Journal,* 42(7), 317–324.

Schultz, P. (1987). When client means more than one: Extending the foundational concept of person. *Advances in Nursing Science,* 10(1), 71–86.

Schumacher, K. and Meleis, A.I. (1994). Transitions: A central concept in nursing. *Image: Journal of Nursing Scholarship,* 26(2), 119–127.

Silva M. (1983). The American Nurses' Association's position statement on nursing and social policy: Philosophical and ethical dimensions. *Journal of Advanced Nursing,* 8, 147–151.

Smith, J.A. (1982). Letters to the editor. *Advances in Nursing Science,* 4(3), xi.

Smith, J.A. (1983). *The idea of health: Implications for the nursing professional.* New York: Teachers College, Columbia University.

Stevens, B. (1989). A critical social reconceptualization of environment in nursing: Implications and methodology. *Advances in Nursing Science,* 11(4), 56–68.

Sullivan, H. (1953). *The interpersonal theory of psychiatry.* New York: W.W. Norton.

Thibodeau, J.A. (1983). *Nursing models: Analysis and evaluation.* Monterey, CA: Wadsworth.

Tornberg, M.J., McGrath, B.B., and Benoliel, J.Q. (1984, April). Oncology transition services: Partnerships of nurses and families. *Cancer Nursing,* 7(2), 131–137.

Torres, G. (1986). *Theoretical foundations of nursing.* East Norwalk, CT.: Appleton-Century-Crofts.

Toulmin, S. (1972). *Human understanding: The collective use and evolution of concepts* (2nd ed.). Princeton, NJ: Princeton University Press.

Travelbee, J. (1971). *Interpersonal aspects of nursing* (2nd ed.). Philadelphia: F.A. Davis.

Tripp-Reimer, T. (1984). Reconceptualizing the construct of health: Integrating emic and etic perspectives. *Research in Nursing and Health,* 7, 101–9.

Walker, L.O. and Avant, K.C. (1995). *Strategies for theory construction in nursing* (3rd ed.). East Norwalk, CT: Appleton & Lange.

White, C. (1984). A critique of the ANA social policy statement. *Nursing Outlook,* 32(6), 328–331.

Wiedenbach, E. (1963). The helping art of nursing. *American Journal of Nursing,* 63(11) 54–57.

Yura, H. and Torres, G. (1975). *Today's conceptual frameworks with the baccalaureate nursing programs* (National League for Nursing Publication No. 15-1558, 17–75). New York: National League for Nursing.

Yura, H. and Walsh, M.B. (1978a). *The nursing process: Assessing, planning, implementing, evaluating.* New York: Appleton-Century-Crofts.

Yura, H. and Walsh, M.B. (1978b). *Human needs and the nursing process.* New York: Appleton-Century-Crofts.

CHAPTER 8

Bedpans and Spinoza: Sources, Resources, and Paradoxes

To Spinoza, a 17th century Dutch philosopher, one of the most significant goals a human being can pursue is knowledge development because knowledge represents power and freedom for humanity. Spinoza considered the pursuit of knowledge and the pleasures of understanding to be precursors to permanent happiness, which in turn leads to healthful living. His philosophy integrates mind, body, and nature in articulating the sources and resources of knowledge. He considered some conditions essential for knowledge development, two of which are of concern to us here. He proposed that a high level of understanding of the sources of knowledge and the availability of human beings who are interested and committed to activities related to the processes of development as two essential criteria for knowledge development.

On the sources of knowledge, Spinoza distinguished among four forms of knowledge. The first is "hearsay knowledge," knowing one's birthday because we were told of the day, the time, the circumstances, and who the parents are; the source of that knowledge is not personal experience. The second type of knowledge is perceived through the source of "vague or confused experience." Here, "general impressions" that something has "usually worked" is the source of a great deal of our knowledge, such as knowing that dogs bark, that we will die and that water extinguishes flame. The third type of knowledge is achieved through "immediate deduction, or by reasoning, one thing is inferred from the essence of another." Specific relationships are absent; therefore, part of the reality is out there to be observed and the other part is logically deduced. Experience may refute this type of knowledge. Hence, the fourth form (which is the highest, incorporates deduction and perception, and combines reality, perception, intuition, and feelings) Spinoza called intuitive knowledge (*scientia intuitiva*). It is not totally unlike the third form of knowledge. It is the kind of knowing that proceeds from "an adequate idea" to the "adequate knowledge of the essence of things" (Copleston, 1963; Durant, 1953).

On human beings in pursuit of knowledge development, Spinoza said a person who is:

> in pursuit of knowledge should be able 1. To speak in a manner comprehensible to the people and to do for them all things that do not prevent us from attaining our

> ends. . . . 2. To enjoy only such pleasures as are necessary for the preservation of health. 3. Finally, to seek only enough money . . . to comply with such customs as are not opposed to what we seek." (Spinoza, cited in Durant, 1953, p. 128).

In this chapter the sources and resources of theory as essential components for theory development are discussed and analyzed. It is assumed that to engage in some form or another in the theoretical development of the discipline, members of the discipline should be aware of the sources and resources for theory, use them, and promote them. The conditions related to the sources and resources are necessary but not sufficient for theory development. Other conditions are the identification and resolution of paradoxes that may be related to theory development. Two paradoxes are identified and discussed here. Additional conditions, such as knowledge of strategies for the development and evaluation of concepts and theories are discussed in Chapters 12, 13, and 14. All these conditions provide contexts for experiencing the processes for knowledge development which support the development of abilities and expertise in developing theories.

Sources: For Theory Development

The Domain Phenomenon

Ideas, questions, and phenomena are the sources of ideas for theory development. Ideas originate in the mind, and it is through the power of the mind that they are analyzed, separated, and sorted into mere passing thoughts or intellectual ideas worth pursuing. Early philosophers differed in their discussions of where ideas come from. John Locke (cited in Nidditch, 1975) used the image of the *tabula rasa*, the "blank slate," to describe the meaning of ideas. To Locke, experience is the source of all ideas, reason, and knowledge. Knowledge is founded in experience and is derived from experience. Locke spoke of observations and reflections as mechanisms for the experiences to be translated into ideas. Experience is not limited to the external senses, although these sensations are extremely important for knowledge development, but also include internal senses, reflections of the mind. It is the combination of the discourse between external and internal senses, between observations and reflections, the internal and external dialogue that creates ideas. The conscious experience, according to Locke, is significant but inseparable from the internal experience.

Although the *tabula rasa* idea has long since died, the inseparability of internal and external sensations is the essence of theory development in nursing. It is through the connection between experience and thinking that ideas may be formed. The mind is ultimately the vehicle through which ideas evolve, yet what external mechanisms exist for the mind to observe? Nurses have many sources of ideas, sources that have gone through three distinct stages.

1. The first stage was the total dependence on other disciplines and paradigms. A scholarly discipline cannot have its needed autonomy and accountability with continuous dependence on other disciplines and paradigms as sources of ideas. Such dependence dictates the significant phenomena or problems instead of allowing the discipline itself to generate its phenomena and problem areas. A focus emanating from

educational paradigms promoted the development of theories that explained and predicted phenomena that better answered questions in the educational field, such as theories regarding modularized instruction or teaching and learning strategies. A medical model allowed for observations related to signs, symptoms, illness, and observations.

2. Second, methodology and functions dominated the idea reservoirs of the discipline of nursing. Ideas related to what nurses do and how nurses conduct research led to conceptualizations of nurses' roles and of methods of research (Gortner and Nahm, 1977). The few dissatisfied scholars who continued to consider sources of ideas such as patients and patient care were rejected. They were thought to advocate a single paradigm in nursing—one single explanation of the world, one system of thought and action that would cover everything. That was perceived to be the route to discipline development. The ideas of these scholars were rejected by the majority, and decades went by in which ideas were methodological and functional—research and theory methodologies—rather than substantive. Some perceived the approach of one paradigm for the entire field to be a method of mind control, a stifling approach conducive to insignificant work.

3. Third, our current stage is the acknowledgment of multiple sources of ideas. This stage allows different philosophical thoughts to exist side by side. This is the stage of looking back at all our sources of ideas and using any and all that help to address the problem areas of nursing to develop nursing theories.

The phenomena of the discipline are the core source for the needed theoretical development. The phenomena stimulate ideas, questions, and explorations. The phenomena related to understanding, explaining, predicting, and prescribing the caring process that happens between clients and nurses are, and should be, the focus of theoretical work in the discipline of nursing. However, the context and the sources of phenomena that have occupied nurses have been numerous. Each source provides a medium for articulating significant theoretical questions and each lends itself to theoretical analysis and development. Because the context and the source influence the type and the nature of the phenomenon to be considered, it is important for nurses to understand the different sources and to make deliberate choices based on the discipline's mission and priorities.

Extant Nursing Practice

One of the earliest sources of theoretical nursing was the recipient of nursing care and the actual nursing care offered. The writings of Florence Nightingale attest to the significance of nurses' experience the care process for those suffering from disease and from the Crimean War in developing her conceptualization of nursing and its mission. Nightingale's conceptualization of environment as the focus of nursing care, and her admonition to nurses that it is not enough to know all about the disease process, are the earliest attempts at differentiation between the focuses of nursing and medicine. Her concept of nursing, which has been considered more carefully in the 1980s, includes the proper use of fresh air, light, warmth, cleanliness, and quiet, and the proper selection and administration of diet, all with the least expense of vital power to the patient. For example, the statement, "Nursing should be to assist the reparative process, and decrease suffering" (Nightingale, 1859), could be subjected to concept development for suffering or the reparative process, or to theory development for the relationship between the reparative process and suffering.

Nightingale's *Notes on Nursing*, in which she articulated phenomena central to the domain of nursing, evolved from extant nursing practice and for experiencing the wholeness of the processes of caring (Nightingale, 1859). The notes were based on her observations and her experience in nursing. They are a living indication of the potential for extant nursing practice to be a source of ideas for theories to describe, predict, and prescribe nursing care. Her focus on environment and health is becoming a more accepted focus of nursing. One cannot help but wonder, if nurses had continued to consider extant nursing practice as the major source of ideas, whether or not the theoretical development of the discipline would have taken a different path. Extant nursing practice as a source of theoretical development was revisited in the late 1980s. The development and analysis of concepts that are related to clinical phenomena are indicators of the acknowledgment of the centrality of nursing practice as a source of theoretical nursing.

Biomedical Paradigm

Those who followed Florence Nightingale in the development of schools of nursing to educate novices in the art of nursing took her advice regarding the necessity of providing education and apprenticeship to young women who wished to become nurses; however, these followers failed to continue to differentiate the focus and goals of nursing and medicine and failed to further Nightingale's theorization of nursing. Somehow the medical domain of practice, better developed and more powerful, replaced what was starting to become a nursing domain of practice (health: hygiene, environment, and care).

Ideas evolving from the medical domain of practice addressed medical phenomena, signs, symptoms, surgery, medication, illness, and diseases. Early textbooks provide documentation of the context provided to students, which was medicine and surgery. The medical domain with its biomedical theories dictated the questions that may have been asked by nurses. The richness of nursing practice did not provide the impetus for a focus on generalizing, describing, and predicting nursing phenomena or for prescribing nursing care interventions.

The era of total dependence on the medical model neglected the patient as a human being and the environment as significant in the care of ill people. This is well described by Norris (1982):

> Nursing knowledge, because of nurses' close alliance with medicine, has been traditionally oriented to symptoms. Symptoms represent processes whose end products are failure of bodily systems unless there is medical intervention. It follows that much of the nursing assessment has arisen out of a process of identifying a problem and tracing it back into the medical model where it is considered from the point of view of failure of the human organism. Much of nursing intervention has emerged from attempts to assist in or complement medical intervention and to provide measures that reduce the discomfort caused by the pathology or medical treatment of it (Norris, 1982, p. 405).

The dependence on the biomedical model has resulted in conceptualizing and developing ideas emanating from and influencing medical care rather than nursing care (Allen and Hall, 1988). The biomedical paradigm as a source for knowledge development in nursing has regained prominence with the increasing number of nurse practitioners who use it extensively in their practice. In addition, questions driven by the advanced practice roles of nurses that combine the nurse practitioner and the clinical specialist roles require integration of different paradigms to answer them fully. The challenge facing nursing in the future is to develop theories that reflect this integration.

Nurses' Experience

Some of nursing care knowledge has been based on personal and group experiences and has been transmitted from generation to generation through apprenticeship, teaching, or textbooks. Ideas generated from experiences of comforting, caring, changing the environment, preparing for hospitalization, preparing for surgery, or preparing for discharge; ideas related to a sense of timing of when to help patients and when not to help patients; and properties and types of interactions are the kinds of ideas that could be developed further into theories. Experiences of patients with certain diseases and surgeries were exchanged between the seasoned and the novice, the educator and the student, and the nurse and a colleague. These rich experiences were not articulated into conceptual entities that would have made them more amenable to wider communication, to generalization, to refinement, or to testing. To "know" from individual experience permits knowledge that is influenced by personal beliefs, personal convictions, and personal experiences to be shared.

It is possible that knowing becomes knowing through a method of "tenacity," in which people hold firmly to their beliefs because of psychological attachment to the thing they presume to know. In the case of nurses, knowing may be repeated experiences, and nurses therefore may refuse to modify their beliefs in the face of new evidence. Fixed beliefs emanating from experiences are then communicated as knowledge through the method of "authority" (Pierce, cited in Kerlinger, 1964, pp. 6–8). To frame ideas and relationships as "authoritative" dictates a decrease in the potential of progress by development or refinement. To develop ideas and relationships as theories allows for further exploration. To speak only from personal experience in patient care is not a scientific sin; but to generalize, to transmit from generation to generation these limited ideas based on personal idiosyncrasies and individual differences, stifles progress in the discipline, limits options for patient care to individuals, and limits experience.

To use experience, however, as a source of ideas to develop concepts and consider relationships prepares those ideas for further exploration, for testing, for generalization, for being challenged and modified. Experiences, when communicated as personal experiences and on an individual basis, do not have the same power of explanation, description, or prediction as experiences that have been raised to a higher level of abstraction and then commitment. Caring for wounds in a certain way, based on one's personal experience, can be an impetus for developing wound-care theory that would describe the wounds, the different modes of caring for them, variables to consider, the proper environment to help the healing process, the materials to use, the outcomes expected, and the relationship between all these.

Experiential accounts of caring have been published over the years in clinical journals (Agan, 1987; Moch, 1990; Rew, 1988). These accounts have been useful for clinicians but ignored by scientists who have claimed a scientific discipline has no place for experiential knowledge. Writings by nurse scholars in the late 1970s and in the 1980s have supported the significance of clinicians' experiences as sources of knowledge. Carper (1978) demonstrated that the nursing literature contains four modes of knowledge, only one of which is empirical; others are aesthetic, personal, and ethical. Benner (1983) acknowledged the clinical know-hows of expert nurses. Nurses' experiences and nursing practice were identified as sources for the discipline's theories and its knowledge (Meleis, 1985). Even when nurses are functioning from a context of a medical model, how that model is modified to become congruent with nursing's mission and goals is a significant question that continues to merit description and investigation.

Extant nursing practice and nursing experience as sources of phenomena for theoretical nursing are different but related. For example, comfort may be described and explained as perceived and experienced by different client populations under different sets of circumstances, resulting in a theory of comfort that addresses the dimensions of comfort, the conditions under which comfort is needed and experienced. The source of this theory is extant nursing practice through nurses promoting comfort to the different populations and nursing experience through nurses observing the different populations' comfort responses to the care delivered. Both sources may increase the scope and the significance of the theory.

Roles

All the sources of ideas mentioned previously evolved from practice and pertained to practice. After that, interest shifted to role preparation, which coincided with the 1950s' conceptualization of nursing as a set of functions. Looking for ideas for preparation of nurses for such functional roles as teachers, administrators, consultants, and clinical specialists prompted a shift to disciplines such as education and business administration. Functions within the context of nursing, but derived from other disciplines' theories, became the impetus for investigations and explorations.

Ideas evolving into theoretical propositions were those related to how to prepare for different roles, the effects of different types of institutional organizations, or the different types and levels of nursing care delivered mostly on nursing personnel. Occasionally patient outcomes were considered, but even then, patient outcomes that were more congruent with other paradigms (eg, conceptualization of team nursing, nurse satisfaction, and patient satisfaction) were the ideas of the time from which nurses conceptualized nursing. Concepts that emanated from the role preparation paradigm described and predicted effective and efficient functioning as a teacher, administrator, or consultant. Role preparation was not conducive to theoretical development of the discipline; it provided, however, a functional framework for graduate education.

Basic Science

Nurses have relied heavily on paradigms from other fields and disciplines in addition to the medical and role preparation paradigms. The education of nurses at the doctoral level in the fields of sociology, psychology, anthropology, and physiology has prompted a healthy proliferation of ideas. A kind of cross-pollination occurred when systems, adaptation, and stress paradigms, among others, were modified to define and explain nursing phenomena. For example, Peplau (1952) developed an interpersonal theory of nursing using ideas from a psychoanalytical paradigm. Another example is the use of Piaget's theory as a source for developing theories in nursing (Maier, 1969).

Because much of nursing care is predicated on establishing a relationship with patients and on interaction, it becomes important to assess cognitive abilities of patients to deliver the appropriate and congruent messages (eg, patient education). Whereas Piaget's work provided the assumptions and major concepts, propositions specific to nursing care will necessitate concept refinement and derivation. They will also necessitate consideration of variables that may influence cognitive abilities in health care situations. Examples within an area that may be the impetus for theory development based on Piaget (1971) are:

- Changes in cognition, before, during, and after nursing or medical interventions
- Effect of intrusiveness of procedures on altered cognition and on patient responses
- Clinical therapeutics to deal with the responses in relation to the cognitive level
- Clinical therapeutics to change the responses in relation to the cognitive level

Thus, a theory of cognitive functioning of adults in acute situations may result from a developmental paradigm (Maier, 1969), but it addresses nursing by explaining, describing, predicting, or prescribing nursing phenomena or questions, such as responses to health/illness situations.

Examples of theories deductively evolving from other paradigms but attempting to address nursing phenomena and nursing problems are Johnson's theory (based on a systems paradigm), Roy's theory (based on adaptation, systems, and interaction theory), and Rogers' theory (using systems and developmental paradigms) (see Chaps. 15 through 18).

Ideal Nursing Practice

One other source of ideas for nursing theories has been what Barnum (1994) called the ought-to-be nursing practice, as opposed to the as-is or extant nursing practice. Some theorists who have developed theories based on the ideal or ought-to-be nursing practice did not use a discovery method, that is, by observing, experiencing, categorizing, and analyzing reality. Instead, they reconstructed reality; they invented what reality should be and how nurses ought to deal with it. When Johnson conceptualized a person as a system of behavior and conceptualized assessment as a process for identifying behaviors, sets, and goals of subsystems, no nurses were assessing reality as such. It was her mental image of what nursing could and should be. A person as an energy field was not a focus of nursing action, nor was a nurse a temporary self-care agent. However, the conceptual images of nursing dealing with a person as an energy field and a nurse as a temporary self-care agent were created by Rogers and Orem, respectively. These nurses combined nonnursing theories, not with actual nursing but with imaginary nursing, or perhaps with nursing as practiced by the few.

Although they were the visionaries in conceptualization, it is this kind of invention that has been problematical for practicing nurses for two decades and may have slowed down the further development and refinement of existing theories and the development of other significant ideas into theories. (Theories developed in the late 1950s and early 1960s were fully acknowledged for discussion and refinement in the 1980s.) Nurses in practice could not reconcile the images of the few with the practice of the many. Theorizing was linked with the ideal (albeit nonexisting) practice, and usefulness of a theory for practice was severely questioned. Both areas, practice and theory, were pushed farther and farther apart.

The Nursing Process

The process of assessment, diagnosis, intervention, and evaluation is another source of ideas for nursing theory. Interest in the nursing process has resulted in numerous conceptualizations of process in nurse–patient relationships and of process in decision making in patient care. Examples are Peplau's, Orlando's, Wiedenbach's, and Travelbee's conceptualizations of components of the nurse–patient interaction process. Other examples are the Harms and McDonald (1966) and Abdellah, Beland, Martin, and Matheney (1961) conceptualization of the decision-making process. Ideas related to problem solving, priority setting, and decision making evolved from a focus on the nursing process and from questions such as: What are the best approaches to identify needs of patients and to deliver nursing therapeutics? What are the similarities and differences between nursing process, clinical judgment process, and other decision-making processes? (Duldt, 1995; Gordon, Murphy, Candee, and Hiltunen, 1994). Frisch (1994) asked the question whether or not we need the nursing process and answered by proposing it as the foundation for practice and teaching to explain and document care.

Nursing Diagnosis and Nursing Interventions

Ideas for theory may emanate from classification systems such as those developed for nursing diagnosis and nursing interventions. *Nursing diagnoses* are defined as labels given to problems that fall within the domain of nursing. "It is a concise summary, a conceptual statement of the client's health status" (Kim and Moritz, 1982, p. 84). A diagnosis states a conclusion that is based on some order and pattern the diagnostician arrived at through nursing investigation (Durand and Prince, 1966). It incorporates a nurse's judgment. The process of developing theories through the use of nursing diagnosis is in agreement with stages in theory development beginning from concepts.

Jacox identified the first step in theory development as a period of specifying, defining, and classifying concepts used in describing the phenomena of the field (Jacox, 1974, p. 5). Therefore, if there is agreement that a first step in theory development is a period of specifying and classifying, and if practice is the arena for theory development, then indeed nursing diagnosis provides a springboard for theory development. Dickoff, James, and Wiedenbach (1968) would classify the result of the process of classifying diagnosis as a step toward a first-level theory. Labeling without description of what is labeled and without propositions for testing is not a theory.

A classification system for nursing diagnosis began with the efforts of the St. Louis University School of Nursing, which sponsored the first conference on diagnosis in 1976 (Gebbie, 1976). The nurses who participated made a decision that theory development in nursing could not begin without the development of and agreement on its terminology. The work of nurses who participated in several of these nursing diagnosis conferences is inspiring and should continue to be the impetus for ideas that could be developed further into theories.

A warning, however, is in order. The taxonomy that evolved out of these three decades of work resulted in a list of diagnoses that some may consider esoteric in language and nonrepresentative of the complexity of human beings. They are nontheoretical or do not emanate from a coherent theoretical perspective, nor is there evidence that they have contributed to clarifying the nursing mission or to improving communication among nurses and with the rest of the health care team (Gordon, Sweeny, and McKeehan, 1980; Shamansky and Yanni, 1983). Nursing diagnoses are only meaningful if we look at diagnosis as a concept denoting a phenomenon (Kritek, 1978). Then questions arise such as:

- When does the phenomenon occur?
- Why does it occur?
- How do we deal with it?
- How do we prevent it?
- What other conditions occur at the same time?

These are questions that help in developing theories based on nursing diagnoses. In addition, the extensive reviews of research related to nursing diagnosis (eg, Gordon, 1985; Kim, 1989) can be the impetus for the development of concepts, validation of concepts, as well as for furthering theoretical synthesis (eg, Burns, Archbold, Stewart, and Shelton, 1993; Dougherty, Jankin, Lunney, and Whitley, 1993; Grant, Kinney, and Guzzetta, 1990).

Another taxonomy was developed during the early 1990s, which could also be used as a source for theory development, and this is the one related to *nursing therapeutics* or *nursing interventions*. Efforts to identify, label, describe, and categorize the interventions and the therapeutics that nurses use in their practice resulted in a three-level taxonomy of nursing interventions or therapeutics (Iowa Intervention Project, 1993). Nursing therapeutics are defined as:

> . . . singular or multiple interventions (actions) by the nurse to alter life processes, life patterns, functional health patterns, and responses in order to alter the health-illness trajectory of a person (Eisenhauer, 1994).

The typology was created to reflect the level of alteration related to either patient responses, patterns, or life processes. The Iowa Intervention Project (1993, 1995) resulted in a three-level taxonomy of nursing interventions, the top level containing six domains, the second level containing 26 classes, and the third level consisting of 357 interventions. There is a pattern of increasing number of interventions in each subsequent publication based on ongoing validation and coding studies.

All these classification systems were driven by nursing practice, and if considered as tentative, dynamic, and evolving, could stimulate growth in the knowledge base for the discipline of nursing (Grobe, 1990). However, if they are perceived and used in practice as static, procedural, and terminal, they may become a constraint to the development of the theoretical aspects of the discipline of nursing (see discussion of Nursing Diagnosis, Nursing Therapeutics, and Theoretical Nursing in Chap. 19).

Concepts Clarified and Classified

Delineated and described concepts central to the field of nursing, other than those dealing with diagnosis and intervention, constitute another source of ideas for theory development. The sources of knowledge discussed here are the already clarified concepts. Norris (1982) and others delineated and described 15 concepts that are significant in acute care nursing. Norris (1982) reviewed and considered common elements in the concepts and looked for an umbrella concept under which she synthesized all classified concepts. Therefore, the concepts comprised the source for the development of a construct, "basic physiological protection mechanisms." The new synthesis, with relationships among all delineated concepts and with a binding label, underscores a new entity, a nursing perspective. This new synthesis allows for viewing each of the clarified concepts (nausea, vomiting, morning sickness nausea without vomiting, thirst, hunger, insomnia, fatigue, immobility, chilling, itching, disorientation, bed sores, diarrhea, constipation, flatulence, urinary frequency, and perspiration) as a "functional behavioral response that attempts to remove threat" by sounding an alarm or an all-out bulletin announcing some aspect of the law of dynamic homeostasis. Each of the concepts has a protective function. Emotions after responding to protective warnings can be observed and delineated. For example, after vomiting there is a great sense of relief. Some common attributes can bind groups of these responses (eg, restlessness and insomnia have the common attribute of increased vigilance). With identification of assumptions, linkages, nursing population, types of nursing therapeutics, and nurses' actions, a theory of protection evolved.

Nurses have identified, defined, and clarified many concepts that could be considered sources of ideas for synthesis and further development of theory beginning in the 1960s and 1970s (Byrne and Thompson, 1978; Carlson and Blackwell, 1978; Kintzel, 1971; Zderad and Belcher, 1968). In the 1980s and 1990s, nurses scholars have made major contributions to the development of the discipline through concept development. (See Chap. 12 for an extensive discussion of concept development.)

Nursing Research and Nursing Theory

A new source of ideas for further development has been available for nurses since the early 1950s. Research already completed and theory already developed are sources of ideas for refinement and further development. Some examples are Barnard's (1980) research on stimulation and development of infants, potentially leading to a set of systematic and coherent propositions, and Lindeman's (1980) work on preoperative teaching, which, together with Johnson's (1972) work, has the potential of becoming a coherent set of propositions about anticipatory guidance. Reviews of research findings related to central nursing concepts or phenomena are significant sources for the development of nursing theory (eg, those published in *Annual Review of Nursing Research*).

Each of the existing nursing theories is a potential source of ideas for further theorizing. For example, Levine stated that she will develop two theories that she calls "therapeutic intention and redundancy." These theories emanate from her existing nursing theory (Fawcett, 1989, p. 156). (See Chap. 13 for more details on research and theory as sources for theory development.)

Combined Sources of Ideas

The complexity and contextuality of nursing practice requires a multiplicity of sources for its theories. These sources include clinicians who encounter phenomena that have not been explicated before, researchers who encounter relationships that have not been accounted for in previously developed theories, historians who get a new insight into the development of nursing knowledge, philosophers who question some of the agreed-on assumptions or who uncover an implicit assumption; all give significant impetus to conceptualization and theorizing. Theory development can proceed from any of those vantage points.

Resources

The sources for theory development are only one essential component in the development of theory. Resources are the second major component. Resources for the theoretical development of the discipline are the nurses themselves and the environment that could nurture and support such development. Each resource is discussed here.

Being Theoretical

Theoretical thinking, theoretical approaches to viewing situations, and the development of a theoretical identity are essential in engaging in the theoretical development of the discipline. Certain myths surround theory development. Some of these are related to who could and should develop theories. One of these myths is that "idea people" are "ivory-tower types of individuals," that only extremely intelligent people can develop theories. Another myth delineates theoreticians and practitioners; the former cannot practice and the latter cannot theorize.

These myths have greatly influenced the process of conceptualizing in nursing. The intent of this chapter is to demonstrate that, even if the myths had been true at one time, perpetuating them at this time does not promote the discipline of nursing or, more importantly, patient care.

There are no theories without ideas, but there are ideas without theories. Theories evolve from ideas and ideas evolve from hunches, personal experiences, insights, inspirations, intuition, and others' work and experiences. New ideas could be based on the discovery of a new phenomenon, the invention of a new theoretical concept, reintegration of old concepts with new realities, a reformulation of an existing idea, or a new way of organizing old concepts. New ideas also may evolve from asking new questions or even from asking old questions but finding that the old answers no longer answer the questions. The context may have changed and therefore the answers may no longer be adequate.

Ideas are all around us; however, only some ideas develop into theories. Ten conditions may assist in the development of theories, and each of these conditions may be subjected to research investigations.

1. An idea is usually generated by one person, although others may help to nourish it, others may be triggered to follow through, or even two people on opposite sides of the globe may get the same idea simultaneously; however, for each one, the "aha" is a personal matter (Reynolds, 1971). Therefore, a creative person should have the capacity to be alone to develop inner resources (Arietti, 1976).
2. Intelligence and intellectual abilities are necessary but not sufficient conditions for developing theoretical thinking (Reynolds, 1971; Roe, 1951, 1963). Theoretical thinkers also need creativity and persistence.
3. Theoretical thinkers have an extra sense by which they can differentiate between a good and a bad idea; therefore, they do not spin their wheels on something that will not materialize or on an idea that has no potential for development (Reynolds, 1971).
4. They have thorough knowledge of the field in which their idea may fit (Meleis and May, 1981). They know the accepted notions surrounding their ideas, and they have a sense of history and context; otherwise, they would not be able to tell whether their discovery, their invention, or their conceptualization is new or whether they have the context within which to place their ideas. "In short, they know when a good idea is a new idea" (Reynolds, 1971, p. 152).
5. These individuals are not particularly committed to all the ideas of the field or to the ideas held by the scholarly community. They are open to new ideas and are able to stand independent and apart from others (Roe, 1951, 1963). They stand alone to support their own convictions (Armiger, 1974).
6. They are in touch with the phenomenon in some way. They are either deeply engrossed in a clinical area, are committed to researching a particular phenomenon, are trying to synthesize some of the concepts in the field, or are involved in an in-depth study of a particular theory. "No matter what the endeavor, the individuals are deeply engrossed in the subject matter, so deeply that an intuitive or uncommunicable organization of new concepts and their relationships may develop a feeling that later takes form as a theory" (Reynolds, 1971, p. 153).
7. Developers of ideas are willing to take risks.
8. A person whose ideas go beyond the initial idea stage possesses a sense of persistence to work, self-discipline, and an ability for developing a sense of satisfaction that goes with the hard work (Arietti, 1976; Roe, 1951, 1963).
9. Ideas flourish and develop when a person is able to articulate and communicate them to others. Communication of ideas allows for a healthy debate and a healthy critique, both of which are essential for continuous clarification and refinement of ideas. Fear of "idea snatching" may have prevented some good ideas from being communicated and therefore may have kept them from the potential of further development.
10. Whether aware of it or not, a person with an idea that is potentially productive may have an intuitive capability, and, furthermore, accepts intuition as a significant asset in the development of ideas. To develop that sense a person needs periods of inactivity to daydream, to think freely with no specific struc-

ture, and also to be able to suspend judgment until ideas develop (Arietti, 1976). Finally, a person whose ideas go far is usually a person with a good sense of timing.

Nurses, wherever they are and in whichever settings, are observing new phenomena, are articulating significant questions and, moreover, may have developed their own personal theories about patient care. Some may not have been aware of the significance or the timeliness of the phenomena they observed, the relationships, or hunches they developed; or they may have not discussed or communicated these hunches to others. Awareness, reflection, and/or discussion of these initial hunches allows them to grow, flourish, and attain more potential for a systematic theoretical development. For example, the observations (or intuition, or both) of a nurse in a kidney dialysis unit who is consistently able to decide, within a few minutes of interaction with patients who come in weekly for dialysis, whether or not that patient's dialysis will be completed efficiently and effectively, without complication, could evolve into the articulation of antecendent variables and outcome criteria that are more predictive. This nurse, then, is able to formulate questions about an important phenomenon and may be able to offer a conceptualization of an important aspect of patient care. Other conditions for theory development, such as communication of this clinical knowledge is a next step to further development of these conceptual ideas. Clinicians with such embodied clinical knowledge need to be provided with opportunities to further develop these ideas through collaboration with others who are experienced in the development of theories pertaining to practice.

Conditions for theory development, therefore, are: the presence of a cadre of individuals who are firm believers in the significance of theoretical thinking for nursing practice and who have and are provided with the conditions outlined above. In addition, they need the availability of a theoretically supportive environment as discussed below.

Theoretically Supportive Environment

Even if a person has the characteristics listed above, she may not be able to engage in the activities and processes inherent in theoretical reflection and development without an intellectually nurturing environment. An intellectually nurturing environment is one that values theoretical nursing, allows time to clarify values, time to articulate and relate ideas, and time to question. It is an environment that permits ambiguity, that does not press for immediate solutions, that allows dissension and does not press for consensus, and that permits philosophical discourse (Jennings and Meleis, 1988; Meleis and Jennings, 1989; Meleis and Price, 1988). What is needed is an environment that acknowledges theoretical abilities and rewards theoretical thinking.

Strategies to develop such environments could evolve from the nature of nursing to complement its natural activities. A team report, for example, could be the medium for questioning and reflecting on clinical phenomena. Members of an administrative team may devote some time for discussing a pressing problem theoretically and from different perspectives. Goals related to theoretical nursing are somewhat different from those related to immediate problem solving. Goals related to theoretical nursing are the development of a concept or the analysis of a theoretical perspective. Problem solving, however, focuses on resolving a problem. Creating a supportive environment should not be analogous to creating an environment that is artificial or foreign to an institution; it should fit within an institution's mission and goals and within its daily experiences and functions.

Identifying Domain Paradoxes

Another condition for theoretical development in a discipline is to identify, acknowledge, and accept or transcend the paradoxes that may be related to theory development. Living with paradoxes in a discipline is as effective in the development of its theories as confronting the paradoxes, making a choice, and then moving on with the business of developing the discipline. What is not effective is to pretend there is only one view or to be immobilized with the paradox and to make resolving it the focus rather than the means.

A commitment to theory development was made in nursing by the American Nursing Association in the mid-1960s. However, the debates related to nursing theory may have delayed the process. Much has been written and debated about nursing theory and about the differences for practice between nursing theories and nonnursing theories. Other debates centered around whether nursing needs theory *in* nursing, *of* nursing, or *for* nursing. Others developed a rather strong case for the lack of need of practice theory. Still others showed that nurses borrow all theory. Another group of debaters demonstrated that other practice fields have no theory of their own, and therefore nursing's quest for theories is an unwarranted one.

Theory is not a status symbol or a special honorary card that nursing needs to remain in the halls of academia or to achieve professional status. Theory provides the mechanism from which we can organize our observations, focus our inquiry, and communicate our findings. Theory helps to explain, describe, and predict the range of phenomena of interest to nurses that are central in meeting the identified goals and in highlighting gaps in our knowledge. Instead of getting on with the business of developing theories related to our substantive area of practice and advancing nursing knowledge, a good part of two decades (1960–1980) has been spent debating whether nurses are capable of developing theories, whether they should develop theories, or whether theories are even necessary to nursing. On the whole, the theories that were developed in nursing have not been developed further or refined. (There are some exceptions; for example, Roy has been systematic in developing her theory and in proposing refinements and theoretical propositions. See Chap. 15 for analysis of Roy's ideas and for citations.)

In general, theories have become subjects of debate about whether they are philosophies, theories, concepts, metaparadigms, paradigms, grand theories, or, even worse, not theories at all. From all these debates more concepts have evolved to describe theoretical thinking in nursing, such as conceptual frameworks, theoretical models, and conceptual models. This evolution only managed to add considerably to the confusion of nurses. The muddle may have delayed the seasoned theoreticians and researchers in their attempts at knowledge development; it has kept the novice from getting involved in the process of theory building, it has confused those outside the discipline who have not understood what nurses are quibbling about, and it has stood in the way of nurses understanding, contributing to, and improving patient care.

In this section, examples of the confusion in the discipline related to its theoretical development are identified and discussed. Only two of the paradoxes that have been the subject of debates in the past are analyzed. These paradoxes were selected for three reasons: they transcend time; their influence on the level of development of theoretical nursing during the 1970s to 1990s is hypothesized to be profound; and understanding these two paradoxes through careful analyses can be useful for analyzing and understanding other contemporary and future paradoxes. These paradoxes symbolize a significant period in the development of the theoretical aspects of the nursing discipline. The full meanings of these debates and their roles in enhancing or constraining the intellectual environment in the discipline have not yet been fully extracted. By reflecting on the meanings of each side of the debates, students of theory and theory development may be able to develop some insights and some visions about forces and constraints in theory development.

Conceptual Models Versus Theory

In one of the first theory classes in the United States, taught at the University of California, Los Angeles in the late 1960s, Dorothy Johnson classified the conceptualizations of nursing that existed at that time as nursing models. It appears that, since then, terms such as *models, frameworks,* or *theories* have been used freely and interchangeably to refer to any conceptualization of nursing reality. An example of a common usage of models is when one is used to denote that the study of a system B is based on the study of a system A, and that all parts of system B correspond to all parts of system A. Then it is said that B is modeled after A, but it does not say there is any causal relationship between A and B. It only means that some of system A's properties are in system B. It also means that the properties of system B that are different from system A's properties need to be identified. Therefore, modeling denotes similarities in most of the pattern and order and in some of the properties. In other words, "when one system is a model of another, they resemble one another in form and not in content" (Kaplan, 1964, p. 263).

Although this is the common use, there are different types of models. The *physical model* duplicates the form and structure but differs in scale; the miniature train and the baby doll who cries, laughs, and sucks are examples of physical models. They are replicas; in other words, laws that govern the original are obeyed by the model. The *semantic model* is built by using similar symbols and could be called a *conceptual analogue.* We use semantic models when we reduce our hypothesis to statistical symbols for the purpose of analysis. A widely used model in nursing is the *formal model.* To develop formal models we resort to deductive logic, deducing from the original theory by using the central components and crucial relationships as a model for data gathering. Formal models exhibit the same properties in components and the same structure, but the context may be different. For example, we may use an epidemiologic theory of disease transmission with its components of incubation, contagiousness, and quarantine to describe how nursing theories are transmitted. Whereas correspondence in the formal model is theoretical, there is abstract correspondence between theoretical ideas and empirical observations in the *interpretive model.* Data may be interpreted using an old theory. The model for interpretation combines both data and the old theory.

The notion that nursing conceptualizations are conceptual models evolved out of ideas representing two different assumptions. In the nursing theory course developed by Johnson in the 1960s, the idea that nursing conceptualizations were modeled after guiding paradigms (systems, adaptation, developmental, and symbolic interaction) was introduced. Other writings and analyses were based on the same premise of guiding paradigms. The second idea, that of models, was based on interpretive models and assumed that nursing is the reality and that each of the existing conceptualizations model that reality at different levels of isomorphism. Early designations of nursing thought correspond to the first idea, that conceptualizations are formally modeled after other conceptual schemata (Riehl and Roy, 1974), and later designations correspond to the second idea, that conceptualizations are based on interpretive models (Fawcett, 1995; Fitzpatrick and Whall, 1989).

Use of models also differs in another respect. In some usage, models correspond more to reality: they are less abstract than theories; they contain all variables of the subject matter; and they describe reality more fully. Theories describe fewer variables and are more abstract, but they also correspond more or less to reality (Kaplan 1964). Others considered models as simplified forms of reality. Chin (1961) defined model as "a constructed simplification of some part of reality that retains only those features regarded as essential for relating similar processes whenever and wherever they occur" (p. 201).

Conceptual models and theories have been used synonymously (Dickoff and James, 1968) or definitions for one were used for the other: a set of concepts that are interrelated into a coherent whole and a set of propositions. Johnson (1968a) viewed a model as an "invention of the mind for a purpose" that "is drawn from reality and pertains to reality, but it does not constitute reality" (p. 2). Both sets of definitions could be used to define one or the other, that is, conceptual framework or theory.

Further confusion has arisen because of other interchangeable terms. Conceptual frameworks have been used by some interchangeably with conceptual models and by others interchangeably with theory. Fawcett (1989), among others, dismissed the matter by equating conceptual framework with conceptual model and blamed the difference on semantics. Dickoff and James (1968) defined theory as a mental image being invented for the purpose of describing, relating, and predicting a desired situation. To them, theories are conceptual frameworks; they do not differentiate between the two.

Some attempts have been made to differentiate between theory and conceptual models on such criteria as level of abstraction, degree of explication, level of specificity, types of linkage, and degree to which concepts and assumptions are interdefined (Fawcett, 1989; Fitzpatrick and Whall, 1989; Klein and Hill, 1972, cited in Rodman, 1980). They argued that conceptual frameworks (or models, as they are used interchangeably) are more abstract than theories. They represent a global view of a field—its main concepts and propositions—and therefore provide the blueprint for practice, education, and research (Johnson, 1968a).

Whether or not conceptual frameworks are necessary steps in the process of developing theories has also been debated. Some contend that the conceptual framework is a stepping stone toward theory development (Hill and Hansen, 1960; Nye and Berardo, 1966), a view that has been adopted by some in nursing (Fawcett, 1993, 1995). Others question the necessity of conceptual frameworks for development of theory and argue that conceptual frameworks are not necessary steps, nor are they likely to promote or hinder theory development (Rodman, 1980).

The interchangeable use of the different concepts such as conceptual frameworks, models, and theories to describe the same thing has been a problem to the pure semanticists in the field. The attempt to differentiate between them has frequently taken on the dimension of splitting hairs and has only added to the confusion. It is just such confusion that may have contributed to the slow progress and, at times, stilted theory development in nursing and has led to an almost exclusive preoccupation with method and process rather than content and consequences. Instead of addressing the central issues in providing quality care to clients, we have had to debate and defend the methodology for theory development. Theorizing is a painstakingly long process, the results of which may be minimized by relegating them to the level of "it is only a conceptual framework." This in itself may decrease the impact of the conceptualizations and may make it less significant. The discipline using only conceptual frameworks tends to be regarded as pretheoretical and, as a result, nursing's contribution to knowledge about patient care processes and outcomes are minimized.

There are other disadvantages to the preference of using conceptual frameworks and models when the use of theory would have been much clearer. One such disadvantage could be understood by examining analogous situations—one in which conceptual frameworks and models were used before the use of theory and one in which theories were used from the outset.

Sociology, particularly family sociology, has been unique in believing that conceptual models are distinct from theories. Sociologists have maintained, and nursing scholars have begun to agree, that conceptual models provide a step in the development of theory. However, modern sociologists have since questioned the wisdom of using a conceptual framework to denote the results of theorizing. The skeptics in sociology have pointed out numerous examples in which conceptual frameworks have resulted in theorizing that lacked specification and definition and the slow process of developing propositions for testing (Rodman, 1980).

Physical and natural sciences, on the other hand, do not use conceptual frameworks and models as steps toward development of theory. Instead, they may use the term *developing theory* versus *tested theory*. Notice that many theories (genetic fat theory of obesity, cholesterol theory of cardiovascular diseases, psychoanalytical theory of neurosis) are at different levels of abstraction and different levels of sophistication and have different scopes, different levels of clarity, and varying degrees of understandable definitions; however, they are all called theories.

To be sure, some differences exist between models, conceptual frameworks, and theory. A model has to model another entity, while a theory may or may not model other properties, structures, or functions. Conceptual frameworks may present a set of discrete concepts that are not as interrelated and linked in sets of propositions as we expect from theory. However, this varies, based on the level of development of the theory. Models tend to evoke the idea of empirical positivism mixed with rationalism as a guiding philosophy or a goal, rather than the tool it ought to be. Functions attributed to models as frameworks or directives for the development of research, frameworks for the generation of a hypothesis, guides for data collection, or depositories for research findings or the further development of theory are the same functions attributed to theory.

It is not entirely clear that nursing theorists, in using different labels for their conceptualizations, have done so in any systematic way. For example, in a 1983 text, eight theorists used four different labels when referring to their conceptualizations: theory, model, science, and paradigm (Clements and Roberts, 1983). Others used theory to describe their conceptualizations and then developed and/or isolated one part of these conceptualizations and defined it as conceptual frameworks and another part that was labeled a theory (King, 1995a, 1995b). The similarities and the differences in degree of specificity, level of abstraction, and number of concepts and propositions are not always consistent with the labels. One option for using these conceptualizations is to attach the label preferred by the theorist; another option is to use whatever label the user prefers, as long as a definition and rationale are given. Some literature could always be found to document any of the uses.

The perspective of this text is to minimize the differences between conceptual models, frameworks, and theories and to relegate most of these differences to semantics and the confusion created by the many nursing scientists and theoreticians who have been educated in a multitude of fields. The rationale for taking this perspective is not to argue for a new position or to initiate a debate, but rather to cast some doubt on the significance of the differences between theories and conceptual models.

"Theory" is sufficient to describe the conceptualizations that have been proposed by our theorists. The three related aspects claimed to differentiate between theory and conceptual model are definitions, interrelationships, and level of abstraction. The first two, which state that concepts should be defined and interrelated, are considered in the present perspective as a necessity for both theory and conceptual models. The third aspect, level of abstraction, remains an important consideration. Because theories could be classified as grand, middle range, or single domain, based on the number of phenomena that the theory addresses, the number of propositions, and the operational level of the definitions, the present perspective proposes this schema to classify nursing theory rather than to relegate the classification system to such different labels as conceptual model, framework, metaparadigm, paradigm, and theory.

Although this perspective is proposed to enhance a common language across disciplines and to divert energy into development and progress in theoretical nursing rather than into circular debates, the final choice of a label is a personal matter and depends on the purpose for which the label is applied. Just as role theory has been proposed and used as a concept, a framework, a model, or a theory in research, practice, and administration in a number of disciplines, and just as the user may consider role theory from a cultural, structural, or intra-actionist perspective, nursing theories could also be used in the same way. The manner and the goal of the utilization may help determine the appropriate label.

Based on the perspective proposed here, *nursing theory* is defined as an articulated and communicated conceptualization of invented or discovered reality pertaining to nursing for the purpose of describing, explaining, predicting, or prescribing nursing care. Nursing theory is developed to answer central domain questions.

Nursing Theory Versus Borrowed Theory

For some time now, nurses have been involved in a debate over the types of theory that ought to be developed. They have taken either practice or basic theory positions. Each side has developed a good case as to why one or the other type is possible. The significance of taking one or the other position lies in the idea that the practice theory position encourages forging ahead with theory development and the borrowed theory position discourages nurses from participating in the seemingly futile attempt to develop theories.

The proponents and supporters of the development of practice theory in nursing (Dickoff, James, and Wiedenbach, 1968; Jacox, 1974; Johnson, 1968a; Wald and Leonard, 1964) view nursing theory as a conceptual framework invented by the theorist for the ultimate purpose of creating situations to meet desired, preferred end results. Therefore, the ultimate goal for theory development in nursing is to produce a change in a nursing client or a nursing situation that is desired by the nurse or the client. Dickoff and James (1968, p. 200) called this a situation-producing theory.

This is a fourth-level theory; theories at other levels are invented and articulated with the purpose of ultimately leading to this level. The first level is factor isolating, a level where theories help delineate and describe a phenomenon. The second level is a correlating theory, where factors or concepts are related to depict theories, and the third level is a situation where theories permit prediction and allow promotion or inhibition of nursing care. Each of these levels brings the theorist closer to the goals of nursing that are demonstrated in prescriptive theories, or by the situation-producing level of theory, the fourth level. The development of fourth-level theory is congruent with the purpose of the profession, which ought to be action oriented as opposed to only academically oriented. Nurses are shapers, not just observers, of reality.

The first-level theory, the factor-isolating theory, helps to articulate and label concepts. The significance of this kind of theory is to enable one to refer back to those concepts that are invented. Without a label we have no concepts; without concepts we have no relationships. Labeling allows for the creation of conceptual entities that become the cornerstones for each subsequent theory level. What Dickoff and James helped nurses to see was the significance of this level of theory, in which they had been engaged long before they began to speak of theory development.

Norris (1975), a "curious nurse clinician," observed numerous incidents of restlessness and noted that, although the term was frequently used in charting, it was not clear how restlessness was identified, when it was identified, why it occurred, and what its consequences were. More importantly, it was not clear what the nursing intervention should be. Norris' descriptive, labeling conceptual work is an excellent example of first-level theory according to Dickoff and James (1968). Other examples are Norbeck's (1981) social support concept, Norris' (1982) classification of 15 concepts related to basic physiologic protection mechanisms, and my own (Meleis, 1975) work on role supplementation and role insufficiency.

Other nurses have proposed organizing nursing around concepts and, in so doing, have provided nursing with numerous identified and labeled concepts (Carlson, 1970; Meltzer, Abdellah, and Kitchell, 1969; Mitchell, 1973). Still others researched labeled concepts in search of validity and reliability (Kim, 1980; Norbeck, 1981; Weiss, 1979). All these are considered first-level theories, an end in their own right, and a beginning of other theory levels when considering Dickoff, James, and Wiedenbach's definitions (1968). (For a review of concept and theory development, see Chaps. 12 and 13.)

Once concepts are delineated and labeled, a theorist is ready to develop relationships. Correlating theories result from theorists inventing relationships between labeled concepts. These theories are second-level, factor-relating theories. Relating preoperative teaching to postoperative behavior, restless and muscular tension under different conditions, social support and health, or role insufficiency and role supplementation could result in a factor-relating theory.

To predict postoperative behavior by varying preoperative teaching is an instance of third-level, predictive theory. Third-level theory depicts and predicts with a time reference. It is not only relational—as is second-level theory—it is causal, as the theorist discovers that certain conditions lead to others. In fact, all three levels incorporate a discovery of reality but not an invention of reality. None of these three levels purports to change or influence reality. Rather, all lead to the development of the most powerful of theories for a professional practice discipline, the situation-producing theory, which is a fourth-level theory.

One of the significant differences between third- and fourth-level theories is in commitment to a goal. A predictive theory describes what happens, such as postoperative behavior with different strategies of preoperative teaching. In a fourth-level theory, there is a commitment to finding out how it happened. An example could be that certain postoperative behavior is conceived as appropriate behavior to bring about. The theory then proceeds to describe what to do preoperatively to bring about that desired behavior. This level of theory, therefore, has several essential components: (1) an aim or goal specified by the theorist as desirable; (2) a prescription to bring about the desired aim; and (3) a "survey list" to use in future prescriptions.

The survey list is designed to respond to six crucial questions for prescriptive theory:

1. Who or what performs the activity? (Agency)
2. Who or what is the recipient of the activity? (Patiency)
3. In what context is the activity performed? (Framework)
4. What is the end point of the activity? (Terminus)
5. What is the guiding procedure, technique, or protocol of the activity? (Procedure)
6. What is the energy source for the activity? (Dynamics) (Dickoff, James, and Wiedenbach, 1968, p. 422)

The activities in a prescriptive theory expected to correspond to these questions are agency, patiency, framework, terminus, procedure, and dynamics. Each incorporates internal and external resources as well as the potential for using theories from other disciplines if deemed useful.

All survey questions are asked from the viewpoint of the goal of the activity and take the prescription into consideration. It is assumed, and practice supports such assumption, that the agent who is expected to perform the prescription does not always hold full jurisdiction over the prescription. A combination of internal resources, such as certain skills, experiences, and techniques, and external resources, such as policies and environment, specifies the agent. In some instances, prescription may be delegated; in others, it may be relegated. A fourth-level theory should include the kinds of agents who are expected to perform the prescription to bring about the desired end result. The authors (Dickoff, James, and Wiedenbach, 1968) proposed a broad concept of *agency* to include all those who have the internal and external resources; they proposed a similar one about patiency. Nurses, physicians, family members, visitors, and so on may be agents performing nursing activities toward nursing goals. Therefore, a theory should specify all possible agents.

Patiency specifies the recipients of the prescriptions with whom agency interfaces for the purpose of bringing about the desired goal. Patiency may designate sick or well people, interacting or noninteracting things or people, animate or inanimate objects, recipients of activities done by registered nurses, and activities done by people other than nurses, but all are bound together by the goal of the activity. Patients are "interactors" with agency and others geared toward the "activity of a desired kind and as possessed of a repertoire of capacities and limitations (much as is the agent) to see a great range of latitude as to ways of producing desired outcomes" (Dickoff, James, and Wiedenbach, 1968).

The agent and the patient in a theory have to be specific in terms of the context within which both occur. The context, called the *framework* by Dickoff and colleagues, requires that the situation-producing theory specify all variables that should be considered to bring about the desired goals through an activity produced by an agent and received by a patient. The end product of the activity is the *terminus*, the situation to be produced.

A situation-producing theory also includes the pattern by which the activity is performed. *Procedure* includes the steps to be taken to bring about the desired goal. Procedure, then, includes the arena, the equipment, the type of charting, the type of follow-up, policies to govern it, timing, and the rules-of-thumb governing activity. Although procedures could be detailed, most often they are guidelines and safeguards.

Finally, a nursing theory of the situation-producing type should consider the aesthetic satisfaction of performing the activity and the desire for self-esteem. These are motivating factors in performing and sustaining activities to realize a nursing goal. The more developed the theory, the more likely these two factors are considered. These factors are grouped under what Dickoff and colleagues called the *dynamics* of the theory. When the dynamics are conceptualized adequately, all factors that relate to the agent, such as education, reputation of institution, and rewards, or to patients, such as insurance, will have to be considered in a situation-producing theory.

To understand, explain, predict, and prescribe nursing phenomena and nursing care, nurses should develop practice theories that emanate from the discipline and guide the discipline's actions. There is one significant feature of theory in a practice discipline. Although descriptive, relating, and predictive theories are equally important, nursing practice theory needs to strive for prescriptive theory. Nurses may develop basic theories that describe discovered concepts, relationships related to human beings, nursing situations, nurse–patient interactions, environments, or health; but the ultimate goal is to develop theories to change situations. Therefore, theories that stress change as their goal are practice theories.

Discovery charts a more probable process for the development of basic theories; invention, on the other hand, is a more probable goal of practice theory. Properties or dimensions of transitions, for example, lend themselves to basic theory that describes and explains when transitions are healthy, under what circumstances transitions in health and illness occur, what the consequences of various types and levels of transitions are, and why the variability of consequences exists. What to do to enhance smooth transitions for nursing clients, how to maintain the person–environment harmony in transition, and how to maintain homeostasis and enhance adjustment are questions that lend themselves to practice theories.

Even when theories developed in other disciplines are used to explain nursing phenomena and nursing problems, the new derivations and new syntheses make them nursing theories. The concept "nursing" does not denote who developed it or where it is used; rather, it reflects the phenomenon that the theory addresses. Nursing theories evolve out of the practice arena or anything that pertains to the practice arena. They are then tested in research. Until the time-consuming job of research is accomplished, face validity of a theory as it pertains to practice should be enough to allow the theory to be one of the blueprints for action.

Some challenge the notion that nursing should develop its theoretical base. Their arguments are based on the premise that nursing is a practice discipline and that practice disciplines depend on other disciplines for their theoretical underpinnings. Beckstrand (1978a, 1978b, 1980), for example, tiij issue with the contention that nursing is concerned with practice theory. For practice theory to be meaningful, practice knowledge should be different from scientific and ethical knowledge. Beckstrand then examined two aspects of practice knowledge, the knowledge of how to control and how to make changes and the knowledge of what is morally good. She examined these aspects with the question in mind of whether it is possible for practice theory to exist as distinct from science and ethics. The first part of the question needs knowledge of science and the second needs knowledge of what is morally good.

Science, to Beckstrand, seeks to develop the knowledge necessary to change and control. This knowledge, containing lawlike relationships, is synonymous with scientific knowledge. Controls are possible in practice situations; however, practice methodology proceeds by valid deductions from scientific laws. Beckstrand then showed that the field of philosophy known as ethics provides the other body of knowledge that is necessary for practice but that substitutes for practice theory. Both normative ethics and metaethics have relevance to practice, and we can easily borrow and co-opt theories to explain moral obligations and moral values in the discipline. The method of obtaining such knowledge and using it is that of logical reasoning, also a borrowed concept.

Nursing uses scientific knowledge and logic to meet its ethical goals—all that constitutes the knowledge base of nursing. So, in essence, there is no need for practice theory (Beckstrand, 1978a, 1978b).

Others who agreed that nursing does not need its own theory made a case for borrowed theories to describe, explain, and predict phenomena significant to nursing. Family theory, systems theory, and psychological theory are examples of theories that could be borrowed. Johnson, who was the first to use the concept of borrowing (1968a, 1974), defined borrowed theory as "that knowledge which is developed in the main by other disciplines and is drawn upon by nursing" and defined unique theory as "that knowledge derived from the observation of phenomena and the asking of questions unlike those which characterize other disciplines" (Johnson, 1968b, p. 3). However, she warned that any attempts at differentiation are hazardous, first of all because the man-made, more or less arbitrary, divisions between the sciences are neither firm nor constant. It appears there is a special unity in knowledge, corresponding to a unity in nature, which defies established boundaries and continuously presses for the larger, more cohesive view. Moreover, knowledge does not innately "belong" to any field of science. It is not exactly happenstance that a given bit of knowledge is discovered by one discipline rather than another, but the fact of discovery does not confer the right of ownership. Viewed in this light, borrowed and unique have no real permanence, or any meaning (Johnson, 1968b, p. 206).

Johnson, however, differentiated between them to make a case for the development of a unique theory of nursing that addresses knowledge of order, disorder, and control and that focuses on phenomena and research questions in a way that is not characteristic of any other discipline (1968a).

Some may agree that applied theory could evolve out of these borrowed theories to describe and explain prediction and prescribe nursing action. These critics make a distinction between basic theory, emanating from other disciplines, and applied theory, based on basic theory, with the exclusive purpose of defining nursing care and patterning interventions with predictable responses. The latter continues to be called borrowed theory by some, which could be considered a fallacy because if we begin with the premise that knowledge is not the exclusive property of any one field and that, eventually, knowledge is for all, "knowledge which we share in common" (Johnson, 1959, p. 199), then knowledge organized into theories in one discipline could freely be used by members of other disciplines. Therefore "borrowing" is really "adapting" or "deriving." Even if we agree that there is such a thing as the borrowing of theories to help in describing, explaining, and predicting phenomena that are significant to nursing, the mere fact that the questions and problems under consideration are nursing questions and problems changes the nature of the so-called borrowed theories. Johnson (1968b) made the point in this way:

> If we continue to observe behavior from the perspective of sociology, anthropology, or psychology; or if we continue to study disease with the aim of elucidating etiologies, properties, or life cycle; or if we continue to inquire into biological functioning or malfunctioning, we will be serving the cause of science but not necessarily the cause of nursing (p. 209).

Therefore, the nursing perspective guides the reconceptualization of existing theories (Donaldson and Crowley, 1978). Synthesis of so-called borrowed theory with a nursing perspective is essential or the focus of nursing will continue to remain within other disciplines, and, therefore, nursing problems will not be addressed (Phillips, 1977). Barnum (1994) supported this position. She stated that theories from other disciplines must be adapted to the nursing milieu and to the nursing image of a human being to be meaningful for nursing.

The so-called borrowed theories, then, are given new meaning within a perspective appropriate for nursing. Barnum supported Johnson's stand and called knowledge used in different disciplines "shared"; perhaps we should also have shared theories. To say that nursing theories are applied theories based on basic theories borrowed from other disciplines is therefore a myth that only serves to further obfuscate nursing theory. Nursing uses "borrowed theories" originating in other disciplines to describe phenomena belonging to those disciplines, when propositions remain in the context of the borrowed theory. Borrowed theories become "shared theories" when used within a nursing context. Nursing theories describe, explain, and predict domain phenomena.

Nursing needs theories to describe and explain phenomena that are significant in the act and process of nursing, to prescribe effective strategies of care, and to predict outcomes. Theories that were developed in other disciplines are also useful for derivation, integration, and synthesis with the nursing perspective. This process yields nursing theories or theories for nursing practice.

Conclusion

The sources of ideas for theory development are numerous and varied, with each inspiring different questions and providing different components to theoretical nursing. Some sources (such as biomedical models) have received more attention form nurses than others (such as nurses' daily experiences). Awareness and knowledge of the various sources may drive the development of theories that address the multidimensional and dynamic nature of nursing care.

In this chapter, I have suggested some ways by which an environment could be developed to nurture critical thinking in nurses. Such a dialogical and affirming environment could nurture and support nurses' abilities to capture their experiences and to reflect their clinical wisdom in theoretical nursing. Once again in this chapter, support is provided for the extent to which clinical nurses are a most significant resource for theory development.

Finally, two major historical debates are discussed and a proposal for their resolution is presented. The two paradoxes are whether nursing conceptualizations are theories or conceptual frameworks and whether nurse scholars should be engaged in developing theories or adapting borrowed theories from other disciplines. Although students of theory should be aware of the nature of these debates, I do not believe that resolving either of them is a crucial step toward knowledge development. Progress in knowledge and in developing theoretical nursing can and must proceed in spite of historical or future paradoxes.

REFERENCES

Abdellah, F.G., Beland, I.L., Martin, A., and Matheney, R.V. (1961). *Patient-centered approaches to nursing.* New York: Macmillan.

Agan, R.D. (1987). Intuitive knowing as a dimension of nursing. *Advances in Nursing Science,* 10(1), 63–70.

Allen, J. and Hall, B. (1988). Challenging the focus on technology: A critique of the medical model in a changing health care system. *Advances in Nursing Science,* 10, 22–34.

Arietti, S. (1976). *Creativity: The magic synthesis.* New York: Basic Books.

Armiger, B. (1974). Scholarship in nursing. *Nursing Outlook,* 22(3), 162–163.

Barnard, K. (1980). Knowledge for practice: Directions for the future. *Nursing Research,* 29(4), 208–212.

Barnum, B.J.S. (1994). *Nursing theory: Analysis, application, and evaluation* (4th ed.). Philadelphia: J.B. Lippincott.

Beckstrand, J. (1978a). The notion of a practice theory and the relationship of scientific and ethical knowledge to practice. *Research in Nursing and Health,* 1(3), 131–136.

Beckstrand, J. (1978b). The need for a practice theory as indicated by the knowledge used in conduct of practice. *Research in Nursing and Health,* 1(4), 175–179.

Beckstrand, J. (1980). A critique of several conceptions of practice theory in nursing. *Research in Nursing and Health,* 3(2), 69–80.

Benner, P. (1983). Uncovering the knowledge embedded in clinical practice. *Image,* 15, 36–44.

Burns, C., Archbold, P., Stewart, B., and Shelton, K. (1993). New diagnosis: Caregiver role strain. *Nursing Diagnosis,* 4(2), 70–76.

Byrne, M.L. and Thompson, L.F. (1978). *Key concepts for the study and practice of nursing.* St. Louis: C.V. Mosby.

Carlson, C.E. (Ed.). (1970). *Behavioral concepts and nursing intervention.* Philadelphia: J.B. Lippincott.

Carlson, C.E. and Blackwell, B. (Eds.) (1978). *Behavioral concepts and nursing intervention* (2nd ed.). Philadelphia: J.B. Lippincott.

Carper, B. (1978). Fundamental patterns of knowing in nursing. *Advances in Nursing Science,* 11, 13–23.

Chin, R. (1961). The utility of system models and developmental models for practitioners. In W. Bennis, K. Benne, and R. Chin (Eds.), *The planning of change.* New York: Holt, Rinehart & Winston.

Clements, I.W. and Roberts, F.B. (1983). *Family health: A theoretical approach to nursing care.* New York: John Wiley & Sons.

Copleston, F. (1963). *A history of philosophy* (Vol. 4) *Modern philosophy: Descartes to Leibniz.* Garden City, NY: Image Books.

Dickoff, J. and James, P. (1968). A theory of theories: A position paper. *Nursing Research,* 17(3), 197–203.

Dickoff, J., James, P., and Wiedenbach, E. (1968). Theory in practice discipline: Part 1. Practice oriented theory. *Nursing Research,* 17(5), 415–435.

Donaldson, S.K. and Crowley, D. (1978). The discipline of nursing. *Nursing Outlook,* 26(2), 113–120.

Dougherty, C.M., Jankin, J.K., Lunney, M.R., and Whitley, G.G. (1993). Conceptual and research based validation of nursing diagnoses: 1950 to 1993. *Nursing Diagnosis,* 4(4), 156–165.

Duldt, B.W. (1995). Nursing process: The science of nursing in the curriculum. *Nurse Educator,* 20(1), 24–29.

Durand, M. and Prince, R. (1966). Nursing diagnostics: Process and decision. *Nursing Forum,* 5(4), 50–64.

Durant, W. (1953). *The story of philosophy: The lives and opinions of the greater philosophers.* New York: Simon & Schuster.

Eisenhauer, L.A. (1994). A typology of nursing therapeutics. *Image: Journal of Nursing Scholarship,* 26(4), 261–264.

Fawcett, J. (1989). *Analysis and evaluation of conceptual models of nursing* (2nd ed.). Philadelphia: F.A. Davis.

Fawcett, J. (1993). *Analysis and evaluation of nursing theories.* Philadelphia: F.A. Davis.

Fawcett, J. (1995). *Analysis and evaluation of conceptual models of nursing* (3rd ed.). Philadelphia: F.A. Davis.

Fitzpatrick, J. and Whall, A. (1989). *Conceptual models of nursing: Analysis and application* (2nd ed.). Bowie, MD: Robert J. Brady.

Frisch, N. (1994). The nursing process revisited [editorial]. *Nursing Diagnosis,* 5(2), 51.

Gebbie K. (Ed.) (1976, March 4–7). *Summary of the second national conference: Classification of nursing diagnosis.* St. Louis: C.V. Mosby.

Gordon, M. (1985). Nursing diagnosis. *Annual Review of Nursing Research,* 3, 127–147.

Gordon, M., Murphy, C.P., Candee, D., and Hiltunen, E. (1994). Clinical judgment: An integrated model. *Advances in Nursing Science,* 16(4), 55–70.

Gordon, M., Sweeny, M.A., and McKeehan, K. (1980). Nursing diagnosis: Looking at its use in the clinical area. *American Journal of Nursing,* 80, 672–674.

Gortner, S.R. and Nahm, H. (1977). An overview of nursing research in the United States. *Nursing Research,* 26(1), 10–33.

Grant J., Kinney, M., and Guzzetta, C. (1990). A methodology for validating nursing diagnoses. *Advances in Nursing Science,* 12(3), 65–74.

Grobe, S.J. (1990). Nursing intervention lexicon and taxonomy study: Language classification methods. *Advances in Nursing Science,* 13 (2), 22–33.

Harms, M. and McDonald, F.J. (1966). A new curriculum design: Part III. *Nursing Outlook,* 14(9), 50–53.

Hill, R. and Hansen, D.A. (1960). The identification of conceptual frameworks utilized in family study. *Marriage and Family Living* 22, 299–311.

Iowa Intervention Project (1993). The NIC taxonomy structure. *Image: Journal of Nursing Scholarship,* 25(3), 187–192.

Iowa Intervention Project (1995). Validation and coding of the NIC taxonomy structure. *Image: Journal of Nursing Scholarship,* 27(1), 43–49.

Jacox, A. (1974). Theory construction in nursing: An overview. *Nursing Research,* 23(1), 4–13.

Jennings, B. and Meleis, A.I. (1988). Nursing theory and administrative practice: Agenda for the 1990s. *Advanced Nursing Science,* 10(3), 56–69.

Johnson, D.E. (1959). A philosophy of nursing. *Nursing Outlook* 7(4), 198–200.

Johnson, D.E. (1968a, April). *One conceptual model of nursing.* Paper presented at Vanderbilt University, Nashville, TN.

Johnson, D.E. (1968b). Theory in nursing: Borrowed and unique. *Nursing Research* 17(3), 206–209.

Johnson, D.E. (1974). Development of theory: A requisite for nursing as a primary health profession. *Nursing Research,* 23(5), 372–377.

Johnson, J.E. (1972). Effects of structuring patients' expectations on their reactions to threatening events. *Nursing Research,* 21(6), 499–504.

Kaplan, A. (1964). *The conduct of inquiry: Methodology of behavioral science.* San Francisco: Chandler.

Kerlinger, F.N. (1964). *Foundations of behavioral research.* New York: Holt, Rinehart & Winston.

Kim, H.S. (1980). Pain theory: Research and nursing practice. *Advances in Nursing Science* 2, 43–59.

Kim, M.J. (1989). Nursing diagnosis. *Annual Review of Nursing Research,* 7, 117–142.

Kim, M.J. and Moritz, D.A. (Eds.). (1982). *Classification of nursing diagnosis: Proceedings of the third and fourth national conferences.* New York: McGraw-Hill.

King, I. (1995a). A systems framework for nursing. In M.A.Frey and C.L. Sieloff (Eds.). *Advancing King's systems framework and theory of nursing.* Los Angeles: Sage Publications, pp. 14–22.

King, I. (1995b). The theory of goal attainment. In M.A. Frey and C.L. Sieloff (Eds.). *Advancing King's systems framework and theory of nursing.* Los Angeles: Sage Publications, pp. 233–32.

Kintzel, K.C. (1971). *Advanced concepts in clinical nursing.* Philadelphia, J.B. Lippincott.

Kritek, P. (1978). The generation and classification of nursing diagnosis: Toward a theory of nursing. *Image,* 10(2), 33–40.

Lindeman, C.A. (1980). The challenge of nursing research in the 1980s. In *Communicating nursing research: Directions for the 1980s.* Boulder, CO: Western Interstate Commission for Higher Education.

Maier, H.W. (1969). *Three theories of child development.* New York: Harper & Row.

Meleis, A.I. (1975). Role insufficiency and role supplementation: A conceptual framework. *Nursing Research,* 24(4), 264–271.

Meleis, A.I. (1985). *Theoretical nursing: Development and progress* (2nd ed.). Philadelphia: J.B. Lippincott.

Meleis, A.I. and Jennings, B.M. (1989). Theoretical nursing administration: Today's challenges, tomorrow's bridges. In H.C. Arndt and M. DiVincenti (Eds.), *Dimensions and issues in nursing administration.* Oxford, UK: Blackwell Scientific Publications.

Meleis, A.I. and May, K.M. (1981). Nursing theory and scholarliness in the doctoral program. *Advances in Nursing Science,* 4(1), 31–41.

Meleis, A.I. and Price, M. (1988). Strategies and conditions for teaching theoretical nursing: An international perspective. *Journal of Advanced Nursing,* 13, 592–604.

Meltzer, L.E., Abdellah, F.G., and Kitchell, R. (Eds.). (1969). *Concepts and practice of intensive care for nurse specialists.* Philadelphia: Charles Press Publishers.

Mitchell, P.H. (1973). *Concepts basic to nursing.* New York: McGraw-Hill.

Moch, S.D. (1990). Personal knowing: Evolving research and practice. *Scholarly Inquiry for Nursing Practice: An International Journal,* 4(2), 155–170.

Nidditch, P. (Ed.). (1975). *An essay concerning human understanding.* New York: Oxford University Press.

Nightingale, F. (1859). *Notes on nursing: What it is and what it is not.* London: Harrison.

Norbeck, J. (1981). Social support: A model for clinical research and application. *Advances in Nursing Science,* 3, 43–59.

Norris, C.M. (1975). Restlessness: A nursing phenomenon in search of meaning. *Nursing Outlook,* 23(2), 103–107.

Norris, C.M. (Ed.) (1982). *Concept clarification in nursing.* Germantown, MD: Aspen Systems.

Nye, F. and Berardo, F. (Eds.). (1966). *Emerging conceptual frameworks in family analysis.* New York: Macmillan.

Peplau, H.E. (1952). *Interpersonal relations in nursing.* New York: G.P. Putnam's Sons.

Phillips, J.R. (1977). Nursing systems and nursing models. *Image,* 9(1), 4–7.

Piaget, H. (1971). *Biology and knowledge.* Edinburgh: Edinburgh University Press.

Riehl, J.P. and Roy, C. (Eds.). (1974). *Conceptual models for nursing practice.* New York: Appleton-Century-Crofts.

Rew, L. (1988). Nurses' intuition. *Applied Nursing Research,* 1(1), 27–31.

Reynolds, P.D. (1971). *Primer in theory construction.* Indianapolis: Bobbs-Merrill.

Rodman, H. (1980). Are conceptual frameworks necessary for theory building: The case of family sociology. *The Sociological Quarterly,* 21, 429–441.

Roe, A. (1951). A psychological study of eminent biologists. *Psychological Monographs,* 65, 1–67.

Roe, A. (1963). *The making of a scientist.* New York: Dodd Mead.

Shamansky, S.L. and Yanni, C.R. (1983). In opposition to nursing diagnosis: A minority opinion. *Image,* 15, 47–50.

Wald, F.S. and Leonard, R.C. (1964). Towards development of nursing practice theory. *Nursing Research,* 13(4), 309–313.

Weiss, S.J. (1979). The language of touch. *Nursing Research,* 28(2), 76–80.

Zderad, L.T. and Belcher, H.C. (1968). *Developing behavioral concepts in nursing.* Atlanta, GA: Southern Regional Education Board.

CHAPTER 9

Patterns of Knowing: The Syntax of the Discipline

Disciplines are characterized by a perspective, a domain, sources for the development of knowledge, and ways by which knowledge is characterized and developed. In this chapter I discuss the different patterns of knowing and the prevailing perspectives on theory development; I argue for the use of those patterns of theoretical formulations that support clinical theories, conceptual theories, and empirical theories. Two metatheoretical models are presented and described.

Ways of Knowing

Knowing includes knowledge based on observations, research findings, clinical manifestations, and scientific approaches. Knowing is more dependent on sense data, but it also includes other types of data. To understand is to connect bits of knowledge in a relational form to other broader statements. For example, we know that women who work outside the household tend to work a double shift, one shift outside their home and the other to take care of their home. We also know that women who work outside the home tend to have better mental health than women who work only inside the home. Inferences could be made about what types of support and health care resources these women need based on this knowledge. Housework, on the other hand, is an activity that was not acknowledged as work or leisure, an activity with no set hours, wages, or rewards, an activity with no retirement benefits (Harding, 1988, p. 87). Considering the findings within this context of meanings may prompt a consideration of the forces and constraints in using resources that are developed especially for promotion of health of women who are primarily engaged in housework. That involves understanding. Understanding, therefore, includes putting the experience and situation of women within historical, gender, and social contexts. It includes a consideration of the norms, values, and the meanings of housework and the barriers that societies impose on women and their work.

Knowing results from careful systematic research or from repeated experiences in clinical practice. Reflecting on that knowledge and interpreting the meanings of relationships, as seen and experienced by all parties concerned, and putting that which is known within a context of feelings, values, and different perspectives is what brings us closer to an understanding of that which is known. One pattern of knowing by itself will not uncover all the knowledge needed for a human and practice-oriented science.

Four patterns of knowing have been identified in nursing; empirical (the science of nursing); aesthetic (the art of nursing); personal knowledge, which is concerned with the quality of interpersonal contacts, promoting therapeutic relationships, and individualized care; and ethics, which includes the moral component of nursing (Carper, 1978). These patterns have received a great deal of attention and were instrumental in alerting nurses that science alone will not answer the significant questions in our discipline (Johnson, 1994). Fry (1988) reminded us that these patterns are neither complete nor static and that other patterns need to be considered and further developed.

Jacobs-Kramer and Chinn (1988) extended knowledge about the four patterns by developing a model that includes five dimensions: creative, expressive, assessment questions, process–context, and credibility index to describe and explain the four patterns developed by Carper. White (1995) supported the four patterns but added a fifth one, sociopolitical knowing, which is considered an essential pattern for the understanding that may evolve from all other patterns of knowing. This pattern focuses on the broader context for the caring processes, it allows and drives inquiry to critically question the status quo of the participants in the caring process. It includes organizational, cultural, and political processes that influence the person, the nurse, the other health care providers, the profession, and other structures involved in the caring processes. This pattern of knowing allows for constructing alternative structures of reality and is expressed through critiques and transformations. It is a pattern predicated on collaboration and on a movement toward more equity in knowledge development.

Patterns of knowing include both theoretical and practical knowing. Sarvimäki (1994) makes a distinction between theoretical and practical knowledge, although she acknowledges their equal significance. Theoretical knowledge includes and reflects the basic values, guiding principles, elements, and phases of a conception of nursing. Its goals are to drive and promote thinking and understanding of that which is the nursing discipline. Its base is intellectual, and it is organized into assumptions, concepts, propositions, and models. Practical knowledge, however, does not have to be organized in the same way because many parts of this knowledge are not yet articulated and because the artistic side of practice may not be amenable to total articulation. The channel of communication for theoretical knowledge may be theories and science, whereas the channel of communication for practical knowledge may be tradition, according to Sarvimäki (1994). Practical knowledge may be achieved through personal and collective means and reflections. Personal knowing, which may be arrived at through one's own practice, reflection, synthesis, and integration of artistic, scientific, and practice components is, according to Moch (1990), essential to the development of nursing knowledge. She identifies three components in personal knowing: experiential, interpersonal, and intuitive knowing. Experiential knowing is achieved through being part of the world of nursing and becoming increasingly aware of the experiences inherent in this participation. Interpersonal knowing results from enhanced awareness about situations resulting from extensive, in-depth interactions with others. These interactions are another source of knowing and they promote the development of knowledge.

When a person knows without the explicit use of scientifically accepted forms of reasoning, it is said that the person achieved the knowing through intuition. It is knowing a whole without resorting to linear reasoning (Polanyi, 1962). It is knowing without knowing how (Benner and Wrubel, 1982; Rew, 1988; Rew and Barrow, 1987). When nurses use intuition to know, they open themselves up to allow sensing and understanding of the patient's responses and situations to occur leading to a better knowledge of the patient's situation (Agan, 1987; Paul and Heaslip, 1995). Intuitive knowing was a neglected pattern of knowing, but it has been gaining more attention as a component in "clinical knowing," as essential in a more holistic understanding of clinical situations and as significant in making more effective therapeutic decisions (Rew, 1990).

Knowing patients allows for more particular and individualistic approaches that may be based on more general knowledge related to patients' situations. Knowing the patients leads to more appropriately selected nursing therapeutics, based on knowing patients' resources, readiness, and current understanding related to their responses.

Several processes have been identified to elucidate the meaning of knowing the patient. These were defined by Jenny and Logan (1992) as perceiving/envisioning, communication, self-preservation, and showing concern. Perceiving and envisioning involve identifying the meaning and significance of patients' responses. Knowing the patient also involves communication and interaction with or about the patient. It includes having the nurse be present for the patient and be trusted by the patient and family. Knowing patients is assumed to be connected to the extent to which a nurse shows and demonstrates concern. To be able to know a patient or a situation is to be open to know what is unknown about this individual. Munhall (1993) made a cogent argument for 'unknowing' as another pattern of knowing that requires reflection on oneself—about whom we have a certain degree of knowledge—and the other (patient) about whom we have a very limited knowledge. Unknowing is another dimension of knowing; without realizing and understanding the degree, the extent, and the nature of what one does not know, knowing is not fully realized.

Nursing phenomena reflect human conditions and situations, and therefore, these phenomena could be developed through different patterns of discovery. Uncovering and describing the art component of nursing is predicated on developing the aesthetic pattern of knowing. Sorrell (1994) described this pattern as embodying the "unique pattern of knowing that offers enrichment to our understanding of nursing experience that is not accessible through other ways of knowing" (p. 61). Aesthetic knowing depends on processes that are imaginative and creative. It allows the knower to be engaged and interpretive and allows for envisioning. It is also expressed through some creative means such as art, music, and expressive writing. Writing to reflect aesthetic knowing is not bound by scientific reporting; it may include poetry, narratives, stories, fiction, letters, and journals (O'Brien and Pearson, 1993; Sorrell, 1994). The knowing that results from these modes of expression integrates sensory perceptions with experiences and acts. Aesthetic knowing requires engagement and distancing from experiences, particularizing and generalizing, abstraction and concretization, objectivity and subjectivity, and separate and united components and experiences.

Experiences such as compassion, suffering, and mourning may best be uncovered through metaphors and may be understood more if scientific methods are used in combination with aesthetic approaches. Younger (1990) provides an example of using the Book of Job in the Bible, and analyzing it as a "literary work" to uncover knowledge of, and the meaning of, suffering. The art of nursing is closely tied to the realities of the practice situation (Timpson, 1996). These aspects of nursing can be somewhat articulated by nurses who value the uniqueness of individual experiences and who can communicate through aesthetic pathways that may fully capture the connection between the different components (Boykin, Parker, and Schoenhofer, 1994). Clinical expertise and its dimensions represent one aspect of nursing art (Hampton, 1994).

Patterns of knowing are not static, nor are they discrete. They are dynamic, evolving, multidimensional, and may be transformed or transforming. It is not always possible to classify knowledge using only one of these patterns. Knowing can and does occur through "nonlinear, meditative thinking that moves in all directions" Therefore, Silva, Sorrell, and Sorrell (1995) called this type of knowing *"the-in-between."* There is also the knowing through *"the beyond,"* which is knowledge that concerns "those aspects of reality, meaning, and being that persons only come to know with difficulty or that they cannot articulate or ever know" (p. 3). Accepting the inexplicable and the unknowable in clients, nurses, relationships, and health and illness may allow exploration of meanings and ways by which some lived experiences cannot be felt or explained by those who never had those experiences. These patterns of knowing bring a nurse closer to a more profound understanding of the complex multidimensional aspects of reality that characterize human experiences related to their health and illness.

Patterns of Understanding

Understanding includes interpretation, a total comprehension of other human beings' responses based on their "feelings, ideas, choices, and purposes" as they experience the situation, and as they express their own meanings and understanding of the situation through their own words and through their own responses (Schwartz and Wiggins, 1988, p. 143). The degree to which we need to develop that understanding depends on the extent to which we want to and how significant our attempt to achieve that level of understanding is. It also depends on the degree to which clients are willing to have their responses and their situations fully uncovered and understood. True understanding not only illuminates the situation, it also uncovers weaknesses and flaws as well as strengths and abilities. In some ways, true understanding may uncover individuals' power as well as areas of vulnerability.

Health and illness situations require a level of understanding that is not required from other situations in which two strangers might come in contact with each other. However, a true understanding of how individuals experience and respond to health and illness mandates an understanding of what a group of people value in life, what priorities they have, how they usually respond to disruptions in their lives, how they prefer to express their discomfort, and what are the most comfortable ways by which they usually prefer to express their feelings.

Knowing about specific groups' perceptions of health and illness, patterns of help-seeking behaviors, and patterns of responses to uncomfortable situations is essential for the level of understanding required to develop an intervention plan, whether that intervention plan is as specific as postoperative deep breathing or maintaining prenatal appointments. Knowing about the extent to which an immigrant is connected to individuals and events in his country of origin may help a nurse clinician understand the out-of-pattern expressions of pain and discomfort to a seemingly less painful experience. Knowing about normal patterns of touch between members of the opposite sex in different social classes may help a health care provider understand when (and when not) to communicate this way.

Understanding includes making connections and achieving syntheses that may go beyond the perception and knowledge of the client or the provider (Habermas, 1971; Schutz, 1967). Understanding has been advocated by interpretive scientists (Allen, 1988, p. 98) as the hallmark for knowledge development in nursing. This understanding includes specific research findings, the experience that evolves from the practice arena, and knowledge awareness from primary theoretical formulations. It includes all these and goes beyond them.

Understanding is predicated on knowing about phenomena, knowing about the contexts in which certain phenomena occur, and knowing about patterns of presentation of these phenomena. Knowing about the different roles women enact; knowing about the stresses, strains, and satisfactions in these roles; knowing role theory; and knowing the relationships between levels of role involvement and number of roles and health status are all important and significant for developing an understanding of why and when women tend to seek care for themselves or for their children and how they choose to maintain or enhance their health. That level of understanding is also achieved through a deliberate effort to reflect theoretically on some of these concepts and put them together in an organized way to describe and explain some central problems in nursing. Examples of central problems are patterns of maintaining and developing health and patterns of seeking health care.

Jaspers, a physician and a philosopher, addressed the laws of understanding as follows (Jaspers, 1963; Schwartz and Wiggins, 1988, pp. 153–155):

1. Empirical understanding is an interpretation. The data provide the impetus for interpretation and therefore interpretation is not absolute but is subject to other interpretations—and therefore may be theoretical.
2. Understanding opens up unlimited interpretations. To have understanding as a goal frees the researcher to consider many different interpretations. These different interpretations should be subjected to more data to gain support or refutation.
3. Understanding moves in deepening spirals. Starting from parts to understand a certain behavior, one goes to the whole to put the behavior in context and then comes back to the part for better understanding. The process increases understanding.
4. Opposites are equally meaningful. The same evidence could be interpreted in two opposite ways. In doing that, we are attempting not to settle for preconceived notions and we are attempting to understand the synthesis between the opposites. Schwartz and Wiggins (1988, p. 154) give an example:

We can understand the stoicism of a patient as stemming from bravery and nobility. But we can also understand this same stoicism as motivated by profound fears and a complete inability to face up to a difficult predicament.

5. Understanding is inconclusive. Not all feelings, meanings, and values can be expressed in understandable ways, and not all interpretations are willingly shared.
6. To understand is to illustrate and expose. To really comprehend, both positive and negative aspects of any group or person have to be exposed. Ethical considerations of the balance between exposure and illumination need to be considered.

Should nursing knowledge help us to know, to understand, or to care? Do each require different approaches to knowledge development? Can these approaches substitute for each other, or do they complement each other to enhance knowledge development? I believe that the predominant goals for research are to know and that the predominant goals for theoretical development of the discipline are to understand. I am not saying that one leads exclusively to knowing and one leads exclusively to understanding. I am using the concept "predominant" to differentiate between goals. Imagine knowing and understanding on two continuums. Imagine each going from none to high. Research findings and theorizing could be plotted on the two continuums. Research findings tend to be toward the higher end of the continuum of knowing and may be the middle of the understanding pole, whereas theorizing tends to be on the higher pole of understanding and may be the middle of the knowing pole.

Perspectives on Knowing

Approaches to knowledge development—including theory development—should also be analyzed against the properties of human science, the mission of a practice-oriented discipline, and the balance among knowing, understanding, and caring. Three perspectives for research have been identified in nursing literature. These perspectives are addressed here in relationship to theory development.

Empiricism is presented here, once again, as a point of departure in comparing it with other perspectives. The rationale for the choice of empiricism as a perspective for the development of theories is obvious in its universality, its vast numbers of followers and supporters, and its appeal as the perspective *sine qua non* with scientific developments. Empiricism is compared with two other perspectives, the feminist perspective and critical theory perspective, as shown in Table 9-1.

Empiricist Perspective

A theory for empiricists is a product of research findings that is used as a framework for further research. The empiricists' observations are not contextual and usually focus on single behaviors, events, or situations. Theorizing for empiricists is based on sense data supported by a set of value-free assumptions. Empiricists develop theories by providing precise, well defined, operationalized concepts—measurable variables. Empiri-

Table 9-1 ***Perspectives on Knowing***

Component	Empiricist	Feminist	Critical Theory
Units of observation	Acontextual Behavior Event Situation	Human beings Gender Experience Totality Uniqueness Perception of meanings	Social structure Power Political structure History Relationships with structure
Strategies for theory development	Multiple research findings	Experience of participants Analysis of situation and context Advocacy	Experience of participants and nonparticipants Analysis of context Action
Assumptions	Axiomatic facts Value-free	Personal Disciplinary Societal values critiqued	Societal values critiqued and selected
Concepts	Precise Operationalized Not acontextual Provide a framework Unit of analysis	Considered within gender orientation Analytical statements Patterns	Not essential
Goals/uses	Theory development Truth-finding for discipline	Theory development Consciousness-raising Awareness of participants Illumination	Emancipation Structural Awareness structure Understanding
Theorist	Objective Separated Distanced Secretive	Engaged Connected	Observer of social structure and proactive participant
Approach	Inductive	Inductive Deductive Retroductive Philosophical analysis	Creation of new structures
Use	Know	Understand	Change
Starting point	Research question	Experience Response	Structure Organization Political
Language	Research-specific	Gender-specific	Philosophical Political

cists are objective, separated, distanced from their theories; they treat the theories as objects and are reluctant to share insights related to findings or evolving ideas with their clients or research subjects. The language they use is research specific and their approach is inductive. Statistical model building is a significant tool for theory development by the empiricists.

Empirical theories are based on careful and impeccable research studies geared to finding relationships between different variables and finding support for a multitude of statements—all geared to answering a set of well defined questions. Empiricists' theories are well understood by colleagues from other disciplines, and when theory development is discussed, it is more likely to be understood in relationship to the development of empirical theories.

Gender Orientation and Feminist Perspectives

The history of nursing attests to how the concept of gender permeates and pervades every aspect of the discipline. Nursing has been predominantly a female profession and continues to be in the 1990s as female nurses claim about 97% membership in the profession (Ashley, 1980; Doering, 1992). Despite some studies' efforts to open the profession more to men and despite the many contributions men have made to nursing, nursing remains a woman's profession and continues to be saddled with all the accompanying issues related to the values of women's work, women's contributions, and the relationship between nursing and other predominantly male professions.

This history could be used to the advantage of the discipline and its clients by attempting to use it as a perspective for the development of gender-sensitive theories. Understanding the constraints inherent in these experiences and the lack of participation in shaping the structure and the goals of inquiry may sensitize nurses to similar experiences of clients.

Gender-sensitive theories are those based on connections between the theorist and the subject matter, the involvement of the theorist with the subjects of the theory in the development and interpretation of the theory (MacPherson, 1983; Sherwin, 1987; Stacy and Thorne, 1985). They are also based on the acknowledgment and affirmation of gender equity, on the premise that women should be affirmed for their own contributions in a patriarchal society, and on the assumption that women should have options and control over their own bodies (Sampselle, 1990). The goal of gender-sensitive theories is understanding rather than just knowing; the goal is based on uncovering and including personal experiences of the nurse and client and evolves from considering the totality of the experiences, responses, and events described theoretically as well as from giving similar consideration to the experience and the context of the theorist (Hagell, 1989).

A feminist perspective could be used not only in understanding issues related to women as clients or women as providers, but as a perspective for developing an understanding of all nursing clients, regardless of sex, gender, race, or culture. It could be used to understand, to explain, to raise consciousness, and to develop theories to bring about needed changes for nursing clients (Duffy and Hedin, 1988; Jagger, 1988).

Whereas the assumptions of the empiricists may lean toward value-free axioms and facts and truths derived from previous research findings, assumptions evolving from feminist perspectives are acknowledged as value laden and include personal, disciplinary, and societal values (Harding, 1986).

Gender-sensitive theories could be based on similar principles that have been discussed in conjunction with gender-sensitive research. Cook and Fonow (1986) defined some guidelines for conducting gender-sensitive research. These guidelines are modified and offered for guiding the development of theories related to recipients of care in nursing. Thus, gender-sensitive theories are theories that

- Consider gender as a basic feature and a central agenda in the theory
- Provide guidelines for raising consciousness about the experiences described within the theory, heighten understanding of the role of a social system or organization in relationship to these experiences
- Challenge any norms of objectivity that create distances between participants or between theory subject matter and participants in the theory development
- Provide a critique of situations and circumstances that may interfere in healthful living
- Enhance empowerment for options, for understanding, for decision making, or for self-care
- Decrease any potential of exploitation
- Enhance advocacy and provide guidelines for advocacy
- Provide guidelines for changes, including institutional and organizational changes

In caring for patients or clients, nurses knowingly or unknowingly have adhered to some of these principles. In fact, some nurse theorists have described nursing using the very principles in the 1960s and 1970s (Paterson and Zderad, 1976; Travelbee, 1963). However, these principles may have been overshadowed by a quest for empiricalization of theories to render the nursing discipline theoretical and scientific. By considering their caring mission, nurses, whether theoreticians or researchers, may be able to synthesize their goals for caring and knowing and thus develop theories that enhance understanding of the situation, the daily experience, and responses of clients.

Gender-sensitive perspective is not to be construed as a substitute for nursing theories. It is a framework that guides the kind of phenomena that nursing theorists may select for development, the approach by which such theories are developed, and the interpretation of findings related to this phenomenon. A gender-sensitive perspective is a framework that guides nurses to study phenomena that represent and emanate from the lives of their clients, phenomena that are important to these clients, phenomena that reflect and are related to the quality of their lives or their health care and that may be seen as problematic from their perspective (Harding, 1987).

Feminist theorizing "seeks to bring together subjective and objective ways of knowing the world" (Rose, 1983, p. 87). It challenges attitudes, beliefs, values, and assumptions that discredit women's sense of ownership of their own selves, and it also empowers nurses and clients (Sampselle, 1990; Sohier, 1992). A nursing theory that is developed using a feminist perspective is one that values the experiences of the developer, values her intuitions and analyses, values the client's world, and values the client's sociocultural and political perceptions. It is one that includes a sensitive understanding of the conditions that impinge on clients' responses and one that is representative of clients from different sociocultural backgrounds. Language is powerful; therefore, a theory from a feminist perspective is one that uses language that is empowering, that is gender sensitive, that values experiences, and that denounces the status quo. For example, Wuest (1993) critically reviewed research on compliance and demonstrated how it was based on patriarchal and oppressive assumptions. Feminist principles may be better suited for enhancing understanding, and developing insights about clients' responses, which might be ultimately more productive. Nursing theories, whether they are guided by a feminist perspective or an empirical perspective, should continue to inform members of the discipline. Therefore, these theories remain closely connected to the domain of nursing with its focus on responses of human beings and their environments to health and illness situation.

Critical Theory Perspective

Critical theory is a philosophical perspective that emanates from the Frankfurt school of thought and was further developed in West Germany by Habermas (1971) and Gadamer (1979).

> Critical social theory begins with a premise . . . [that] a fully rational social decision must be made in a context in which participation is not distorted by internal or external constraints (Allen, 1988, p. 93).

To Habermas (1971), there are three distinct but connected approaches to scientific inquiry. These approaches are empirical/analytical, historical hermeneutic, and critical oriented. The three approaches include the technical, practical, and emancipatory interests. All three types of knowledge and approaches to knowledge development are essential for the development of knowledge for human sciences. Habermas (1971) further proposed that technical problems are best understood through an empirical/analytical approach, practical problems through an historical hermeneutic approach, and problems that include issues critical to human beings through emancipatory approaches. The latter incorporates both the empirical/analytical and the historical hermeneutic approaches in a higher-order synthesis. The goal of the critical-oriented inquiry is an active reflective stand that includes changes that are emancipatory (Allen, 1985; Habermas, 1974; Holter, 1987).

The feminist theorists focus on gender inasmuch as the critical theorists focus on power and emancipation through reflection and action. Theories developed through this perspective provide ways of understanding the sociopolitical structure and patterns of oppression of clients within such a structure and also provide guidelines for a reflective approach to the situation and ways by which the subjects of theory are transformed and emancipated from unequal power structures (Bernstein, 1978; Habermas, 1979). The goal of a theorist here is to develop some means by which the participants can be put on the road toward emancipation from oppressive social structures. The goal is not only to understand, but to change and to do so drastically. Reflection, understanding, and action are the hallmarks of a nursing theory developed within this perspective.

A nursing theory developed within this perspective offers a focus on social structure, power, and political structure as units of analyses, a "critique of power and ideology" in existing societal structures in which the nursing client interacts (Allen, Benner, and Diekelmann, 1986). It is a theory that incorporates an understanding of a phenomenon or a situation by all involved parties; it provides insights about the health/illness situation and a framework of what is to be done about it. Therefore, an equal partnership between the subject matter of a theory and the developer of the theory has to be maintained.

Critical theory is not a substitute for nursing theory; rather, it is a framework or a perspective that informs the phenomena to be considered theoretically, guides the approaches for developing them, provides ways by which the phenomena are to be interpreted, and suggests approaches for handling these phenomena.

Patterns of Theorizing

Three patterns of theoretical formulations were proposed by Schultz and Meleis (1988), who maintained that the development of theory could not be, and in reality is not, dependent on any particular source or perspective. Practice, theory, and empirical findings could all be theory sources, and empiricism, feminism, and critical perspectives could all drive the development of nursing theory. (See Chap. 8 for sources of theory and Chaps. 12 and 13 for strategies for concept and theory development from related sources.) Therefore, they identified clinical, conceptual, and empirical theories as the types of theories to develop in nursing. The three patterns of theorizing are not totally distinct or mutually exclusive; they should only be treated as prototypes. The emphasis on the differences does not preclude hybrid theorizing that is developed from knowledge emanating from any or all sources. Table 9-2 compares these three types of theories.

Thus, theorizing in nursing evolves from extending other theories, abstracting from practice, or synthesizing research findings, or any combination of these types. The differences are in how the phenomena are identified, the nature of concepts, and the origins of the propositions. Although all theory may be developed to describe, explain, prescribe, or predict, there are differences in the purposes of each type as well as in the approaches to the development of each type. Evaluation and testing of each theory type would be expected to correspond with its nature and use. The challenge for members of the discipline is in the development of patterns of establishing credibility for each type. Each type of theory is briefly described next.

Clinical Theories

Clinical knowledge results from engaging in the gestalt of doing and caring. Florence Nightingale developed her ideas from her work with the wounded soldiers in the Crimean War; her theory of environment evolved from clinical work. Clinical knowl-

Table 9-2 ***Patterns of Theorizing***

Component	Clinical	Conceptual	Empirical
Phenomena	Discovered	Discovered	Created
Concepts	Emerge from phenomenon	Used as per theory or redefined	Used as is redefined Modified due to research
Propositions	Linkages evolve from experience	Theoretical properties evolve from theory	Deduced from theory
Theory	Descriptive/explanatory Prescriptive	Descriptive Explanatory	Descriptive Predictive
Purpose	Explain Prescribe Development of theory Clinical practice	Explain Development of theory	Explain Development of theory Researcher
Approach	Clinical experience	Conceptualization	Measurement testing
Evaluation	Guided by practice situation	Guided by theory	Guided by research

edge could be the result of personal and subjective knowing. Numerous examples in the literature, particularly in the clinical literature, describe clinical examples that are the sum total of the wisdom of clinicians. The question is how we can enhance that knowledge and establish its credibility. This credibility may have been based in the past on the fact that it worked! However, because we are trying to establish a case for the significance of this knowledge, perhaps we need to think of some established ways that will render some of this knowledge acceptable.

Clinical theories use what feminist psychologists call "connected knowing," that is, developing theories collaboratively through interpersonal relations with clients and through being connected with what another person may be experiencing. These theories have been described in different ways by different authors. They have been defined as narrative, naturalistic, or clinical concepts. Theories that evolve from a clinical setting have richer clinical context and a longer span; their credibility may be enhanced for other clinicians, and they are developed from concrete experiences.

Conceptual Theories

The second type of theory is one that is abstracted and generalized from other theories and goes beyond personal experiences. Nursing theorists have provided us with many examples of this type of theorizing. Their work is a product of their reflecting about phenomena they consider central to the discipline of nursing; their theories are products of theoretical reflections based on other prototype theories. The criteria for accepting theories have been described by a number of metatheorists as falling within the norms of coherence and corroboration. The criteria for accepting theories that are developed from conceptual knowledge involve the extent to which members of the discipline find them useful in illuminating the discipline of nursing. Therefore, a set of criteria for evaluating these theories are expected to evolve from their origins and objectives.

Empirical Theories

The third type of theory is knowledge that results from research, whether that research is historical, phenomenological, interpretive, or empiricist. Criteria for establishing the credibility of theories that evolve from each of these research traditions have yet to be developed. Theories that are empirical are among the most accepted types and are usually the better established.

Ways of Knowing and Models for Metatheory

The combination of philosophical perspectives discussed in this chapter, ways of knowing, and the different perspectives on knowing suggest the evolving of two central complementary models for the development of nursing theories. These models evolved from our history, our mission, our propensity to knowing, and our gender orientation. These models are not inclusive of all approaches to theory development; rather they appear to represent evolving disciplinary approaches. They do not correspond to any particular philosophy in its totality; for example, model 1 is not to be equated with an empirical, neopositivist philosophical stance nor should model 2 be exclusively equated with phenomenological approaches. These models are modified to represent the nature of knowing and understanding in nursing. I propose that we think of these models as intrinsic to the discipline of nursing and as emerging from its needs and goals. The use of these models could provide support for the kind of knowing and understanding needed in the discipline of nursing. Both models can be analyzed against the social policy statement defining nursing, the nature of nursing as a human science, and the phenomenon that represents the nursing focus.

The premise on which these two models are developed is that both are equally essential for the development of the discipline of nursing. To avoid labeling that may cast shadows on either model, I prefer to call them model 1 and model 2. Table 9-3 compares them.

Model 1

The unit of observation for model 1 is more definable than that for model 2; it is more concise, operational, and amenable to being reduced to variables. An example is support. Support is further defined and operationalized into tangible or intangible support, which is further operationalized into tangible daily support for family members. Each of these concepts is carefully defined. The assumptions on which the theory is developed are carefully delineated and support for each is provided.

Model 1 theory development evolves from a research tradition, whatever that tradition may be; therefore, theories are carefully and immediately connected with existing or evolving research. A theorist using model 1 will not venture sharing her theory until completed and supported and, when it is shared, it is provided to the scholarly community. Its theory development derives its support through documentation of its central questions and answers. The criteria used for evaluating it are its ability to explain

Table 9-3 ***Models for Metatheory***

Unit of Analysis	Model 1	Model 2
Unit of observation	Defined, concise, operational Predefined A particular aspect	Behaviors, events, or situations embedded in a context Human being and environment
Assumptions	Axioms Value free	Context Value laden, beliefs, action
Concepts	Defined, operationalized *a priori*	Emerge from clinical, research, or theory
Propositions	Operationalized	Descriptive, explanatory statements
Theory development	Relationship between concepts Theory evolves from a research tradition	Theory evolves from theory, practice, research
Conditions	Conciseness, source, facts	Perceptions, meanings, patterns, context
Tools for development	Observation Research designs Research findings	Collaboration Dialogue Intuition Experiences Diaries Self
Reasoning	Logical development	Connective
Context	Documentation of justification	Documentation of discovery
Theorist	Distanced, objectified, not active participant	Engaged, attached, acting, developing
Purpose	Explain, predict	Describe, explain, understand
Theory use	Congruency with evidence	Congruency with human values
Focus	Knowing	Understanding Caring
Criteria for evaluation of phenomena	Centrality and closeness to cutting edge in discipline	Significance to discipline, to theorist, to humanity
Evaluation	Validity, reliability Critique Testing	Description Analysis Testing
Criteria for analysis	Validity and reliability of concepts Operationalizability	Theorist experiences
Criteria for testing	Research Empirical evidence Statistical methods Corroboration	Social structure Values Understanding Usefulness Intuition Coherence Comprehensiveness Support from experience Diversity of exemplars
Validity	Universality Replicability	
Norms	Stands the test of time Universal Observation Ordered	Contextual Reflection

(continued)

Table 9-3 ***Models for Metatheory*** *(Continued)*

Unit of Analysis	Model 1	Model 2
Time	Defined time period Transcends time	Time and historically embedded
Approach	Analysis of findings Not contextual	Reflection Analysis Forward leaps Historical and structural context
Language	Evidence Generalizability Replicability	Understanding Intersubjectivity Consistency Consensus
Goals	Probability Prescription	Pattern Identification Liberation Change Consciousness-raising
Dissemination	Professional audience	Subjects Policy makers

and predict phenomena, the centrality of the questions and answers to the discipline's cutting edge, and its potential for more universal use.

Model 1 is still based on some shared assumptions that nursing is a human science and that its mission as a practice-oriented discipline is to care for people. Therefore, theories developed as a result of the model 1 approach are not the same type of theories that may evolve from empiricist, neopositivist, phenomenologist, or any other traditions that may be more appropriate for other disciplines. Model 1 represents the nature of nursing phenomena, nurses' ways of knowing, and the mission of nursing. It may represent a synthesis of other disciplines, or it may represent a new whole, tailored for nursing. It is a model awaiting discovery, created from our history and created for our future.

Model 2

The units of observation for theorists who choose model 2 are behaviors, events, or situations that are embedded in a context. This may include but is not limited to the person–environment relationship. The theorist is an actively engaged participant, and her theory evolves from theory, practice, and research arenas. The reasoning is connective, the process is collaborative, and the theorist uses dialogues, diaries, experiences, and the self in developing the theory. The goal of the theory is to enhance understanding of and action for changes, and its evaluation is based on the central questions significant to humanity, to the theorist, or to the discipline. The goals for theory development for model 2 are to increase the visibility of the community reflecting the theory and to provide them with a voice, either their own or that of someone speaking for them.

Some of the same comments made about model 1 are also appropriate for model 2. Model 2 does not emanate from one tradition, such as feminist, interpretive, or critical theory. Rather it is informed by these traditions inasmuch as it is informed by nursing history, by nurses' ways of knowing, by the nature of nursing's mission, by the properties of nursing as a human science, and by the practice orientation of the discipline. Model 2 needs to be created to represent nursing.

Conclusion

Nursing's identity as a human science and as a practice-oriented discipline has emerged. We are establishing our unique approaches to knowledge development—approaches that represent our identity as a human science and a practical discipline and approaches that acknowledge the nurses' different propensities for knowing.

It is time for synthesis of the different knowledge identities and the many routes for knowledge development. It is time for further development, utilization, and support of the different models for knowledge development. Models that enhance knowing and understanding, models that evolve from our caring traditions, are mechanisms that support the emerging identity of nursing.

Two models were proposed for the development of knowledge. Some may call these models "paradigms" to guide the formation of communities of scholars and the kind of knowledge developed and structured by them. I prefer to call them models and to offer them as a stimulus for a dialogue about the two major routes in the theoretical journey of theoreticians, researchers, and clinicians. Either could be selected in pursuit of knowledge development in general and theoretical development in particular. They are also offered to consolidate our efforts, to enhance the potential of our speaking with each other in an understandable language, and to focus our knowledge development activities.

As we nurture and support our emerged identity, we need to support more coherent approaches to knowledge development, ones that encompass knowing, understanding, and caring; ones that support the development of models for knowledge development congruent with our mission. Support of such identities includes tangible support from granting agencies as well as publishing support from editors of nursing journals.

By being clear about our mission, our values, and the models we choose to use for knowledge development, we are empowering ourselves to empower our consumers. To become clear and to consolidate efforts, we are challenged to further develop and structure knowledge using each model. I believe both models will continue to exist side by side during the decade of the 1990s and perhaps beyond.

REFERENCES

Agan, R.D. (1987). Intuitive knowing as a dimension of nursing. *Advances in Nursing Science*, 10(1), 63–70.

Allen, D. (1985). Nursing research and social control: Alternative models of science that emphasize understanding and emancipation. *Image: The Journal of Nursing Scholarship*, XII(2), 58–64.

Allen, D. (1988). The challenge of gender for the development of nursing science. In V.C. Bridges and N. Wells (Eds.), *Proceedings of the fifth nursing science colloquium: Strategies for theory development in nursing: V.* Boston: Boston University.

Allen, D., Benner, P., and Diekelmann, N. (1986). Three paradigms for methodologies to understand the concept of health. In P. Chinn (Ed.), *Nursing research methodology: Issues and implementation.* Rockville, MD: Aspen Publications.

Ashley, J.A. (1980). Power in structured misogyny: Implications for the politics of care. *Advances in Nursing Science*, 2(3), 3–22.

Benner, P. and Wrubel, J. (1982). Skilled clinical knowledge: The value of perceptual awareness. *Nurse Educator*, 12(5), 11–17.

Bernstein, R.J. (1978). *The restructuring of social and political theory.* Philadelphia: University of Pennsylvania Press.

Boykin, A., Parker, M.E., and Schoenhofer, S.O. (1994). Aesthetic knowing grounded in an explicit conception of nursing. *Nursing Science Quarterly*, 7(4), 158–161.

Carper, B. (1978). Fundamental pattern of knowing in nursing. *Advances in Nursing Science/Practical Oriented Theory, Part 1*, 1(1) 13–23.

Cook, J.A. and Fonow, M.M. (1986). Knowledge and women's interests: Issues of epistemology and methodology in feminist sociological research. *Sociological Inquiry*, 56(1), 2–29.

Doering, L. (1992). Power and knowledge in nursing: A feminist post-structuralist view. *Advances in Nursing Science*, 14(4), 24–33.

Duffy, M.E. and Hedin, B.A. (1988). New directions for nursing research. In N.F. Woods and M. Catanzaro (Eds.), *Nursing research: Theory and practice.* St. Louis: C.V. Mosby.

Fry, S.T. (1988). The nature of knowledge. In V.C. Bridges and N. Wells (Eds.), *Proceedings of the fifth nursing science colloquium: Strategies for theory development in nursing: V.* Boston: Boston University.

Gadamer, H. (1979). The problem of historical consciousness. In P. Robinson and J. Sullivan (Eds.), *Interpretive social science—A reader.* Berkeley: University of California.

Habermas, J. (1971). *Knowledge and human interests.* Boston: Beacon Press.

Habermas, J. (1974). *Theory and practice.* Boston: Beacon Press (original work published in 1971).

Habermas, J. (1979). *Communication and the evolution of society.* Boston: Beacon Press.

Hagell, E.I. (1989). Nursing knowledge: A sociological perspective. *Journal of Advanced Nursing*, 14, 226–233.

Hampton, D.C. (1994). Expertise: The true essence of nursing art. *Advances in Nursing Science*, 17(1), 15–24.

Harding, S. (1986). *The science question in feminism.* Ithaca, NY: Cornell University Press.

Harding, S. (1987). Introduction: Is there a feminist method? In S. Harding (Ed.), *Feminism and methodology.* Bloomington: Indiana University Press.

Harding, S. (1988). Feminism confronts the sciences: Reform and transformation. In V.C. Bridges and N. Wells (Eds.), *Proceedings of the fifth nursing science colloquium: Strategies for theory development in nursing: V.* Boston: Boston University.

Holter, I.M. (1987). *Critical theory.* Oslo, Norway: Unpublished Master's thesis.

Jacobs-Kramer, M.K. and Chinn, P.L. (1988). Perspectives on knowing: A model of nursing knowledge. *Scholarly Inquiry for Nursing Practice: An International Journal*, 2(2), 129–139.

Jagger, A.M. (1988). *Feminist politics and human nature.* Sussex, UK: Rowman & Littlefield.

Jaspers, K. (1963). *General psychopathology.* J. Hoenig and M.W. Hamilton (Trans.). Chicago: University of Chicago Press.

Jenny, J. and Logan, J. (1992). Knowing the patient: One aspect of clinical knowledge. *Image: Journal of Nursing Scholarship*, 24(4), 254–258.

Johnson, J.L (1994). A dialectical examination of nursing art. *Advances in Nursing Science*, 17(1), 1–14.

MacPherson, K.I. (1983). Feminist methods: A new paradigm for nursing research. *Advances in Nursing Science*, 5(2), 17–25.

Moch, S.D. (1990). Personal knowing: Evolving research and practice. *Scholarly Inquiry for Nursing Practice: An International Journal*, 4(2), 155–170.

Munhall, P.L. (1993). 'Unknowing': Toward another pattern of knowing in nursing. *Nursing Outlook*, 41, 125–128.

O'Brien, B. and Pearson, A. (1993). Unwritten knowledge in nursing: Consider the spoken as well as the written word. *Scholarly Inquiry for Nursing Practice: An International Journal*, 7(2), 111–127.

Paterson, J.G. and Zderad, L.T. (1976). *Humanistic nursing.* New York: John Wiley & Sons.

Paul, R.W. and Heaslip, P. (1995). Critical thinking involving nursing practice. *Journal of Advanced Nursing*, 22, 40–47.

Polanyi, M. (1962). *Personal knowledge.* New York: Harper & Row.

Rew, L. (1988). Nurses' intuition. *Applied Nursing Research*, 1(1), 27–31.

Rew, L. (1990). Intuition in critical care nursing practice. *Dimensions of Critical Care Nursing*, 9(1), 30–37.

Rew, L. and Barrow, E. (1987). Intuition: A neglected hallmark of nursing knowledge. *Advances in Nursing Science*, 10(1), 49–62.

Rose, H. (1983). Hand, brain, and heart: A feminist epistemology for the natural sciences. *Signs: Journal of Women in Culture and Society*, 9(1), 73–89.

Sampselle, C.M. (1990). The influence of feminist philosophy on nursing practice. *Image: Journal of Nursing Scholarship*, 22(4), 243–206.

Sarvimäki A. (1994). Science and tradition in the nursing discipline. *Scandinavian Journal of Caring Sciences*, 8, 137–142.

Schultz, P.R. and Meleis, A.I. (1988). Nursing epistemology: Traditions, insights, questions. *Image: Journal of Nursing Scholarship*, 20(4), 217–221.

Schutz, A. (1967). *The phenomenology of the social world.* G. Walsh and F. Lehnert (Trans.). Evanston, IL: Northwestern University Press.

Schwartz, M.A. and Wiggins, O.P. (1988). Scientific and humanistic medicine: A theory of clinical methods. In K.L. White, *The task of medicine: Dialogue at Wickenburg.* Menlo Park, CA: The Henry J. Kaiser Family Foundation.

Sherwin, S. (1987). Concluding remarks: A feminist perspective. *Health Care for Women International*, 8(4), 293–304.

Silva, M.C., Sorrell, J.M., and Sorrell, C.D. (1995). From Carper's patterns of knowing to ways of being: An ontological philosophical shift in nursing. *Advances in Nursing Science*, 18(1), 1–13.

Sohier, R. (1992). Feminism and nursing knowledge: The power of the weak. *Nursing Outlook*, 40(2), 62–93.

Sorrell, J.M. (1994). Remembrance of things past through writing: Esthetic patterns of knowing in nursing. *Advances in Nursing Science*, 17(1), 60–70.

Stacy, J. and Thorne, B. (1985). The feminist revolution in sociology. *Social Problems.* 32(4), 301–315.

Timpson, J. (1996). Nursing theory: Everything the artist spits is art? *Journal of Advanced Nursing,* 23, 1030–1036.

Travelbee, J. (1963). What do we mean by "rapport"? *American Journal of Nursing,* 63(2), 70–72.

White, J. (1995). Patterns of knowing: Review, critique, and update. *Advances in Nursing Science,* 17(4), 73–86.

Wuest, J. (1993). Removing the shackles: A feminist critique of non-compliance. *Nursing Outlook,* 41(5), 217–224.

Younger, J.B. (1990). Literary works as a mode of knowing. *Image: Journal of Nursing Scholarship,* 22(1), 39–43.

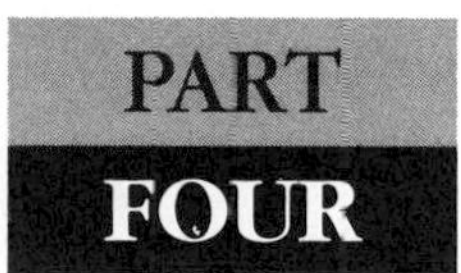

Our Scholarship

Part Two described and analyzed internal and external factors that have influenced the development and progress of theoretical nursing. Part Three described our discipline and its structure as known to its members during the last decade of the century. Part Four is about the agents and the producers of knowledge—the scholars in the discipline. It is also about the theories that were articulated by the early theorists who helped shape the theoretical aspects of nursing. In Chapter 10, a discussion is offered about scholarship as defined as well as redefined in more contemporary writing. Questions related to the congruency of frameworks for scholarship that emanated from other disciplines and their relationship with scholarship in the discipline of nursing are raised and discussed. Norms, tools, and strategies to support scholarliness are proposed and defined. There is a growing support that scholarship must be more sensitive to sociopolitical forces and constraints and that scholarship must be driven by the mission of the discipline and reflect the members' passion for making a difference in the lives of the communities they serve.

In Chapter 11, the discussion revolves around the many ways and options by which theories in nursing may be viewed. It includes two methods of viewing nursing theories. The first is to analyze theories in terms of their paradigmatic origins, time, and period of development, central questions, and central concepts. The second method considers the theories in terms of the current agreed-on central concepts that characterize our discipline.

CHAPTER 10

Hypatia, Hatshepsut, and Nurses as Scholars

Hypatia was a renowned Greek philosopher and scholar during the fourth century AD (Osen, 1974), and Hatshepsut was the only ruling queen among the pharaohs of Egypt in 2500 BC (Wells, 1969). Both demonstrated commitment, persistence, innovation, leadership, and intelligence. Both were true scholars. Both followed similar paths in their lives—different from the universal and mainstream paths that existed at their respective times. Both met death violently and may have been tortured because they charted different paths for their people, were forceful in expressing their views, and succeeded in making changes.

Hypatia left her mark on the world in the form of innovative devices to study astronomy and to determine the specific gravity of liquids—devices that were praised highly by Socrates. Hatshepsut left her mark in the form of architecturally beautiful temples for her people, peace within her country and between her country and the neighboring countries, and new artifacts in her land. Both women demonstrated a unique brand of scholarship; however, scientists had to dig hard to learn about their work and their stories. Was that because they were women? Can they be judged by the same criteria used to evaluate and judge male mathematicians and male pharaohs?

Is nursing scholarliness different from scholarliness in other disciplines? Do nurse scholars have the same attributes as other scholars? Do some differences exist? What might they be? In this chapter, these questions are raised and discussed. Answers, however, are dynamic and are evolving and changing, reflecting new experiences for nurses and redefined goals of the discipline.

There are some indications now that the nature of disciplines that are oriented to human responses and the nature of disciplines that focus on clinical matters may differ considerably from other disciplines that focus on physical phenomena or are only theoretical in nature (Holmes, 1990; Sarvimäki, 1988; Watson, 1990). There are also historical indications that women's history and their lived experiences may provide them with different voices, different cognitive styles, and different ways of knowing (Belenky, Clinchy, Goldberger, and Tarule, 1986; Gilligan, 1984). The discipline of nursing is defined by its perspective, domain, as well as by its historical association with women, and the propensities of members of most societies to assign the work and labor of caring to women. These definitional characteristics may be reflected in the philosophical perspectives adopted by its members. They also drive the way by which members of the discipline approach the framework they develop or use for defining the curricular content and the educational strategies used. These characteristics may also define the ethical decision making frameworks that govern knowledge development and utilization.

It is also expected that disciplines oriented to human responses may require a different set of criteria to judge their scholarly progress and development. These criteria would evolve from the people-oriented nature of the clinical and human sciences and from the struggles that women have endured to achieve equity and receive acknowledgment for their work and respect for their credibility. Scholarliness in such disciplines may, by necessity, provide different routes and different destinations. Nursing falls into this category of disciplines, and nurses (women and men), may represent scholarliness that is more congruent with the nature of nursing and less with the nature of other disciplines.

Scholarliness in Nursing

A scholarly discipline has a focus that is evident and significant. Scholarship in a discipline refers to the degree to which its mission is defined and based on rigorous and credible research and on well-developed, supported, and significant theories. Scholarship is evident in disciplines in which knowledge and its progress are easily articulated, and in which research and philosophical inquiries explore, examine, and answer significant domain questions. Theory is an essential component of scholarly disciplines; it provides members of the discipline with the means to articulate their focuses. Scholarliness combines theory, research, philosophy, and, in disciplines such as nursing—practice—and it is reflected in the synthesis between a discipline's different components. A characteristic of the stage of scholarliness in a discipline is that the relationships between theory, research, philosophy, and practice become more apparent, and it is that clinical scholarship is expected, practiced, and differentiated from clinical research (Diers, 1995). Nursing is in a stage of scholarliness. It would not have been able to reach this current stage without having gone through the many previous stages discussed throughout this book.

In the early 1960s, nursing theorists developed theories in isolation, researchers pursued questions of interest only to educators or administrators, investigators asked isolated questions, and practitioners pursued their practices while remaining somewhat oblivious to what the other two groups were doing. Yet significant changes have occurred in the relationships between educators, researchers, theoreticians, and practitioners. They are now talking to each other, writing for each other, and working with each other. Note the increasing involvement of clinicians in educational programs, the increasing commitment of academics to practice, and the emerging research collaboration between both groups. They are crossing the boundaries to work together and, more important, most of them believe that practice is the *raison d'etre* of nursing. Therefore, middle-range and situation-specific theories are being developed to answer clinical questions. These may include more inclusive questions such as: Who are our nursing clients? When does a client need nursing care in addition to or instead of medical care? When do we discharge a client from our care? Or they may include more specific questions pertaining to ways in which we make our patients comfortable, strategies for pain relief, symptom management, care of wounds, culturally competent nursing therapeutics, and transitions and health promotion.

These questions should be compared with questions about strategies for teaching (such as those related to modular or individualized instruction) or with questions about styles of leadership (such as those related to maintenance or developmental styles of leadership). Both sets of questions were the forms of inquiry in the past and led to knowledge that was not as central to clinicians' concerns about providing quality nursing care. These questions could be practice oriented if they focused on the discovery of the effects of teaching strategies and leadership styles on practice. The current generation of scholars in nursing is asking questions central to practice and exploring phenomena emanating from and influencing practice. New generations of scholars are being prepared educationally to provide answers that could drive and shape the future of nursing practice.

Nursing theories to describe, explain, and predict the quality and consequences of nursing practice have been developed during the decades of the 1960s to the 1980s to attempt to answer broad questions that were central to the field of nursing. Although they evolved from interest in the curriculum, they nevertheless addressed practice in its broadest sense. These questions concerned what knowledge is essential for students, how to organize curricula, and what to include and what not to include in a nursing curriculum. Answers came back in the form of theories that addressed the nursing client, environment, transitions, health, nursing process, nursing therapeutics, and strategies for nursing care. The theories attempted to describe the phenomenon of nursing and attempted to chart a theoretical course for nursing actions. So, the beginnings of a scholarly discipline were created.

There are more indications that nursing scholarliness characterizes the 1980s and 1990s (Table 10-1). Theory and practice were beginning to be interrelated. In clinically oriented meetings, there was an outgrowth of presentations that were theory based and there were discussions of questions that lent themselves to theory and theory development. A review of nursing practice literature demonstrated a growing awareness of a stronger relationship between theory and practice. We moved away from "how to" to "why," "what if," and "when" in an attempt to generalize, document, and verify phenomena in nursing practice.

The existing nursing theories tended to address imaginative and ideal nursing practice. These theories were visions of what nursing ought to be and what care should be;

Table 10-1 Characteristics of the Stage of Scholarliness

- Relationships between theory, research, practice, and philosophy become more apparent.
- Pluralism in paradigms is encouraged.
- Boundaries of domain become more identified.
- Domain guides nursing practice, research, and theory.
- Knowledge is developed that makes a difference in health care.

they were necessary visions of how nursing should move forward to establish its identity and its boundaries. Once the ideal goals were established, these theories were modified as nurses described and documented what exists and what goals are attainable. Nurses became more comfortable with looking at their own practice, describing it, and allowing theoretical formulations to emanate from it (Benner, 1984).

Indications are that professional organizations speak a language congruent with that spoken by theorists and clinicians. One example is the social policy statement issued by the American Nurses Association (ANA) in 1980. The statement provided nursing with a national definition of nursing and a direction for practice and was another indication of agreement on nursing concepts and issues. Nursing was defined as "the diagnosis and treatment of human responses to actual or potential health problems," which is congruent with the focus that emerged on human beings' responses (versus nurses' functions, interactions, or relationships, and versus symptoms, signs, and behavior) (ANA, 1980, p. 9). This definition was reviewed, affirmed, and supplemented by an ANA task force (ANA, 1995). The policy statement states, "The nursing profession remains committed to the care and nurturing of both healthy and ill people, individually or in groups and communities" (p. 6).

The definition of nursing provided in the policy statement acknowledges several essential features of nursing practice; these are the full range of human responses, less emphasis on problem-focused evaluation, the integration of knowledge based on objective data as well as knowledge that reflects subjective experiences, application of knowledge related to diagnosis and intervention processes, caring relations, and the goal of facilitating and promoting health and healing.

The definition of human responses to health and illness includes need, condition, concern, event, dilemma, difficulty, occurrence, fact—as well as lived human experiences that can be described within the target area of nursing. It considers the diversity of human responses in the health/illness situation. One can see the influence of the different theories on the concepts selected in the social policy statement (ANA, 1995). These responses provide us with phenomena on which to base further research and theory development.

A positive relationship between theory and research is not as foreign and unattainable as it was in previous stages. More specifically, research went through a stage of limited relationship with theory (Batey, 1977). The links between theory and research preceded links between theory and practice and are becoming more apparent. The literature is replete with suggestions of ways in which nurses can use theory to guide research and of ways in which they can use research to build theories (Fawcett and Downs, 1986).

Different philosophical premises infiltrated nursing from the 1960s and throughout the 1990s. Questions about truth drew on the writings of such diverse philosophers as Popper and Kaplan and spanned the gamut of empiricists, rationalists, pragmatists, existentialists, feminists, and critical theorists. Some questioned the received view as a guiding framework; others proposed to incorporate intuitive thinking and combine it with the more traditional Baconian approach to nursing science. Silva (1977) and Benoliel (1977) supported the idea that nursing should not lose sight of the significant notion that truths gained from intuition are as important as truths gained through more traditional research methods.

In the late 1980s, writing in nursing demonstrated a passion for knowledge, a search for the meaning of truth, and an exploration of values guiding practice as well as knowledge; it also indicated that changes occurred in the outlooks of nursing's pacesetters. As a result, areas of nursing that during a prior generation were not deemed worthy of investigation enticed a new generation of scholars. An examples of this is comfort as an area worthy of investigation (Arruda-Neves, Larson, and Meleis, 1992; Morse, 1983).

Norms of Scholarliness

An analytical view of the normative structure of nursing supports the notion of scholarliness in nursing. Education and practice came back together during the 1970s and 1980s. Some institutions tried, and succeeded, in having their faculty maintain joint appointments. Theory infiltrated practice, and from practice, theories evolved. Instead of occurring within the curriculum, tests of theories were done in practice. Research findings demonstrated significant consequences for nursing care through changes in morbidities, mortalities, and quality of life (Fagin, 1981). There was not only tolerance for multiple theories in nursing but there was in addition an evolving view that pluralism in nursing theory is essential (Newman, 1983).

The use of many theories and the acceptability of pluralism was accompanied by an attempt to derive meaning from their relationship to nursing. Representative examples of excellent theoretical frameworks of nursing phenomena appeared increasingly in the nursing literature (Mercer, 1981; Millor, 1981; Mischel, 1990; Norbeck, 1981; Tilden, 1980; Weiss, 1979; Younger, 1991). These conceptualizations represented openness to multiple approaches (Armiger, 1974; Schlotfeldt, 1981); they comprised a pluralism that was neither addressed nor advocated during the previous stages.

Authors of these new conceptualizations combined the traditional view that concepts were not accessible to empirical testing with the view that concepts generated variables that are testable. Other nursing concepts, such as maternal role attainment, touch, and temperament in battered children, were based on research and premises from interactionist and developmental models and were drawn from natural and physical science. The new propositions allowed for the divergences that were essential for the development of further testable propositions and, eventually, the development of theories.

This process was analogous to other processes in the history of science. Johannes Kepler, for example, developed the four laws of planetary motion by using careful observations painstakingly collected by Tycho Brahe (Bernstein, 1978). By doing so, Kepler opened up new avenues and brought up new questions. Therefore, he used a convergence of Brahe's data and his own ideas to evolve the laws and to allow for more questions and propositions to develop. Extensions and refinements of early data produced refined and usable laws.

Another property of scholarliness in nursing is that of collaboration. The essence of collaboration is that each member of the team has a major contribution to make and that without that contribution the collaborative act has no meaning (Gortner, 1980). All established disciplines require collaboration within and between disciplines. Our discipline demonstrated increased collaboration by leaps and bounds during the 1990s in both research and publications. The establishment of research centers such as the Women's Health Research Center at the University of Washington and the Research Center for Symptom Management at the University of California, San Francisco, are examples of collaborative research endeavors.

Just as the nature and premises guiding the intellectual discipline of nursing are interdisciplinary, there is also synthesis of truth in nursing. Existing notions of truth in nursing are truth as corroboration through verification and by falsification, in the Popperian sense, and as logical coherence of arguments in the Aristotelian sense. It is also the prestige and power that prompt members of the discipline to agree on its main concepts, parameters, and units of analysis that are the focal features of the discipline in the sense that Kuhn advanced. It is introspection, conception, and derivation of meaning in the Kantian sense.

Nurses used all these meanings to constitute multiple truths, combining subjectivity and objectivity. Because nurses deal with complex phenomena, with human beings, with behaviors, cognitions, and perceptions, the discipline cannot use one meaning of truth to the exclusion of others. Because of the consideration of the relationship between science and humanity during the 1980s, and because of the close relationships between philosophy and science and science and ethics, nursing realized that a singular theory of truth was inadequate and would defy the essence and purpose of nursing. Theories and research in nursing considered the problems that have motivated the construction of the intellectual systems of nursing, such as the use of self in caring and the need for the total involvement of clients in their care.

As we increasingly accepted the shifts from the received to the perceived view, and as we began to acknowledge the uniqueness of our progress (the integrative processes discussed in Chap. 5), we looked at questions of truth as archaic, traditional, and useless. Questions of truth were beginning to be replaced by such questions as the degree to which theories are able to solve scientific problems. The basic unit of analysis for progress became "the solved problems" in nursing (Laudan, 1981; Silva and Rothbart, 1984) instead of relying on confirmation and verification only.

Tools of Scholarliness

Scholarliness requires creativity. Creativity in nursing is manifested in many ways. Rogers, in the late 1960s and early 1970s, used electromagnetic concepts to explain human beings' reactions to health and illness and to give philosophical guidelines to nurses' interventions. She talked about holism before holism became part of our health care language (Rogers, 1970). Orem (1971) spoke of self-care before the initiation of the self-care movement. Travelbee (1966) pioneered the role of a nurse as explorer of perceived meanings of suffering and discussed the significance of spirituality in nursing care. The humanists in the discipline articulated the meaning of the experience of loss and death before it became part of our media lexicon, and clinicians used creative therapeutics such as touch, imagery, and acupressure as alternative health care interventions before the National Institute of Alternative Health Practices was instituted to legitimize these practices.

Creativity is the ability to link seemingly unrelated concepts and to link seemingly unrelated variables (Bronowski, 1956), just as Einstein linked time with space and mass with energy. To Newton, gravity was the concept he created to describe his data. Creativity is the discovery of hidden likenesses. Bronowski (1956) said that the act of creation is original but does not stop with the originator. Kepler's laws that describe the movements of the planets were not arrived at by mounds of corresponding facts that he collected himself or by corresponding readings, although both are significant. He speculated, dreamed, used metaphors, and made analogies (eg, with music), all of which helped to give conceptual order to the data. In the same fashion, Rogers (1970) used the analogy of symphonic harmony to describe a human being's relations with his environment. Creativity is a leap of imagination, and scholarliness is characterized by leaps that enhance explanation and understanding of phenomena.

Scholarliness is a process and state that encompasses the norms and tools of science and the norms and tools of theorizing and philosophizing. It includes not only creativity but also the communication of ideas through teaching to enhance the scholarly socialization of its members. Over the decades, nursing added the necessary pieces to the puzzle of scholarliness. Nursing continues to have a high commitment to improve its curricula, its teaching and learning strategies, its methods of evaluation, and its administrative styles. It is one of few disciplines that isolates the components of research design and methodology and helps students to develop necessary skills to undertake a research career.

Scholarliness is a hallmark of the 1990s because research and theory help explicate major agreed-on nursing phenomena; because nursing is able to articulate its mission in theoretical terms and with scientific data (Fagin, 1981); because nursing has well established organizations, scientific journals, and scientific arenas in which to express its views using both scientific and philosophical methods; because it has authoritative reference groups—all of which helped in establishing agreed-on, well defined intellectual goals; because it believes in the autonomy of its clients; because it has a pluralistic view of truth that encompasses internal coherence of premises and propositions, external correspondence of truth through sense, and pragmatic truth through metaphysical processes; because it deals with significant problems; because it deals with humanity and is therefore a stage for humanity; because its constituents have both a passion for knowledge and a flair for practice and finally, because it offers cumulative wisdom. Nursing goals are generally congruent with those of the recipients of its care; nursing operates from a health and holistic approach and purports to enhance coping and harmony with one's environment.

Indicators of Scholarliness in Nursing

Several indicators serve as examples of the scholarly maturity of nursing. *First,* scholarliness is demonstrated through *continuity.* Continuity is manifested by the important and fundamental questions in the field that are addressed within a conceptual or theoretical scheme to refine and modify ideas over generations of scholars (Gortner, 1980).

Answers are not the isolated incidents nursing deals with. The relationship of mechanostimulation on primary or secondary pain; therapeutic touch as a modality for communication, assessment, and intervention; or the consequences of reality testing on the elderly are linked to other answers to form a whole that belongs to a theory of stimulation or person–environment interaction.

Scholarliness is the ability to delineate the premises on which one's decisions and questions are based; the ability to engage in, complete, and communicate the results of research projects that are supported and documented; the ability to critically assess the objective and subjective components in their inquiry; and the ability to relate the results to existing theory and to participate in the development of theories. Our scholarly efforts are concentrated on sharpening and refining our knowledge of the process identified as central to the discipline and using the frameworks that define a nursing perspective.

Scholars in nursing use quantitative and qualitative analyses to define, refine, sharpen concepts, and test basic propositions for the purpose of adding to the substantive knowledge. We must not forget, however, that a significant mission of the discipline is not only better care of the patients but the emergence of our clients from the transition situation equipped with the tools to cope with similar or different transitions in life, equipped with ways to promote their health, equipped with means to prevent further illness episodes, and equipped with techniques to deal with stress in life. Thus, we would be helping to merge research, theory, and practice—the concatenation realized as we handle clinical problems more and more with the same ease we handle theoretical and research problems (Barnard, 1980).

The *second* indicator, therefore, is demonstrated through nursing theories that evolve from practice and are used in education. As practice is joining with education (Schlotfeldt, 1981), the distance between creation of knowledge, corroboration, and use of knowledge in practice is diminishing. This process I called *concatenation*. Concatenation is the condition under which that shortening of distances is occurring. Concatenation also involves joining with the public media to inform the public of nursing's mission and to modify its goals based on public needs. Our local and national media are cooperating in modifying the negative image the public had of nursing experts, and more importantly, nurses are speaking up, their messages are loud and clear, and they are being heard (Reemtsma, 1981).

The *third* indicator of scholarliness is the *development of the National Institute of Nursing Research,* which was authorized under the Health Research Act of 1985 and was established in 1986. This represented a significant milestone in nursing scholarliness, and it affirmed two significant aspects of the discipline of nursing. First, quality nursing care depended on a careful and systematic program of investigation; and second, nursing defined its domain and its thematic characteristics. It made us hopeful that there will be increased support and commitment to knowledge development.

The *fourth* indicator of nursing's growing scholarly maturity is the cumulative work through research and theory that is being done on the central concepts in nursing. For example, health of environment is considered as the patients' environment, as the sociopolitical environment, as the administrative environment, and as the environment for students. Studies were developed to explain different components of environment that add to our understanding of environment. The concept may be the same; the different settings help in the development of all components and all properties of the concept. In an innovative study related to environment, Holzemer and Chambers (1986) found a significant relationship between faculty perceptions of the environment's scholarly excellence, available resources, student commitment, and motivation and faculty productivity. They helped us conceptualize properties of health environments for students in the same way we conceptualize healthy environments for patients.

The *fifth* indicator is that the nursing domain became more recognizable by nurses in many of their special clinical and functional fields and is used as the organizing framework for education, clinical practice, and research.

Nurses as Scholars

Although nursing is a field of study open for men and women, the predominance of women in nursing must not be ignored when considering nursing scholarship. Scholarship is based on knowledge and women are agents of knowledge whose characteristic activities provide a grounding that is different from and in some respects (in some disciplines based on human science) preferable to men's grounding (Harding, 1988). Harding makes this argument:

> What it means to be scientific is to be dispassionate, disinterested, impartial, concerned without abstract principles and rules, but what it means to be a woman is to be emotional (passionate), interested in and partial to the welfare of family and friends, concerned with concrete practices and contextual relations (Harding, 1988, p. 83).

The question that forms the basis for this section is: Are nurses' approaches to knowing, understanding, and formulating conceptualizations unique? There are indications in the literature of the 1980s and 1990s of the uniqueness of women's developmental processes and women's ways of describing their experiences, and the unique ways by which experts tend to make decisions.

The unique ways by which experts in general analyze, judge, and make decisions about situations were discussed and defined by Dreyfus and Dreyfus (1985). In using this framework, Benner and Tanner (1987) demonstrated how nurses use intuition in expert clinical judgment. Six key aspects of intuitive judgment were identified and discussed in a study that included 21 nurses who were defined by their colleagues as experts. Nurses demonstrated their ability to make judgments by using their intuitive expertise to recognize patterns of relationships in situations that are not readily recognizable by others, by detecting similarities between situations through common-sense understanding, by "knowing how" in a way that is not definable in common scientific terms, by having a "sense of salience" (ie, recognizing priorities), and by using "deliberative rationality" (shifting perspectives for better understanding) (Benner and Tanner, 1987). These processes involved a level of intuition that has been devalued by nurses for its lack of scientific bases. Are any of these characteristics for caring congruent with those needed for knowing and understanding? The uniqueness of nurses' capacity to know and the unique ways by which they demonstrate that knowing and understanding are proposals that should be seriously considered.

That there are different processes of knowing is a proposal that has been supported by a number of key publications in the 1980s. For example, Belenky, Clinchy, Goldberger, and Tarule (1986) identified five different types of knowers. Schultz and Meleis (1988) theorized that these types could be found in nursing. Types of theories and levels of development of theories may be influenced by the ability of nursing theorists to uncover knowledge of the different types, to be able to hear and reflect the voices of the different knowers in theoretical development.

If the five types of knowers identified by Belenky and colleagues (1986) are defined from a nursing perspective, the following is what we might find:

1. **Silent knowers** are nurses who tend to accept the voices of authority and thus learn to be silent. These nurses know their practice, their teaching, or their administrative practice, but they may not be able to articulate what they know through abstract thought for theoretical development and may not have the language to express their analysis or interpretation of the phenomenon. Their work, insights, and wisdom are invisible because they are not represented or because theorists have not been able to retrieve them for further theoretical development. Could these silent knowers conceptualize their understanding of phenomenon in ways that are more congruent with their propensity to develop theories?
2. **Received knowers** believe others are capable of producing knowledge that they can follow and reproduce. They believe in external authorities' abilities to generate knowledge, but not in their own or their peers' abilities to do the same. These people depend on and value the expertise of others. Many nurses have contented themselves in using the works of others, believing those works to be far superior to anything they themselves could create. Examples are the different theories and paradigms that we have bought into and used for years without questioning.
3. **Subjective knowers** depend on their personal experiences. These knowers believe and depend on their own inner voices and inner feelings. Knowledge to them is "personal, private, and subjectively known and intuited," and truth "is an intuitive reaction—something experienced, not thought out, something felt rather than actively pursued or constructed" (Belenky, Clinchy, Goldberger, and Tarule, 1986, p. 69). Although these knowers find it difficult to articulate the processes used to arrive at the knowledge, they have the wisdom that holistically looks and explains complete situations. Knowledge from nursing practice as articulated by subjective knowers could inform the discipline of nursing in ways that no other knowledge could. This is the knowledge that Carper (1978) referred to as personal knowledge and Benner (1984) as expert knowledge.
4. **Procedural knowers** depend on careful observations and procedures. They are the rationalists among us. These are the people who communicate proce-

dures, rules, and regulations, and thus may be best suited for developing empirical or procedural theories.

5. **Constructed knowers** view all "knowledge as contextual, they experience themselves as creators of knowledge and value both subjective and objective strategies of knowing." These knowers integrate the different ways of knowing and the different voices (including the silent voice). To them, "all knowledge is constructed, and the knower is an intimate part of the known" (Belenky, Clinchy, Goldberger, and Tarule, 1986). To subscribe to this view is to accept the never-ending process of knowledge development, to accept that theories are always in process, to accept that frames of reference are constructed and reconstructed, and to accept that situations as well as knowledge are contextual and subject to different interpretations (Schultz and Meleis, 1988).

Are there different types of scholars in nursing? In considering the major theoretical and research literature from the 1970s through the 1990s, patterns of scholarship emerge. These patterns are tentative and are continuously evolving; however, I think they represent patterns of scholarship in nursing. I use several concepts to reflect the nature of the different patterns that may be found among nurses.

The synthesizers are conceptualizers who are able to connect already developed ideas, analyze them, and arrive at new wholes. These new wholes make for a more effective explanation and interpretation of already existing knowledge.

The leap theorizers are those who amass research or clinical data and reduce these data to abstract ideas. They are the conceptualizers who are able to make leaps to generalizations to create challenging theoretical questions and answers.

The bush describers are those who know how to describe relationships that have been empirically identified and verified They usually are reluctant to go beyond these specific findings.

The out-of-discipline theorizers are those who see the world of nursing through the glasses tinted by other disciplines. Therefore, when engaging in conceptualizing and answering questions, they select those that are more accepted and more central to other disciplines. At the same time, however, their findings and conceptualizations shed some light on nursing problems, however minor those problems are to the core of nursing.

The conceptualizers are those who are discovering, identifying, and exploring the discipline's concepts. These concepts may be central or tangential.

The integrated theorizers are those who are as comfortable with theorizing as with researching or practicing. More importantly, these are individuals who have synthesized the different aspects of their problem of interest and have been able to develop conceptualizations in which clinical, research, and theoretical insights are contained.

Scholarliness Redefined

Scholarliness has been described by many writers, with some slight variations in the definition. The common themes are that a scholar is a person who has a high intellectual ability, is an independent thinker and an independent actor, has ideas that stand apart from others, is persistent in her quest for developing knowledge, is systematic, has unconditional integrity, has intellectual honesty, has some convictions, and stands alone to support these convictions. A scholar is a person who is flexible and who respects all divergent opinions (Armiger, 1974; Diers, 1995; Meleis, Wilson, and Chater, 1980; Parse, 1994; Roe, 1951). In addition, of course, a scholar is a person who is deeply engaged in the development of knowledge in the field (Johnson, Moorhead, and Daly, 1992). Not all scientists are scholars, nor are all scholars scientists. Scholarliness concerns having a sense of history about a discipline and knowing how one's work fits within the larger framework and goals of the discipline.

The definition of scholarship has changed. Rules once were clear. Scholarship meant research and research meant one type of research. Scholars were defined as:

> Academics who conduct research, publish and then perhaps convey their knowledge to students or apply what they have learned (Boyer, 1990, p. 15, Carnegie Foundation).

Scholarship was confined only to those involved in the discovery of knowledge and was limited to innovative discovery that made contributions to knowledge development and progress. Scholarship within this prevailing framework was defined as having an academic rank and as engaged in basic research and in publications. Furthermore, the sentiment prevailed that those who applied knowledge were not scholars; rather, they were practice-oriented folks who must leave scholarship aside and focus on their own practice.

Nurses have always known something is missing in this definition. It robbed nurses of their rich clinical heritage and it stifled the processes needed to integrate knowledge and relate it to practice. And practice, we suspected, was the heart and the soul of the discipline. As nurses, we were, however, afraid to rock the halls of "ivory towers" and attempt to change these definitions. After all, we were just the new kids on the block with no clout and with a lot of vulnerability. Beginning rumblings were manifested in the writings of many nurses who questioned this status quo. But these rumblings became louder in the Carnegie Foundation report described above (Boyer, 1990), which urged that scholarship must be redefined. The proposal of this document was for accepting other types of scholarships, such as *scholarship of integration.* Scholars who excel more at the *integration of knowledge* rather than the discovery of knowledge tend to focus on conceptualizing and theorizing; they not only describe findings, but also interpret and ascribe meanings to these findings within the context of the discipline. Their scholarship is thus manifested in presenting thoughtful analyses of profound, philosophical, and theoretical changes in the discipline.

Another form of scholarship was identified that acknowledges the fine and necessary practice-oriented work done in our discipline, and that is the *scholarship of application.* Work that is considered scholarly in a practice field is service oriented and evolves guidelines that shape policies related to practice, which in turn shape theory.

This type of scholarship of application is defined by Palmer (1986) as:

> . . . a complex activity and synthesis of observations of clients and patients . . .
> a complex activity that has as its purpose, the discovery, organization, analysis, synthesis, and transmission of knowledge resulting from client-centered nursing practice (p. 318).

Diers (1995) also defines clinical scholarship (or scholarship of application in Boyer's report) as:

> . . . certain habits of mind. Clinical scholarship modifies the noun only by focusing on observations in and of the work, including the perception of one's own participation in it. To these observations are applied disciplined habits of analysis (including careful attention to sources) and analogy, that are carefully described and even more carefully edited so that, when written, the activity produces new understanding, new knowledge (p. 25).

Clinical scholarship is reflected in careful analyses of situations and critical assessment of responses; it requires a certain intellectual maturity that comes from expertise and repeated experiences. The explanations and reflections offered by the clinical scholar are contexted in her personal history and are enhanced by her well supported interpretations.

The Carnegie report also acknowledged an area of scholarship that nurses, for a long time, suspected should be deemed as scholarly. That is the *scholarship of teaching*. Teaching was set aside also as an application of knowledge, accepted as secondary to knowledge discovery. We all spent hours developing innovative curricula, creative teaching strategies, learning modules, and we discovered new ways to help students understand their practice roles, defined ways by which we could create synthesis and integration in student's knowledge, watched with admiration how seasoned clinicians assisted the inexperienced to become transformed. We wished there were some ways we could articulate how the productive researchers managed to inspire and guide the beginning researchers. But we were reluctant to consider all this as scholarship.

I believe what has begun in nursing decades ago, what nurses have attempted to demonstrate as scholarship is now acknowledged as such. The question before us today is: In what ways will these redefinitions of scholarship reshape scholarship in nursing?

These redefinitions of scholarship are more friendly to the nature of the discipline, the practice of nursing, and the mission of nursing. They allow for the complex and diverse knowledge base that nurses need to educate, to practice, to administer, to consult, and to discover new knowledge. They acknowledge the need for nurses to have a "group of fields" that are related to nursing but are outside of nursing (Diers, 1995).

Our discipline is scholarly if it engages in the development of knowledge that has some significance to humanity and to human beings, if it has a conviction, if it opens doors for those who have the most difficulty in accessing the health care system, and if it encompasses and includes the underserved population. Nursing scholars deal with human beings, and they not only pursue explanation and prediction, they also address understanding of clinical phenomena that may result from clinical knowledge as well as theoretical knowledge.

Unlike other disciplines that may have promoted competition and distancing as hallmarks of their scientific development, the nature of nursing, with its gender orientation, respect, and use of feminist approaches in viewing the discipline (see Chap. 9), would necessitate the promotion of cooperation and collaboration over competition and separation. Scholarliness in the discipline means flexibility regarding its theoretical base. Finally, a scholarly discipline is predicated on the soundness of its theoretical base.

Scholarliness in nursing includes the *collaborative efforts* of all the resources within nursing to work together to develop critical and reflective thinking in students, academicians, and clinicians. According to Dewey (1922), *critical thinking* is defined as the ability to suspend judgment on matters of interest. Critical thinking should be fostered by cognitive and affective approaches in the educational and the clinical arenas. The cognitive approach is enhanced by the provision of frameworks for teaching, for discussion, and for clinical practice. The affective approach is enhanced by providing frameworks that allow for dialogue, analysis, and reflection on experience.

Examples of critical thinking in nursing included the awareness and inclusion of a focus on systems of patriarchy and domination and their influence on knowledge development (Thompson, 1987). Scholarship in nursing must reflect the type of critical thinking that generates awareness of unequal resources, of relationships that are distorted because of domination, and of the influence of marginalization on members of the discipline and on those who are the recipients of care (Hall, Stevens, and Meleis, 1994; Thompson, 1987). A scholar in nursing demonstrates a *passion for making a difference,* for dismantling old patterns that are based on unequal power and reconstructing patterns that are based on equity, resources, shared power, and on collaboration in decision making.

There should be a balance between *providing a framework* that enhances critical thinking and one that may lead to other created frameworks. If only one framework is provided, it could be a stifling act that prevents a person from seeing other potential avenues in understanding the situation. Critical thinking lies in the balance between framework thinking and flexible viewing of a situation. Critical thinking can also be enhanced by using affective approaches, for example, through the creation of dialogues about patient care situations that are open to debates and critiques. Critiquing existing theories or research is also appropriate for developing critical thinking. Scholarship includes the creativity needed to consider ways to develop knowledge in a human science, ways that do not stifle the richness of its phenomena.

Scholarliness necessitates the use of *local models of excellence* and the promotion of sponsorship of novices by experts or mentors and mentorees as essential. To preach scholarship without demonstrating it in a close working relationship between mentor and mentoree leaves a lot to the imagination of the mentoree that may not be tangible and attainable (Meleis, Hall, and Stevens, 1994). Participation in a mentorship relationship with a person who is pursuing scholarship in practice, theory, or research tends to promote the potential of the development of the same characteristics in the mentorees. Scholarliness in a discipline not only depends on the definition of the discipline by those who are inside it; it also depends on how the discipline is viewed by those outside it. We need to make our discipline more *public*—demonstrate its significance to the health and care of the public. We also need to become involved in the political and policy-making processes and to make a point of speaking to the public directly.

Conclusion

One does not develop knowledge to gain scholarliness in a discipline. Being a scholar is a means toward an end and not an end in itself; it is a means toward the empowerment of nursing as a profession, and of nurses as scientists, clinicians, educators, and policymakers. The end goal is patient care that is based on socially relevant knowledge that is developed with social consciousness. It is to provide, to enable, and to empower nurses to make the changes they want to make in the quality of patient care. It is to participate in the development of policies that affect the care that is given. That influence is possible only if it comes from a socially relevant knowledge base. Such a knowledge base can be developed only if reflective attention is given to patterns of knowing in nursing, and to the phenomena relevant to nursing, within a values system that accepts and respects a nursing perspective.

Acknowledgements

This section, dealing with scholarliness, norms of scholarliness, and tools of scholarliness, was adapted, with extensive revisions, from the Helen Nahm Lecture I delivered at the University of California, San Francisco, in 1981; and from (by permission) Meleis, A.I. (1983). The evolving nursing scholarliness. In Chinn, P.L. (Ed.), *Advances in nursing*. Rockville, MD: Aspen Systems.

REFERENCES

American Nurses Association. (1980). *Nursing: A social policy statement* (Publication No. NP-63). Kansas City, MO: Author.

American Nurses Association (1995). *Nursing's social policy statement* (Publication No. NP-107). Washington, DC: Author.

Armiger, B. (1974). Scholarship in nursing. *Nursing Outlook*, 22(3), 162–163.

Arruda-Neves, E., Larson, P., and Meleis, A.I. (1992). Comfort: Immigrant Hispanic patients' views. *Cancer Nursing*, 15(6), 387–394.

Barnard, K. (1980). Knowledge for practice: Directions for the future. *Nursing Research*, 29(4), 208–212.

Batey, M.V. (1977). Conceptualization: Knowledge and logic guiding empirical research. *Nursing Research*, 26(5), 324–329.

Belenky, M.F., Clinchy, B.M., Goldberger, N.R., and Tarule, J.M. (1986). *Women's ways of knowing: The development of self, voice, and mind.* New York: Basic Books.

Benner, P. (1984). *From novice to expert: An excellence and power in clinical nursing practice.* Menlo Park, CA: Addison-Wesley.

Benner, P. and Tanner, C. (1987). Clinical judgment: How expert nurses use intuition. *American Journal of Nursing*, 87(1) 23–31.

Benoliel, J.Q. (1977). The interaction between theory and research. *Nursing Outlook*, 25(2), 108–113.

Bernstein, J. (1978). *Experiencing science.* New York: Basic Books.

Boyer, E. (1990). *Scholarship reconsidered: Priorities of the professoriate* [special report]. Princeton, NJ: The Carnegie Foundation for the Advancement of Teaching.

Bronowski, J. (1956). *Science and human values.* New York: Harper Colophon Books.

Carper, B. (1978). Fundamental pattern of knowing in nursing. *Advances in Nursing Science/Practical Oriented Theory, Part 1*, 1(1) 13–23.

Dewey, J. (1922). *Human nature and human conduct.* New York: Henry Holt.

Diers, D. (1995). Clinical scholarship. *Journal of Professional Nursing*, 11(1), 24–30.

Dreyfus, H. and Dreyfus, S. (1985). *Mind over machine: The power of human intuition and expertise in the era of the computer.* New York: Free Press.

Fagin, C. (1981, September). *Nursing's pivotal role in achieving competition in health care.* Paper presented at American Academy of Nursing meeting, Washington, D.C.

Fawcett, J. and Downs, F.S. (1986). *The relationship of theory and research.* East Norwalk, CT: Appleton-Century-Crofts.

Gilligan, C. (1984). *In a different voice: Psychological theory and women's development.* Cambridge, MA: Harvard University Press.

Gortner, S.R. (1980). Nursing science in transition. *Nursing Research*, 29(3), 180–183.

Hall, J.M., Stevens, P.E., and Meleis, A.I. (1994). Marginalization: A guiding concept for valuing diversity in nursing knowledge development. *Advances in Nursing Science*, 16(4), 23–41.

Harding, S. (1988). Feminism confronts the sciences: Reform and transformation. In V.C. Bridges and N. Wells (Eds.), *Proceedings of the fifth nursing science colloquium: Strategies for theory development in nursing: V.* Boston: Boston University.

Holmes, C.A. (1990). Alternatives to natural science foundations for nursing. *International Journal of Nursing Studies*, 27(3), 187–198.

Holzemer, W. and Chambers, D. (1986). Healthy nursing doctoral programs: Relationship between perceptions of the academic environment and productivity of faculty and alumni (research). *Research in Nursing and Health*, 9(4), 299–307.

Johnson, R.A., Moorhead, S.A., and Daly, J.M. (1992). Scholarship and socialization: Reflections on the first year of doctoral study. *Journal of Nursing Education*, 31(6), 280–282.

Laudan, L. (1981). A problem solving approach to scientific growth. In I. Hacking (Ed.), *Scientific revolutions*. Oxford, UK: Oxford University Press.

Meleis, A.I., Hall, J.M., and Stevens, P.E. (1994). Scholarly caring in doctoral nursing education: Promoting diversity and collaborative mentorship. *Image: Journal of Nursing Scholarship*, 26(3), 177–180.

Meleis, A.I., Wilson, H.S., and Chater, S. (1980). Toward scholarliness in doctoral dissertations: An analytical model. *Research in Nursing and Health*, 3, 115–124.

Mercer, R. (1981). A theoretical framework for studying factors that impact on the maternal role. *Nursing Research*, 30(2), 73–77.

Millor, G.K. (1981). A theoretical framework for nursing research in child abuse and neglect. *Nursing Research*, 30(2), 78–83.

Mischel, M.H. (1990). Reconceptualization of the uncertainty in illness theory. *Journal of Nursing Scholarship*, 22, 256–262.

Morse, J.M. (1983). An ethnoscientific analysis of comfort: A preliminary investigation. *Nursing Papers*, 15(3), 6–19.

Newman, M. (1983). The continuing revolution: A history of nursing science. In N. Chaska (Ed.), *The nursing profession: A time to speak*. New York: McGraw-Hill.

Norbeck, J. (1981). Social support: A model for clinical research and application. *Advances in Nursing Science*, 3, 43–59.

Orem, D. (1971). *Nursing concepts of practice*. New York: McGraw-Hill.

Osen, L.M. (1974). *Women in mathematics*. Cambridge, MA: MIT Press.

Palmer, I.S. (1986). The emergence of clinical scholarship as a professional imperative. *Journal of Professional Nursing*, 2, 318–325.

Parse, R.R. (1994). Scholarship: Three essential processes [editorial]. *Nursing Science Quarterly*, 7(4), 14.

Reemtsma, J. (1981, May). *Nurse, where are you?* Television news documentary, CBS.

Roe, L. (1951). A psychological study of eminent biologists. *Psychological Monographs*, 65, 1–67.

Rogers, M.E. (1970). *An introduction to the theoretical basis of nursing*. Philadelphia: F.A. Davis.

Sarvimäki, A. (1988). Nursing as a moral, practical, communicative, and creative activity. *Journal of Advanced Nursing*, 13, 462–467.

Schlotfeldt, R.M. (1981). Nursing in the future. *Nursing Outlook*, 29, 295–301.

Schultz, P.R. and Meleis, A.I. (1988). Nursing epistemology: Traditions, insights, questions. *Image: Journal of Nursing Scholarship*, 20(4), 217–221.

Silva, M.C. (1977). Philosophy, science, theory: Interrelationships and implications for nursing research. *Image*, 9(3), 59–63.

Silva, M.C. and Rothbart, D. (1984). An analysis of changing trends in philosophies of science on nursing theory development and testing. *Advances in Nursing Science*, 6(2), 1–13.

Thompson, J.L. (1987). Critical scholarship: The critique of domination in nursing. *Advances in Nursing Science*, 10(1), 27–38.

Tilden, V. (1980). A developmental conceptual framework for the maturational crises of pregnancy. *Western Journal of Nursing Research*, 2, 667–677.

Travelbee, J. (1966). *Interpersonal aspects of nursing*. Philadelphia: F.A. Davis.

Watson, J. (1990). Caring knowledge and informed moral passion. *Advances in Nursing Science*, 13(1), 15–24.

Weiss, S. (1979). The language of touch. *Nursing Research*, 28(2), 76–80.

Wells, E. (1969). *Hatshepsut*. Garden City, NY: Doubleday.

Younger, J.B. (1991). A theory of mastery. *Advances in Nursing Science*, 14(1), 76–89.

CHAPTER 11

Nursing Theory: An Elusive Mirage or a Mirror of Reality

Nursing theories mirror different realities. Throughout their development, they reflected the interests of nurses of the time, the sociocultural context, and the theorists' educational and experiential backgrounds. When we consider all the theories together and hold them up to the realities of nursing practice, a number of other images are then formulated. The images are not always distinct images, well formulated images, or true mirror images; however, they are not mirages or figments of the imagination of the theorists either. They reflect some realities of nursing at the time of development, and they are helping to shape the realities of nursing care over time.

This chapter provides several ways in which theories can be viewed. These ways are neither mutually exclusive nor inclusive. They are presented to stimulate other innovative ways in which to view and classify nursing theories. The purpose of these different views and classifications is twofold. First, the more ways in which we can analyze any phenomenon, the more potential we have for seeing different images and details that are not readily apparent when only viewed from one perspective. The second purpose is related to the first: using theories for different purposes is enhanced by the many different perspectives from which we view the theories. It is like seeing the image of a garden in a mirror with many flowers, many colors, and many beds, then moving the mirror closer to a bed of California poppies and seeing the rich orange-yellow cups swaying in the fine breeze, then keeping the mirror in position and stepping back a few feet to get another look, to discover the different shades of color blending with the green of the stems. Each image depends on the position of the mirror in relation to the garden and the location of the viewer in relation to the mirror and the garden.

The first section of this chapter provides an analysis of nursing theories that were developed between 1950 and 1970 according to the images of nursing of that time (Fig. 11-1). In the second section, theories are classified according to their primary focus and according to how they will be evaluated in this book. In the third section, theories are classified according to images of nurses and the roles that nurses may play. Roles played by nurses are to a large extent determined by the theoretical perspective guiding their practice. In the fourth section, areas of agreement among and between theories are presented. Whether these are the same images or the same classifications that the theorists saw when they developed their theories is neither discussed nor debated here. What is

		1950	
		—	
		—	H. Peplau
		—	
		—	
	V. Henderson	1955	
		—	
		—	
D. Johnson		—	
	D. Orem	—	
	F. Abdellah	1960	
	L. Hall	—	J. Paterson & L. Zderad
		—	I. Orlando
		—	
		—	J. Travelbee
		1965	E. Wiedenbach
M. Levine		—	
		—	
		—	I. King
		—	
M. Rogers		1970	
C. Roy		—	
		—	
		—	
		—	
B. Neuman		1975	
		—	
		—	
		—	
		—	
		1980	

Figure 11–1 Chronology of nursing theories.

becoming apparent is that the theories together offer a number of images—translated into concepts—that both the images and the concepts are reflected in the theories and that they reflect nursing practice simultaneously. The classification systems sometimes reflect the hindsight of the critics rather than the theorists themselves. One of the earliest classification of theories was done by Johnson in her teaching in the 1960s. She classified them by their paradigmatic origins as those theories that reflect the developmental theory premises, which are:

> . . . models based on the developmental theories of Erikson (1963), Freud (1949), Maslow (1954), Peplau (1952), C. Rogers (1959), and Sullivan (1953) and based on the behaviorist school (Bijou and Baer, 1961). Among the systems models are found the adaptation system model of Roy (1970), the triad system of Howland and McDowell (1964), the life process system of M. Rogers (1970), and Johnson's behavioral system model (1968). . . . Then, in addition, there is another type of model for nursing practice, called an interaction model, since its conceptual system is dependent on symbolic interaction theory. The most well-known models in this group are those of Orlando (1961) and Wiedenbach (1964) (Johnson, 1974, p. 376).

Nursing theories were also analyzed and classified using other dimensions. In the first section of this chapter, 30 years of theorizing are analyzed using several other dimensions for classification of theories. One of the dimensions is credited for Dorothy Johnson's insights—paradigmatic origins of theories as described above. Others include the chronological time for the development of theory, temporal dimensions focusing on different sociocultural contexts, central theory questions, and central concepts. The purposes of these proposed analyses along the different dimensions are twofold: to provide opportunities for critical thinking about theoretical nursing and to stimulate the development and use of a variety of analytical frameworks. Each analysis uncovers different aspects and different explanations within and about the theories, and each different analysis and explanation could drive and further the development of theoretical nursing. The analyses of theories using these dimensions resulted in three distinct patterns or schools of thought (Table 11-1). Each school of thought is presented and discussed below. Members of each school of thought are compared in terms of their views of nursing, focus of nursing, goals of nursing, nursing problems, and nursing therapeutics. The images of nurses and the central roles that nurses are expected to play when adopting a particular school of thought to practice are also compared and contrasted in this chapter.

Images of Nursing, 1950–1970

The First School of Thought: Needs

This school of thought includes theories that reflect an image of nursing as meeting the needs of clients and were developed in response to such questions as:

What do nurses do?
What are their functions?
What roles do nurses play?

Answers to these questions focused on a number of theorists describing functions and roles of nurses. Conceptualizing functions led theorists to consider a nursing client in terms of a hierarchy of needs. When any of these needs are unmet and when a person is unable to fulfill his own needs, the care provided by nurses is required. Nurses then provide the necessary functions and play those roles that could help patients meet their needs.

Table 11-1 ***Schools of Thought in Nursing Theories—1950–1970***

Needs Theorists	Interaction Theorists	Outcome Theorists
Abdellah	King	Johnson
Henderson	Orlando	Levine
Orem	Paterson and Zderad	Rogers
	Peplau	Roy
	Travelbee	
	Wiedenbach	

Peplau preceded Henderson by providing a theoretical construct of what nursing is. Hers was a theory designed to give focus to psychiatric nursing. Therefore, although intrapsychic needs play a major role in her theory, her interest and experience in psychiatric nursing prompted her introduction of nurse–patient interpersonal relationships as a focus in nursing. Henderson's theory, in keeping with the intraperson focus of the time and not deviating completely from medical science, was conceived to describe all nursing care goals in terms of the needs of patients, and in terms of activities that are motivated and driven by patients' hierarchy of needs.

This school of thought, of need deficits or nurse functions, also included Abdellah and Orem. One may refer to this group as the *need* or *deficit school of thought*, which is based on Maslow's hierarchy of needs and influenced by Erickson's stages of development (with a neo-Freudian orientation). Although proponents of this school of thought were the first to promote nursing functions as distinct from medical functions, the theories developed within this school were still greatly influenced by the biomedical model. Because most of the theorists who focused on needs and need deficits in patients either graduated from or worked at Columbia University in New York, this school of thought could also be called the *Columbia school of thought.* Although the theorists may not attribute the development of their theories to their work or association with Columbia, by noting that they have a common educational background, we may be able to consider themes of shared assumptions as well as shared goals, and therefore explore the influence of Columbia Teachers College on nursing theory development and the development of early scholars. Judging from the number and caliber of international students who graduated from the institution, Columbia Teachers College may have had a significant influence on the development of theoretical nursing in other countries as well. The extent of the influence of this school on the development of schools of thought, on the development of nursing education and practice nationally and internationally, is yet to be examined.

As Tables 11-2 through 11-6 indicate, the needs theorists provided us with a view of a human being that was slightly different but close to the view provided by the biomedical model. The hierarchy of needs begins with physiologic needs and safety needs and progresses to include other higher-level needs, such as belonging, love, and esteem needs. Neither Henderson nor Abdellah considered self-actualization needs as within the province of the nurse (as manifested in the omission rather than the commission); Orem added the development of self-care requisites as she continued to develop her theory.

Table 11-2 Needs Theorists—A View of Nursing

Theorists	Definition of Nursing
Abdellah	Use of problem solving approach to deal with 21 problems related to needs of patients
Henderson	Helping with 14 activities contributing to health or recovery, help the individual become independent of assistance
Orem	Self-care agency to meet individual's need for self-care action in order to sustain life and health, recover from disease or injury, and cope with the effect

Table 11-3 ***Needs Theorists—Focus of Nursing***

Theorists	Focus of Nursing
Abdellah	Problem solving approach to 21 nursing activities, sustenal, remedial, restorative, preventive, self-help, need deficit or excess
Henderson	Assistance with 14 daily activities or needs
Orem	Deficit between self-care capabilities and self-care demands of patients

Table 11-4 ***Needs Theorists—Goals of Nursing***

Theorists	Goals of Nursing
Abdellah	Help individual meet health needs and adjust to health problems
Henderson	Completeness or wholeness and independence of patient to perform daily activities
Orem	Eliminate deficit between self-care capabilities and demand

Table 11-5 ***Needs Theorists—Nursing Problems***

Theorists	Nursing Problems
Abdellah	Condition faced by patient for which a nurse can assist, overtly and covertly (21 problems)
Henderson	Patient's lack of knowledge, strength, or will to carry out 14 activities
Orem	Deficiency in 8 universal, 2 developmental, and 6 health deviation requisites/needs

Table 11-6 ***Need Theorists—Nursing Therapeutics***

Theorists	Nursing Therapeutics
Abdellah	Preventive care (hygiene, safety, exercise, rest, sleep, body mechanics) Sustenal care (psychosocial care) Remedial care (provision of oxygen, fluid, nutrition, elimination) Restorative care (coping with illness and life adjustment)
Henderson	Complementing and supplementing knowledge, will, and strength of patient to perform 14 daily activities and to carry out his medical prescriptions
Orem	Wholly compensatory system (nurse performs all self-care for patient) Partly compensatory system (nurse and patient perform patient self-care) Supportive-educative system (nurse helps in overcoming any self-care limitations)

A summary of the needs theorists' conceptualization of nursing is presented in Table 11-7. The focus of this school of thought, then, is on problems and needs of patients as seen by health care providers and on the role of nurses to assess these needs, to fulfill the need requisites. When lower needs are met, more mature needs may emerge (Peplau, 1952). Perceptions of clients, a focus on environment, and the role of nurse–patient interactions in dialogues and intervention are not fully developed.

Table 11-7 ***Needs Theorists—A Summary***

Focus	Problems Nurses' function
Human being	A set of needs or problems A developmental being
Patient	Need deficit
Orientation	Illness, disease
Role of nurse	Dependent on medical practice Beginnings of independent functions Fulfill needs requisites
Decision making	Primarily health care professional

A Second School of Thought: Interaction

A second set of questions was then beginning to be formulated, based on a view of nursing as supporting and promoting interactions with patients. The theorists in this group did not totally ignore the first set of questions; rather, the new sets of questions complemented the first. Whereas the first questions that guided earlier theorists were related to the central one—"What do nurses do?"—the second set of questions evolved from the Yale University School of Nursing and was related to another central question—"How do nurses do whatever it is they do?" Answers to the "how" question focused on the interaction process. Peplau was the pioneer in that group (1952); yet her answer was more congruent with the prevailing interest at the time in psychoanalytic theory and closer to the biomedical model. It is significant when studying the history of ideas to note the connection between the first school of thought at Teachers College and the second one at Yale. The Yale or *interactionist school of thought* grew out of the needs approach, with some of the concepts still prevailing in both; this will be demonstrated in the following discussion. The conceptualization of Imogene King, also a graduate of Teachers College, evolved out of interest in the "how" of nursing care.

Interaction theories were conceived in the late 1950s and early 1960s by theorists who viewed nursing as an interaction process with a focus on the development of a relationship between patients and nurses. These theories grew out of a social milieu in the United States that included the following:

- This was the post-Sputnik era.
- There was a focus on such values as human integrity, as promoted by President Kennedy.
- The Cuban missile crisis may have promoted return to focus on humanity and relationships in fear of outside invasion.
- The beginning formation of hippie groups, communal living, and the flower children indicated a definite need for intimacy and human relations.
- Technological advances continued but with a growing distaste for mechanization and dehumanization.

These theories also reflected the sociocultural forces within the profession of nursing. Nursing was undergoing some significant changes; among them were two that had a direct impact on the development of the interactional theories:

- Federal monies to improve curricula and education of nurse researchers were available.
- A need for integrated curricula arose, freeing psychiatric nurses to identify core concepts and to integrate these concepts throughout nursing curricula, and allowing them to observe and reflect on the process of nursing care in all nursing subspecialties.

Tables 11-8 through 11-13 present theories of the interactionists. Although some of these theorists continued to address the needs of the patient, all the interactionist theorists focused their attention on the process of care and on the ongoing interaction between nurses and clients. Their theories were based on interactionism, phenomenology, and existentialist philosophy.

What did we learn from the interactionists? (See Table 11-13 for a summary of the major components of the interaction theories.)

- Nursing is a deliberate process that can be elucidated.
- Nursing encompasses help and assistance.
- Nursing is an interpersonal process occurring between a person in need of help and a person capable of giving help.
- The nurse, to be able to give help, should clarify her own values, use the self in a therapeutic way, and be involved in the care.
- Care is not a mechanistic act but a humanistic act.
- The humanistic interactionist nurses used existential philosophy, symbolic interaction, and developmental theories to develop their conceptions of nursing.

Table 11-8 ***Interaction Theorists—A View of Nursing***

Theorists	Definitions
King	A process of action, reaction, and interaction whereby nurse and client share information about their perceptions of the nursing situation and agree on goals
Orlando	Interaction with patients who have a need or response to suffering individuals or those anticipating helplessness Assistance to individual to avoid, relieve, diminish, or cure sense of helplessness
Paterson and Zderad	A human dialogue, intersubjective transaction, a shared situation, a transactional process, a presence of both patient and nurse
Peplau	Therapeutic interpersonal, serial, goal-oriented process A health-focused human relationship
Travelbee	An interpersonal process, an assistance to prevent, cope with experiences of illness and suffering, and to find meaning in these experiences
Wiedenbach	Sensing, perceiving, validating patients need for help, ministering help needed in a deliberate, goal-oriented way

Table 11-9 ***Interaction Theorists—Focus of Nursing***

Theorists	Focus of Nursing
King	Nurse–patient interactions that lead to goal attainment in a natural environment
Orlando	Care for the needs of the patients who are distressed, with consideration for perception, thought, and feeling through deliberate action
Paterson and Zderad	Patient is a unique being Patient's perception of events Both patient and nurse are the focus
Peplau	Nurse–patient relationship and its phases Orientation, identification, exploitation, and resolution Harnessing energy from anxiety and tension to positively defining, understanding, and meeting productively the problem at hand
Travelbee	Interpersonal relations, finding meaning in suffering, pain, and illness Self-actualization
Wiedenbach	Patient's perception of condition, care, action

- They defined illness as an inevitable human experience; if one learns to find meaning in it, it will become a growing experience. In this, they differ from the previous group of theorists who defined illness as a deviation that must be corrected.
- They defined nursing as caring, assisting (all other health care professionals), and helping patients to find meaning and actions that increase human potential and better well-being.
- They all indicated that the nurse needs systematic knowledge to help her in assessing, diagnosing, and intervening.
- The nursing process is well developed by these theorists.

Table 11-10 ***Interaction Theorists—Goals of Nursing***

Theorists	Goals of Nursing
King	Help individuals maintain their health so they can function in their role
Orlando	Relieve distress, physical and mental discomfort Improve sense of well-being
Paterson and Zderad	Develop human potential, more well-being for both patient and nurse
Peplau	Develop personality, making illness an eventful experience Forward movement of personality and other ongoing human processes in the direction of creative, constructive, productive personal and community living
Travelbee	Cope with an illness situation and find meaning in the experience Assist patient to accept humanness
Wiedenbach	Meet the needs of an individual experiencing need for help

Table 11-11 Interaction Theorists—Nursing Problems

Theorists	Nursing Problems
King	When nurse and patient do not perceive each other, the situation, or communicate information, transactions are not made, goals are not attained
Orlando	Distress due to unmet needs
Paterson and Zderad	Persons with perceived needs related to the health/illness quality of living
Peplau	Unsuccessful or incomplete learning of life tasks
	Energy used in tensions and frustrations due to unmet needs, opposing goals—giving rise to conflict, aggression, anxiety
	Discomfort, anxiety, doubt, guilt, obsession, compulsion
Travelbee	Lack of support in nurse–patient relationship
	Not finding meaning in illness, transitory discomfort, anguish, malignant despair, apathetic indifference
Wiedenbach	Person with need for help (unmet needs due to physical or inadequate environment)

- Properties, antecedents, and consequences of interactions are advanced by this group of theorists, and all the theories reflect the relationships that are formed to relieve distress as well as those formed to enhance trust.
- These theories mark the beginning of a movement that led toward the patient becoming an equal partner in the nursing process.
- The interactionist nurse considers uniqueness, dignity, and worth values of patients as important in the development of wellness. A view of an autonomous individual with individually established norms was beginning to emerge. Help, it was emphasized, was to be tailored to individual needs.
- Properties of interaction as validation (Wiedenbach), as meeting the needs of patients (Orlando), as being totally present, and as relating to others (Paterson and Zderad) are delineated and defined by this group of theorists.
- The theories concede that perception of the patient is important in assessing illness and its meaning.

Table 11-12 Interaction Theorists—Nursing Therapeutics

Theorists	Nursing Therapeutics
King	Goal attainment, transaction, perceptual validation
Orlando	Deliberate nursing process not automatic
Paterson and Zderad	Humanness—use of nurse's self, existentially nurturing, being, relating, meeting, maximum participation
Peplau	Development of problem-solving skills through the interpersonal process (educational, therapeutic, and collaborative)
Travelbee	Use of nurse's self, original encounter, emerging identities, empathy, sympathy, rapport
Wiedenbach	Ministration of help, validation, rational, reactional, and deliberate

Table 11-13 ***Interaction Theorists—A Summary***

Focus	Nurse–patient interactions Illness as an experience
Human being	Interacting being A set of needs Can validate needs Human experience with meanings
Patient	Helpless being A human experience with meaning
Orientation	Illness/disease
Role of nurse	Deliberate helping process Self as a therapeutic agent Use of the nursing process
Decision making	Primarily health care professional Validated by clients

- The major nurse–patient interaction relationship goal is derived from their observation that the person in need of help becomes distressed; the purpose is to prevent or deal with this distress.
- The interactionist theorist reminds us that the nurse is a human being who needs to self-reflect to understand her own values. Without such understanding, the nurse will not be able to be a human being who cares, gives care, establishes connections, and helps patients relieve their distress.
- The theorists tentatively introduced the notion of effect of environment on patients. To them, unmet needs of the patient develop because of:
  - Physical limitations (from incomplete development, temporary or permanent disability, or restrictions in environment)
  - Adverse reactions to inadequate environment (Orlando)
- This group of theorists reintroduced the significance of nurses' intuition and subjectivity in the nursing act.
- Some common assumptions guided the development of the interactionist theories. These are:
  - The integrity of an individual has to be maintained.
  - Individuals have self-awareness and are therefore able to identify their needs.
  - Individuals strive toward actualization.
  - Events in life are human experiences inevitable and essential in helping to move to the next stage in development.
  - The nurse cannot separate herself as an individual from the act of care—the nurse is an integral part of care.
- Interaction theorists provided nursing with a new perspective:
  - There is a reciprocal assessment process.
  - Patient perspective is significant in health care.
  - Situation determines needs and care.
  - Patients are helpless and suffer due to illness.

A number of concepts were identified by the interaction theorists as central to nursing. These concepts remain significant components of interaction in nursing:

Sensing
Perceiving
Validating
Existential transactions
Goal orientation of interaction
Nurses' self-development

Interaction theories neither addressed nor focused on:

A more complete view of a human being (human beings are interacting beings with a minimal focus on biopsychocultural focus)
A view of the environment, except tangentially in some instances

A Third School of Thought: Outcomes

The third set of questions that nurse theorists asked was related to the central question—the "why" of nursing care. Although not ignoring the "what" and "how" questions, this group of theorists attempted to conceptualize the outcome of nursing care and then described the recipient of care. The image of nursing as portrayed by this group of theorists is that of concern over outcomes and end results of the caring processes. Two of the most influential theorists in this group are Dorothy Johnson and Martha Rogers. They graduated from Harvard and Johns Hopkins, respectively, but did most of their work at opposite ends of the North American continent—New York and Los Angeles. This East/West school of thought is referred to in this book as the outcome school of thought.

Johnson influenced theoretical thinking in nursing, and her theory will influence nursing more in the future than it did in the past as the goals of nursing become more congruent with stability than change (Hall, 1983). Rogers, on the other hand, has helped to shape nursing research that is based on theoretical thinking. Neither theory is as developed as that of Sister Callista Roy who, as nursing director of Mount St. Mary's (Los Angeles, California), had the faculty resources to implement her theory into courses and content, thereby helping in turn to operationalize the theory further. Both Johnson and Rogers, with faculty members of the University of California, Los Angeles, and New York University, respectively, have also partially operationalized their theories, but not to the same extent. The publications of Roy on uses of theory in practice have enhanced the use of her theory in several schools of nursing. Myra Levine, who views the goals of nursing as conservation of energy, also belongs in this group.

This group of theorists (Tables 11-14 through 11-18) conceptualized the goal of nursing care as bringing back some balance, stability, and preservation of energy or enhancing harmony between the individual and the environment. They based their conceptualizations on system, adaptation, and developmental theories. They directed their focus on the outcome of care. Their view of a human being and the nursing client incorporated the need theorists' conceptualization of the human being. (The goals of sub-

Table 11-14. ***Outcome Theorists—A View of Nursing***

Theorists	Definitions of Nursing
Johnson	External regulatory force acting to preserve the organization and integration of patient's behavior at an optimal level when behavior is a threat to social, physical health or illness
Levine	Patient advocacy, devotion to humanity and self-respect of patient, perception and support for personal and individualized needs, compassion, commitment, and protection
Rogers	Humanistic science for maintaining and promoting health, preventing illness, caring for and rehabilitating the sick and disabled
Roy	Theoretical system of knowledge viewing client as biopsychosocial being (ill or potentially so) who adapts to changing environment Nurse acts through nursing process to promote adaptation

Table 11-15 ***Outcome Theorists—Focus on Nursing***

Theorists	Focus of Nursing
Johnson	Man as a behavioral system with subsystems, each having a structure, a function, and functional imperatives (drive, set, behavior) and each requiring protection, stimulation, and nurturance
Levine	Four principles guide conception of human being (energy, personal, structural, and social integrities) and their organismic responses (fear, inflammation, stress, sensory) Nursing is conservation of energy and integrities
Rogers	Life processes of human beings, unitary person–environment energy fields, complementarity, resonance, and helicy
Roy	Focal, contextual, and residual stimuli and their effect on the cognator and regulator mechanisms, in turn effecting four adaptive modes: physiologic, self-concept, role function, and interdependence

Table 11-16 ***Outcome Theorists—Goals of Nursing***

Theorists	Goals of Nursing
Johnson	Behavioral system balance, subsystems that function efficiently and effectively
Levine	Conservation of energy and integrities (personal, structural, social), restoration of well-being and independent activity
Rogers	Promote symphonic interaction and harmony between man and environment Strengthen coherence and integrity of human field
Roy	Promote person's adaptation in physiologic needs, self-concept, role function, and interdependence

systems of behavior of Johnson's theory and adaptive modes by Roy have parallels in the hierarchy of needs by Henderson, nursing functions by Abdellah, and universal needs by Orem.) Although they spoke of harmony with the environment, stability, conservation of energy, and homeostasis as potential outcomes, the consequences are at a high level of abstraction, limiting utility of theories in outcome measures. The outcome theories provide nursing with a well articulated conception of a human being as a nursing client and of nursing as an external regulatory mechanism (Table 11-19).

Table 11-17 ***Outcome Theorists—Nursing Problems***

Theorists	Nursing Problems
Johnson	Structural functional stress in one subsystem (insufficiency, discrepancy) and between subsystems (incompatibility, dominance)
Levine	Response to fear, response to stress, inflammatory response, sensory response
Rogers	Disruptions in organization and structure of interacting human environment fields
Roy	Ineffective coping mechanisms causing ineffective responses that disrupt the integrity of the person

Table 11-18 ***Outcome Theorists—Nursing Therapeutics***

Theorists	Nursing Therapeutics
Johnson	Inhibition, constriction, supplementation, protection, nurturing (supportive/maintenance, teaching, counseling, and behavior modification)
Levine	Therapeutic—alter course of adaptation Supportive—maintain course of adaptation
Rogers	Repatterning of human environment fields or assistance in mobilizing inner resources
Roy	Manipulation of focal, residual, and contextual stimuli with patient's zone of positive coping

Table 11-19 ***Outcome Theorists—A Summary***

Focus	Energy Balance, stability, homeostasis presentation Outcome of care
Human being	Adaptive and developmental being
Patient	Lack of adaptation Systems deficiency
Orientation	Illness, disease
Role of nurse	External regulatory mechanism
Decision making	Primarily health care provider

Theories' Primary Focus

Nursing theories are further classified in this text in terms of the primary focus in the theory. In classifying theories for analysis, it is assumed that each classification system adds more understanding to each theory. Correspondence between each of the classification systems is neither presented nor discussed in this text. You may wish to consider the relationship between the different classification systems.

In reviewing the theories for classification, central domain concepts, central questions the theory addresses, and the areas that seem to be most developed were some of the conditions used as a guideline for theory classification. Four central focuses emerged from this review: clients, person–environment interactions, interactions, and nursing therapeutics. Although theories may appear to fit in more than one of these areas, my decision to place a theory in a particular area in this text was based on the *primary* focus in the theory.

Johnson, Roy, and Neuman focused their theoretical development on the *client* or the client system. These theories provide a comprehensive analysis of the client as seen from a nursing perspective. Although health and environment may have been discussed in various degrees, these concepts do not appear to be as well developed or as central to these theories. Hence, Johnson, Roy, and Neuman were classified as client-focused theories, and they appear in Chapter 15.

Rogers' central focus is on the relationship between clients and their environment. In fact, clients in Rogers' theory are the environment, and one cannot be assessed in isolation from the other. Rogers' theory is one of the most supportive of the centrality of environment in the mission of the discipline of nursing. Hence, it was classified under person–environment interactions and is analyzed in Chapter 16.

The properties, the components, and the nature of the interactions between clients and nurses were the focus of several theoretical formulations. King, Orlando, Paterson and Zderad, Travelbee, and Wiedenbach concentrated on nurse–patient interactions and considered them the focus of nursing. These theories are evaluated in Chapter 17.

What nurses should do and under what circumstances these actions should be delivered were the focus of theoretical formulations in Levine's and Orem's theories. These theories are therefore evaluated as theories that could provide nurses with frameworks for *intervention*. Unlike client-oriented theories that are more effective in providing nurses with a framework for assessment, intervention theories provide nurses with guidelines for intervention. These theories are evaluated in Chapter 18.

Images of Nurses and the Roles They Play

The preceding analyses suggest that nurses focus on different aspects of care at different times or for different purposes. Nursing is not exemplified by one group of theories more than another at all times. Rather, the situation may dictate when nursing should focus on needs, interaction, or outcomes. Newman (1983) makes the following point:

> One of the factors determining the applicability of a theory is the temporal frame of reference. For example, if one is viewing a relatively short time frame, the adaptation model might apply, whereas in a longer time frame, phenomena would be apparent that could not be explained by adaptation alone (p. 391).

Nurses play different roles at different times and project different images, and the nursing theories have helped to suggest the different images and the roles that nurses play. Need-oriented nurses are actively doing and functioning; they rely on problem solving, they carefully plan their interventions, and they evaluate their work mainly (but not only) by the activities performed.

Interaction-oriented nurses rely on the process of interaction and include themselves in the sphere of other actions; they use themselves therapeutically and evaluate their actions primarily in terms of interactions. Interaction-oriented nurses rely more on counseling, guiding, and teaching—helping clients find meanings in their situations—and less on doing and functioning. Among the interactionists are the existentialists who focus on the support and development of the human potential. That potential includes, for both the nurse and the client, the goal of authentic being, the process of creating options, and an openness to present and future experiences.

Outcome-oriented nurses focus on the goals of maintaining and promoting energy and harmony with the environment and on enhancing the development of healthy environments. Outcome nurses do not include themselves as therapeutic agents; they enact the healing roles but do not necessarily consider authentic being as essential in the healing processes. The roles and images of nurses that are reflected in the different groups of nursing theories are summarized in Table 11-20.

Areas of Agreement Among and Between Theorists and Schools of Thought

Nursing theories have been considered in terms of their contrasting and competitive views. In the first section of this chapter, an attempt was made to address how they may complement each other as theories and as different schools of thought. In this section, areas of agreement among the various schools of thought are identified.

- Nursing theories offer a beginning articulation of what nursing is and what roles nurses play.
- Nursing theories offer a view of the philosophical underpinnings in nursing (eg, interaction, phenomenology, and existentialism).
- Nursing theories provide descriptions of how to help patients become comfortable, how to deliver treatment with the least damage, and how to enhance high-level wellness.
- Nursing theories offer a beginning common language and a beginning agreement about who the nursing care recipients are.
- It is obvious that we should not view the recipients only through biologic glasses (as biologic systems) or psychological glasses (as id, ego, and superego), but rather through holistic glasses. Nursing clients are more than the sum total of their psychological, sociological, cultural, or biologic parts.
- Recipients of care respond to events in a holistic way.
- The recipient is a member of a reference group set, and interventions are only meaningful if the whole unit is considered.
- Recipients have needs, and nursing assists them in meeting those needs.

The theories have other themes in common. These emerge when one considers images evolving from the theories when compared with nursing realities. In this process, several concepts emerge as central to nursing. These are addressed in the following conclusion.

Table 11-20 ***Roles and Images of Nurses in Different Categories of Theories***

Theorists	Roles Nurses Play	Image
NEEDS THEORISTS		
Abdellah	Problem solver and performer of 21 physiologic and psychosocial activities for the patient	They provide an image of a nurse who is active and busy working and a patient who is striving for independence. The nurse's work is focused on doing a deliberate and well planned activity.
Henderson	Complementing, supplementing knowledge The will to perform daily activities	
Orem	Temporary self-care agent for universal health deviation and development of self-care needs	
INTERACTION THEORISTS		
King	Goal attainer or else! Teach, counsel, guide, give care, gather information, set mutual goals	They provide an image of a nurse as a present-oriented, situational, a humanist, a process-oriented professional whose interest is the interaction and, for some, also the person. The nurse, to some, is also important in the interaction.
Orlando	Deliberate, repetitive, and situational interactions	
Paterson and Zderad	Existentialist and phenomenological nurturer of the human potential (self and patient)	
Peplau	Freudian helper Stranger who works hard to become a surrogate	
Travelbee	Meaning finder (more than a dictionary meaning) and existentialist	
Wiedenbach	Deliberate helper who focuses on extrasensory perception and does not forget to validate the process	
OUTCOME THEORISTS		
Johnson	The external manipulator: external regulatory force to preserve organization and integration of patient's behavior Controller	They provide an image of the nurse as goal setter, a futurist, environmentalist, who has extrasensory and energy preservation powers.
Levine	Conservator of all	
Rogers	The environmental nurse, the symphony player: promotion of person–environment interaction The healer without touch	
Roy	The pace setter: external regulatory force to modify stimuli affecting adaptation to create four modes of adaptation	

Conclusion

The domain of nursing deals with people who are assumed to be in constant interaction with their environment and yet have unmet needs, are not able to care for themselves, or are not adapting to the environment due to interruptions or potential interruptions in health. The domain of nursing focuses on therapeutics to help in meeting the needs of the person and to enhance adaptation capability, self-care ability, health, and well-being. Nursing theories capture and reflect different visions of this domain; they mirror different aspects of nursing realities as they are and as they ought to be. The mission of nursing, the processes by which nursing care is provided, and the images of nursing portrayed in these theories continue to be shared by nurses around the globe. Considering the theories in the categories presented in this chapter may lead to many productive explorations and explanations of the processes of clinical judgment and clinical decision making.

REFERENCES

Bijou, J.W. and Baer, D.M. (1961). *Child development: A systematic and empirical theory.* New York: Appleton-Century-Crofts.

Erikson, E.H. (1963). *Childhood and society* (2nd ed.). New York: W.W. Norton.

Freud, S. (1949). *An outline of psychoanalysis.* New York: W.W. Norton.

Hall, B. (1983). Toward an understanding of stability in nursing phenomena. *Advances in Nursing Science,* 5(3), 15–20.

Howland, D. and McDowell, W.E. (1964). Measurement of patient care: A conceptual framework. *Nursing Research,* 13(1), 4–7.

Johnson, D.E. (1968). *One conceptual model of nursing.* Paper presented at Vanderbilt University, Nashville, TN.

Johnson, D.E. (1974). Development of theory: A requisite for nursing as a primary health profession. *Nursing Research,* 23(5), 372–377.

Maslow, A.H. (1954). *Motivation and personality.* New York: Harper & Row.

Newman, M. (1983). The continuing revolution: A history of nursing science. In N. Chaska (Ed.), *The nursing profession: A time to speak.* New York: McGraw-Hill.

Orlando, I.J. (1961). *The dynamic nurse—patient relationship.* New York: G.P. Putnam's Sons.

Peplau, H. (1952). *Interpersonal relations in nursing.* New York: G.P. Putnam's Sons.

Rogers, C. (1959). A theory of therapy, personality, interpersonal relations as developed in a client-centered framework. In J. Koch (Ed.), *Psychology: A study of a science* (Vol. 3). New York: McGraw-Hill.

Rogers, M.E. (1970). *An introduction to the theoretical basis of nursing.* Philadelphia: F.A. Davis.

Roy, C. (1970, March). Adaptation: A conceptual framework for nursing. *Nursing Outlook,* 18, 42–48.

Sullivan, H. (1953). *The interpersonal theory of psychiatry.* New York: W.W. Norton.

Wiedenbach, E. (1964). *Clinical nursing: A helping art.* New York: Springer-Verlag.

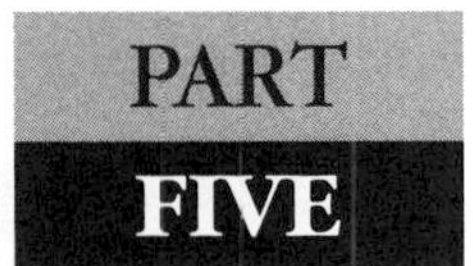

Our Epistemology

Many strategies for the development of theory have been identified, discussed, and presented in the nursing literature. In the beginning, these strategies were borrowed without modifications from other disciplines. We have become more comfortable with our own identity and with the nature of our discipline, and as a result, we have considered our own discipline-specific epistemological approaches while engaging in ontological analyses of the discipline.

In this part of the book, you will find both historical and more current approaches to theory development. In Chapter 12 strategies and processes for the development of concepts are delineated and discussed. Examples are provided for the use of each one of the strategies as they appeared in the nursing literature during the 1980s and 1990s. Because of the nature of nursing and its connections to clinical practice, a more integrated approach to the development of concepts is also described.

Chapter 13 describes and analyzes four strategies that have been used in the development of theories in nursing. These are: (1) the theory–practice–theory strategy, (2) the practice–theory strategy, (3) the research–theory strategy, and (4) the theory–research–theory strategy. The chapter ends with a proposed strategy offered as another option, a modified practice–theory–research–theory strategy. Exemplars are offered for each strategy to help you better understand the strategy in actual use.

Chapter 14 reviews previous models used in describing, analyzing, critiquing, and testing theories and proposes a model congruent with current trends and philosophies in nursing.

CHAPTER 12

Strategies for Concept Development

The theoretical development of the discipline of nursing began with the broad question of "What is nursing?" and resulted in numerous inclusive theories that attempted to answer the question by identifying the mission and the goals of nursing. This was followed by the attempts of metatheorists to define the structure of the discipline, the strategies, and the tools for the development of knowledge. One important stage that followed is concept development. The development of concepts is a significant stage in a discipline's progress. Processes used in the development of concepts in nursing have received considerable attention during the last two decades of the 20th century and, in turn, the use of these strategies made major contributions to advancing the development of concepts that reflect the nature of the discipline of nursing (Rodgers and Knafl, 1993; Walker and Avant, 1995).

One important premise is that concepts guide what we see and are essential in giving some order to situations and events. Evolving concepts result from early experiences; their definitions and meanings reflect the theorists' educational background and the theoretical bases for their work. The interactionist theorists look at a nurse–patient situation and focus on interaction, role taking, symbols, and roles. Another theorist who has a psychoanalytical lens may explain the same situation through such concepts as denial, repression, latent hostility, and maternal or paternal conflict. Before we had a concept called "burnout," we did not see burnout, even though the syndrome may have existed in one form or another. We did not have a label to give to that constellation of behaviors; we did not have a reservoir in which we could connect and deposit those seemingly discrete feelings of apathy, demonstrations of irritability and impatience, and the urge to flee and change one's life. Therefore, describing the varied behaviors and actions related to them may have been limited and somewhat ineffective. For example, there is no burnout described by people living in the Middle East; that is, there is no such concept even though the experiences and the responses may exist and may have always been there, but it may not be described as concisely or be dealt with as effectively. Labeling a concept should not be considered permanent or static. It should be a dynamic process that is responsive to new knowledge, experiences, perceptions, and data. In a human science discipline, participants should be able to articulate and label new concepts or redefine existing concepts.

Some confusion has surrounded concept development, and it has been used interchangeably with concept analysis and concept clarification. The beginnings of concept analysis in nursing can be traced to Wilson (1963, 1969), whose processes were used as the only guidelines for nurses' attempts at identifying and describing concepts. Walker and Avant's (1988, 1995) thoughtful strategies for concept and theory development, derivation, and integration further clarified the process and demonstrated its multidimensionality. These pioneering efforts were followed by the introduction of other options that made the processes of concept development more congruent with the nature of the discipline of nursing as a human and caring science (Rodgers and Knafl, 1993). Each new strategy was developed to reflect the perspective of nursing as holistic and interactive and with the natural domain of nursing and its dynamic concepts (Rodgers, 1989; Schwartz-Barcott and Kim, 1986; Wuest, 1994). The introduction of options in the development of concepts allowed for more congruency with style and format of the agents of knowledge development, as well as goals and levels of existing knowledge in the discipline of nursing.

In this chapter, I provide a framework for the different strategies and approaches used for the development of concepts. I also discuss the different components of concept development and describe the strategies for concept development that are useful for future development of concepts, particularly those that are more suitable for developing phenomena from clinical practice.

The three major strategies for concept development are concept exploration, concept clarification, and concept analysis. These strategies are used in the development of concepts in nursing. Each strategy uses different processes to achieve its goals. Each is described below.

Concept Exploration

Concept exploration is one strategy for concept development used when new concepts are identified and before they become an accepted component of the nursing lexicon. Similarly, a concept may have been accepted in the dailiness of nurses' experiences, yet because of its embeddedness in the nursing experience, its existence and properties are normalized, camouflaging and limiting its growth and meanings. Concept exploration is a strategy used when a concept has only recently been introduced in the literature and it is too early to articulate its definite properties and potential explanatory power. Exploration of a concept presupposes that it is an unknown concept to the readers of nursing literature or that it is such a familiar concept that it has been taken for granted, to the extent that members of the discipline are not aware of its significance to the development of knowledge. Concept exploration is also appropriate for concepts that have been uncritically adopted in nursing from other disciplines without consideration for the values, assumptions, and missions of a discipline (eg, see the concept of empathy in Morse, Anderson, Bottorff, Yonge, O'Brien, Solberg, and McIlveen [1992]). It is the process by which a phenomenon is identified and introduced to colleagues to raise their consciousness about the phenomenon, to claim its importance and significance for nursing, and to stimulate the members of the discipline to consider it further in their research. Another goal for concept exploration is to nurture curiosity about a particular concept. When a concept is introduced into the literature through concept exploration, the author should be raising and answering questions about its relevance to nursing and its meaning to nursing clients. Concept exploration is used when concepts are still ambiguous and the relationship to the discipline of nursing is still at the preliminary stages of consideration.

Concept exploration includes identifying the major components and dimensions of the concept with appropriate questions raised about each component, and triggers are proposed to continue the exploration process. Advantages to the discipline or nursing practice are identified and defined. The ultimate goal in concept exploration is to demonstrate whether or not there is the potential for further development of this concept. It is also to build a case for reasons to continue or discontinue with such explorations. Concept explorations are essential in a dynamic and changing discipline that is responsive to global, societal, and individual changes. It maintains the dynamism and the responsiveness of the discipline.

Two examples of concept exploration are Norris's (1985) proposal of the concept of "primitive pleasure" as the basic human need and as a possible goal for nursing to nurture, preserve, and attend to in human beings. In proposing to give attention to primitive pleasure, she questioned physiologic homeostasis as a goal for nursing practice. She explored primitive pleasure as sensual, sensory, and carnal as compared to cognitive and aesthetic. She defined pleasure as bodily pleasure at the basic and reflexive level and less at the intellectual level. Although it may call on some cognitive processes to perceive these pleasures, it reflects a certain level of awareness and consciousness and does not require any cognitive processes to experience it or to modify it. Norris explored the meaning of this concept and its relationship to nursing, indicating that nurses' work has always included a focus on enhancing patients' pleasure by helping them to feel comfortable through touch and through other sensory stimuli. By offering a clinical exemplar to demonstrate the potential of better understanding patients' needs through the concept of primitive pleasure, she further supported her claim for the need to explore the development of this concept. However, because her goal was to raise nurses' consciousness to the competing goal of heightened pleasure as compared with maintaining homeostasis, the major questions that she was answering were what it is and what potential it has for nursing. She proposed that the range of patterned experiences to demonstrate it must be identified and examined. She also looked at other writings in nursing to document and support her arguments for developing the constellation of subconcepts related to primitive pleasures. She further explored the concept by examining others' seminal writing such as Nightingale, who almost a century earlier proposed promoting pleasure of the Crimean War patients. The ultimate goal for concept exploration is for a reader or a listener to say "this is worth considering and developing further."

Another example of exploration is provided by Laborde (1989) who proposed to consider the concept of torture as a nursing concern. She described the nature of the concept and situated the concept within the domain of nursing and within health care. In reviewing this exploration, a reader realizes that nurses can have different experiences of torture; they can be the subjects of torture, they may participate in torture, either willingly or unwillingly, and they may care for patients who have been tortured. Therefore, there is a need for further development of knowledge related to this concept, its implications in health care of tortured individuals, and the roles that nurses play.

These two examples demonstrate what I mean by concept exploration. In neither example was the concept ready for a full-fledged concept analysis nor for the development of any propositions. Both raised consciousness, both made the reader curious about their meanings and implications, both connected the concepts of nursing to the proposition, both challenged some levels of the status quo about what nurses need to know, and both provided support for why the concept is worth further development. These processes are essential for concept exploration and concept exploration is a strategy for concept development.

Concept Clarification

Concept clarification may be used to refine concepts that have been used in nursing without a clear, shared, and conscious agreement on the properties or the meanings attributed to the concept. The goal of concept clarification is to refine existing definitions, refine theoretical definitions, consider interrelationships between the different elements of the concept, and discover new relationships and discuss these relationships to resolve existing conflicts about meaning and definitions. Concept clarification was defined by Kramer (1993) as "a highly creative, rigorous, and intuitive process that can generate multiple useful meanings for a single concept" (p. 407). This strategy includes processes of inclusion and exclusion where attempts are made to define what could be included and what could be excluded in the foundation, the meaning, and the attributes of the concept. One useful process is to clarify boundaries, to define contexts, and to define other subconcepts surrounding concepts that are being clarified. Concept clarification reduces ambiguity; yet clarification includes a critical review of the properties of a concept, illuminating new dimensions to it that had not been considered beforehand, widening the sphere of the concept beyond previous views, while narrowing the boundaries for better definition to support its further development. Processes in concept clarification include comparing, contrasting, delineating and differentiating, providing exemplars, identifying assumptions and philosophical bases, identifying what events trigger the phenomena, and proposing questions from a nursing perspective. Answers to these questions further develop the concept. In concept clarification, the implications for nursing research, theory, and practice are carefully discussed.

According to Norris (1982), concept clarification has five steps:

1. After identification of the concept from within the discipline, as well as consideration of how it could be considered through the lens of other disciplines, repeatedly describe the phenomenon inherent in the concept.
2. Systemize the observations and the descriptions of the phenomenon. Establish categories and hierarchy, continue to observe, discover, communicate, think about the concept, and develop insights. Look for patterns and sequences of events. Ask and answer such questions as: What events trigger the phenome-

non? What happened before to inspire the phenomenon? What happened as a result of the phenomenon?

3. Develop operational definitions and ask yourself and others: How will I know the concept when I see it?
4. Construct a model.
5. Develop hunches and hypotheses.

All strategies and processes for concept development are based on the ability of the developer to use critical thinking skills. Kramer (1993) and Chinn and Kramer (1991) made a compelling argument for the connection between critical thinking and concept clarification and for the rationale that concept clarification is a strategy that could enhance critical thinking. They identified several steps toward clarifying concepts, each with several processes; these are: formulating the purposes of clarification, selecting and synthesizing data sources, and developing a conceptualization. In clarifying concepts, the theorist identifies and examines assumptions, identifies and analyzes contexts, provides multiple interpretations and engages in reflective analysis of the results.

Concept clarification does not require the development of contrary cases, propositions, hypotheses, antecedents, or consequences, which are essential processes in concept analysis. A clarified concept stimulates thinking and explains an aspect of nursing (Mairis, 1994). Concept clarification in nursing must be connected to health and to the goals of nursing. Concept clarification includes literature reviews and analysis of the literature to identify values and attributes and to compare and contrast the properties that may have been defined.

I believe that the processes of concept clarification described above may have contributed to the identification of the different meanings and conceptualizations of caring. Morse, Solberg, Neander, Bottorff, and Johnson (1990) explored caring and described the different ways in which it appeared in the literature. They clarified caring by its epistemological perspectives, which resulted in five conceptualizations: caring as a human trait, as an emotion, as a moral imperative, as a mutual endeavor, or as a therapeutic intervention.

Hall, Stevens, and Meleis (1994) introduced a concept to the nursing literature that had been taken for granted, was accepted and used, yet its conscious use was limited. They defined marginalization as "the process through which persons are peripheralized on the basis of their identities, associations, experiences, and environments" (p. 25). Marginalization is defined as being away from the center, being at the borders or the periphery. It is being a part of the periphery of social networks. They defined its properties as intermediacy, differentiation, power, secrecy, voice, and liminality (perceptions of time, world, and self-image and its relationship to experiences). Each of these properties is defined, discussed, and related to the concept as a whole. They clarified the central components (peripheralization), some salient properties (associations), and some conditions (it is a process). They differentiated it from alienation (focused on subjective experience), from stigmatization (one aspect), and from segregation (more physically oriented). Furthermore, marginalization is differentiated from vulnerability and from oppression.

Absent from this analysis were those processes used in developing exemplars and contrary cases. However, the authors made a case for the significance of the concept for nursing research, nursing practice, and the theoretical development of the discipline. The concept is studied in the discipline of nursing, and a case was made for its relevance to further knowledge development. One significant aspect of this concept is its origin and the process by which it is clarified. It is not a new concept. It has been used interchangeably with a number of other concepts including vulnerability; therefore, the authors set out to clarify it and to propose its centrality in nursing. It evolved from individual research programs dealing with low-income women or women without incomes and their access to health care, patterns of self-care, lesbians' patterns of responses and relationships in the health care system, lesbians living with or dealing with substance abuse, low-income women with human immunodeficiency virus, and lesbians dealing with sexual abuse. The common thread in all of these programs of research was the intense marginalizing experiences of women, which prompted the authors to take a closer look at the concept and its meanings and potential for further development. The other important aspect of this example of concept clarification is the collaborative effort of the authors/researchers and its influence on clarifying a concept transcending time, geography, and setting.

A third example of concept clarification is provided by Beeber and Schmitt (1986) in their clarification of the concept of group cohesiveness. Although this is a concept that has been previously described, discussed, and studied, the authors developed a case for its relevance to nursing, for reexamining and redefining the potential contribution of nurses to the development of theory related to this concept. In clarifying the concept, they added a new perspective that allowed the questioning of the positive values that were automatically granted to this concept. Their critical examination of a broader view of its meaning, allowing the exploration of both the negative and positive, made the process more of a clarification process and less of an analysis process. The authors provided a history of the definition, identified the diffusion of the concept and the ambiguities inherent in the existing definitions, defined its properties, reviewed relevant literature in other disciplines, critically analyzed the use of group cohesiveness in the nursing literature, and provided alternative uses for it in nursing research and theory building for introducing students to group work, for further developing precise measures, and for the development of clinical indicators among other uses.

Concept Analysis

In using concept analysis processes for the development of concepts, the assumption is that the concepts have been introduced in the literature, that they have been defined and clarified, but they are in need of further analysis to move them to the next level of development. Concepts are analyzed when their significance is established and their relationship to the discipline of nursing has been clarified. Analysis implies breaking down to well defined components; it reflects building and rebuilding and presumes the essential components are identified and defined. The goal of the analysis is to bring the concept closer to use in research or clinical practice. Concept analysis contributes also to instrument development and theory testing (Davis, 1992). Processes inherent in concept analysis include answering some significant questions and raising some new pertinent questions.

Several strategies have been used in the nursing literature for analyzing concepts: the Wilson method, the simultaneous concept analysis strategy, the hybrid, and the integrated strategy for concept development. Each is described briefly.

Wilson's Method of Concept Analysis

One of the most cited references for concept analysis is Wilson's (1963/1969) method. The variations on this method have been described by Chinn and Kramer (1991) and Walker and Avant (1995) among other scholars in nursing. Wilson identified eleven steps to use in concept analysis.

1. Identify what the questions are for the concept. He describes three different sets of questions. The first set is questions related to facts. He proposes that these questions should be answered by existing knowledge about the concept. The second set of questions involves those related to values about the concept. These need to be answered based on moral principles of the 'shoulds' and 'should nots' as determined by society or other important bodies that influence moral judgment in a discipline. The third set of questions is related to meanings; these are best considered in terms of concepts. Questions related to concepts are of this third type; they do not concern facts or values.
2. Consider the possible answers to the questions and identify the essential elements of these questions. The goal here is clarity of communication of answers and elements.
3. Identify and describe exemplars to reflect the different critical and essential characteristics of the concept. Identify the typical features as well as those that may not be so typical. The question he proposes answering here is: "If that is not an example of it, then nothing is."
4. Identify "contrary cases," that is, those exemplars that do not include any of the properties of the concept. Just as with exemplary cases, the contrary cases may be the extreme opposites of the exemplars in that the concept is not readily visible or apparent. These are cases in which the concept and its properties are absent.
5. Identify, describe, and use some related cases in which the concept may be connected or similar in some way, or as it occurs in similar texts. Analyze which features are essential and which are not.
6. Provide borderline cases as exemplars. Select exemplars that may have some features or attributes of the concept and in which ambiguity exists about whether the case belongs to the concept or not. Particularly consider cases that are difficult to classify. The purpose of these cases is that they help in further development of the concept.
7. Develop and present invented cases. Wilson promoted the idea of developing a situation that is an invention to exemplify the typical features and properties

for the concept. The context for the invented case may be different, the exemplar may be totally out of the ordinary, and the method for recounting the case should be innovative. These invented cases are developed to highlight or enhance the major features of the concept. Examples may be found in poetry and in fables.

8. Identify and define the social contexts and analyze concepts as to who may use it, why it may be used, and how it could be used.
9. Beware of underlying anxiety related to concepts or generated by the concepts. Wilson encourages identifying, describing, and analyzing the feelings attached to the concept. What he means is identifying any controversy related to the concept, whether it has any stigma attached to it, and what debates exist related to it.
10. Define and explain the potential practical results related to the concept. The practical uses of the concept need to be defined and identified, and a breakdown of its essential elements and their relationship to practice should be defined.
11. Choose the language for describing the results and the label carefully. Finally, Wilson recommends a decision on the best words to use to reflect the concept and its meaning.

There are many variations in nursing to Wilson's method (Avant, 1993). An example is analysis of pain management. Pain management is accepted in nursing as an integral component of nurses' mission in providing nursing care to clients. The meaning of this concept is varied and the goals are numerous. It could be based on a value system of reciprocity, patriarchy, or collaboration. Davis (1992) used a concept analysis strategy to identify the role of involvement of patients in managing their own pain. Based on Walker and Avant's (1995) strategies, she examined the patients' perceptions of pain management, explored the different definitions offered in the literature, defined the concept's attributes, developed an exemplary case, identified border and related cases, and identified ways by which pain management could be empirically referenced in clinical situations. The analysis led to providing the bases for patient involvement in the caring processes.

Similarly, Hawks' (1991) analysis of power resulted in identifying the properties of power as "power to" versus "power over" and in the development of a conceptual map that contains the different components inherent in power (sources, skills, orientation) and the role of self-confidence in attaining the goals. The systematic analyses for both these concepts may result in giving direction for further development of the concepts and the potential for more systematic research. The ultimate result is developing theories that are client sensitive and client responsive.

Simultaneous Concept Analysis

Many concepts in nursing are interrelated and overlapping; notice, for example, interaction, communication, relating, and reciprocity, among others. The concepts of change, transition, coping, and adapting also have many common and uncommon attributes. One innovative and discipline-congruent strategy for analyzing concepts is the simultaneous analysis strategy used by Haase, Britt, Coward, Leidy, and Penn (1992) in analyzing spiritual perspective, hope, acceptance, and self-transcendence. This strategy is based on collaboration, critical thinking, expertise of participants, complementarity, mutual trust building, and mutual consensus building. These are attributes congruent with the nature of nursing as a human science and a caring discipline.

Colleagues interested in similar or different concepts may join efforts to clarify their concepts in relationship to a larger whole, and in the process, they clarify others' concepts and increase the clarity of the concept based on the common root of the related concepts. Although most other strategies used a more individual approach to concept development, the simultaneous concept analysis is based on a value system of connectedness and collaboration (Haase, Britt, Coward, Leidy, and Penn, 1992). Individual analysis, thinking, and conceptualizing form the first building blocks for this strategy. Antecedents, critical attributes, and outcomes for each concept are first identified and defined. Similarities and differences in attributes, antecedents, and consequences are then identified to create what the authors called a validity matrix.

The group reviews, compares, and contrasts the result of their development of the similar components with each original concept and engages in critical assessment with particular attention to language, semantics, meanings, and goals. This process continues until some shared agreement is achieved and a visual diagram or table is constructed to reflect this agreement. This strategy supports the potential of refining concepts and developing them further.

The Hybrid Strategy

This strategy synthesizes empirical approaches with theoretical approaches. Schwartz-Barcott and Kim (1986, 1993) developed this method. This is another strategy more congruent with the evolving nature of methodology in nursing research that combines quantitative and qualitative methods. The hybrid strategy is also based on Wilson's (1963, 1969) concept analysis strategy and Schatzman and Strauss's (1973) grounded theory approaches.

Schwartz-Barcott and Kim identified three major phases. The first is the theoretical phase, the second is the field work, and the third is the analytical phase. These phases are not sequential or linear; work can be ongoing in each one and in all simultaneously. In the theoretical phase, the theorist defines a concept, searches the literature, identifies meaning and measurement issues, and selects a working definition. In the field work phase, the theorist sets the stage for the proposed work, negotiates, selects participants, and collects and analyzes data. Comparing, contrasting, and weighing the results, allowing time to revisit the theoretical and field work phases, constitute the final analytical phase. Some similarities exist between the simultaneous and the hybrid strategies. Both could deal with clusters of related concepts and both are multidimensional.

Madden (1990) used this strategy to develop the concept of therapeutic alliance and supports its utility in distinguishing the properties of one concept from other similar and related concepts.

An Integrated Approach to Concept Development

All the above strategies, in addition to the foresight of metatheorists who pioneered the movement toward developing knowledge in nursing (eg, Walker and Avant [1995] and Chinn and Kramer [1991]), have made major contributions to elucidating the most appropriate strategies to use in a human science discipline. New strategies continue to evolve (Rodgers, 1989). Most of them have been based on Wilson's approach to concept development. Over the years, I have worked with colleagues and students to develop concepts, narratives, and theoretical propositions by using an integrated approach to concept development.

This approach evolved over the years through teaching, mentoring, researching, and theorizing. Since the late 1960s and early 1970s, I have presented students in graduate theory classes with the request/requirement to participate in developing concepts from phenomena that have captured their interest and attention.

In reflecting on some of my rationale for not using existing strategies, three reasons become apparent. The first is well analyzed by Wuest (1994). Existing strategies appear limited in capturing the context and are less direct about biases (sexism, politicism, racism) that exist in the social structure in which health care is embedded. The strategies provide little framework to uncover oppression, to analyze the status quo, or to reflect on the different realities and ways by which to shatter unresponsive realities.

The second reason is limited guidelines for approaching concept development from the perspective of clinical practice or experience. The strategies, I believed, were limited in their acknowledgment and affirmation of the experiences that the students, clinicians, researchers, and theoreticians bring with them.

The third rationale is inherent in the "recipe" approach to concept development that reduces the process to a series of ingredients, steps, and phases—rather than critical thinking, consciousness raising, and value clarification—which are components of knowledge development. The question is how to build into the strategy opportunities for raising consciousness about what is and what ought to be for concept development (Henderson, 1995). Reed and Leonard (1989) admonished nurses to "move beyond conceptual ruts" (p. 51) by ethically questioning the frameworks used in analyzing problems and allowing the process of concept analysis and development to raise more questions than it may answer (Rodwell, 1996). The selection of the concept itself is a process of consciousness raising. These are the rationales that have prompted the development and refinement of the following strategy over the years.

From Phenomenon to Theory

In this section I propose a strategy for developing concepts from phenomena and I demonstrate the process from concept to theory development. There are no recipes for the development of theory; there is no one way of doing it, nor is there a way by which the richness and the haphazardness of the process can be fully captured. Theorizing is not reducible to a linear set of components or to neat and tidy sets of processes. A conceptualization could happen all at once, or it could take years and never quite evolve into a useful integrated view of reality. There are, however, six stages and several processes that are useful in engaging in the whole activity of theorization, whether theorization is used as a framework for research, for data interpretation, for concept development, for statistical model building, or for the development of a theory. The stages are: (1) taking in, (2) describing the phenomenon, (3) labeling, (4) concept development, (5) statement development, (6) explicating assumptions, and (7) sharing and communicating. Although these stages and processes are presented here linearly and consequentially, they could occur simultaneously, out of sequence, or in conjunction with other yet undelineated stages. It is useful for students of theory to deliberately and consciously experience each of these stages, even when such experiences are based on just rehearsals.

Taking In

Taking in is a process of sizing up a situation that has attracted our attention for whatever reason, whether that reason is cognitive, affective, objective, or subjective, whether it is a hunch or just an uneasy feeling. Taking in has several characteristics. A phenomenon may attract and hold the attention of the observer, making her pause to think about it and reflect on its nature. This *attention grabbing* may happen when the phenomenon is occurring or it may evolve retrospectively. A clinician may air the room whenever she changes a dressing without pausing to think about the relationship of increased fresh air in the room and healing. That action or its consequences may have been occurring regularly but, because it has not grabbed her attention, she has not been able to develop it further. Attention grabbing includes observations, mental labor, and personal involvement, all so closely intertwined that it is hard to reduce them to linearity as to what happens first and what happens second.

Observation is a complex process, more of a sensory experience than merely seeing. Accurate observation is difficult because of the tendency for selective observations and selective inattention. To know when one is observing with the eyes and when one is observing through mental activity helps to clarify and distinguish dimensions of observation (Zderad and Belcher, 1968). Both activities are part of attention grabbing and are essential in developing theories, but they need to be distinguished. We cannot totally separate what we observe from what we want to see or what we observe from our experiences; nor do we want to. However, we can allow ourselves to observe what we do not know, what we, at this time, do not understand, and what is out of the realm of our experience. Observation occurs both with the "naked eye" and within a "matrix of theory." Beveridge (1957) reminds us that:

> Accurate observation of complex situations is extremely difficult, and observers usually make many errors of which they are not conscious. Effective observation involves noticing something and giving it significance by relating it to something else noticed or already known; thus it contains both an element of sense-perception and a mental element. It is impossible to observe everything, and so the observer has to give most of his attention to a selected field, but he should at the same time try to watch out for other things, especially for anything odd. . . . Powers of observation can be developed by cultivating the habit of watching things with an active, inquiring mind. (pp. 104–105)

A deliberate attempt needs to be made to experience and practice naked-eye observations as well as observations within the matrix of theory or those guided by a paradigm. Observation is not a new skill to nurses; it has been the cornerstone of practice. As King (1975) put it:

> Direct observation has been a primary function of nurses for centuries. Nurses collect voluminous data in their daily activities to gain immediate factual information to plan and give nursing care. They have been trained to make observations and to measure selected physiological and behavioral parameters of human beings to answer immediate questions. (p. 26)

After the initial serendipitous identification of a phenomenon from a clinical setting or from careful review of research studies, the attention grabbing is followed by *attention giving*. Attention giving is a more deliberate process. It is a process that includes careful delineation of situations or events that have the potential of demonstrating the phenomenon under consideration. Situations or incidents selected for observation should vary to consider different aspects of phenomena. An example may illustrate this process. A primary health care worker in Cali, Colombia noticed over the years that *per diem* maids tended to ignore all attempts to bring them to the clinic early in their pregnancy for prenatal care. She also noticed that they tended to bring their sick children to the emergency room with the very first sign of any mild illness. The discrepancy between getting prenatal care and getting pediatric care caught her attention. The health care worker may then choose to give this matter her attention and deliberately look into the differences between the two clinics, the meanings attached to pregnancies and offspring and to preventive and curative care, or she may choose to consider the environment of both clinics or a number of alternatives depending on the interest, the goals, and the previous experiences of the theorist.

> Sometimes a question—a patient's, a colleague's, one's own—may call attention to some phenomenon and provoke thinking. The beginning may be the absence of an expected response experienced by the nurse with surprise, anger, disappointment, or relief. These subjective responses may be used as clues to the nature of the phenomenon itself. (Zderad, 1978, p. 40)
>
> It is looking at the experience with wide-open eyes, with knowledge, facts, theories held at bay; looking at the experience with astonishment. Concentrating on the experience is absolutely necessary. Becoming absorbed in the phenomenon without being possessed by it is equally important. (Oiler, 1982, p. 180)

During the taking-in stage, a dialogue with oneself, with one's theoretical journal, with others, or with all these may be helpful in delineating the phenomenon to further pursuit. The dialogue may include the following questions:

What is it that is attracting the attention of the observer?
Where does it happen?
Is it similar to or different from happenings under different sets of circumstances?
Under what conditions does the observer sense it, see it, hear it, observe it, read it, or touch it?
Can the observer describe it? What is the description?
Can the observer document it with model cases and prototype situations?

The objective of completing the taking-in stage with the two processes of attention grabbing and attention giving is to delineate a phenomenon for further theoretical development.

Describing the Phenomenon

The interest in some problem, question, situation, or event—theoretical or clinical—gnaws at the observer for some time. Our early theorists began their theoretical formulations with a nagging problem based on experience, observation, and thinking related to organization of nursing curricula and the nature of the substantive knowledge that should be included in nursing courses. Some specific questions that baffled them were: What is nursing? and What is nursing's mission? The combination of their questions and their clinical backgrounds resulted in several theories that have helped us distinguish the boundaries of our discipline. These theories have attempted, and succeeded in some ways, to provide some abstract concepts and propositions that can be generalized to different areas of specialization in nursing.

Nursing has gone beyond the beginnings of being concerned only with the global questions that preoccupied our colleagues in theory. The discipline of nursing is capable of focusing its inquiry and the goals for developing theories to phenomena surrounding health, transitions, interactions, nursing clients, and nursing therapeutics.

The observer should attempt to respond to the following questions in defining the phenomenon:

What is the phenomenon?
When does it occur?
What are the boundaries of the phenomenon?
What does it share with a larger class of phenomena?
Does the phenomenon vary? Under what circumstances?
Is the phenomenon isolated in reality?
Does it have a function? Are there multiple factors associated with it? Does it serve an explanatory purpose?
Does it refer to a long-term behavior, to characteristic or habitual modes of behaving, or to patterns of behavior detectable in repeated or similar acts?
Is the phenomenon related to time and place?
Is the phenomenon related to some theoretical framework, to one's basic philosophy of nursing or manner of being? In what way?

This sums up what the phenomenon is and where and when it occurs. All this will help in describing a phenomenon.

A description of a phenomenon may be first articulated in question form. An interest in sleeplessness in intensive care units may prompt one of the following questions (Landis, 1983):

Why do patients experience periods of lack of sleep in intensive care units?
What are the properties of sleeplessness or wakefulness in intensive care units?
Is sleeplessness an adaptive coping style or a maladaptive one?

Others' interests or clinical focuses may prompt other types of questions, such as:

What processes do nurses go through to decide whether or not to provide pain medication for patients experiencing pain?

What are the properties of effective transition into the sick or well role?

What are effective and ineffective transitions?

What are the predictors of occurrence of premenstrual stress?

What is a stressful menopausal experience?

Why do certain immigrant groups seem to be more consistently "satisfied" with health care than others?

What types of social support do different subcultural groups need during illness?

Once the general problem area is identified, questions are then asked to determine whether the problem of interest falls within the domain of nursing. They include:

In what way is the phenomenon related to nursing's substantive knowledge process?

In what way would understanding the phenomenon help in explaining some aspect of nursing care?

Can you think of some questions around that phenomenon, the answer to which would be significant to nursing?

How is the phenomenon related to the social policy statement of what nursing is?

Are there some biases that you could identify: background of the researcher, presence of the researcher?

Did the investigator provide contrasting observations, thereby demonstrating contexts in which phenomena are observed or not observed?

Are there repetitive patterns?

A phenomenon is not a thing in itself; it is not what exists, but rather it is organized around perceptions. When experience and sensory and intuitive data become coherent as a whole, and prior to attachment of any meaning, we have a phenomenon. A phenomenon, then, is an aspect of reality colored by the perception of the viewer of that reality. A phenomenon remains merely a phenomenon as long as we attach no cognitive, intuitive, or inferential interpretation. For example, separate and repetitive observations of the appearance of newly immigrated groups occurring more often in emergency rooms than in the regularly scheduled outpatient clinics is a beginning observation that may evolve into a phenomenon. When one observes that individuals belonging to the immigrant group tend to miss scheduled appointments and appear at unscheduled times, a vague pattern begins to emerge. When the observer further hears an individual from the same or another immigrant group rejecting the pace of life in the United States and complaining about having to plan activities and events so far in advance, then the vague pattern begins to form into a shape. The form could be concerns about planning, disenchantment with structured existence, or various abilities to deal with emergencies in preference to maintenance. The observer can then ask questions, can observe, can read, can structure situations in which planning is considered a norm (eg, birthing preparation, rehabilitation, and discharge), and can therefore ascertain whether indeed a pattern is still apparent.

Delineation of phenomena is achieved through the analysis of models or exemplars. Model situations are vivid examples of the phenomenon and help to describe it. A model situation depicts reality in its prototype, its ideal form, and it allows demonstration of what the phenomenon is and where it exists (Chinn and Jacobs, 1987).

Labeling

Labeling is a stage that comes somewhere in the process of theorizing, and the label may change several times in the process. The function of labeling is to communicate succinctly, to relate to the written literature, to help to delineate what further observations to obtain, and to reduce a phenomenon that is usually described in a paragraph to a concept or statement. Labeling is more than selecting a Label X to describe Phenomenon Y. Labeling allows for semantic analysis (Scheffler, 1958). Semantic analysis permits the theorist to consider the normative use of the term as well as other more esoteric uses of it. Labeling is associated with a kind of defining that ranges from a dictionary definition to a more complex definition that takes the perspective of the theorist into consideration. The label, "preference for spontaneity," emerged from further consideration of Middle Eastern immigrants' health and illness behaviors to denote their lack of enthusiasm about planning, preference for dropping in over making appointments, preference for missing appointments, and preference for showing up in the delivery room with no prenatal care (Olesen and Meleis, 1990). A label and semantic analysis bring the theorist closer to concept development.

Some criteria must be considered in labeling concepts. Lundberg (1942) suggests Eubank's (1932) criteria, which are using precise labels that contain only one idea and that are consistent in their meaning whenever they are employed.

Labeling a concept is a highly individualized experience involving interpretations of the phenomenon. It includes hunches, opinions, and speculations. A labeled phenomenon is a concept or a statement, but it is predefined theoretically and operationally.

Concept Development

Somewhere in this process of theorizing, and not in linear progression, a concept begins to emerge. Concepts evolve out of a complex constellation of impressions, perceptions, and experiences. Conception in Kantian terms is an organized perception. Phenomena are perceived, and only when they are organized and labeled do they become concepts. Concepts are a mental image of reality tinted with the theorist's perception, experience, and philosophical bent. They function as a reservoir and an organizational entity and bring order to observation and perceptions. They help to flag related ideas and perceptions without going into detailed descriptions.

Several processes are useful in concept development. These are defining, differentiating, delineating antecedents and consequences, modeling, analogizing, and synthesizing. *Defining* depends on the label given to the phenomenon. Therefore, the labeling stage should be carefully considered; premature labeling may prompt the theorist to review unrelated literature. Defining a concept helps to delineate subconcepts and dimensions of the concept. During the process of defining concepts theoretically and operationally, the theorist is smoothing rough edges, clarifying ambiguities, enhancing precision, and relating concepts to some empirical referents.

Lundberg (1942) also suggests that:

> Operational definitions, then, are merely definitions which consist as far as possible of words clearly designating observations of events and performable and observable operations subject to corroboration. Thus, they may consist of (1) "physical manipulations," such as reading the weight on a weight scale, (2) "objective verbal designations of these manipulations," or (3) "verbal designations of symbolical or mental operations," such as the definition of "preference for spontaneity."

Operational definitions of concepts in nursing have to be referenced in practice and put into context in reality. Otherwise, they would not be useful for nurses (Jacobs and Huether, 1978). Human responses, one of the units of analysis for nursing theorists, may not always lend themselves to the same corroboration expected in the physical sciences and strived for by social scientists, nor should they.

Differentiating is a process of sorting in and sorting out similarities in and differences between the concept being developed and other like concepts. In developing the concept of transition as a central concept in nursing, Chick and Meleis (1986) discussed the similarities and the differences between the priorities of the concepts of transition and change. Similarly, Reed and Leonard (1989) described how they saw the differences between self-neglect, the concept under development, and suicide and noncompliance. The importance in using the process of differentiation is in accessing related bodies of literature and in further refining the attributes of the concept under development.

In *delineating antecedents*, the theorist is attempting to define the contextual conditions under which the concept is perceived and is expected to occur. Antecedents to transitions that are of interest to the domain of nursing have been defined as events such as recovery, death, immigration, amputation, diagnoses of chronic illnesses, pregnancy, and admission to hospital (Chick and Meleis, 1986). The theorist may ask "So what?" in attempting to identify the consequences of the concept. Consequences are those events, situations, or conditions that are related to and preceded by the concept under development.

To *delineate consequences*, a theorist can practice listing every concept or statement that, in her opinion, or as manifested in research findings, may result from the concept. It is important to deliberately attempt to delineate positive as well as negative consequences. Consequences of transition may be disorientation, confusion, growth, changes in body image, changes in self-concept, and role sufficiency (Meleis, 1975).

Modeling is the process of defining and identifying exemplars to illustrate some aspect of the concept. Exemplars could be clinical referents or research referents. Several types of models are used, each to illustrate different aspects of a concept. A same model is one that illustrates the concept in its entirety. A contrary model is a situation, a group, or an incident in which a contrasting aspect of the concept is absent or is present under a different set of contextual conditions. A population that is not in some major transition may be compared with one that is undergoing a significant transition, which may provide the contrary model. A like model and a contrary model help the theorist in articulating, demonstrating, and highlighting the differences between situations, events, and clients in which the phenomena related to the concept are demonstrated and not demonstrated, thus increasing the potential for clarifying it further. Paterson and Zderad (1988) described a technique of explanation through negation to help in describing the phenomena. Presenting another related phenomenon that does not describe the phenomenon under development helps in sharpening the clarity of that phenomenon.

> A phenomenon cannot be described completely by negation but it may be clarified to some extent by saying what it is not. For instance, empathy is not sympathy; it is not projection; it is not identification. (p. 90)

Analogizing is a process by which a deliberate choice is made to describe the concept under development through another concept or phenomenon that is sufficiently like the one under study but that has been studied more extensively, explored more systematically, and therefore is better understood than the concept under study. If the phenomenon an the concept are alike but represent different domains, and we understand one more than the other, then perhaps the better understood phenomenon will help shed some light, raise better questions, and offer greater insight into the lesser understood phenomenon. An example of analogizing is the use of fables or fictional stories to illustrate the concept. One example of analogizing that I used is of aliens from other times and planets to illustrate the need for international collaboration in knowledge development (Meleis, 1987).

Synthesizing is a process of bringing together findings, meanings, and properties that have been amplified by each of the processes described previously. Synthesizing includes, but is not limited to, describing future steps in theorizing.

Statement Development

The development of a concept may be an end result for some theorists and an interim stage for others that leads to further development through statement development, or research implementation. However, concept development may not be possible because the situation requires statement development. The questions that we may be facing in nursing as a human science are: Is concept development the only avenue to development of theory? Is it possible that the building block for nursing theories are statement development?

Statement development is a stage during which explanations related to the phenomenon are provided. The explanations link the concepts, antecedents, consequences, and assumptions. Statements are developed to describe, explain, prescribe, or predict. They are developed as an end result or to synthesize other statements for research purposes.

To develop statements, several questions may be helpful. Examples are:

In what ways can we further explicate the concept being considered?
In what ways are nursing clients' health and environment affected by the concept?
What are some potential consequences of the concept?

What are some corollaries of the concept?

Propositions are tentative statements about reality and its nature. They describe relationships between events, situations, or actions. Propositions could be developed to describe the properties of the concepts; these descriptive propositions are called *existence propositions* (Zetterberg, 1963). They are factor-isolating propositions (Dickoff, James, and Wiedenbach, 1968), and the end result is therefore descriptive theory, as essential to science as any other theory. Consider, for example, descriptive theory of the atom and its significance to our knowledge of the atom.

Propositions may also be relational, describing the association between concepts or causal relationships between concepts (Reynolds, 1971). The process of developing propositions is also a process of identifying the central questions related to the concept. Propositions provide the central answers that help to explain, describe, or predict nursing reality. The more refined, developed, and advanced the relationship statements are, the more they are able to describe and predict the nature of the relationship, the direction of the relationship, and the strength of the relationship (Chinn and Jacobs, 1987).

Organizing propositions is one of the processes in the propositional stages. Organization of propositions could be accomplished through different channels. Propositions may be arranged to represent process of concept discovery and process of formation of a proposition. In this case, a chronological organization is achieved. A second way is to organize propositions around the central concepts in the theory. A third method is to organize propositions in terms of significance for testing, beginning with those whose test represents the central questions of the theory. Other ways are to organize around independent variables or around dependent variables. Ordering propositions enhances their usefulness and their aestheticism (Zetterberg, 1963).

Explicating Assumptions

During every stage of the process the observer pauses, reflects, and questions both implicit and explicit assumptions. To regard periods of wakefulness as sleeplessness, the observer has made an assumption that certain periods of wakefulness are disruptive and that disturbed behavior may result in sleeplessness. Imagine that the observer is beginning from an opposite point of view (ie, that wakefulness promotes healing); observation will be more open to positive consequences, to what promotes wakefulness, and so on. Therefore, reflection on and analysis of one's views, beliefs, and theoretical underpinnings will help delineate assumptions of the developing theory.

Sharing and Communicating

None of these stages and processes are entirely new to nurses, whether they are clinicians, theorists, or researchers. What may have made it appear new in the 1980s was the growing acceptance of conceptualization as a significant aspect of knowledge development in nursing. This acceptance is demonstrated in the journals devoted to conceptual development of the discipline and in the increasing productivity in metatheory and theory writing. No theorization process is complete without opportunities to share and communicate it with colleagues. Theorizing may happen in isolation, but it does not grow in isolation. Sharing and communicating goes beyond writing and publication. It should be defined as a daily happening in the lives of clinicians, theorists, and researchers.

Instead of staging opportunities for sharing and communicating conceptualizations, redefining existing opportunities and resources may enhance this process of sharing and communicating. Clinical conferences may be redefined to include a theoretical journal sharing hour. Faculty meeting time may be reorganized to permit discussion for evolving concepts or statements; students may use part of their class time for a juice or sherry hour to freely discuss phenomena of interest.

Conclusion

Concepts are the building blocks of theories and the cornerstones of every discipline. The rate of progress in the discipline of nursing can be measured by the extent to which members of the discipline are able to uncover and develop concepts that reflect the phenomena related to nursing care. These phenomena, neglected in the past because of the focus on more biomedical phenomena, are being identified, defined, and developed by nursing scholars. Strategies used in developing concepts that reflect these phenomena were initially borrowed from other disciplines. In the process of using these strategies, nursing scholars refined and further developed them. This chapter has described major strategies for the development of concepts, providing examples to ground each strategy in the experience of developing concepts. The strategies were also compared and contrasted.

As you select one of these strategies to use in developing a concept of your choice, remember to use it as a guideline and not as a blueprint that must be implemented as is. The nature of the phenomena, the creativity of the user, the experience of the clinician, and the findings of the research should shape the nature of the concept. Do not sacrifice the substance for the method. The substance of nursing should continue to shape and drive the methods used. You, the reader, should also remember that you have a vital role in further developing and refining any and all strategies used in developing concepts.

REFERENCES

Avant, K.C. (1993). The Wilson method of concept analysis. In B.L. Rodgers and K.A. Knafl (Eds.), *Concept development in nursing* (pp. 51–60). Philadelphia: W.B. Saunders.

Beeber, L.S. and Schmitt, M.H. (1986). Cohesiveness in groups: A concept in search of a definition. *Advances in Nursing Science*, 8(2), 1–11.

Beveridge, W.I.B. (1957). *The art of scientific investigation.* New York: W.W. Norton.

Chick, N. and Meleis, A.I. (1986). Transitions: A nursing concern. In P.L. Chinn (Ed.), *Nursing research methodology.* Boulder, CO: Aspen.

Chinn, P.L. and Jacobs, M.K. (1987). *Theory and nursing: A systematic approach* (2nd ed). St. Louis: C.V. Mosby.

Chinn, P.L. and Kramer, M.K. (1991). *Theory and nursing: A systematic approach.* St. Louis: Mosby-Year Book.

Davis, G.C. (1992). The meaning of pain management: A concept analysis. *Advances in Nursing Science*, 15(1), 77–86.

Dickoff, J., James, P., and Wiedenbach, E. (1968). Theory in practice discipline: Part 1. Practice oriented theory. *Nursing Research*, 17(5), 415–435.

Eubank, E.E. (1932). *The concepts of sociology.* Lexington, MA: D.C. Heath.

Haase, J.E., Britt, T., Coward, D.D., Leidy, N.K., and Penn, P.E. (1992). Simultaneous concept analysis of spiritual perspective, hope, acceptance, and self-transcendence. *Image: Journal of Nursing Scholarship*, 24(2), 141–147.

Hall, J.M., Stevens, P.E., and Meleis, A.I. (1994). Marginalization: A guiding concept for valuing diversity in nursing knowledge development. *Advances in Nursing Science*, 16(4), 23–41.

Hawks, J.H. (1991). Power: A concept analysis. *Journal of Advanced Nursing*, 16, 754–762.

Henderson, D.J. (1995). Consciousness raising in participatory research: Method and methodology for emancipatory nursing inquiry. *Advances in Nursing Science*, 17(3), 58–69.

Jacobs, M.K. and Huether, S.E. (1978). Nursing science: The theory-practice linkage. *Advances in Nursing Science*, 1(1), 63–74.

King, I.M. (1975). A process for developing concepts for nursing through research. In P.J. Verhonick (Ed.), *Nursing Research* (Vol. 1) Boston: Little, Brown.

Kramer, M.K. (1993). Concept clarification and critical thinking: Integrated processes. *Journal of Nursing Education*, 32(9), 406–414.

Laborde, J.M. (1989). Torture: A nursing concern. *Image: Journal of Nursing Scholarship*, 21(1), 31–33.

Landis, C. (1983). Sleeplessness in intensive care unit: A developing concept. Paper presented in the course Theory Development in Nursing at the University of California, San Francisco.

Lundberg, G.A. (1942). *Social research*. New York: Longman's Green.

Madden, B.P. (1990). The hybrid model for concept development: Its value for the study of therapeutic alliance. *Advances in Nursing Science*, 12(3), 75–87.

Mairis, E. (1994). Concept clarification in professional practice—dignity. *Journal of Advanced Nursing*, 19, 947–953.

McIlveen, K.H. (1992). Exploring empathy: Fit for nursing practice? *Image: Journal of Nursing Scholarship*, 24(4), 273–280.

Meleis, A.I. (1975). Role insufficiency and role supplementation: A conceptual framework. *Nursing Research*, 24(4), 264–271.

Meleis, A.I. (1987). Pandemic images: Knowledge development for empowerment. Keynote address given at Sigma Theta Tau, San Francisco.

Morse, J.M., Anderson, G., Bottorff, J.L., Yonge, O., O'Brien, B., Solberg, S.M., and McIlveen, K.H. (1992). Exploring empathy: Fit for nursing practice? *Image: Journal of Nursing Scholarship*, 24(4), 273–280.

Morse, J.M., Solberg, S.M., Neandor, W.L., Bottorff, J.L. and Johnson, J.L. (1990). Concepts of caring and caring as concept. *Advances in Nursing Science*, 13(1), 1–14.

Norris, C.M. (1982). *Concept clarification in nursing*. Rockville, MD: Aspen Systems.

Norris, C.M. (1985). Primitive pleasure as the basic human state. *Advances in Nursing Science*, 8, 25–43.

Oiler, C. (1982). The phenomenological approach in nursing research. *Nursing Research*, 31(3), 178–181.

Olesen, V. and Meleis, A. (1990). Spontaneity: A social phenomenon observed in Middle-Eastern immigrants. Unpublished manuscript.

Paterson, J.G. and Zderad, L.T. (1988). *Humanistic nursing* (2nd ed.). New York: National League of Nursing.

Reed, P.G. and Leonard, V.E. (1989). An analysis of the concept of self-neglect. *Advanced Nursing Science*, 12(1), 39–53.

Reynolds, P.D. (1971). *Primer in theory construction*. Indianapolis: Bobbs-Merrill.

Rodgers, B.L. (1989). Concepts, analysis and the development of nursing knowledge: The evolutionary cycle. *Journal of Advanced Nursing*, 14, 330–335.

Rodgers, B.L. and Knafl, K.A. (1993). *Concept development in nursing*. Philadelphia: W.B. Saunders.

Rodwell, C.M. (1996). An analysis of the concept of empowerment. *Journal of Advanced Nursing*, 23, 305–313.

Schatzman, L. and Strauss, A.L. (1973). *Field research: Strategies for a natural sociology*. Englewood Cliffs, NJ: Prentice-Hall.

Scheffler, I. (1958). *Philosophy and education*. Boston: Allyn and Bacon.

Schwartz-Barcott, D. and Kim, H.S. (1986). A hybrid model for concept development. In P.L. Chinn (Ed.), *Nursing research methodology: Issues and implementations* (pp. 91–101). Rockville, MD: Aspen Systems.

Schwartz-Barcott, D. and Kim, H.S. (1993). An expansion and elaboration of the hybrid model of concept development. In B.L. Rodgers and K.A. Knafl (Eds.), *Concept development in nursing* (pp. 107–133). Philadelphia: W.B. Saunders.

Walker, L.O. and Avant, K.C. (1988). *Strategies for theory construction in nursing* (2nd ed.). New York: Appleton-Century-Crofts.

Walker, L.O. and Avant, K.C. (1995). *Strategies for theory construction in nursing* (3rd ed.). East Norwalk, CT: Appleton-Lange.

Wilson, J. (1963/1969). *Thinking with concepts*. New York: Press Syndicate of the University of Cambridge.

Wuest, J. (1994). A feminist approach to concept analysis. *Western Journal of Nursing Research*, 16(5), 577–586.

Zderad, L.T. (1978). From here-and-now to theory: Reflections on how. In J.G. Patterson (Ed.), *Theory development: What, why, how?* New York: National League for Nursing.

Zderad, L.T. and Belcher, H.C. (1968). *Developing behavioral concepts in nursing*. Atlanta, GA: Southern Regional Education Board.

Zetterberg, H.L. (1963). *On theory and verification in sociology* (Rev. ed.). Totowa, NJ: Bedminster Press.

CHAPTER 13

Strategies for Theory Development

The aim of nursing science is to develop theories to describe, explain, and understand the nature of phenomena, and anticipate the occurrence of phenomena, events, and situations related directly or indirectly to nursing care. Theories are also developed to provide nurses with the rationale and the guidelines by which to control unwanted aspects of phenomena as well as with frameworks for prescriptions. These emerging explanatory and prescriptive theories reflect abstract representations of response patterns of human beings to health and illness to environments, to treatments, and to health care professionals. They also represent patterns of how and under what conditions and within what contexts are healthy and unhealthy relationships formed in the health care system. In nursing, a human science, such descriptions and explanations are developed within a context of time, history, environment (social sanctions and obligations), and human conditions (including human rights). These aims for the development of theories in human science are congruent with the aims of other human sciences that are focused on human beings and their lives (Schensul, 1985).

The nature of nursing science and the potential in its growth require a close relationship between theory, practice, and research. Theoreticians, clinicians, and researchers in nursing share one ultimate goal—understanding the health care needs of clients and communities for the purpose of enhancing their sense of well-being, promoting their health status, facilitating their transitions, and increasing their access and options for health care most appropriate for their situation.

Despite this shared goal, few would deny that in the history of the discipline there has been some tension between theorists, clinicians, and researchers. This tension has been caused by myths and confusion about each others' intentions, methods, and goals. Nurses who primarily hold one of these roles believe many myths about each other. For example, the clinicians believe that theorists are only "ivory tower" philosophers who dream up ideas unconnected with practice or research. Researchers, the theorists counter, focus on those small research projects using empirical approaches to the development of nursing knowledge, which may confirm or refute propositions that are disconnected and that do not reflect a coherent whole needed for illuminating phenomena. Clinicians believe that researchers and theorists are too far removed from clinical practice, so how can they possibly develop theories that could be helpful in understanding clinical phenomena. How could they presume that they can describe, explain, or predict outcomes of clinical practice when they have not seen a client for a while?

There are some truths in all these positions, but none represents all truths of any of the positions in their entirety. The theorists have provided the discipline—and continue to do so—with a coherent vision of the core of its domain: the focus on human beings, the interactional nature of clients, nurses, environment, and the primacy of health and well-being. The goals of self-care, adaptation, homeostasis, expanded consciousness, balance, and harmony with environments were articulated by theorists. They proposed concepts that have become the cornerstones of the discipline and about which there has been more agreement than was anticipated in the 1970s. The researchers, on the other hand, have developed instruments for some central concepts, such as wound healing, levels of confusion, social support, pain intensity, and symptom distress. The researchers also have tested some theoretical propositions related to clinical practice, such as the determinants of maternal role development, or the determinants of recovery in cardiovascular patients. Clinicians have used theory as the bases for their actions, even when they were not able to articulate what theories they use and under which circumstances.

In the 1980s, attempts were made to complete the practice–theory–research cycle. Mercer, for example, systematically worked on identifying responses to mothering in adult women, in adolescent women, and in women undergoing cesarean and vaginal deliveries (Mercer, 1984; Mercer, Ferketich, May, and de Joseph, 1987; Mercer, Ferketich, May, de Joseph, and Sollid, 1987). Mercer identified clinical issues related to mothering, such as ways in which new mothers establish mothering role cues and timing in the development of these cues. Benoliel's work on psychosocial responses of patients to cancer is another example. Benoliel is a researcher who was engaged in studying clinically relevant questions that are embedded in a theoretical tradition and has developed theoretical propositions from her clinical and investigative work. She also provided guidelines to using her findings and theoretical guidelines in holistic caring for clients who have life-threatening diseases or who are bereaving from losses related to terminal illness (Benoliel, 1977; Benoliel and De Valde, 1975; Benoliel, Tornberg and McGrath, 1984). She bridged the gaps between education, research, and practice by providing guidelines for educators for curricular development related to transitions and life-threatening diseases (Benoliel, 1982, 1983). These are only two examples that support the belief that progress in the discipline of nursing is predicated on actualizing the relationship between the research, theoretical, clinical, and educational bases.

One assumption that members of the discipline agree on is that disciplines develop through scientific discoveries, and scientific discoveries are useful when they are organized into some coherent wholes. These wholes could be theories or theoretical statements. Theories provide the frameworks that help in describing, explaining, predicting, and prescribing. Therefore, theory construction and development are activities that are essential in all disciplines. In fact, the progress of any discipline is measured by the scope and quality of its theories and the extent to which its community of scholars is engaged in theory development. Completing isolated research projects that are not cumulative or that do not lead to development or corroboration of theories has limited usefulness. Kuhn (1970) contends that disciplines that are in the preparadigmatic stage demonstrate a pattern of research equated with haphazard problem solving; the central questions of the field are not well identified, and results of the individual research projects do not lead to theoretical formulations that may explain phenomena, may predict events, situations, or responses, and may help in prescribing interventions.

Activities of theory development are not new to nurses, despite another existing myth that nurses began to learn how to develop theories only in the mid-1970s and early 1980s. Whether they were aware of it or not, clinical nurses have actively participated in conceptualizing many aspects of the domain of nursing. These conceptualizations demonstrate different approaches to theory development. The earliest attempts at conceptualizing are well illustrated by Florence Nightingale, who, through the wisdom she gained from her work in the Crimean War, linked health with environmental factors, linked care with systematic data collection, and linked hygiene with well-being. Her efforts resulted in conceptual views of patients as physical, spiritual, and intellectual beings needing warmth, nutrition, and quiet environments. She conceptualized the environment as external to the patient and that it is comprised of air, water, drainage, light, and cleanliness. Her writings have components of theories about data collection, graphics and statistics, and health and illness that have been tested by epidemiologists. Other aspects of her conceptualization, such as the relationship between health and clean environments, have been used in the development of other theories such as Rogers' theory of unitary human beings.

Many more attempts at theory development followed Nightingale's. Some are reported in the literature, and many more may have gone unreported. Any time that concepts are delineated, hunches are developed by linking concepts together to help describe, explain, predict, or prescribe, and those hunches are communicated and used in a number of situations (the genesis of generalization), the beginnings of a theory are formulated. The developer of those hunches has been engaged in a process of theory development. In most instances, the process and product go unreported; therefore, the process is not complete and a theory does not formally develop. A theory is an articulation and communication of a mental image of a certain order that exists in the world, of the important components of that order, and of the way in which those components are connected. The mental image is an abstract representation of order that exists in reality as perceived by the theorist. It includes abstract concepts that then provide the potential of being generalized to a number of categorical events or situations. Some efforts in theory development go unrecognized, most probably because of a lack of communication and a limited potential for generalization beyond the one experienced situation. But perhaps it is also because of lack of awareness of nurses of their potential to articulate aspects of the discipline theoretically or a reluctance to accept the potential for theorizing in a practice discipline.

The construction of theory in nursing occupied select members of the discipline from the mid-1950s to the late 1970s. Then metatheoretical writings attracted another select group of nurses and they focused on suggestions about formulating theories, defining types of theories, and identifying sources for theories. Subsequently conceptualizing nursing phenomena commanded the attention of a wider circle of members of the discipline. Several major features have characterized writing on theory and the development of theory:

1. There was an assumption that processes of theory development were essential for the development of nursing science.
2. There was an assumption that the process of theory development was new to nursing and that nurses had not participated in such activity (Hardy, 1974; Harris, 1971).
3. Most of the writing about theory development discussed what ought to happen and what strategies should be used. To my knowledge, until late in the 1990s, there has been no analysis of the strategies that actually have been used.
4. The tendency was to describe processes that were based on other sciences, mainly the physical and social sciences (Dubin, 1969; Gibbs, 1972; Hage, 1972; Wilson, 1963).
5. An implicit assumption was that there should be one single strategy for theory development; this was particularly evident in the early writings (Hardy, 1978; Jacox, 1974; Johnson, 1974; Newman, 1979). Although I doubt that any of these distinguished authors would have argued against a multiple route to theory development, their written work at that period of time appeared to give that impression.
6. An implicit assumption was that theory development was an elitist activity to be engaged in only within the halls of academia. Furthermore, there was an explicit assumption by clinicians that what goes on within the halls of academia had no resemblance to the clinical work that goes on in real life. (Notice the many comments over the years about nursing theory and the lack of clinicians' need for such theory.)
7. Some believed that nursing had always borrowed its theory and that nursing was an applied field. To them, nursing practice theory was not needed because theories from science and ethics were enough to guide nursing (Beckstrand, 1978a, 1978b). Therefore, theory development was an unnecessary process. These people would have disagreed that the redevelopment, resynthesis, and reintegration of theories were also processes of theory development. Fortunately for nursing, others disagreed with them (Barnum, 1990; Walker and Avant, 1995).

The 1980s were characterized by a multiplicity of strategies for theory development. For example, Walker and Avant (1988, 1995) proposed different beginning points for theorizing concepts, statements, or theories and different approaches for derivation, synthesis, or development. The 1980s also were characterized by multiplicity of research approaches that would inevitably lead to different types of theories (Allen, Benner, and Diekelman, 1986). The development of concepts important to nursing and central to its domain was another significant feature of the decade. Examples of these concepts are self-neglect (Reed and Leonard, 1989), environment (Stevens, 1989), dyspnea (Carrieri, Janson-Bjerklie, and Jacobs, 1984), cachexia (Lindsey, Piper, and Stotts, 1982), and comfort (Neves-Arruda, Larson, and Meleis, 1992).

There is more agreement and a shared view among those who have discussed theory development that the proper domain for theory development in nursing is nursing practice and situations or events related to responses or anticipated responses to health and illness. Current and future theoretical work will focus on further development of concepts emanating from the domain of nursing and its mission and the practice and actions of nurses. Central domain concepts are environment, sense of well-being, interaction, coping with transitions, and nursing therapeutics, among others. Theory development may also occur in the functional areas of administration and teaching and learning.

Theory Development: Existing Strategies

A review and analysis of the literature of theory in nursing yields four major strategies of theory development. These are differentiated primarily by their origin theory, practice, and research, and by whether in addition to their origin, other sources were used to develop the theory. These are: (1) theory–practice–theory; (2) practice–theory; (3) research–theory; and (4) theory–research–theory. A fifth strategy, an integrated approach to theory development, is recommended as an ought-to-be strategy, to be used by itself or in combination with any of the others. Each of the strategies is presented and discussed in this chapter.

Theory–Practice–Theory Strategy

The theorist who uses this strategy begins the process of theorizing by selecting a theory to use in practice. This strategy is based on several premises:

- There is an existing theory that can help in describing and explaining nursing phenomena; however, the theory assumptions are not completely congruent with the assumptions that guide nursing.
- The theory is not entirely useful in helping nurses meet their goals in nursing practice. The theory does not define phenomena in ways that are useful for the integrity of the nurse practice act definitions.
- The theory does not directly help in defining actions for nurses. The focus of the theory is different from the focus needed for nursing practice.
- The theory does not provide adequate definitions of the central concepts of nursing.

A theorist using this strategy attempts to explain and describe a clinical situation through the selected theory, discovers the need for modification of concepts, redevelopment of others, and possible reconsideration of other definitions that better reflect the practice situation. She may also consider relationships between concepts that were not proposed in the original theory or ones that interpret these relationships from a nursing perspective. This strategy for theory development speaks only to circumstances in which we see the world through an established theory with delineated concepts. It is a particular theory then that guides actions and dictates how we see nursing and how we act in the world.

Many examples in the nursing literature demonstrate the use of this strategy in theory development (Table 13-1). Peplau's (1952) theory of interpersonal relations in nursing was based on psychoanalytical theory that she used as a framework to describe psychiatric nursing practice. Her theory of nursing reflects psychoanalytical concepts and her psychiatric nursing clinical expertise. Johnson's (1980) view of the client as consisting of subsystems of behavior and her theory about assessments and diagnoses of nursing problems as occurring due to imbalance, overload, or deprivation are based on biomedical and systems paradigms. Her background in pediatric care, her continuous interest in clinical nursing, and the paradigms guiding her nursing world resulted in her theory of nursing. Johnson's view of a client with subsystems of behavior is analogous to, but not equal to, the biomedical system. Her notion of homeostasis as a goal of nursing is parallel to Parsons' (1951) idea of homeostasis of social systems. The structure and function of Johnson's subsystems are modeled after the structure and function of Parson's social systems. The result is a theory of nursing that describes a nursing client, explains some of the actions of the client and the nurse, and, perhaps, could in the future predict further action. Another example of this strategy is Benner's theory of novice and expert practice (1984) based on her clinical observations through the Dreyfus and Dreyfus model of skill acquisition of aircraft pilots (1986).

Some may say these are borrowed theories. Barnum (1990) disagreed. She stated that "borrowed theories remain borrowed as long as they are not adapted to the nursing milieu and the nursing image of human beings. Once such theories have been adapted to the nursing milieu, it is logical to refer to these boundary overlaps as shared knowledge rather than as borrowed theories" (p. 95). The strategy discussed here is based on deriving nursing theories from theories developed in other disciplines. These derived theories reflect the unique nursing knowledge and its practice field. Dickoff and James (1968) contended that theories from biology, psychology, and sociology are "building blocks . . . in the mansion of nursing theory" (p. 202). A new meaning is given to the guiding theory or paradigm, a new meaning that is pertinent to nursing. Norbeck (1981), Mercer (1981), Millor (1981), and Meleis (1975) used a theory or viewed nursing through another paradigm and developed a conceptualization of social support,

Table 13-1 ***Examples of Theory–Practice–Theory: Clinical and Paradigmatic Origins of Selected Nursing Theories***

Theory	Practice	Theory
Psychoanalytic theory	Psychiatry	Peplau
Systems theory	Pediatrics	Johnson
Adaptation theory	Pediatrics	Roy
Existentialist	Psychiatry	Travelbee
	Adult/Med Surg	Paterson and Zderad
Biomedical systems	Med Surg	Orem
		Henderson
		Abdellah
		Maslow

maternal role attainment, child battering, and role supplementation, respectively, describing and explaining behaviors related to nursing care.

Other modifications of this strategy are exemplified by Roy and Roberts (1981) and Paterson and Zderad (1988). Roy viewed nursing from systems, adaptation, and interactionist paradigms. Her theory combines those paradigms with nursing practice and the result is the person as an adaptive system or with two internal control systems, the regulator and the cognator subsystems. The activities of these subsystems are demonstrated through four adaptive modes (effectors): the physiologic mode, the self-concept mode, the role–function mode, and the interdependence mode. The development of the modes, particularly the self-concept, the role–function, and the interdependence modes, is derived from an interactionist sociological paradigm as exemplified by self-concept, role, and symbolic interactionist theories. Paterson and Zderad's (1988) uniqueness evolved from using existentialist philosophy as the paradigm for the development of their nursing theory. There are several common processes in the development of theories through this strategy:

- Knowledge of nonnursing theories and of a practice field
- Analysis of theory and practice area (analysis is a process by which the object of analysis is reduced into components and each component is defined and evaluated, theories are reduced to assumptions, concepts, and propositions, and practice is described through exemplars and case models)
- Use of assumptions, concepts, and propositions of theory to describe the clinical area
- Redefinition of assumptions, concepts, and propositions to reflect the domain of nursing (redefining may also include modifications of some aspects of theory)
- Construction of theories involving the development of explanation of exemplars representing the redefined assumptions, concepts, and propositions (assumptions, concepts, and propositions reflect a centrality in original theory)

An example of these processes is provided by considering Johnson's theory of behavioral subsystem. Johnson used Parson's concept of behavioral system, redefined it from a nursing perspective as "all patterned, repetitive and purposeful ways of behaving that characterize each man's life, are considered to comprise his behavioral system" (Johnson, 1980, p. 209). She then identified seven subsystems, labeled each, and discussed the relationship between each subsystem and the whole system. Several characteristics of a theory evolve from this strategy. The parent theory is well described and parallels the new practice-based theory. Concepts, attributes, properties, and descriptions are similar in both theories. The context for the evolving theory is differentiated from the context of the parent theory.

Finally, it might be helpful to differentiate between the *clinical theorist* and the *clinician who uses theory.* The clinical theorist is the person whose goals include the refinement and development of theory. The clinician who uses theory has a goal of application of theory. The clinical theorist is engaged in practice and in the development or refinement of theory. She uses such processes as analyses, syntheses, comparisons, refinements, extensions, and reflections as well as other mental processes. She uses the process of theory development to understand, to know, or to further develop some coherent generalizations that go beyond the present situation. The clinician who uses theory uses mainly clinical strategies to apply theories for the purpose of understanding and knowing. The differences and similarities are presented in Table 13-2.

Practice–Theory Strategy

Some theories are driven by clinical practice situations and are inductively developed. They reflect experiences that evolve from practice and are based on clinical situations and on the experiences of theorists in practice. This strategy is built on several premises:

1. Whatever theories that exist are not useful in describing the phenomenon of interest to the person. We may not know, for example, what is providing comfort to nursing clients, how comfort is defined, how it is achieved, who is expected to participate in providing it, what are the different ways in which it is manifested, and what is feasible and what is not feasible in comforting patients in various stages of health–illness. Answers to these questions could be articulated conceptually by clinical experts through descriptions of models of comforting acts derived from their practice.
2. The person is able to develop theories; there are resources to support the process of developing theories.
3. The phenomenon is significant enough to pursue, as developing knowledge about a phenomenon is a long process.
4. There may be clinical understanding and wisdom about the phenomenon, but that understanding has not been articulated into a meaningful whole.

The clinician begins the process of theory development with a nagging question that evolves from a practice situation. The insight is grounded in the practice situation,

Table 13-2 ***The Clinical Theorist (Theory–Practice–Theory) and the Clinician Who Uses Theory (Theory–Practice)***

Theory–Practice–Theory	Theory–Practice
GOAL	
Development; strategies for development	Application; strategies for application
STRATEGIES	
Analyses; synthesis; comparison; refinement; extension; mental processes; reflection; creation	Analyses; description; interpretation; application
USES	
Understand; know; develop	Understand; know
EVALUATION	
Authenticity; congruency; context for discovery; context for justification; other criteria for evaluation of theory	Authenticity; congruency; context for justification
PERSON	
Clinical theorist	Clinician

and the result has the potential for understanding other similar situations through the development of a set of propositions. The strategy depends on observations of new phenomena in a practice situation; development of sensitizing concepts; and labeling, describing, and articulating properties of these concepts. The properties are the subconcepts included in them, the boundaries, the definitions, the examples, the meaning, and so forth.

The development of theory using this strategy is heavily based on the work of Glaser and Strauss (1967). While collecting data, the researcher keeps diaries, observes, analyzes similarities and differences, compares and contrasts responses, and develops concepts and then linkages. The grounded theory approach is credited to sociologists Schatzman and Strauss (1973) and Glaser and Strauss (1968), who have done a great deal to articulate the process and share its nuances, providing us with a multitude of examples to demonstrate its utility. It is a strategy not entirely foreign to nursing; the Yale school of thought in nursing produced many examples of theoretical development that are parallel to the work done by Glaser and Strauss. Theories evolving from the Yale approach are those related to interpersonal relations and interactions in nursing, as viewed by Orlando, Travelbee, and Wiedenbach (see Chap. 17). These theorists developed their ideas by being totally immersed in clinical work, either giving care themselves or observing care being given. They used a variety of methods to collect their clinical data, such as case studies, interviews, and observations. It appears that they then isolated the central phenomenon of nursing related to the client's interaction with the nurse and those phenomena related to the development of nurse–patient relationships. Categories emerged, concepts were labeled, and beginning propositions were developed.

These were theories based on and evolving from clinical practice, with the intention of describing and explaining extant nursing practice. One may presume that the theorists did not use any existing paradigm or theories. This may or may not be true. An equal presumption may be that these theorists had an interactionist background, prompting them to see nursing practice in one particular way. This strategy is most useful for clinicians, particularly when they deliberately begin to use the process to develop theories and articulate and communicate them. (Backscheider [1971] offers a useful example of this process.)

One of the most significant processes used by the pre-1980s theorists who demonstrated this strategy is their knowledge of their clinical areas. They had the resources to identify exemplars and to compare and contrast different exemplars. They may have used the same components defined and discussed in this chapter under the heading "practice–theory–research–theory strategy." However, without more information published about their strategies, it is not possible to use their work as an example of the modified practice–theory method.

Theorists using this strategy in the late 1980s tended to describe the clinical situation and processes that supported and/or inspired the evolving theories. An example of the use of this strategy is that provided by theorists who were interested in describing noncompliant behaviors. Clients who do not follow and "comply" with prescribed regimens have been labeled noncompliant or difficult. Some nursing scholars provided analyses demonstrating that neither concept adequately described the roles of intention and environment in not adhering to a regimen. Therefore, Reed and Leonard (1989) proposed instead the concept of *self-neglect*, which is defined as intentional neglect despite available resources. The authors described a clinical situation that prompted their conceptualization, reviewed existing theories, compared and contrasted self-neglect with other like concepts, such as suicide and noncompliance, and provided more clinical exemplars to refine the properties and attributes of the concept. This strategy is also exemplified by Maeve's (1994) "carrier bag theory of nursing practice." Her theory of nursing practice was modeled after Fisher's (1979) carrier bag theory of human evolution positing that human beings evolved not through developing weapons, tools, and hunting, but through collecting, gathering, and accumulating. Instead of viewing human evolution as based on "man the hunter," she proposed "women as the carriers," and suggested that instead of viewing evolution through the innovation of hunting, that we consider the spectacular development of containers by women the heroines, as the impetus for evolution and development. Maeve (1994) used this theory to reflect everyday practices of nurses that evolve from story telling of lived experiences in practice situations. She proposes that theories should be the result of capturing practice through articulating ideas that represent nursing phenomena. The theory components are bedside nurses sharing their experiences, the process of sharing and articulating these experiences, and the outcome of the narrative is practice-driven theories.

The processes used in developing practice-driven theoretical formulation are dynamic and changing to reflect the participants in the development of theories. Keeping journals, writing notes, reflecting in diaries, writing stories about clinical practice, talking with others, exposing our ideas for discussion, uncovering meaning, challenging assumptions, and most importantly, using critical thinking throughout these processes are methods to develop theories (Benner, 1984; Gadow, 1988; Habermas, 1984).

Research–Theory Strategy

The most acknowledged and accepted strategy for theory development by scientists in other fields as well as by many within the discipline of nursing is this strategy, which is developing theories that are based on research. In fact, for empiricists, postempiricists, and postpositivists, theory development is considered exclusively as a product of research. Therefore, according to this perspective, the strategy *par excellence* is research–theory. Theorists who adhere to this strategy believe that theories evolve from replicated and confirmed research findings. From this perspective, theories are referred to as scientific theories, and the purpose for developing such theories as described by Jacox (1974) is because

> . . . isolated facts are of little interest to scientists, they try to put the knowledge of their respective fields together in such a way that the various events or phenomena with which they are concerned are systematically related to one another. A biologist, for example, wants to know not only about cells, species, and adaptation, but also how all of these are related to each other and to other biological phenomena. Scien-

tific knowledge is systematically organized into 'theories.' The purpose of a scientific theory is to describe, explain, and predict a part of the empirical world. (p. 4)

Reynolds (1971) refers to this strategy in the construction of theories as the "Baconian approach." It is also most commonly known as the inductive method. Reynolds proposed four steps to this strategy.

1. Select a phenomenon that occurs frequently and list all the characteristics of the phenomenon.
2. Measure all the characteristics of the phenomenon in a variety of situations (as many as possible).
3. Analyze the resulting data carefully to determine if there are any systematic patterns among the data worthy of further attention.
4. Once significant patterns have been found in the data, formalization of these patterns as theoretical statements constitutes the laws of nature (axioms, in Bacon's terminology). (p. 140)

The strategy presupposes two significant conditions: (1) that there is agreement in the field on the major concepts that should concern its community of researchers and (2) that each research concerns itself with a manageable number of variables with easily detectable patterns. Social science research could not guarantee these conditions (Reynolds, 1971); nursing is similar in some ways. Until the 1980s, there was very little agreement on the central questions in the field. Therefore, isolated research projects were launched to explore questions that were either tangentially related to the mission of nursing or the answers to which were central to other disciplines.

As nurse scholars began to agree that nursing deals with human beings who are constantly influencing and being influenced by their environment, there was more appreciation of the complexities inherent in the phenomena central to the care processes. Therefore, although some theories may evolve from research findings, others may continue to capture nursing practice and still others may be derived from other theories. In a dynamic science all strategies for theory development will continue to inform the discipline.

The development of theory from research will be enhanced by completing research projects that answer questions that are central to the discipline and that are driven by common and shared conceptualizations. Often, we find that research findings were designed to answer questions that are either not central to nursing or are not translatable to connect with other findings to form a coherent conceptualization. This limitation in potential coherence results from lack of articulated theory to drive the questions and therefore the consequences may be research findings but not theory development.

This strategy is built on the assumption that there is truth out there in real life that can be captured through the senses and that this truth can be verified or falsified. Repeated verification is an indication of the existence of this truth and repeated support of a hypothesis leads to the development of scientific theories. There are numerous examples in the literature of nurse researchers who have used this strategy in developing theories; among them are Johnson (1972), Barnard (1973), Lindeman and Van Aernam (1973), and Johnson and Rice (1974).

Not all proponents of this method advocate sensory data as the basis of truth, and not all of them speak of validation and falsification. The grounded theorists have proposed another approach within this strategy that is based on the discovery of concepts and on identification of patterns, processes, and explanations. The research design proposed by Glaser and Strauss (1968), and further developed by Strauss and Corbin (1994), is that of field study, in which not only theories evolve from research but the research question also evolves from the data gathered. The sole purpose of research, as proposed by this group of field researchers, is the development of theory. Numerous theories have been developed using this second approach, the grounded theorists' approach (Fagerhaugh, 1974; Stern, 1981). A similar approach was used by Smith (1981) in conceptualizing health. She identified four modalities to describe how her research participants tended to view health. These were clinical, role-performance, adaptation, and eudaemonistic modes of viewing and conceptualizing health.

Two examples will be offered here of the steps to use in the research–theory strategy. The first is by Lindeman (1980), who advocated the development of theory from research in her keynote address to the Western Society for Research in 1980. Lindeman used her own research to illustrate the research–theory process and to identify the steps to use in developing theory from research.

The Research–Theory Method: Exemplar by a Researcher: Carole A. Lindeman (1980):*

> The first study, designed to determine the value of preoperative teaching, led to the conclusion that structured preoperative teaching significantly improved the adult surgical patient's ability to cough and deep breathe postoperatively and also significantly reduced the mean length of hospital stay.
>
> A second study was conducted to determine the most efficient way to implement a structured preoperative teaching program. That study, 'The Effects of Group and Individual Preoperative Teaching,' led me to conclude that group teaching was as effective and more efficient than individual teaching. These findings and those from the first study were consistent with educational research and theory. However, other results from that second study could not be explained by existing theory and continued to trouble me. Those results were:
>
> 1. Site of incision does interact in a significant way with teaching method. Subjects receiving group instruction and having 'other' incisions had a shorter length of hospital stay than the same group receiving individual instruction. Ventilatory function scores were not different for the two groups. Interpretation required consideration of psychosocial factors in contrast to the physiological factors associated with the stir-up regime.
> 2. Age, per se, does not alter postoperative ventilatory function when preoperative teaching and practice are provided. Mean postoperative values on ventilatory function tests were not significantly different for subjects in the various age ranges. In fact, older subjects having major procedures did significantly better than their younger counterparts.

*Quoted by permission from the author and publisher. Lindeman, C.A. (1980). The challenge of nursing research in the 1980s. In *Communicating nursing research: Direction for the 1980s*. Boulder, CO: Western Interstate Commission for Higher Education.

3. Smoking history, per se, does not affect postoperative ventilatory function, length of hospital stay, or number of analgesics administered when preoperative teaching and practice are provided. There were no significant differences between smokers and nonsmokers.

According to the medical literature, these were factors associated with high risk groups. However, when these so-called 'high risk' patients received structured preoperative teaching, their postoperative ventilatory function measures were comparable to other patients. The conceptual/theoretical framework for the research did not explain these results. I was left with a big unanswered 'Why?'

Before pursuing those unanswered questions, I conducted a third study dealing with the effects of preoperative visits by operating room nurses. Although a large array of dependent variables were included, the data led to the conclusions that the preoperative visit was useful to the operating room nursing personnel for creating a safe, effective, and efficient intraoperative experience, but it did not produce measurable health status benefits for the patient. Coming from an educational psychology framework, I focused on the content of the teaching encounter as a way to explain why the one intervention, structured preoperative teaching, produced measurable benefits and the second intervention, preoperative interview, did not. I concluded that patients could learn and recall psychomotor behaviors taught in the preoperative period, but material that only served a cognitive structuring process, if learned, would not be retained.

However, I was then involved in a fourth study that refuted my interpretation and led me to propose a different set of theoretical statements. The fourth study was a descriptive study of significant nursing interventions in the preoperative and intraoperative periods and postoperative welfare. The study used Donabedian's structure, process, and outcome framework; however, due to observations made in our pilot study, we added patient baseline data to the overall framework. Much to my surprise, the data showed that patient baseline and organizational data were more strongly correlated with patient welfare than were specific nursing interventions.

I continued to mull over the conclusions from these various studies in an attempt to bring order to the data. Although each study by itself had been useful in making decisions about nursing practice, it seemed that they would be more useful if the results—the expected and the unexpected—could be tied together in some meaningful way in the form of nursing practice theory.

It is difficult, if not impossible, to describe one's thought processes as data and concepts are analyzed. Let it suffice to say that I continued to focus on three concerns:

1. A nursing intervention relating to skill development had a significant impact; a nursing intervention involving cognitive structuring did not.
2. Interactions between the patient and the intervention were not totally predictable and, in fact, were quite surprising.
3. Interactions between the institution and the intervention were not totally predictable.

Emerging from these data, from observations made during the research, and from my further analysis was the conclusion that patient welfare is [affected] by three major sets of variables: organizational, content of care, and patient characteristics. It also seemed clear to me that the critical variable is the patient, with nursing care only effective to the extent that it facilitates the patients' management of their own care.

Having identified the major concepts, the next step in this inductive process involves formulation and validation of relational statements.

The following statements have validity in terms of the research cited earlier:

1. The recipient of health care is the single most important variable in determining actual health status.

> 2. Those organizations having a potential for enhancing self-health-care management are most likely to have a positive influence on actual health status.
> 3. Those interventions having a potential for enhancing self-health-care management are most likely to have a positive influence on actual health status.
> 4. Characteristics of the care-giver as a person are not significant in determining actual health status.
> 5. The presurgical nursing interventions designed to enhance the self-health-care management abilities of the patient will influence postoperative health status.
>
> Within this inductive process, I am now at the point of theory construction. To complete this step of the process I have had to reconsider the nature or definition of nursing. Without this broader perspective, any theory would exist in limbo. Its ability to predict and its test in reality would remain unknown. Again, for my own efforts, I have conceptualized nursing as a profession that exists because society has needs for health care. These needs generate from three factors: environmental and social factors, disease factors, and health factors. Those health issues or needs that arise because of the interaction of these three factors are the primary focus of nursing. Included are such issues as child abuse, maternal attachment, teenage suicide, the chronically ill, and so forth. Nursing may also assist other professionals by coordinating or implementing components of their plan of care. The social workers, nutritionists, physicians, psychologists, and others all have a role in dealing with issues generating from one or more of these three factors. I personally believe that nursing does have a unique and independent practice role, and it is defined in terms of the point of interplay of these factors.
>
> Now, back to theory development. My next step is to analyze already completed research in terms of the five relational statements presented earlier. I need to consider patients other than presurgical. I need to explore settings other than acute care. I need to explore further interventions—those that relate to health maintenance more than disease prevention. I need to re-examine my major construct, 'self-health-care management,' in terms of the label—does it truly and clearly communicate the nature of the variable? Is it really the variable producing the observable effects? Only when a review of this nature is completed will I be ready to construct a formal theory that can then be tested, modified, and expanded by other researchers and scholars.

A second example is Dluhy's (1995) proposal for a method to map pluralistic knowledge for the purpose of generating theory. She proposes to identify the core elements, the implicit and explicit assumptions, the relationship between variables from studies that have been done in nursing and other disciplines. The purposes of knowledge mapping are to answer the questions of what are the best explanations of a central question in the discipline and what are the optimal ways by which these explanations tend to complement each other. Mapping findings is a strategy to integrate massive amounts of knowledge by linking multiple variables and considering these variables from within multiple contexts. Developing theory from research, particularly theory that could inform the discipline of nursing requires knowledge of the discipline of nursing, knowledge of its mission and its perspective, knowledge of philosophical views of science, and knowledge of the various theoretical perspectives that drive the kind of questions explored.

Several steps support the processes needed for integrating research knowledge into theoretical wholes. These steps are used to develop a coherent map of findings (Blalock, 1979; Dluhy, 1995):

1. Know well the substantive area for which mapping is proposed by identifying all relevant literature, findings, and dialogues.

2. Identify the different ontological beliefs and epistemological approaches used in this area of research.
3. Identify major philosophical and theoretical issues that can clearly divide the findings related to the question under review.
4. Develop a grid reflecting the ontology on one axis and epistemology on another axis.
5. Identify major concepts that evolve as core in the literature. This process may entail counting the number of times that a concept may have been the focus of an investigation, or it may require a qualitative analysis of the centrality of the concept. The context of the particular question may dictate the ways by which a concept is declared central. Identify and analyze similarities and differences between the evolving central concepts.
6. Analyze the core concepts and the findings to reflect patterns and themes by placing them at different points on the four quarters of the grid.
7. Engage in scholarly dialogues to identify assumptions, conceptual areas, and epistemological approaches.
8. Validate axes of grid and placement of conceptual themes and areas through some established methods of validation, such as constant comparisons, Q-sort, or use of different validation teams.

Dluhy (1995) mapped knowledge related to chronic illness by identifying two ontological vertical axes representing the ability to control and be controlled (determinism to free will), and the nature of person (reductionism to idealism). She then identified the horizontal axis as the epistemological axis ranging from positivism to subjectivism. She placed conceptual areas in each quadrant that resulted from a review of over 300 research and theoretical references. Placement in a particular quadrant was based on the conceptual area within the context of the related ontology and epistemology. Examples of conceptual areas are: fatigue, dyspnea, pain, defense mechanisms, or support, among others. A large cluster of conceptual areas in any quadrant is an indication of the predominance of conceptual areas within a context of a certain set of ontological assumptions and epistemological approaches.

Determining agreements on concepts, or findings related to these concepts, on translating findings that reflect diverse contexts are steps toward developing coherent conceptualizations that may lead to developing theory from research.

Several variations of processes for integrating knowledge have been used to develop theories. Lenz, Suppe, Gift, Pugh, and Milligan (1995) pooled their individual work and collaborated in developing a middle range theory to describe "unpleasant symptoms." The processes they used are similar to the processes used in mapping with the difference that this group primarily worked on mapping their own findings.

Theory–Research–Theory Strategy

In this strategy, theory drives the research questions and the results that answer these research questions inform and modify the theory. The difference between this strategy and research–theory strategy lies in the use or nonuse of theory as a guiding framework for the research questions. Theorists who begin the research by defining a theory and determining propositions for testing and then go steps further to modify and develop the original theories are considered users of this strategy. Although many researchers use processes similar to the ones that theorists may use, some significant differences are apparent between researchers and theorists using this strategy. The researcher using theories aims at testing, confirming, refuting, or replicating theories. She uses theory as a framework for operational definitions for variables and statements, and she uses mental processes, problem solving, and interpretive processes to describe findings. The theorist who uses research as a means for the development of theory ends investigation with a refined, modified, or further developed coherent theoretical explanation of theory. The impact on the discipline is different and is needed for different purposes. The theorist researcher's findings are specific to selected phenomena and selected findings, whereas the theorist's impact may be through integrated theoretical statements that explain and predict a wider range of phenomena (Table 13-3).

The processes used for theory–research–theory are:

1. A theory is selected that is compatible with the domain of nursing to explain the phenomenon of interest.
2. Concepts of the theory are redefined and operationalized for the research.
3. Findings are synthesized and used to modify, refine, or develop the original theory.
4. In some instances, the result may be a new theory.

Table 13-3 ***Differences Between Theory–Research–Theory Strategy and Theory–Research Strategy***

Theory–Research–Theory	Theory–Research
GOAL	
Test, refine, develop theory; openness to options for further developments	Test, accept, refute, replicate; aim to conclude
USES	
A framework for research and for modification of theory; define concepts for future use; generate new propositions; explain, define questions	A framework for research; define variables and questions; prove/disprove
STRATEGIES	
Mental processes; creative, abstract, reflective thoughts; interpretation; synthesis; intuitive leaps	Mental processes; problem solving; interpretation
EVALUATION	
Theoretical thinking; conceptual definitions; other theory analyses criteria	Variable definitions; validity; reliability; other research criteria
IMPACT ON DISCIPLINE	
Through integrated theoretical statements that explain and predict with a wider scope	Through selected scientific findings that explain and predict specifics
FUTURE	
Generates more propositions; inspires	Provides support for existing propositions and for clinical actions

An Integrated Approach to Theory Development

Nursing practice has been one of the most significant sources for theory development that was neglected for many decades. Theorists who use this strategy assume the significance of the relationship between practice, theory, and research and assume that each plays a role in the development of nursing theory. The theorist also assumes, implicitly or explicitly, that clinical situations are viewed with the cumulative wisdom of previous clinical situations as well as with whatever theories or frameworks the individuals may have in their repertoires. The person, theorist, clinician, or researcher in a human science is also an integral part of these experiences. Even when an attempt at distancing between the nursing theorist and client is premeditated and carefully implemented and guarded, the infiltration of previous experiences or theories in shaping the clinical situation is inevitable. These previous experiences are part of a nursing perspective. All these factors are the context that shapes what we see, how we see it, and how we analyze it.

Phenomena seen from a nursing perspective are not seen in exactly the same way as phenomena seen from a sociological perspective. A nursing perspective is focused on considering the phenomenon holistically and dynamically and within a context. Nurses are concerned with such phenomena as health, comfort, care, the nursing process, and other domain concepts, and those that will eventually make a difference in some aspect of health care. Phenomena are described or explained through the interaction of health/illness events, person–environment relationships, and human responses perspective. Different perspectives provide different sets of glasses through which phenomena are viewed. Each perspective identifies the limits within which inquiries are made (Donaldson and Crowley, 1978; see also Chap. 6 for a discussion on perspectives). Another assumption for this strategy is that there is some kind of reality that exists out there, and there is a pattern and order in the universe around us, as well as paradoxically, a certain degree of uniqueness. Because we live in an orderly, nonrandom world, this order is comprehensible to a certain extent and within a context. That concept of uniqueness deserves a pause.

If each event or process of a phenomenon were absolutely unique or occurred randomly, without order or pattern, there could be no generalization, albeit a contextual one. Without some degree of generalization there is no science because all sciences attempt to generalize about recurrent phenomena. Scientists, unlike philosophers, must also assume some logical connection between perceivable events as well as a certain degree of predictability. Nurses have been focusing on uniqueness of individuals in practice for the purpose of individualizing care. However, we must consider seriously Ellis' (1982) admonition against using the uniqueness of man as a crutch to avoid patterning and order, the essential components of theory and science. Uniqueness reminds us to consider patterns of diversity and individuality, which, when considered, could add to the complexity and richness of theory. Therefore, uniqueness and patterning are also significant premises on which this strategy is based.

With this caveat and with the necessity of considering the rich contextual background in mind, it may seem difficult to isolate a beginning point for this strategy. However, like the previous strategies, some essential, but not sufficient, stages and processes may facilitate theorizing attempts. The most significant processes used in contemporary nursing are those used to clarify and develop concepts. These processes are discussed in Chapter 12. Any one of the strategies used for clarifying and developing concepts could be used in a process of developing theory from practice.

Nursing as a human and caring science has many properties inherent in the caring processes themselves, which cannot be fully explored using the strategies described above because these research strategies are carried out in isolation from others. Theories that tend to be rich in explaining responses, in illuminating situations, in enhancing wisdom about events, and in providing directions for actions are theories that have evolved through an integrated approach. Such theories may have emerged primarily from any one source; however, the complexity of situations that give rise to these theories compels the theorists to gather clinical evidence, identify exemplars, collect solutions, and garner support from other sources. An integrated approach to theory development has some essential components, such as clinical grounding that drives the basic or clinical questions, opportunities for clinical involvement and for conceptually thinking about the health/illness responses, the situations, the environment, the relationships, and the questions themselves. The beginning hunches and conceptual schemes are then shared and communicated through dialogues with others to allow for critique and further development. An integrated approach requires the development of a framework and a theoretical vision, as well as opportunities to test these hunches or evolving conceptualizations with colleagues and other participants. Other components of this integrated approach are research (different designs) and different methods to clarify, support, or test some of the evolving hunches. That research documentation may be gathered from different sources. An integrated approach to theory development uses skills and tools from clinical practice, research, reflective clinical diaries, descriptive journals, and dialogues about analyses, among other sources and approaches. An example of a theory that is evolving in which the theorists used an integrated approach is a "theory of human relatedness" (Hagerty, Sauer, Patusky, and Bouwsema, 1993). The authors of the theory experienced situations in clinical practice that prompted them to think of various states of connectedness and disconnectedness. They dialogued, observed, kept notes, conducted research in the library, and identified the social processes inherent in relating, as well as the different states of relatedness including connectedness, disconnectedness, parallelism, and enmeshment. The evolving theory explains, describes, and has the potential of clarifying situations in which nurses relate to others (which is most of the time). The potential power of this theory in enhancing understanding of situations is directly related to its integrated approach of development.

Tools for Concept and Theory Development

Theory development includes mental processes that incorporate analysis, discovery, formulation, and validation of uniformities. These may come as a result of sensory observation or as a consequence of logical or rational analysis of the problem or the phenomenon. They may also result from intuitive reasoning, from an insight that occurs over an extended period of time, or from a "click" that comes as quick as lightning. The thought processes can be spontaneous or premeditated—the timing is never predictable (Sorokin, 1974)—but a conscious effort to look at the phenomenon or the questions is infinitely more helpful in bringing the process to closure. It does not guarantee the "click," but it increases the chances.

Just as the process of researching is enhanced by knowledge of substantive content, knowledge of research methodology, experience, and ability to critique research, all processes of theory development are supported and enhanced by knowledge of what constitutes theory, knowledge of what major issues are confronting theorizing, the ability to critique theory, knowledge of existing theories, and knowledge of major pitfalls in the development of theory. Knowledge of the context for theory such as the clinical area is essential. Theorizing is a process that is refined through a deliberate experience. The processes of reflecting, analyzing, questioning, relating, thinking, writing, changing, and communicating are integral parts of philosophical analysis, essential to theory development, and a prelude to and a consequence of research. Keeping a theory diary or journal, in which observations, reflections, and relationships are systematically logged, helps the theorist to sort out thoughts, develop documentation, and synthesize empirical reasoning with intuitive reasoning (Zderad, 1978).

Norms used to enhance science are useful in enhancing theory development and drive the utilization of other tools. Merton (1968, 1979) identified a number of these norms, two of which are pertinent here: the norms of communality and organized skepticism. Communality encourages nurses to share developing ideas and expose beginning theories for review by peers to help sharpen the theory and to allow the norm of organized skepticism to prevail. This latter norm "requires detached scrutiny of work according to empirical and logical criteria" (Meleis and May, 1981). Dialogues with colleagues in practice, in theory, and in research promote other ways of looking at concepts—other angles and other perspectives.

Collaboration is another significant tool for theory development. In a human science such as nursing, theory development will become more of a collaborative effort. Collaboration allows constant comparison of evaluating competing ideas, provides the medium for a scholarly dialogue to refine concepts, and enhances integration of seemingly disperse findings all of which are important processes in developing coherent theories. Theorists of the future are not individual workers; they are team participants (Meleis, 1992). There is support for this new generation of collaborative theorists, for example, the team that proposed the use of simultaneous concept analysis in the development of concepts started from the assumption of collaboration (Haase, Britt, Coward, Leidy, and Penn, 1992). Other examples of collaborative theories are the evolving theory of unpleasant symptoms (Lenz, Suppe, Gift, Pugh, and Milligan, 1995) and the conceptualization of symptom management (University of California, San Francisco, School of Nursing Symptom Management Faculty Group, 1994).

Another essential tool that has been discussed in the nursing literature is that of intuition. *Intuition* is defined as reaching some decision or conclusion without the conscious or apparent availability of information (Rew, 1986; Westcott, 1968). Rew (1986) defines the attributes of intuition as follows: "Knowledge of a fact or truth, as a whole; immediate possession of knowledge; and knowledge independent of the linear reasoning process" (p. 23). Whether this tool is intuition or the expert speaking (Benner, 1984), recent writings encourage allowing that inner voice to surface, to believe in it, and to trust it (Agan, 1987; Rew, 1986; Rew and Barrow, 1987).

Closely related to intuition are introspection and reflection. Silva (1977) reminded us "to value truths arrived at by intuition and introspection as much as those arrived at by scientific experimentation" (p. 62). Reflection is a process of thinking that may or may not be bound by the need for problem solving.

Conclusion

Knowing and experimenting with strategies for theory development increases theorizing abilities but does not guarantee the development of theory, nor should it. A probable result of such knowledge is the integration of philosophical processes with empirical processes, resulting in a more integrated knowledge. The rift between scientists and philosophers that marked the era of empirical positivism is decreasing. Our early philosophers believed that science is based totally on philosophical processes; our scientists believed that it is based on the intellectual labor inherent in the philosophical processes. This chapter demonstrated this later process as an essential one for embarking on research, for interpreting research. Both processes are processes of theorizing. The end result may or may not be a theory; the end result may be clarification of a concept or the articulation of a number of propositions that may be an extension of another theory. Systematic research is an essential step in the process to complete the practice–theory–research loop. Eventually, a theory will have to respond to the analytical and critical evaluative criteria presented in the next chapter.

REFERENCES

Agan, R.D. (1987). Intuitive knowing as a dimension of nursing. *Advances in Nursing Science*, 10(1), 63–70.

Allen, D, Benner, P., and Diekelman, N.L. (1986). Three paradigms for nursing research: Methodological implications. In P.L. Chinn (Ed.), *Nursing research methodology: Issues and implications.* Rockville, MD: Aspen Systems.

Backscheider, J. (1971). The use of self as the essence of clinical supervision in ambulatory patient care. *Nursing Clinics of North America*, 6(4), 785–794.

Barnard, K. (1973). The effect of stimulation on the sleep behavior of the premature infant. In M.V. Batey (Ed.), *Communicating nursing research, collaboration and competition.* Boulder, CO: Western Interstate Commission of Higher Education.

Barnum, B.J. (1990). *Nursing theory: Analysis, application, and evaluation* (2nd ed.). Boston: Little, Brown.

Beckstrand, J. (1978a). The notion of a practice theory and the relationship of scientific and ethical knowledge to practice. *Research in Nursing and Health*, 1(3), 131–136.

Beckstrand, J. (1978b). The need for a practice theory as indicated by the knowledge used in conduct of practice. *Research in Nursing and Health*, 1(4), 175–179.

Benner, P. (1984). *From novice to expert: Excellence and power in clinical nursing practice.* Menlo Park, CA: Addison-Wesley.

Benoliel, J.Q. (1977). Social characteristics of death as a recorded hospital event. *Communicating Nursing Research*, 8, 245–265.

Benoliel, J.Q. (1982). Educating nurses for community-based care of advanced cancer patients. AACE Abstracts. *Medical and Pediatric Oncology*, 10(1982), 30A–31A.

Benoliel, J.Q. (1983). The historical development of cancer nursing research in the United States. *Cancer Nursing*, 6(4), 261–268.

Benoliel, J.Q. and De Valde, S. (1975). As the patient views the intensive care unit and the coronary care unit. *Heart and Lung*, 4(2), 260–264.

Benoliel, J.Q., Tornberg, M.J., and McGrath, B.B. (1984). Oncology transition services: Partnerships of nurses and families. *Cancer Nursing*, 7(2), 131–137.

Blalock, H.M., Jr. (1979). Measurement and conceptualization problems: The major obstacle to integrating theory and research. *American Sociological Review*, 44, 881–894.

Carrieri, V.K., Janson-Bjerklie, S., and Jacobs, S. (1984). The sensation of dyspnea: A review. *Heart and Lung*, 13(4), 436–447.

Dickoff, J. and James, P. (1968). A theory of theories: A position paper. *Nursing Research*, 17(3), 197–203.

Dluhy, N.M. (1995). Mapping knowledge in chronic illness. *Journal of Advanced Nursing*, 21, 1051–1058.

Donaldson, S.K. and Crowley, D. (1978). The discipline of nursing. *Nursing Outlook*, 26(2), 113–120.

Dreyfus, H. and Dreyfus, S. (1986). *Mind over machine: The power of human intuition and expertise in the era of the computer.* New York: Free Press.

Dubin, R. (1969). *Theory building*. Toronto: Free Press.

Ellis, R. (1982). Conceptual issues in nursing. *Nursing Outlook*, 30, 406–410.

Fagerhaugh, S.Y. (1974). Pain expression and control on a burn care unit. *Nursing Outlook*, 22, 645–650.

Fisher, E. (1979). *Women's creation: Sexual evolution and the shaping of society.* Garden City, NJ: Anchor Press/Doubleday.

Gibbs, J. (1972). *Sociological theory construction.* Hinsdale, IL: Dryden Press.

Glaser, B.G. and Strauss, A.L. (1967). *The discovery of grounded theory: Strategies for qualitative research.* Chicago: Aldine.

Glaser, B.G. and Strauss, A.L. (1968). *Time for dying.* Chicago: Aldine.

Gadow, S. (1988). Covenant without cure: Letting go and holding on in chronic illness. In J. Watson and M. Ray (Eds.), *The ethics of care and the ethics of cure. Synthesis in chronicity* (pp. 5–14). New York: National League for Nursing.

Haase, J.E., Britt, T., Coward, D.D., Leidy, N.K., and Penn, P.E. (1992). Simultaneous concept analysis of spiritual perspective, hope, acceptance, and self-transcendence. *Image: Journal of Nursing Scholarship*, 24(2), 141–147.

Habermas, J. (1984). *The theory of communicative action: Vol. 1. Reason and the rationalization of society.* London: Heinmann.

Hage, J. (1972). *Techniques and problems of theory construction in sociology.* Toronto: John Wiley & Sons.

Hagerty, B.M., Lynch-Sauer, J., Patusky, K.L., and Bouwsema, M. (1993). An emerging theory of human relatedness. *Image: Journal of Nursing Scholarship*, 25(4), 291–296.

Hardy, M.E. (1974). Theories: Components, development, evaluation. *Nursing Research*, 23(2), 100–107.

Hardy, M.E. (1978). Practice oriented theory: Part 1. Perspectives on nursing theory. *Advances in Nursing Science*, 1(1), 37–48.

Harris, I.M. (1971). Theory building in nursing: A review of the literature. *Image: Journal of Nursing Scholarship*, 4(1), 6–10.

Jacox, A. (1974). Theory construction in nursing: An overview. *Nursing Research*, 23(1), 4–13.

Johnson, D.E. (1974). Development of theory: A requisite for nursing as a primary health profession. *Nursing Research*, 23(5), 372–377.

Johnson, D.E. (1980). The behavioral system model for nursing. In J.P. Riehl and C. Roy (Eds.), *Conceptual models for nursing practice* (2nd ed.). New York: Appleton-Century-Crofts.

Johnson, J.E. (1972). Effects of structuring patients expectations on their reactions to threatening events. *Nursing Research*, 21(6), 499–504.

Johnson, J.E. and Rice, V.H. (1974, May/June). Sensory and distress components of pain. *Nursing Research*, 23, 203–209.

Kuhn, T.S. (1970). The structure of scientific revolutions. In Neurath, O. (Ed.), *International encyclopedia of unified science* (2nd ed., Vol. 2). Chicago: University of Chicago Press.

Lenz, E.R., Suppe, F., Gift, A.G., Pugh, L.C., and Milligan, R.A. (1995). Collaborative development of middle-range nursing theories: Toward a theory of unpleasant symptoms. *Advances in Nursing Science*, 17(3), 1–13.

Lindeman, C.A. (1980). The challenge of nursing research in the 1980s. In *Communicating nursing research: Direction for the 1980s* Boulder, CO: Western Interstate Commission for Higher Education.

Lindeman, C.A. and Van Aernam, B. (1973). Nursing intervention with the presurgical patient: The effects of structured and unstructured preoperative teaching. In F. Downs and M. Newman (Eds.), *A source book in nursing research.* Philadelphia: F.A. Davis.

Lindsey, A., Piper, B., and Stotts, N. (1982). The phenomenon of cancer cachexia, review. *Oncology Nursing Forum*, 9(2), 38–42.

Maeve, M.K. (1994). The carrier bag theory of nursing practice. *Advances in Nursing Science*, 16, 9–22.

Meleis, A.I. (1975). Role insufficiency and role supplementation: A conceptual framework. *Nursing Research*, 24(4), 264–271.

Meleis, A.I. (1992). Directions for nursing theory development in the 21st century. *Nursing Science Quarterly*, 5, 112–117.

Meleis, A.I. and May, K.M. (1981). Nursing theory and scholarliness in the doctoral program. *Advances in Nursing Science*, 4(1), 31–41.

Mercer, R. (1981). A theoretical framework for studying factors that impact on the maternal role. *Nursing Research*, 30(2), 73–77.

Mercer, R. (1984). Predictors of maternal role attainment at one year post birth. *Western Journal of Nursing Research*, 6(3), 52.

Mercer, R., Ferketich, S., May, K., and de Joseph, J. (1987). A comparison of maternal and paternal responses during pregnancy. *Proceedings—Council of Nurse Researchers Conference*, Arlington, VA, October 13–16, American Nurses Association.

Mercer, R., Ferketich, S., May, K., de Joseph, J., and Sollid, D. (1987). Maternal and paternal responses in high- and low-risk pregnancies. Symposium. *Proceedings Sigma Theta Tau International Biennial Conference*, San Francisco, November 10, Sigma Theta Tau International.

Merton, R.K. (1968). On sociological theories of the middle range. In *Social theory and social structure.* New York: Free Press.

Merton, R.K. (1979). *The sociology of science: An episodic memoir.* Carbondale and Edwardsville, IL: Southern Illinois University Press.

Millor, G.K. (1981). A theoretical framework for nursing research in child abuse and neglect. *Nursing Research,* 30(2), 78–83.

Neves-Arruda, E.N., Larson, P.J., and Meleis, A.I. (1992). Comfort. Immigrant Hispanic cancer patients' views. *Cancer Nursing,* 15(6), 387–394.

Newman, M.A. (1979). *Theory development in nursing.* Philadelphia: F.A. Davis.

Norbeck, J. (1981). Social support: A model for clinical research and application. *Advances in Nursing Science,* 3, 43–59.

Parsons, T. (1951). *The social system.* New York: Free Press.

Paterson, J.G. and Zderad, L.T. (1988). *Humanistic nursing* (2nd ed.). New York: National League of Nursing.

Peplau, H.E. (1952). *Interpersonal relations in nursing.* New York: G.P. Putnam's Sons.

Reed, P.G. and Leonard, V.E. (1989). An analysis of the concept of self-neglect. *Advanced Nursing Science,* 12(1), 39–53.

Rew, L. (1986). Intuition: Concept analysis of a group phenomenon. *Advances in Nursing Science,* 8(2), 21–28.

Rew, L. and Barrow, E.M. (1987). Intuition: A neglected hallmark of nursing knowledge. *Advances in Nursing Science,* 10(1), 49–62.

Reynolds, P.D. (1971). *Primer in theory construction.* Indianapolis: Bobbs-Merrill.

Roy, C. and Roberts, S. (1981). *Theory construction in nursing: An adaptation model.* Englewood Cliffs, NJ: Prentice-Hall.

Schatzman, L. and Strauss, A.L. (1973). *Field research: Strategies for a natural sociology.* Englewood Cliffs, NJ: Prentice-Hall.

Schensul, S.L. (1985). Science theory and application in anthropology. *American Behavioral Scientist,* 29(2), 164–185.

Silva, M.C. (1977). Philosophy, science, theory: Interrelationships and implications for nursing research. *Image,* 9(3), 59–63.

Smith, J. (1981). The idea of health: A philosophical inquiry. *Advances in Nursing Science,* 3(3), 43–50.

Sorokin, P. (1974). How are sociological theories conceived, developed and validated. In R.S. Denisoff, O. Callahan, and M.H. Levine (Eds.), *Theories and paradigms in contemporary sociology.* Itasca, IL: F.E. Peacock.

Stern, P.N. (1981). Solving problems of cross-cultural health teaching: The Filipino child-bearing family. *Image,* 13, 47–50.

Stevens, P.E. (1989). A critical social reconceptualization of environment in nursing: Implications for methodology. *Advances in Nursing Science,* 11(4), 56–68.

Strauss, A. and Corbin, J. (1994). Grounded theory methodology: An overview. In N.K. Denzin and Y.S. Lincoln (Eds.), *Handbook of qualitative research.* Thousand Oaks, CA: Sage.

University of California, San Francisco School of Nursing Symptom Management Faculty Group. (1994). A model for symptom management. *Image: Journal of Nursing Scholarship,* 26(4), 272–276.

Walker, L.O. and Avant, K.C. (1988). *Strategies for theory construction in nursing* (2nd ed.). Norwalk, CT: Appleton-Century-Crofts.

Walker, L.O. and Avant, K.C. (1995). *Strategies for theory construction in nursing.* (3rd ed.). East Norwalk, CT: Appleton-Lange.

Westcott, M.R. (1968). *Antecedents and consequences of intuitive thinking.* Final report to U.S. Department of Health, Education, and Welfare. Poughkeepsie, NY: Vassar College.

Wilson, J. (1963). *Thinking with concepts.* New York: Press Syndicate of the University of Cambridge.

Zderad, L.T. (1978). From here-and-now to theory: Reflections on how. In J.G. Patterson, *Theory development: What, why, how?* New York: National League for Nursing.

CHAPTER 14

A Model for Evaluation of Theories: Description, Analysis, Critique, Testing, and Support*

Nurses have always evaluated theories. They evaluated theories to apply to practice, to develop curricula, to use in teaching, to operationalize for research, or to use in daily decision making. These evaluations may be deliberate, systematic, criteria based, objective, conscious, and elaborate, or they may be subjective, experiential, quick, and based on a limited set of criteria. Both types of evaluations are essential; neither type is sufficient by itself.

Evaluation of theory is an essential component of nursing practice and of knowledge development, for the following reasons.

1. To decide which theory is more appropriate to use as a framework for research, teaching, administration, or consultation
2. To identify effective theories in exploring some aspect of practice or in guiding a research project
3. To compare and contrast different explanations of the same phenomenon
4. To enhance the potential of constructive changes and further theory development
5. To identify epistemological approaches of a discipline through attention to the sociocultural context of the theorist and the theory
6. To assess the ontological beliefs in a discipline
7. To identify schools of thought in a discipline
8. To affect changes in clinical practice, to define research priorities, and to identify content for teaching and guidelines for nursing administration
9. To have nursing frameworks to justify nursing to the public
10. To identify strategies for theory development
11. To define a discipline's domain
12. To be a critical consumer of theories

* This chapter is adapted, with considerable changes, from an earlier manuscript written by A.I. Meleis and published in Chaska, N. (1982). *The nursing profession: Time to speak.* New York: McGraw-Hill, 1982.

Before going any further in reading this chapter, you should take a few minutes to identify one or two theories (nursing or nonnursing) that you have used in your work or personal life. For example, you may identify role theory as a framework for your research on women's daily activities in a nursing home and their health; endorphin theory linking stress with exercise; or Maslow's theory in understanding a patient's needs. The next set of questions to ask and reflect on are: Why did you select to use these theories in your work? Why not other theories that may provide a different set of equally plausible explanations? To complete this exercise, you should be able to identify the criteria you used in making a decision about what theory to use.

Over a 30-year span of teaching, I have asked students, faculty, clinicians, and administrators in the United States as well as in many other countries the questions outlined above. In reviewing the answers and analyzing their content, a number of criteria emerged. Now, compare your criteria with those identified next.

Personal: Individuals who use this criterion discuss their personal comfort in using the theory, their intuitive choices, and the theory's congruency with their philosophical view of life.

Mentor: There are those who use a theory because they were mentored by a theorist, or they were exposed to the teaching of a theorist who profoundly influenced and transformed them. They spoke of personal influence, respect, personal contact, and educational experience.

Theorist: Who the theorists are, their standing in the field, their status, and how well they are recognized were among the reasons that a theory was selected.

Literature support: Others identified the availability of extensive writings about the theory that gave them assurance of the level of significance of the theory and the status it holds.

Sociopolitical congruency: The congruency between the theory implementation process and the sociopolitical as well as the economic climate was another criterion often identified by audiences. These people spoke of a climate that supports one theory over another because, for example, it did not necessitate structural changes, it required minimal preparation, or it was imposed by administration.

Utility: The ease by which theory was understood and applied prompted a group of users to select a certain theory over another.

Although these criteria are neither all inclusive nor representative of all nurses, definite themes evolved and are experientially supported. The decision to use one theory and not another involves both subjective and objective processes. The decision process could be considered as falling on two continua, each ranging from low to high. Thus, a decision could be both highly objective and highly subjective, low on subjectivity and on objectivity, or could be one of numerous other combinations of levels of objectivity and subjectivity and the many options in between.

The subjectivity in the selection of a theory is as important as is the objectivity in the selection. We can select a theory by using a number of well defined criteria and by systematically evaluating the theory using each of these criteria; therefore, the decision becomes highly objective. However, if the theory's assumptions are not congruent with ours, or if we are not convinced by the theorist's experiential background, or if we are not comfortable with other work done by the theorist, the decision process becomes subjective. On the other hand, a selection may be based on one's having worked with the theorist and, without making a decision per se, on one's continuing to use the theory. A highly objective decision with low subjectivity could result in theory use that is not as true to the theory premises and propositions; and perhaps vice versa.

The objective evaluation and critique of theories is as complex as the subjective evaluation. To simplify any evaluation, we must break it down into components. For example, when a research project is critiqued, the analysis is done along structural criteria, such as the introduction, conceptual framework, research questions and hypotheses, methodology, results, discussion, conclusions, and limitations. The critique is then completed by looking for clarity, significance, timeliness, and documentation, among other criteria. To analyze and critique theories objectively, numerous criteria have been recommended by a number of authors. In fact, analysis and critique of theories have preoccupied many nurse metatheorists over a period of time that even preceded the diligent theory development efforts.

Two disciplines have profoundly influenced evaluation of nursing theory: sociology and psychology. The result has been a synthesis of criteria from these disciplines, at times too empirically based and at other times too critical of the theories that were developed by nurses, and those driven by our own nursing phenomena. When we adhered to some of these criteria, we tended to discount nursing theories, relegating them to the category of individual subjective philosophical expositions. Although some of these criteria are appropriate for the discipline of nursing, many were not and did not reflect the nature of nursing and the goals of our discipline. Others have emerged that directly relate to and represent nursing. The rationale for developing a different set of criteria is embedded in the nature of nursing care, the assumptions on which the discipline of nursing is built, and the quality of its scientific and humanistic bases. The domain of nursing encompasses human beings' experiences and interactions and deals with complex sets of contextual variables; therefore, the criteria for theory evaluation must consider ways by which its theories reflect and represent these contexts.

Each one of the evaluation models offered in nursing literature addressed one aspect of a theory to the exclusion of others. For example, Johnson (1974) focused on a congruence of theory mission with goals relegated by society to nurses (social congruence, utility, and significance). Earlier, in an unpublished manuscript on requirements of an effective model, Johnson (1970) offered a set of requirements that focused on the mission of nursing practice: goals of action, patience, the actor's place and role, source of difficulty, intervention focus, and mode and consequences of care. Although Johnson also addressed the necessity of explicit and consistent structure (assumption and values) and content (nursing's unique goal, ability to be generalized, restrictiveness, continuity, and specificity), other utility criteria were not included, such as research utility and potential for theoretical propositions. Johnson pioneered the development of a set of objective requirements for effective models in nursing and the use of internal and external requirements. Her evaluation model was not published, however, and was therefore limited in exposure and refinement.

Barnum (1994) proposed evaluative criteria that are appropriate for internal criticism (internal construction of theory) and external criticism (which considers theory in its relationships to human beings, nursing, and health). The criteria for internal criticism are clarity, consistency, adequacy, logical development, and level of theory development. The criteria for external criticism are reality conversion, utility, significance, discrimination, scope of theory, and complexity (Barnum, 1994, pp. 180–191). These criteria represent one framework for critiquing theories that could be used independently or in junction with the descriptive and analytical criteria offered in the model proposed in this chapter.

A similar framework was offered by Ellis (1968), who delineated seven criteria for what she considered significant theories. Significant theories according to Ellis have a broad scope, are sufficiently complex to consider different propositions reflecting the wide scope, and contain propositions that are testable and useful. Significant theories are also those that have explicit values and in which implicit values are carefully delineated. These theories must have well defined and meaningful terminology and they provide opportunities for further generation of information (Ellis, 1968). Hardy (1974) organized her criteria around the concept of "adequacy": meaning, logic, operationalization, empirical evidence, and pragmatism. She also believed that adequate theories should have the ability to be generalized, should contribute to understanding, and should be able to predict. It is indeed a challenge to find theories in any discipline to meet all these criteria simultaneously; however, these criteria provide serious theory developers with milestones toward which they should strive.

Lest theory developers get discouraged by the rigorous criteria, Duffey and Muhlenkamp (1974, p. 571) offered the following modest set of questions by which theories can be evaluated:

Does the theory generate testable hypotheses?
Does the theory guide practice?
How complete is its subject matter?
Did the theorist make her biases explicit?
Does the theory have propositions and are relationships explicit?
Is it parsimonious?

Chinn and Jacobs (1987) offered a refreshingly different approach to evaluating theories that was based more on criteria for evaluation of psychological theory. They recommended evaluating theories by considering five criteria: clarity (semantic clarity, semantic consistency, structural clarity, and structural consistency), simplicity, generality, empirical applicability, and consequences. A list of questions was offered to help the evaluator make an objective decision about the level of the criteria (pp. 137–147).

Fawcett (1993, 1995), dissatisfied with previously developed evaluation criteria because of the seeming overlap between criteria for evaluating theories and those more appropriate for evaluating conceptual frameworks, offered one analytical and evaluative framework for conceptual models as well as one for theories. The framework for conceptual models (Fawcett, 1995) separates questions for analysis from those intended for evaluation. For analysis, Fawcett proposed a consideration of the historical evolution of the model, and the unique focus and context of the model (pp. 52–55). For the evaluation, she proposed evaluation (judgment based on criteria) of the origins of the model, the degree of comprehensiveness of content, the logical congruence of its internal structure, the ability of the model to generate and test theories, the degree to which it is credible as demonstrated in its social utility (use, implementation), social congruency, significance to society, and its contributions to the discipline of nursing (Fawcett, 1995, pp. 55–62). Although these were proposed as criteria for evaluating conceptual models, the same criteria could be used in analyzing and evaluating theories. However, Fawcett proposed another set of criteria for theory critique that she believed to be more congruent with her definition of theory. Critique of theories was also divided into analysis and evaluation. For theory analysis she proposed similar criteria to other metatheorists, such as consideration of the scope of the theory, the context of theory and its attention and consideration of major concepts in nursing and the conceptual frameworks derived from the context. The last criteria to consider in theory analysis are examinations of the theory content (Barnum, 1994, pp. 21–29; Fawcett, 1993, pp. 37–39). Fawcett also proposes an evaluation of theories to complement the analysis described above. The content of theories, she says, could be evaluated in terms of the congruency of its internal structure, the extent to which the theory is stated clearly and concisely (parsimony), and the potential testability of its propositions. Theories must also be evaluated through the adequacy of their empirical evidence and their utility for practice (pragmatic adequacy) (Fawcett, 1993, pp. 39–44).

I encourage you to review as many of these proposals for evaluation as possible. The criteria reflect the level and sophistication of our knowledge at different stages of development of nursing as a scientific discipline. In reviewing the different criteria, several trends emerge:

- Theories are described, analyzed, and tested.
- There are internal and external criteria for evaluating theories.
- The internal descriptive criteria include assumptions, concepts, relationships, and definitions.
- The internal critical criteria include some areas of agreement, such as consistency, clarity, and logical development.
- Evaluation criteria consider the fit between the theory and external criteria (human beings, society, prevailing paradigms) and not only the intrinsic criteria.
- A more accepting attitude has evolved toward a shift from the rigor of empiricism to the more realistic rigor of potential for testability.
- There is wider acknowledgment of the complexity of evaluation criteria (the two sides of simplicity, the many meanings of complexity, etc) and, therefore, wider acceptance of multiple criteria.
- There is less prejudice toward descriptive theories.

The model proposed here considers these trends, draws on many of the previously delineated criteria, and further acknowledges that even when systematic criteria are advanced to ensure objective analysis and critique, objectivity is not guaranteed or required in critiquing theories for one's use in research or practice. Furthermore, individuals may differ on how they use the critique criteria, and the perceptions of the meaning of each of these criteria may be influenced by individual variations and by context variations. It is also acknowledged here that some criteria may be conflicting; that to enhance simplicity, complexity may suffer; and that to advocate a wider scope, accuracy for deviant cases or opposing situations may be jeopardized and generalization may not be as desirable as it once was.

The proposed model defines *evaluation* as encompassing description, analyses, critique, testing, and support. By using this model, a reviewer acknowledges extant evaluations that have been completed by nurse theorists, researchers, and clinicians, among others. The model is also based philosophically more on an historical view of science than on an empirical view. Therefore, it proposes to analyze the central questions that are solved by the theory, the role of the background of the theorist in the development of the theory, and the sociocultural context of the theory, the theorist, and the discipline. In other words, human processes are considered an integral part of theory description, analysis, critique, testing (Laudan, 1977), and support (Meleis, 1995).

Description

Before embarking on theory evaluation, the reviewer should recognize and identify the boundaries of the review. Boundaries include degree of exposure to theory, length of time devoted to understanding theory, and type of work done with theory (eg, having taught theory, used it in practice, used it in research, worked with the theoretician, or any number of other alternatives). In doing so, the reviewer attempts to separate objective and subjective rationales.

An initial thorough reading and scanning of the central work of a theorist helps to identify the central questions the theorist is attempting to answer. For example, a central question for developmental theorists is how human beings mature. More often than not, it is not entirely clear in nursing theory what questions the theorists are attempting to answer. The central questions of the theory are answered in the form of the theory propositions. Propositions are the crux of a theory. From propositions, questions emerge that guide exploration and research. Identification of propositions at the outset helps make the job of delineating assumptions and concepts easier. It is not a linear process, but a cyclical one in which concepts may be identified, followed by pertinent propositions, followed by more concepts and pertinent assumptions, and so on. This entire process of identifying assumptions, concepts, and propositions addresses the structural components of the theory. Table 14-1 offers a summary of theory description.

Structural Components

A theory begins with a set of "givens" that either have been empirically tested or accepted by a number of other theories or previous research. These "givens" are the *theory assumptions.* They could evolve from a philosophical standpoint, from ideological positions, from ethical considerations, from cultural heritage, from social structure, or from previously tested and supported hypotheses. Assumptions also represent one's values. Assumptions of a theory are not subject to testing by the same theory; rather, they lead to a set of propositions that are to be tested. They are the basis from which

Table 14-1 ***Theory Description***

Criteria	Unit of Analysis
Structural components	Assumptions
	Concepts
	Propositions
Functional components	Focus
	Client
	Nursing
	Health
	Nurse–patient interactions
	Environment
	Nursing problem
	Nursing therapeutics

we can determine the viewpoint of the theorist. In nursing theories, there are assumptions about nursing, human behavior, life, death, health, and illness.

Early writing in theory provides *implicit assumptions*; these are statements that are not identified as *explicit assumptions* by the theorist. Explicit assumptions are identified by authors as their assumptions. Implicit assumptions are imbedded in the writings; they are statements not identified as assumptions, yet they are central for the development of theory propositions or answers to questions. They are statements considered by the reviewer to be significant in the development of the theory. The idea that a patient has the right to learn about the gravity of his illness is an implicit assumption in our Western society, whereas the reverse is an implicit assumption in Middle Eastern cultures. A proposition built on this assumption responds to the question of what is the most effective way to impart the information about the grave diagnosis to the patient. Another proposition would question whether a relationship exists, for example, between certain strategies for giving information about diagnosis and rate of recovery. The rationale for the proposition is only understood when assumptions underlying it are delineated.

As theorists in nursing become more systematic in their theory development efforts, more explicit assumptions are stated, and fewer assumptions are left implicit. The plethora of literature that has discussed theory critique and theory development should be credited with the constructive changes demonstrated in the updated, further developed, or new theories evolving in nursing. Roy, for example, in further developing her theory, followed a more systematic approach in which she identified assumptions and carefully related many of the concepts to the assumptions, thereby providing theoretical propositions with better potential for testability (Roy and Roberts, 1981).

When identifying the internal structure of a theory, one should use a description that involves a careful search of the inherent assumptions; at the same time, one should not overlook the implicit ones. The more effective theories are those in which authors explicitly state the assumptions guiding their thinking. The more explicit the premises of the theory are, the less ambiguity there is when interpreting its conditions and goals.

The internal structure of a theory could be further described by delineating the concepts on which the theory is built. Descriptive properties used in relation to concepts are clarity, conceptual definitions, observable properties, and boundaries; concepts are also described as being primitive (ie, concepts that originated in this particular theory) or derived (ie, concepts that were derived from other theories). Hage (1972) provided criteria to help determine whether concepts in a theory are primitive or derived. The introduction of a concept in theory with no definition—because the concept has an agreed-on meaning, has simple definitions, has an intuitively obvious definition, or has been defined elsewhere—designates a primitive concept. The definition of the derived concept is within the theory and is based on the primitive terms. The definitions of the primitive terms are outside the theory (Hage, 1972, pp. 111–115).

The usage of primitive and derived concepts in this book differs from Hage's usage. *Primitive concepts* are those concepts introduced in the theory as new and therefore defined within the theory. *Derived concepts* are concepts from outside the theory that have taken on a different meaning within the theory. For example, in Meleis (1975), role is a derived concept, and role supplementation is a primitive concept, that is, a new concept with a new definition.

Concepts are also evaluated along the abstract/concrete dimension. The degree of generality determines the abstract/concrete level. The more general a concept is, the more it transcends time and geography, the higher the level of abstraction. Concepts have also been classified along the general variable/nonvariable dimension (Hage, 1972). Nonvariable concepts in nursing are sex, ethnic background, religion, and marital status. Examples of variable concepts (general variables) are sex-role orientation, level of well-being, degree of cultural identity, and level of sick role. It becomes apparent that each nonvariable could be converted into a general variable.

There are several advantages to having general variables (Hage, 1972). General variables allow more precise classification and allow for variations that are more congruent with variations in reality. Classification of a patient as male or female yields some significant data and a certain degree of predictability of structure and function of a few of the biologic systems. However, sex-role orientation, a general variable, may help us to more precisely describe clients and predict their patterns of rehabilitation.

Just as assumptions and concepts are delineated, sometimes simultaneously and at other times cyclically, theory propositions also should be delineated and described. A *proposition* is a descriptive statement of the properties and dimensions of a concept or a statement that links two or more concepts together. Propositions provide the theory with the powers of description, explanation, or prediction. A theory that has more assumptions than propositions is a theory with limited power. It indicates that we have to agree to too many conditions for a few descriptions or predictions. If we consider the relationship of assumptions and propositions in a ratio form, an inverse relationship (with the number of propositions being higher than the number of assumptions) allows for more explanatory power.

There are different types of propositions, each type having a different purpose. *Existence propositions* are constructed around one phenomenon and therefore only describe and assert the existence of this one phenomenon. Propositions with the power of explanation, on the other hand, link concepts; therefore, they are expected to have two or more concepts. They are formulated to explain and assert something pertaining to the reality embodied in the theory. These are *relational propositions*, which encompass many types of propositions, such as those that just describe the existence of a relationship, those that describe the direction of such a relationship, and those that can predict the relationship, the direction of the relationship, and the conditions under which that relationship may or may not occur.

Further description of a proposition could be done along dimensions specified by Zetterberg (1963, pp. 69–71). This is best illustrated by using an example of a two-concept proposition derived from Johnson's subsystem theory:

> The higher the level of met functional requirements of the affiliated subsystem of the Middle Eastern immigrant, the greater the recovery rate.

A *reversible proposition* would have "and vice versa" at the end of the statement, therefore requiring two testings, one with the condition of "met functional requirements" and prospectively considering recovery rate, and the other beginning with different levels of recovery rate and then retrospectively considering levels of "met functional requirements."

A second dimension is whether the proposition is *deterministic* or *stochastic.* Nursing has a predisposition toward more stochastic propositions that incorporate a probability condition, rather than "if X then always Y," which is deterministic and improbable in a humanistic science. A stochastic proposition, albeit a probabilistic one, would be:

> The higher the level of met functional requirements of the affiliated subsystem, the more probable is a greater recovery rate.

A third dimension is whether the proposition is *sequential* or *coexisting.* A sequential proposition assumes that one variable occurred before the other variable. Propositions in nursing lend themselves more to coexisting propositions when describing existing relationships and to sequential propositions when engaged in theorizing about interventions and consequences of intervention. This dimension characterizes theorizing that is central and essential to nursing.

A fourth dimension is demonstrated in the relationships between concepts. This relationship may be sufficient (if X, then Y, regardless of anything else) or contingent (if X, then Y, but only if Z) (Zetterberg, 1963, p. 71). Humanistic sciences cannot strive to produce sufficient propositions. Propositions in nursing theory include numerous variables and probabilistic relationships.

A last dimension identifies whether the relationship is necessary or can be substituted. A necessary relationship is "if X, and only if X, then Y." A substitutable relationship is "if X, then Y; but if Z, then also Y." Like other concepts in nursing, greater recovery rate is contingent on a number of variables and not only on "met functional requirements of one subsystem"; therefore, a substitutable proposition is more appropriate. To increase the explanatory power of such a proposition and then the predictive power, all other concepts related to recovery rate could be identified. For example:

> The higher the level of met functional requirements of the affiliated subsystem of the Middle Eastern immigrant, the greater the recovery rate. The higher the level of met functional requirements of the aggressive subsystem, the greater the recovery rate.

Thus, propositions in nursing may be reversible, stochastic, coexisting, contingent, and substitutable. Attention to each dimension provides for a way to describe the propositions and for deliberately developing propositions along these dimensions; this may help in enhancing the power of contextual explanations, if that is what the theorist wishes to do. This labeling also allows appropriate assessment of the propositions and their power of explanation and predictability. The clarity and systematization of propositions are also considered when we analyze the selected ordering and sequencing of propositions.

This first level of description is structural. The next level involves description of theory in terms of the function of the theory. This level considers the concepts of the nursing domain.

Functional Components

Unlike a structural analysis of a theory, a functional assessment of a theory carefully considers the anticipated consequences of the theory and its purpose. A functional analysis is focused on the relationship between the theory's assumptions, concepts, and propositions and those of the domain. (Again, refer to Table 14-1 for a summary of theory description.)

Concepts of the Domain

Theory is described around questions central to the discipline of nursing, including the following:

- Who is acted on? This is the major question that begins to address the function of theory. Does the theory identify the focus of the theory as the client, family, community, or society, or does the theory consider the target as one to the exclusion of others? The target of action here denotes both the target of assessment and the target intervention; the target in nursing should be the client (in the broadest sense) in health or illness.
- What definitions does the theory offer for nursing, client, health, nursing problems, environment, and nurse–patient interactions? Are definitions explicit and clear?
- Does the theory offer a clear idea of what the sources of the nursing problem are, whether the sources lie within or outside of the individual?
- Does the theory provide any insights in the form of intervention for nursing? Are the variables to be manipulated well delineated? Is it clear what the points of entry are for a nursing intervention? Is the focus of intervention justifiable within the theory? Points of entry could vary from manipulating outside stimuli (Johnson, 1968) to interactions and transactions between client and nurse (King, 1971) to behaviors within systems (Auger, 1976).
- Are there guidelines for intervention modalities? Are they specified? Is there potential for the evolution of such intervention modalities?
- As a nursing theory, does it provide guidelines for the role of the nurse?
- Are the consequences of nurses' actions articulated in the theory? Are they intended or unintended, positive or negative, anticipated and delineated? Is there a plan for dealing with such consequences?

These criteria are generally consistent with those offered by others, including Dickoff, James, and Wiedenbach (1968) and Barnum (1994).

Analysis

Analysis is defined as a process of identifying parts and components and examining them against a number of identified criteria. Analysis includes concept and theory analysis.

Concept Analysis

Concept analysis is a useful process in the cycle of theory development as well as in theory evaluation. Concept analysis may occur at many different points in the process of evaluation and development. Wilson (1969) proposed several steps and techniques in analyzing concepts. These steps do not necessarily have to be completed in this order.

1. Definition, identification, and description of the different dimensions and components of the concept. For example we proposed "transitions" as a central concept in nursing; we have defined the concept as "those periods in between fairly stable states, a passage from one life phase, condition, or status to another" (Chick and Meleis, 1986). We have identified some of its components and dimensions as process, disconnectedness, perception of transition, and patterns of response.
2. Comparison of the concept to others with similar properties and dimensions to establish its boundaries (Norris, 1982; Walker and Avant, 1995). Transition, for example, can be differentiated from the general concept of change sufficiently to make it useful in alerting nurses to relevant aspects of the life contexts of clients. In this case, transition is seen as a special case of the general phenomenon of change (Chick and Meleis, 1986).
3. Description of some of the antecedents to the concept and of some of the consequences (Lindsey, Piper, and Stotts, 1982), and matching some of these descriptions with what occurs in nursing practice. Examples of antecedents of transition are illness, recovery, loss, birthing; examples of consequences are distress, role performance changes, and disorientation.
4. Development, description, and analysis of exemplars or model cases. This step may include empirical results that are related to the concept.
5. Development, description, and analysis of contrary cases to normative cases. Situations in which the concept appears only occasionally or appears under a new set of conditions are called borderline cases and are also useful in analyzing concepts. (See Chap. 12 for a more comprehensive discussion of concept analysis.)

The process of concept analysis may include *semantic analysis,* which is analysis of linguistic meanings of the label given the concept; analysis of *logical derivation,* which is the logical progression of identifying, supporting, and labeling a concept; and *context analysis* of the concept, which includes the conditions under which the concept is manifested. Any inferences about concept should be analyzed for their sources, whether they are logically or empirically derived.

Each one of these steps is a test of the occurrence of the concept. These tests are both conceptual and clinical, but they are not tests as defined by empiricists. They are, however, equally necessary tests and equally important steps in the process of testing concepts that involve the development of empirically valid and reliable research instruments.

Theory Analysis

Whereas concept analysis is a process that could occur early in the process and cycle of theory development and theory testing, theory analysis is a later process. (Table 14-2 compares theory analysis and concept analysis.) Theory analysis involves considering important variables that may have influenced the development of the theory and its current structure. In analyzing theories, consider several criteria: the theorist, paradigmatic origins, and internal dimensions. These criteria provide for a better under-

Table 14-2 ***Analysis***

Analysis	Criteria	Units of Analysis
Concepts	Differentiation from others	Definitions
		Semantic
		Logic
		Context
		Antecedents
		Consequences
		Exemplars
Theories	The theorist	Educational background
		Experimental background
		Professional network
		Sociocultural context
	Paradigmatic origins	References, citations
		Assumptions
		Concepts
		Propositions
		Hypotheses
		Laws
	Internal dimensions	Rationale
		System of relations
		Content
		Beginnings
		Scope
		Goal
		Context
		Abstractness
		Method

standing of choices of central theory questions, goals of theory, the theory phenomena, and strategy of theory development; these criteria also set the stage for the critique.

The Theorist

A comprehensive analysis of theories includes a careful consideration of the author of the theory. Areas for exploration include experiential background, educational background, employment, and reconstruction of the professional and academic networks that surrounded the theorist while the theory was evolving. Such an analysis may include mentors, students, and sponsors when appropriate. This analysis helps in identifying influencing factors on the theory's inception and on its further development. Often, clarification in a theory, redefinitions, or extensions are directly or indirectly related to a new mentor relationship, a new degree, an employment move, or other variables that contribute to shifts in orientations. Analysis helps to uncover external and internal factors influencing a theorist, such as beliefs held by the theorist, the patterns of reasoning, and their origins. This may lead to a better understanding of the human parameters involved in theory development, an essential component of a historic's conception of science (Silva and Rothbart, 1984).

This segment of analysis could be done in a number of different ways, including a thorough review of all that has been written by the theorist and all that has been written by others about the theorist, direct communication with the theorist, and communication with mentors and students. A review may also focus on only one aspect or more of the theorist (Fulton, 1987). Analyzing the theorist's background will help to clarify internal dimensions, which follows as the next order of business in analyzing theories.

Consideration of who the theorists are as people, as nurses, as educators, as clinicians, and as theorists was the subject of analyses during the 1980s. Theses analyses took the form of short reviews (for example, Marriner-Tomey, 1989) or elaborate videotapes (see Chap. 21). These analyses are indications of the value the discipline places on the contributions of these theorists, the significance of knowing the theorist behind the theory for further understanding of the theory and for enhancing the potential for others to model theory theoretical work and actions.

Paradigmatic Origins of Theory

Theoretical thinking in nursing evolves from a prototype theory or can be traced to theories used in other fields. Examples of such theories are those of Johnson, who derived her theory from the premises of the systems paradigm (Parsons, 1949; Riehl and Roy, 1980, pp. 207–216), and Paterson and Zderad (1988), who based their work on the existentialist philosophy. Therefore, for a careful consideration of this component, the theory analyst should become conversant with paradigmatic origins of the theory under consideration and address those origins in the analysis.

To identify the paradigm from which the theory may have evolved or other theories that may have influenced the development of the current theory, the review considers the following:

References, bibliography provided
Background of theorist, educationally and experientially
Sociocultural context that may have influenced the development of the theory

Analysis of the theory in relationship to these components provides answers to three major questions:

1. Is the theory derived from and built on a specific paradigm?
2. What are the origins of the paradigm?
3. Why was this particular paradigm used?

More specifically, on what prototype theory or paradigm did the theorist build the conceptual structures? How extensively is the original paradigm or theory used?

Is the use of paradigm obvious to the reviewer, made explicit or implicit by the writer? Does the theorist present the rationale for selection of the theory or parts of the theory used? From where do theory inadequacies originate, prototype theory or nursing theory? Are the problems detected those of borrowed theory or are they the result of translation? Does nursing theory improve on prototype theory? How congruent or incongruent is the use of components of prototype theory with nursing theory? How different or similar are the definitions to prototype theory definitions? Are goals the same? Is justification for variance included? Are other nursing theories derived from the prototype theory? What are they?

Internal Dimensions

The components of the internal structure act as guidelines to describe a theory, as discussed under Theory Description. Dimensions described in this section help in analyzing theories to enhance understanding of the approaches used to develop the theory, in delineating gaps in the theory, and in giving perspective to why some omissions are not necessarily gaps in the theory but in some instances are merely what the theory intended to be. This will soon become clear. The dimensions described next provide the necessary lexicon to describe a theory.

The first dimension to consider is the *rationale on which the theory is built.* Questions to consider in describing the theory along this dimension include: Are components of the theory united in a chain-link fashion? Is it a theory of the factor type? Is the theory developed around concepts and thus a concatenated theory? Or is it based on certain sets of relationships that are deduced from a small set of basic principles and therefore hierarchical in nature? The concatenated theory has fewer explanations that converge on a central point and therefore embodies existence propositions, whereas the set of relationships theory embodies an interpretive model (Kaplan, 1964).

The second dimension to consider is that of *system of relations.* Questions to be asked are: Do relations explain elements or do elements explain relations? A monadic approach in theory construction considers single irreducible units, as opposed to a field approach, which considers its unit of analysis in terms of a number of other miniunits. An example of the monadic approach is cell theory, and an example of the field approach is a theory of personality in terms of roles. A monadic approach is one in which the attributes and properties of the phenomenon are the focus of the theory. A field approach focuses on the relationships between the phenomena and thus explains the phenomena by the relationships. Therefore, a theory of a human being as a subsystem of behavior would be monadic and a theory of human environmental interaction would be a field theory.

Content of the theory is a third descriptive dimension (Kaplan, 1964). Content is distinguished by the range of laws and group of individuals to which the theory refers. A theory could be classified as molar or macrotheory, or as molecular or microtheory. Organizational theories in sociology are macro in content, whereas rule theory is micro. This dimension considers the range of relationships in the theory and the set of individuals to which the relationships refer. When a theory considers the human being in totality, it is macro theory. When the theory address needs during illness, it is a microtheory. Therefore, Rogers' work (1970) is an example of macrotheory, whereas Orem's (1985) is an example of microtheory.

At what point a theorist begins articulating ideas and whether a theorist addresses a theory of extant nursing practice or one of ideal nursing practice specifies another dimension, namely that of *theory beginnings* (Kaplan, 1964). A constructive beginning is hypothetical and is intended to build up a picture of more complex phenomena, whereas a principle theory beginning is more empirically grounded (discovered). A theory with a constructive beginning tends to be more complete, clear, and adaptable and tends to consider relationships hypothetically; the latter is more analytical and addresses the "is" rather that the "ought to be." It is more perfect and better substantiated.

A theory with a constructive beginning is also called a deductive theory because it emphasizes a conceptual structure deduced from another conceptual structure (Duffey and Muhlenkamp, 1974). Its laws are logically interrelated. It is through such deductive logic that some theories are derived. The major criticism of deductive theories is the lack of empirical support until they are tested in research. The principle theory beginning is also called the inductive beginning. It, on the other hand, consists essentially of summary statements or empirical relations. An example of the former (deductive theory) in nursing is Rogers' (1970) theoretical conceptualization of man in his symphonic harmony with the environment. Her theory evolved from principles of physics, thermodynamics, and evolution, among others. An example of the latter (inductive theory) is a conceptualization of issues surrounding dying, evolving from Glaser and Strauss's (1965) and Benoliel's (1967) work, even though these have not been formally labeled a nursing theory.

Many theorists have addressed the *scope of theory* and its significance in describing the capability of the theory. The basic question that considers a theory's scope is: How many of the basic problems in nursing or any of its specialities could be addressed by the same theory? The significance of scope stems from the notion that theories having wider scope tend to be more general and last longer (Kuhn, 1970). In addition, the significance of a theory increases as its scope broadens (Ellis, 1968). Therefore, to answer questions related to scope, we also address generality. Theories with a wide scope are also called "grand theories," as opposed to "single-domain theories," which could be placed at the other end of a scope continuum.

The major criticism associated with both ends of the scope continuum (ie, grand theories and single-domain theories) involves the attempts of grand theories to explain everything surrounding a set of phenomena, which is also why they may be limited in their power to explain (a major criticism of Parsons' [1949] attempts at a theory of sociology). *Single-domain theories* address only simple, abstract, isolated factors and principles. The empiricist and methodologist, Robert Merton (1964), is credited with advocating middle-range theories, thus avoiding those criticisms. *Middle-range theories* consider a limited number of variables, have a particular substantive foc··s, focus on a limited aspect of relationship, are more susceptible to empirical testing ··ld be consolidated into more wide-ranging theories.

In nursing, Jacox (1974), following Merton's ideas, urged the middle-range theories for limited aspects within the discipline of nur alleviation or promotion of sleep. A major criticism of middle-range t lead to fragmentation of a discipline when the discipline has no a non. Middle-range theories are more appropriate now in nursing, have identified and broadly agreed on the boundaries of nursing ing domain concepts.

Questions to ask when considering the *goal of a theory* a developed? What is its aim and intent? Theories are constructe to predict, or to proscribe. A descriptive theory gives inform ena under consideration but does not make a claim beyond t to expect in the future. When a beginning linkage and between derived concept are provided, the theory become relative studies to test explanatory theories provide emp these theories. Another goal explicated in some theori dictive theory encompasses propositions of an "if . . . t manner. The ultimate goal in nursing is to prescribe; t theory goal. Theories might have all of these goals, or or another. At this time in the developmental histo that a theory represent each of the goals.

The *context of a theory*, in which the centr another dimension for theory evaluation. Johnso in nursing for theories addressing knowledge knowledge of control. The knowledge of orde to objects, events, and interactions in a healt such phenomena. They describe the normal provide baseline data. An example of such her explication of Johnson's (1968) normal tems of behavior. Knowledge of disorder r nurses deal. An attempt to develop such oretical schema, was manifested in the fi nosis (Gebbie, 1976) and in subsequer that, when implemented, could chang have knowledge of control. Examp Orem's self-care theory (1985) and M supplementation (1980) theories, a

Relationship Between Structure and Function

In critiquing a theory according to the criteria listed next, the critic considers the relationship between and structure and function (Table 14-3). This is accomplished by making a critical assessment and judgment of the relationship between the different components of the theory, such as assumptions, concepts, propositions, and domain concepts. In doing so, the critic cannot judge the logic inherent in the development of a dialectic theory by the same criteria used when judging a logical theory; rather, the method used dictates the critique. Several criteria could be considered, such as clarity, consistency, simplicity/complexity, and tautology/teleology.

Clarity

Clarity is defined on a continuum ranging from high to low. It denotes prec boundaries, a communication of a sense of orderliness, vividness of meanin sistency through the theory. Clarity is also defined by Chinn and Jacobs ness and consistency" (p. 137). Clarity is demonstrated in assump propositions as well as in domain concepts. To have clarity in oretical and operational definitions that are consistent thro in a parsimonious way, and are consistent with theo Questions such as Are concepts operationally de tent and construct validity? help to determi manifested in a coherent and logical pr ages between the theory concepts high clarity to low clarity.

Consistency

The boundarie to which its co

field approach focuses on the relationships between the phenomena and thus explains the phenomena by the relationships. Therefore, a theory of a human being as a subsystem of behavior would be monadic and a theory of human environmental interaction would be a field theory.

Content of the theory is a third descriptive dimension (Kaplan, 1964). Content is distinguished by the range of laws and group of individuals to which the theory refers. A theory could be classified as molar or macrotheory, or as molecular or microtheory. Organizational theories in sociology are macro in content, whereas rule theory is micro. This dimension considers the range of relationships in the theory and the set of individuals to which the relationships refer. When a theory considers the human being in totality, it is macro theory. When the theory address needs during illness, it is a microtheory. Therefore, Rogers' work (1970) is an example of macrotheory, whereas Orem's (1985) is an example of microtheory.

At what point a theorist begins articulating ideas and whether a theorist addresses a theory of extant nursing practice or one of ideal nursing practice specifies another dimension, namely that of *theory beginnings* (Kaplan, 1964). A constructive beginning is hypothetical and is intended to build up a picture of more complex phenomena, whereas a principle theory beginning is more empirically grounded (discovered). A theory with a constructive beginning tends to be more complete, clear, and adaptable and tends to consider relationships hypothetically; the latter is more analytical and addresses the "is" rather that the "ought to be." It is more perfect and better substantiated.

A theory with a constructive beginning is also called a deductive theory because it emphasizes a conceptual structure deduced from another conceptual structure (Duffey and Muhlenkamp, 1974). Its laws are logically interrelated. It is through such deductive logic that some theories are derived. The major criticism of deductive theories is the lack of empirical support until they are tested in research. The principle theory beginning is also called the inductive beginning. It, on the other hand, consists essentially of summary statements or empirical relations. An example of the former (deductive theory) in nursing is Rogers' (1970) theoretical conceptualization of man in his symphonic harmony with the environment. Her theory evolved from principles of physics, thermodynamics, and evolution, among others. An example of the latter (inductive theory) is a conceptualization of issues surrounding dying, evolving from Glaser and Strauss's (1965) and Benoliel's (1967) work, even though these have not been formally labeled a nursing theory.

Many theorists have addressed the *scope of theory* and its significance in describing the capability of the theory. The basic question that considers a theory's scope is: How many of the basic problems in nursing or any of its specialities could be addressed by the same theory? The significance of scope stems from the notion that theories having wider scope tend to be more general and last longer (Kuhn, 1970). In addition, the significance of a theory increases as its scope broadens (Ellis, 1968). Therefore, to answer questions related to scope, we also address generality. Theories with a wide scope are also called "grand theories," as opposed to "single-domain theories," which could be placed at the other end of a scope continuum.

The major criticism associated with both ends of the scope continuum (ie, grand theories and single-domain theories) involves the attempts of grand theories to explain everything surrounding a set of phenomena, which is also why they may be limited in their power to explain (a major criticism of Parsons' [1949] attempts at a theory of sociology). *Single-domain theories* address only simple, abstract, isolated factors and principles. The empiricist and methodologist, Robert Merton (1964), is credited with advocating middle-range theories, thus avoiding those criticisms. *Middle-range theories* consider a limited number of variables, have a particular substantive focus, focus on a limited aspect of relationship, are more susceptible to empirical testing, and could be consolidated into more wide-ranging theories.

In nursing, Jacox (1974), following Merton's ideas, urged the development of middle-range theories for limited aspects within the discipline of nursing, such as pain alleviation or promotion of sleep. A major criticism of middle-range theories is that they lead to fragmentation of a discipline when the discipline has no agreed-on phenomenon. Middle-range theories are more appropriate now in nursing, particularly after we have identified and broadly agreed on the boundaries of nursing knowledge and nursing domain concepts.

Questions to ask when considering the *goal of a theory* are: Why was the theory developed? What is its aim and intent? Theories are constructed to describe, to explain, to predict, or to proscribe. A descriptive theory gives information related to phenomena under consideration but does not make a claim beyond that, nor does it tell us what to expect in the future. When a beginning linkage and description of relationships between derived concept are provided, the theory becomes an explanatory theory. Correlative studies to test explanatory theories provide empirical evidence in support of these theories. Another goal explicated in some theories is that of prediction. A predictive theory encompasses propositions of an "if . . . then" nature in a consequential manner. The ultimate goal in nursing is to prescribe; therefore, prescription is another theory goal. Theories might have all of these goals, or they may explicate only one goal or another. At this time in the developmental history of nursing theory, it is essential that a theory represent each of the goals.

The *context of a theory*, in which the central phenomenon is addressed, is yet another dimension for theory evaluation. Johnson (1959) called attention to the need in nursing for theories addressing knowledge of order, knowledge of disorder, and knowledge of control. The knowledge of order addresses phenomena that are central to objects, events, and interactions in a healthy context. They describe regularities in such phenomena. They describe the normal state and natural scheme of things. They provide baseline data. An example of such knowledge is provided by Auger (1976) in her explication of Johnson's (1968) normal patterns of a person's behavior within systems of behavior. Knowledge of disorder recognizes a context or disorder within which nurses deal. An attempt to develop such knowledge, not yet bound together in a theoretical schema, was manifested in the first conference on classification of nursing diagnosis (Gebbie, 1976) and in subsequent conferences. To prescribe a course of action that, when implemented, could change the sequence of events in a desired way is to have knowledge of control. Examples of theories addressing such knowledge are Orem's self-care theory (1985) and Meleis (1975) and Meleis, Swendsen, and Jones' role supplementation (1980) theories, among others. Theories could also address knowledge of process, which included the nursing process and nurse–patient interactions (Paterson and Zderad, 1988).

Abstractness, another theory dimension, is evaluated by length of reduction and deduction between its propositions. A highly abstract theory requires more steps to reduce the chain "connecting the theoretical terms with the observable ones" (Kaplan, 1964, p. 301). It is a theory with wide spaces between its proposition and conceptual schema that is highly removed from reality but still pertains to it. If abstractness is put on a continuum from high abstractness to low abstractness, Rogers and Johnson would be at the high end and Orem at the low end.

Finally, the *method of theory development* should be carefully assessed. Barnum (1994) proposed that there are four methods used in developing theories. One can assess these methods by considering the reasoning on which the theory is built, the system of action, and the plan for progression. A dialectical method is exemplified by Rogers' work (Barnum, 1994) and is based on Hegel's dialectical process. It speaks to the fusion of opposites (Newman, 1979) It emphasizes relationship with a whole and, in fact, each whole explains parts and each part is a whole explaining other parts. A dialectical method encompasses contradictions, apposition, and dilemmas, but order evolves from the interaction among all of them. Erickson's developmental theory (1963) is an example of resolution of conflict and crisis in the process of moving into the next level of development. A dialectical method defies Aristotelian logic, which is another method of theory development—the logical method. This is a method in which the parts are organized to described the whole systematically and categorically. A theory of this nature offers a description of each part, and the whole is more than and different from the sum total of all parts. Barnum (1994) considers the theories of Johnson and Roy in this category.

The other two methods of theory development, according to Barnum (1994), are problem theories and operational theories. Both appeal more to common sense, use persuasion in supporting ideas, and use their experiences in theory development. Problem theories (Henderson, 1966; Nursing Theories Conference Group, 1980) are organized around nursing problems, whereas operational theories (Orem, 1985) are organized around methods of intervention.

Critique of Theory

Critique is defined by *Webster's Third New International Dictionary* as "critical examination or estimate of a thing or situation with the view to determining its nature and limitations or its conformity to standards."* Several criteria are essential in critiquing theory. These are relationships between structure and function, diagram of theory, circle of contagiousness, usefulness, and external components. Each is defined and presented below.

Relationship Between Structure and Function

In critiquing a theory according to the criteria listed next, the critic considers the relationship between and structure and function (Table 14-3). This is accomplished by making a critical assessment and judgment of the relationship between the different components of the theory, such as assumptions, concepts, propositions, and domain concepts. In doing so, the critic cannot judge the logic inherent in the development of a dialectic theory by the same criteria used when judging a logical theory; rather, the method used dictates the critique. Several criteria could be considered, such as clarity, consistency, simplicity/complexity, and tautology/teleology.

Clarity

Clarity is defined on a continuum ranging from high to low. It denotes precision of boundaries, a communication of a sense of orderliness, vividness of meaning, and consistency through the theory. Clarity is also defined by Chinn and Jacobs (1987) as "lucidness and consistency" (p. 137). Clarity is demonstrated in assumptions, concepts, and propositions as well as in domain concepts. To have clarity in concepts is to have theoretical and operational definitions that are consistent through the theory, are presented in a parsimonious way, and are consistent with theory assumptions and propositions. Questions such as Are concepts operationally defined? and Do they seem to have content and construct validity? help to determine concept clarity. Propositional clarity is manifested in a coherent and logical presentation of propositions and systematic linkages between the theory concepts. The criterion of clarity varies within a range from high clarity to low clarity.

Consistency

The boundaries between clarity and consistency are not easily determined. The degree to which a congruency exists between the different components of a theory describes its consistency. The fit between the different components of a theory describes its con-

Table 14-3 ***Theory Critique—Relationship Between Structure and Function; Diagram of Theory; and Circle of Contagiousness***

Criteria	Units of Analysis
Relationship between structure and function	Clarity Consistency Simplicity/complexity Tautology/Teleology
Diagram of theory	Visual and graphic presentation Logical representation Clarity
Circle of contagiousness	Geographical origin of theory and geographical spread Influence of theorist versus theory

sistency. The fit between assumptions and concept definitions, between concepts as defined and their use in propositions, and between concepts and clinical exemplars can all be considered determinants of consistency.

Simplicity/Complexity

Another criterion with which to critique a theory is its level of simplicity/complexity. The more phenomena the theory considers, the more potential relationships it could generate, and the more complex the theory is (Ellis, 1968). Simplicity of a theory is more desirable if it focuses on fewer concepts and few relationships that may enhance its utility. Complexity of a theory may be a desirable criterion if the complexity enhances the number of explanations and predictions the theory offers. Therefore, simplicity in the face of complex contextual reality is as unadvisable as complexity in theory would be when the theory explains a limited number of relationships. Chinn and Jacobs (1987) advocate simplicity in theory that has been tested and as a means for generating ideas and hypotheses, but question the value of simplicity in untested theory.

Tautology/Teleology

Clarity, consistency, and simplicity/complexity of a theory could also be described through tautology and teleology. A general assessment of *tautology* is done by considering the needless repetition of an idea in different parts of the theory. Tautology decreases the clarity of the theory. A careful consideration of the extent and the care by which causes and consequences are kept separate ensures that the theorist avoids teleology. *Teleology* occurs when the definition of concepts, conditions, and events uses consequences rather than properties and dimensions. When defining concepts by consequences only, the theorist introduces new concepts to define existing ones. This practice leaves the original concept undefined. Teleology is another dimension in the relationship between structure and function. The critic, therefore, should consider questions such as: Does the theory have logical coherence? Are definitions of nursing phenomena concise? Is it a teleological theory?

Diagram of Theory

Clarity of theories and models are further enhanced by visual representation of the theory. Major questions to be addressed in relation to this component are: Was the theory visually and graphically presented? Did the graphic presentation enhance understanding of different components of the theory? More specifically: How clear is the visual representation? Is it an accurate representation of the text? Does it include major concepts? Are linkages clear? Are linkage directions indicated? Is representation logical? Are there overlaps? Are there gaps? Is representation a substitute for words and explanation or is it a supplementation? Is the diagram clear and well defined? Is there a correspondence between diagram and concepts and propositions in the text? Do the diagrams enhance understanding of the text?

Circle of Contagiousness

The final test of any theory is whether or not is it adopted by others (see Table 14-3). The units of analysis here are geographical location and type of institution. Theories in nursing have been used within the geographical areas from which they emanated. Rogers' theory is used at New York University and tested by Rogers' students; Johnson's is used in Los Angeles and tested by her students. Therefore, when the theory begins to cross several concentric circles from its origin, its circle of contagiousness increases, and we can infer that the theory is receiving more acceptability, uninfluenced by the theorist.

The critic should review the literature, indexes, and citations for answers to questions such as: Where has the theory been developed and used? Where is it being used both geographically and institutionally? What is it used for (research, education, administration, clinical practice, etc)? How influential was the theorist in prompting the implementation of the theory? Where was it first introduced? What happened in the interim? Has the theory been considered and used cross-culturally and transculturally? A critique of the circle of contagiousness of a theory is made in conjunction with the usefulness of theory.

Usefulness

A critique of the usefulness of a theory encompasses four areas: its potential for usefulness in practice, research, education, and administration (Table 14-4).

Usefulness in Practice

A thorough review and assessment of theory has to consider its potential for operationalization and utilization in nursing practice. A practitioner who is considering using a theory in some practice area should assess the theory in terms of its function: its goals,

Table 14-4 ***Theory Critique—Usefulness***

Criteria	Units of Analysis
Practice	Direction Applicability Generalizability Cost effectiveness Relevance
Research	Consistency Testability Predictability
Education	Philosophical statement Objectives Concepts
Administration	Structure of care Organization of care Guidelines for patient care Patient classification system

consequences, and potential for practice. Therefore, the theory should be able to respond to these questions or have a framework to help the clinician respond to them: Does the theory provide enough direction to affect practice? Does it have a framework for prescription? Does the theory include abstract notions that are not applicable to practice? Does the level of abstraction or understandability render it applicable or inapplicable? Does the theory cover all areas of nursing? Should it? Does the theory currently apply to practice? Who pays for use of the theory in practice? Is it cost effective? Is it a timely nursing practice theory? Does it have relevance for the way nursing is practiced today? Where does the theory fit in terms of nursing process? Is the theory understandable to the practitioner? What is the assessment of practitioners of the theory as to its uniqueness and its esoteric language? How does it relate to diagnosis-related groups (DRGs)?

Usefulness in Research

The *raison d'etre* of theories is to guide and be guided by research; therefore, a critique of a theory should include questions related to assessment of a theory's potential for testability. The concepts and propositions should eventually be related in a consistent manner to a systematic set of observable or testable data. Otherwise, if a theory remains untested, its usefulness is in question. Schrag (1967) emphasizes the significance of a theory's potential for research, which he calls "the empirical adequacy" of a theory, and this potential is realized through congruence between "theoretical claims and empirical evidence." He asserts that credibility refers to the "goodness of fit between claims and existing evidence, while predictability estimates how well the claims will hold true in the future" (Schrag, 1967, p. 250).

Theories are established on current information; it usually is up to the future to provide evidence that corroborates them. Although the aim of research is not to establish the absolute truth of the theoretical propositions, it is essential that it begins to indicate a degree of confidence based on empirical evidence. It is noteworthy that to the unsophisticated reviewer, any supportive corroboration between theory and data uncovered through research may be interpreted as giving support to the entire theory structure, however premature that might be. The reverse could also be true. Therefore, the type and extent of empirical corroboration should be skeptically considered by answering several questions, including: What specific theory propositions did the research consider? Were these central or peripheral propositions? Was the research undertaken to provide validity to concepts or relationships? Was theory used to test propositions or to interpret findings? Were explicit theory assumptions considered in designing methodology?

Although it is significant to the theory critic to note that theories are tested on a piecemeal basis, the critic should still consider finding responses to the following questions: Does the theory build on previous research? Was research done using the theory? What propositions were being tested? How reproducible is the research? Can the findings be generalized? What research designs have been used? Why? How appropriate are they? Can proscriptive and predictive (experimental and quasiexperimental) studies be designed? Are the research results relevant to other fields? Is the research used appropriately? Do the theories state what research is to be completed to support central theory propositions? Has there been empirical verification of its properties? How consistent are its propositions with other theories and laws? Is there evidence for corroboration (Schrag, 1967)? Finally, one can detect any spuriousness in the theory's components as manifested in logical or research determination of whether or not dependent variables are potentially related to other independent variables.

The research potential or testability of a theory should not be critiqued lightly. As Berthold (1968) and Ellis (1968) stressed, the ultimate criteria for evaluating a theory's usefulness are whether it generates predictions or propositions concerning relevant events and whether it stimulates new observations and insights that could subsequently be corroborated. Units of analysis for testability are theoretical and operational definitions, theoretical propositions, ongoing research, and completed research.

Usefulness for Education

The beginning evaluation of nursing theories for their potential to offer guidelines for nursing curricula and programs coincided almost completely with the development of most of the theories that we now consider to be nursing theories. In fact, as we analyze the rationales and the goals of a good number of the nursing theories, we find that nursing education invariably prompted their development through the search for a coherent presentation of what nursing is about, to guide and structure the curriculum. Nursing theories grew out of dissatisfaction with what Barnum (1994) called the disease/body systems curriculum model. Invariably, a growing uneasiness prompted a shift to a needs orientation, such as that offered by Henderson (1966) and Abdellah (1969), and with it a rejection of biologic systems and a disease orientation as frameworks. Unfortunately, the shift to a nursing conceptualization was premature because it occurred simultaneously with the theory being developed, and therefore many faculty members suffered from the pitfalls of attempting to operationalize a theory while still evolving it.

The National League for Nursing criteria for accrediting and adopting a conceptual framework to guide curricula was both a blessing and a menace to nursing curricula and to theory development. The blessing was the reorientation of faculty to nursing theory; the menace emanated from the prematurity of the use of nursing theories in nursing education. Nursing theories could provide the major premises on which a curriculum is built, yet I believe that it was not feasible to develop an entire program on just one conceptualization of nursing. For example, theories about teaching and learning, about the learner, and about the environment are complementary to nursing conceptualizations in defining and sructuring curricula.

Usefulness in Administration

Use of nursing theory in administration is considered in terms of the structure and organization of care. Theories ought to provide the potential for guiding and describing nursing care. Nursing theories are expected to guide care of clients and are not expected to provide the administrator with guidelines for administration or for leadership style.

Analysis shows how useful theory can be for provision of guidelines in patient care on a large scale. Does it help the patient classification system? How congruent is the mission of nursing as articulated by theory with the mission as articulated by different nursing organizations? Does the theory provide any specific guidelines for theory implementation on an organizational scale? Does it provide assistance in determining criteria for quality control?

Other criteria for evaluation of theories for nursing administration were identified by Buchanan (1987). These include the congruency of theory with professional standards such as licensing requirements, as well as standards stipulated by such accrediting bodies as the American Nurses Association and the American Hospital Association. Theories selected by administrators should also be congruent with the legal structure governing nursing functions in the different countries.

External Components

Finally, the theory should be assessed against several external criteria. These are: personal values, other professional values, social values, and social significance (Table 14-5).

Personal Values

Ellis (1968) and Johnson (1987) emphasized the importance of recognizing values inherent in theories and in making them explicit. A critical consideration of values should account for those values of the theorist and the critic. In the latter, the fit between the theorist's and critic's personal and professional values should be considered. It is through such careful assessment that biases can be delineated.

Congruence With Other Professional Values

A similar assessment of the values espoused in the theory should be made of the values of other professions. Health care professionals will be able to enhance patient care through collaboration and complementarity of value systems. Awareness of such complementarity or competition in professional values enhances the potential of the devel-

Table 14-5 Theory Critique—External Components of Theory

Criteria	Units of Analysis
Personal values	Theorist implicit/explicit values Critic implicit/explicit values
Congruence with other professional values	Complementarity Esotericism Competition
Congruence with social values	Beliefs Values Customs
Social significance	Value to humanity

opment of a collaborative working schema to close the professional value gaps (Johnson, 1974).

Congruence With Social Values

Beliefs, values, and expectations of different societies and cultures within societies shape and direct the type of theory that is most useful. Although self-help, self-care (at its different levels), and individuality are goals congruent with some cultures' value systems, they are the antithesis of those espoused in others. Therefore, theories with such goals and consequences would be incongruent and inappropriate to some societies and should be avoided. Careful critical assessment of societal values and theory values is an integral part of a thorough theory critique. Questions should be addressed such as: Is the role of the nurse within the model congruent with the role of the nurse as perceived by society? Are actions and outcomes congruent with societal expectations of nursing? (Johnson, 1974, 1987)

Social Significance

In our attempt to enhance nursing science and articulate the discipline of nursing, we must not neglect the significance of its practice to humanity and society. The philanthropic Bacon's profound words of the 18th century still hold true today:

> Lastly, I would address one general admonition to all; that they consider what are the true ends of knowledge, and that they seek it not either for pleasure of mind, or for contention, or for superiority to others, or for profit, or fame, or power, or any of these inferior things, but for the benefit and use of life; and that they perfect and govern it in charity. For it was from lust of power that the angels fell, from lust of knowledge that man fell; but of charity there can be no excess, neither did angel or man ever come in danger by it. (Bacon, in Ravetz, 1971, p. 436)

A critic should ask philosophically whether the goals and consequences of theory make a substantial and valued difference in the lives of people. (Consider questions from the perspective of clients and from the perspective of other health professionals.) The critic should also ask whether intended and unintended consequences are carefully considered (Johnson, 1974, 1987).

Theory Testing

The definition of theory testing has been the subject of many discussions and dialogues in nursing (Chinn, 1984, 1986; Silva and Sorrell, 1992). It has also been equated with evaluation of theories and considered the most significant goal in developing, accepting, and using theories. It is considered here as only one component of a comprehensive evaluation of theories in the discipline. To equate testing with evaluation and to consider it the only significant goal for theory development is to ignore all the descriptive, analytical, and critical commentaries on theories that have been published and that have added to our understanding of theories and are significant for knowledge development. (Refer to writings in *Advances in Nursing Science*, *Nursing Outlook*, *American Journal of Nursing*, and *Journal of Advanced Nursing* during 1970–1990 for extensive examples of writings describing, analyzing, and critiquing theories and theoretical thoughts.) To equate testing with evaluation is also to reduce theoretical knowledge to the context of justification and to exclude the context of discovery with its process orientation.

Theory testing is a systematic process of subjecting theoretical propositions to the rigor of research in all its forms and approaches, and consequently the use of the results to modify or refine the research propositions. Theory testing presumes the complete cyclical relationship between theory, research, and theory. Theory testing is neither a static process nor an end result. The dynamic testing process begins with theory development and continues with testing and more development of theory, pausing long enough to reflect and go through the cycle again.

Theory testing is not a single entity. It has many dimensions needing many different approaches. Silva and Sorrell (1992) reviewed tests of nursing theories and identified three alternative approaches:

- Tests to verify theories through critical reasoning
- Tests to verify theories through the description of personal experiences
- Tests to verify theories through application to nursing practice

Earlier, in a review of 62 studies in which the use of theories of Johnson, Roy, Orem, and Rogers guided the studies, Silva (1986) found three ways in which theory testing was used. In 24 studies, there was a *minimal* use of the theory other than in identifying it as a framework for the study. She labeled 29 of the studies, which used the theories as a way to organize their review of literature or to select their instruments, as *insufficient*. Only 9 of the 62 studies qualified in the third category of *adequate* use of theories. These were studies in which the hypothesis testing and findings were integral to the theory and actually provided evidence to modify, accept, or reject theory propositions.

Silva proposed that this third category, which she labeled *adequate* use of the theory, is an integral part of problem identification, analysis, and interpretation. It is the type of test that should be the goal of nurse scientists in the development of knowledge in the discipline. She further attributed the lack of empirical testing to the pressure on nurse investigators to use a conceptual framework for their studies without clear guidelines on what is involved in testing, to the use of highly abstract theories, to the lack of precise measures, to the subsequent "lack of tolerance to methodological imperfections," and finally to an inability to systematically retrieve theory-based research (Silva, 1986).

Testing of theory in nursing is more complex than mere proposition testing. Considering the types of theories nurses have and will develop, that is, theories that attempt to explain responses of clients, of environments, and of the nursing therapeutics to enhance the health of clients, it would be inadvisable to limit the investigative processes and goals to a limited definition of testing Meleis (1995) proposed to consider theory testing through six principles. Each of these six principles could be used to judge the appropriateness of the tests used for the theory. The principles are: gender sensitivity of the testing, the extent to which a diverse population was used, whether or not the theory was tested on populations that are considered vulnerable and marginalized, whether the questions and the methods reflect cultural competence, whether the theory testing was done nationally or internationally, and finally what philosophy of health care provided a framework for the testing (curative care or primary health care). Currently, there are at least six approaches to theory testing in nursing. These are:

1. Testing the utility of nursing theory: Research developed to evaluate the use of theory in practice, teaching, or administration falls under this category. Units of analysis for this category are the individual nurse, teacher, student, or administrator. The intent of this type of research is to determine the feasibility of the use of theory by the group of individuals using the theory. This research tests the learner's ability to recall, comprehend, evaluate, and use the theory. Results of such tests relate to and enhance adult learning theories or cognitive theories rather than nursing practice theories (eg, Jacobson, 1984).

   A variation of this category is testing the difference between the use of the different existing theories. Jacobson (1984), for example, used a semantic differential scale to define some of the differences among the King, Orem, Rogers, Roy, and Wiedenbach theories as perceived by users. Eight factors emerged to account for 49% to 56% of the variation between the theories as perceived by users. The factors are sophistication, dynamism, clarity, usefulness, focus, utility, scope, and scientific rigor. This approach to testing a model was critiqued conceptually and methodologically by Nicoll, Meyer, and Abraham (1985). Pertinent to the current discussion, suffice it to say that, in their view, nursing models are to be evaluated individually in terms of their content. An external evaluation, from their perspective, is incongruent with the nature of models as specific to a certain context and thus ineffectual in advancing nursing knowledge.

   Tests designed to compare the feasibility of implementing different theories are useful if they are problem and context specific. For example, using Johnson's theory and King's theory to assess and diagnose the nursing care needs of an immigrant patient undergoing a kidney transplant, then comparing the processes and contents of assessment, could help in understanding learners' abilities to use the theories and to compare the efficiency and effectiveness of the theories in defining the priority needs of the patient.
2. Testing propositions from other disciplines: Research in this category is designed to test propositions from theories that were developed in other disciplines. Nursing literature has numerous examples of this type of research. Tests related to theory utilization also fall under this category because they are designed to address proposition related to educational theory. Other examples are research to test propositions evolving from systems theory, adaptation theory, role theory, and stress theory. An example of a test of theories from other disciplines is that of Maslow's theory (Davis-Sharts, 1986).
3. Testing propositions from other disciplines as they relate to nursing: Research in this category involves, more specifically, testing propositions as they relate to a nursing phenomenon or testing propositions that are of interest to nursing. Examples of this research include studies designed to test role strain in nursing

faculty (Meter and Agronow, 1982; O'Shea, 1982) and in women (Woods, 1985a, 1985b), based on role theory, and studies to test concepts from other disciplines (Wewers and Lenz, 1987).

4. Testing nursing concepts: Research in this category is designed to develop a measurable concept by identifying corresponding variables. The objective of testing in this category is to develop a valid and reliable means by which the concept is tested. Validity means that the instrument, the tool, or the means by which the concept is measured indeed measures that concept, and the extent to which it is used provides data compatible with other relevant evidence (Diers, 1979). Reliability means that these instruments consistently measure the same concept. The development of valid and reliable instruments, tools, or means by which concepts could be measured is one of the priorities in the development and testing of nursing theories. Examples include Lush, Janson-Bjerklie, Carrieri, and Lovejoy (1988); Nield, Kim, and Patel (1989); Carrieri, Janson-Bjerklie, and Jacobs (1984); and Derdiarian and Forsythe (1983).
5. Testing nursing propositions: Research in this category is designed to test theoretical propositions that are derived from nursing theories. There are three major types of propositions tested in nursing:
   - Existence propositions: These relate two or more concepts to demonstrate their existence. Research designed to test existence propositions merely demonstrates that the two concepts exist concurrently. Descriptive studies of levels of self-care of oncology patients are one example, others may relate levels of self-care to degree of anxiety. Correlational tests are most suitable analytical models for this type of research.
   - Predictive propositions: Tests designed to explore predictive propositions demonstrate the effect of one concept on another. Such propositions are modeled after the question: What will happen if . . . ? For example, studies designed to test interactional theories propositions asked: What will happen if patients are given an opportunity to express their feelings of anxiety before surgery? (Dumas and Leonard, 1963)
   - Prescriptive propositions: Research designed to test nursing interventions use principles from evaluation research. The objective is to find out how effective is the intervention in bringing about the desired goals. Examples are Smith (1986) who tested Rogers' principle of integrality and Mentzer and Schorr (1986) who tested Newman's proposition linking situational control and perception of duration of time.
6. Testing through interpretation: Theory may also be tested by using it as a framework for interpretation. This may support, refine, or extend a theory.

Theory Support

One other evaluative component for theories is the extent to which the theory is supported. This component of evaluation addresses the extent to which the theory has garnered support, has attracted a dedicated and loyal audience, and for which there is an identifiable community of scholars who are using the theory in their own work and in a variety of situations.

Theory support is a broader concept than testing, more friendly to alternative ways of theory validation, and more congruent with the nature of the discipline (Meleis, 1995). It is not only the validation of a theory that should be considered in evaluating theory—we need to think of support and affirmation of parts of theories, and we need to think of components of theories. Even if we cannot generalize from a theory, about individuals' health and illness situations and experiences, it is still extremely useful to understand the experience of the few who experience health and illness in certain unique ways, particularly in sciences that deal with human experiences and with practice-oriented issues. What other criteria can affirm or support a theory? Accounts, exemplars, and stories can be used as tests of credibility of theories and could bolster a theory's validity. Theory support includes increased advocacy for central statements, goodness of fit with some central problems in the discipline, and new insights about nursing phenomena. Support for a theory could also be obtained through networks formed to evaluate the theory's potential and capability, and by determining what other criteria can affirm or support a theory. Scholars in the discipline of nursing, and I mean by scholars both scientists and clinicians, can provide support for theories through a number of approaches. The following are different ways by which the extent of support for a theory could be determined:

1. Supporting nursing theory through philosophical analyses
2. Supporting nursing theory through conceptual analysis
3. Supporting nursing theory through existing data
   - Analytical synthesis of single utilization studies
   - Component-based meta-analyses
   - National and regional data bases
4. Supporting nursing theory through new data
   - Narrative studies based on clinicians' experiences, assessment of clients' situations, and therapeutics used
   - Interpretive studies based on clients' experiences
   - Predictive studies of stress and wellness
   - Studies to support the utility of nursing therapeutics and through further development of predictive theory studies

Conclusion

Theory development and evaluation are cyclical, continuous, and dynamic processes. One cannot exist without the other. Theory evaluation includes description, concept analysis, theory critique, theory testing, and theory support. These processes are based on the view that science is a human process that includes not only valid findings but also observations, agreements, useful solutions to problems, and the theorists, their experiences and credibility.

Theory evaluation is central to the development of theory; it is the responsibility of every clinician, academician, and administrator. If each does her share, we are then assured of the continuous growth of a body of knowledge to guide research and practice.

The theory evaluation model provided here could be used as a whole or in parts to evaluate theories. One evaluator could not complete a full theory evaluation by using all components of the model. An evaluator may choose to focus on any one of description, analysis, critique, or testing or on one part of any of these components. A careful analysis of the theorist and her contributions is as valuable in advancing knowledge as testing one proposition of a theory. Each offers members of the discipline different findings. Analyses focused on the theorist provide strategies for the development of theories and theorists, as well as forces and constraints that promote scholarship. Tests focused on accepting or rejecting propositions or generating propositions help in explaining, describing, and predicting substantive content of the field.

Despite the many critics who have been skeptical of Kuhn's attempts to delineate criteria that govern choices of good theory and have labeled them as futile, and because "the decision of a scientific group to adopt a new paradigm cannot be based on good reasons of any kind, factual or otherwise," (Shapere, 1966) Kuhn continued to assert that, indeed, we can delineate such criteria and that accuracy, consistency, broad scope, simplicity, and fruitfulness in research are essential as objective criteria for judging competing theories (Kuhn, 1977, p. 321). However, Kuhn also maintained that "every individual's choice between competing theories depends on a mixture of objective and subjective factors, or of shared and individual criteria" (p. 325). The subjective factors are based on idiosyncratic factors and are therefore dependent on individuals' preferences and personalities. Both subjective and objective factors have a place in our understanding of the philosophy of science.

The discussion provided here acknowledged subjective criteria and emphasized objective criteria. It provided criteria for theory description, analysis, critique, testing, and support, in an attempt to decrease the margin of subjectivity and to enhance that of objectivity. The goal is not to avoid subjectivity altogether, but to continue in the attempts to develop and refine components of theory evaluation and of the criteria used in these evaluations. The model of theory critique (Fig. 14-1) is designed not only to provide the basis for understanding the internal structure of theory but also the social, intellectual, and structural context that surrounds its development. It delineates a comprehensive framework for all the norms and parameters against which theories ought to be analyzed and critiqued.

When using the delineated criteria for evaluating theories, it is important to note that theories may be superior in some points and evolving in other aspects. No one theory will satisfy or be able to address all criteria. Styles of inquiry and personal preferences for theory design affect the configuration and function of theory. Throughout the analysis, one should not lose track of the ultimate purpose of theory, which is to systematize data and provide its users with a unique insight into the matter at hand. Nor should we underestimate the test of time. It is finally the temporal dimension that will determine which theory is adequate and useful and therefore survives and dominates. It is ultimately the strength of support a theory receives and the extent to which the theory is useful that leads to an expansion of understanding and enhanced interpretations of situations.

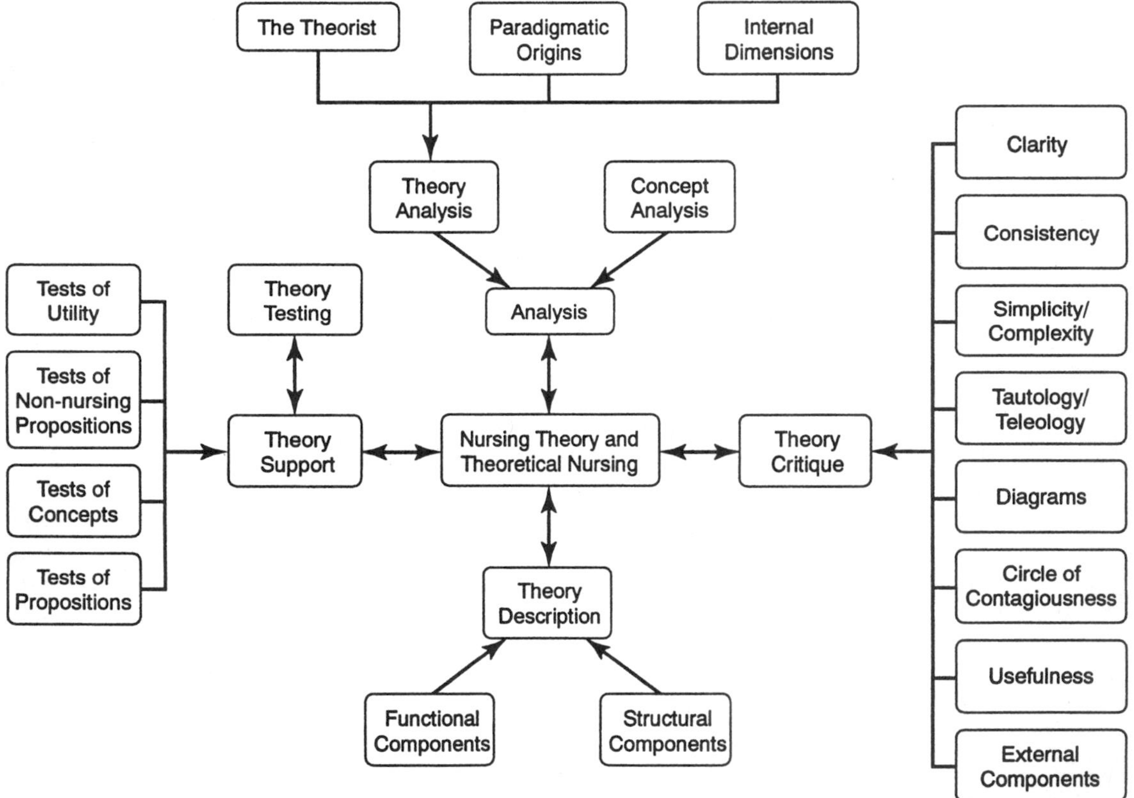

Figure 14–1 A model for theory evaluation

REFERENCES

Abdellah, F.G. (1969). The nature of nursing science. *Nursing Research*, 18, 390–393.

Auger, J.R. (1976). *Behavioral systems and nursing*. Englewood Cliffs, NJ: Prentice-Hall.

Barnum, B.J.S. (1994). *Nursing theory: Analysis, application, and evaluation* (4th ed.). Philadelphia: J.B. Lippincott.

Benoliel, J.Q. (1967). *The nurse and the dying patient*. New York: Macmillan.

Berthold, F.S. (1968). Symposium on theory development in nursing. *Nursing Research*, 17(3), 196–197.

Buchanan, B.F. (1987). Conceptual models: An assessment framework. *Journal of Nursing Administration*, 17(10), 22–26.

Carrieri, V.K., Janson-Bjerklie, S.J., and Jacobs, S. (1984). The sensation of dyspnea: A review. *Heart Lung*, 13(4), 436–447.

Chick, N. and Meleis, A.I. (1986). Transitions: A nursing concern. In P.L. Chinn (Ed.), *Nursing research methodology*. Boulder, CO: Aspen.

Chinn, P.L. (1984). From the editor. *Advances in Nursing Science*, 6(2), ix.

Chinn, P.L. (1986). From the editor. *Advances in Nursing Science*, 6(2), viii.

Chinn, P.L. and Jacobs, M.K. (1987). *Theory and nursing: A systematic approach*. St. Louis: C.V. Mosby.

Davis-Sharts, J. (1986). An empirical test of Maslow's theory of need hierarchy using hologeistic comparison by statistical sampling. *Advances in Nursing Science*, 9(1), 58–72.

Derdiarian, A.K. and Forsythe, A.B. (1983). An instrument for theory and research development using the behavioral systems model for nursing: The cancer patient. Part 2. *Nursing Research*, 32(5), 260–266.

Dickoff, J., James, P., and Wiedenbach, E. (1968). Theory in practice discipline: Part 1. Practice oriented theory. *Nursing Research*, 17(5), 415–435.

Diers, D. (1979). *Research in nursing practice*. Philadelphia J.B. Lippincott.

Duffey, M. and Muhlenkamp, A.F. (1974). A framework for theory analysis. *Nursing Outlook*, 22(9), 570–574.

Dumas, R.G. and Leonard, R.C. (1963). The effect of nursing on the incidence of postoperative vomiting. *Nursing Research*, 12(1), 12–15.

Ellis, R. (1968). Characteristics of significant theories. *Nursing Research*, 17(3), 217–222.

Erikson, E. (1963). *Childhood and society* (2nd ed.). New York: W.W. Norton.

Fawcett, J. (1993). *Analysis and evaluation of nursing theories*. Philadelphia: F.A. Davis.

Fawcett, J. (1995). *Analysis and evaluation of conceptual models of nursing* (3rd ed). Philadelphia: F.A. Davis.

Fulton, J.S. (1987). Virginia Henderson: Theorist, prophet, poet. *Advances in Nursing Science*, 10(1), 1–17.

Gebbie, K. (Ed.). (1976, March 4–7). *Summary of the second national conference: Classification of nursing diagnosis*. 1310 South Boulevard, St. Louis, MO 63104.

Glaser, B.G. and Strauss, A.L. (1965). *Awareness of dying*. Chicago: Aldine.

Hage, J. (1972). *Techniques of problems of theory construction in sociology*. New York: John Wiley & Sons.

Hardy, M.E. (1974). Theories: Components, development, evaluation. *Nursing Research*, 23(2), 100–107.

Henderson, V. (1966). *The nature of nursing*. New York: Macmillan.

Jacobson, S.F. (1984). A semantic differential for external comparison of conceptual nursing models. *Advances in Nursing Science*, 6(2), 58–70.

Jacox, A. (1974). Theory construction in nursing: An overview. *Nursing Research*, 23(1), 4–13.

Johnson, D.E. (1959). The nature of a science of nursing. *Nursing Outlook*, 7(5), 291–294.

Johnson, D.E. (1968). One conceptual model of nursing. Paper presented at Vanderbilt University, Nashville, TN.

Johnson, D.E. (1970, Winter). *Requirements of an effective model* [For N203, Class in Theory]. Unpublished manuscript, University of California, Los Angeles.

Johnson, D.E. (1974). Development of theory: A requisite for nursing as a primary health profession. *Nursing Research*, 23(5), 372–377.

Johnson, D.E. (1987). Evaluating conceptual models for use in critical care nursing practice. *Dimensions of Critical Nursing Care*, 6(4), 195–197.

Kaplan, A. (1964). *The conduct of inquiry: Methodology of behavioral science*. San Francisco: Chandler.

King, I. (1971). *Toward a theory for nursing*. New York: John Wiley & Sons.

Kuhn, T.S. (1970). The structure of scientific revolutions. In Neurath, O. (Ed.), *International encyclopedia of unified science* (2nd ed., Vol. 2). Chicago: University of Chicago Press.

Kuhn, T.S. (1977). *The essential tension*. Chicago: University of Chicago Press.

Laudan, L. (1977). *Progress and its problems: Toward a theory of scientific growth*. Berkeley: University of California Press.

Lindsey, A.M., Piper, B.F., and Stotts, N.A. (1982). The phenomenon of cancer cachexia: A review. *Oncology Nursing Forum*, 9(2), 38–42.

Lush, M.T., Janson-Bjerklie, S., Carrieri, V.K., and Lovejoy, N. (1988). Dyspnea in the ventilator-assisted patient. *Heart Lung*, 17(5), 528–535

Marriner-Tomey, A. (1989). *Nursing theorists and their work* (2nd ed.). St. Louis: C.V. Mosby.

Meleis, A.I. (1975). Role insufficiency and role supplementation: A conceptual framework. *Nursing Research*, 24(4), 264–271.

Meleis, A. I. (1995). Theory testing and theory support: Principles, challenges, and a sojourn into the future. In Betty Neuman (Ed.), *The Neuman systems model* (pp. 447–457). East Norwalk, CT: Appleton & Lange.

Meleis, A.I., Swendsen, L., and Jones, D. (1980). Preventive role supplementation: A grounded conceptual framework. In M.H. Miller and B. Flynn (Eds.), *Current perspectives in nursing: Social issues and trends*. St. Louis: C.V. Mosby.

Mentzer, C.A. and Schorr, J.A. (1986). Perceived situational control and perceived duration of time: Expressions of life patterns. *Advances in Nursing Science*, 9(1), 12–20.

Merton, R. (1964). *Social theory and social structure* (Rev. ed.). London: Free Press of Glencoe.

Meter, M.J. and Agronow, S.J. (1982). The stress of multiple roles: The case for role strain among married college women. *Family Relations*, 31(1), 131–138.

Newman, M.A. (1979). *Theory development in nursing*. Philadelphia: F.A. Davis.

Nicoll, L.H., Meyer, P.A., and Abraham, I.L. (1985). Critique: External comparison of conceptual nursing models. *Advances in Nursing Science*, 7(4), 1–9.

Nield, M., Kim, M.J., and Patel, M. (1989). Use of magnitude estimation for estimating the parameters of dyspnea. *Nursing Research*, 38(2), 77–80.

Norris, C.M. (1982). *Concept clarification in nursing*. Rockville, MD: Aspen Systems.

The Nursing Theories Conference Group. (1980). *Nursing theories: The base for professional nursing practice*. Englewood Cliffs, NJ: Prentice-Hall.

Orem, D.E. (1985). *Nursing. Concepts of practice* (3rd ed.). New York: McGraw-Hill.

O'Shea, H.S. (1982). Role orientation and role strain of clinical nurse faculty in baccalaureate programs. *Nursing Research*, 31(5), 306–310.

Parsons, T. (1949). *The structure of social action*. New York: Free Press.

Paterson, J.G. and Zderad, L.T. (1988). *Humanistic nursing*. New York: National League for Nursing, Publication No. 41-2218.

Ravetz, J. (1971). *Scientific knowledge and its social problems*. New York: Oxford University Press.

Riehl, J.P. and Roy, C. (Eds.). (1980). *Conceptual models for nursing practice* (2nd ed.). New York: Appleton-Century-Crofts.

Rogers, M. (1970). *An introduction to the theoretical basis of nursing*. Philadelphia: F.A. Davis.

Roy, C. and Roberts, S.L. (1981). *Theory construction in nursing.* Englewood Cliffs, NJ: Prentice-Hall.

Schrag, C. (1967). Elements of theoretical analysis in sociology. In L. Gross (Ed.), *Sociological theory: Inquiries and paradigms.* New York: Harper & Row.

Shapere, D. (1966). Meaning and scientific change. In R.G. Colodny (Ed.), *Mind and cosmos: Essays in contemporary science and philosophy.* University of Pittsburgh Series in the Philosophy of Science (Vol. 3) Pittsburgh: University of Pittsburgh Press.

Silva, M.C. (1986). Research testing nursing theory: State of the art. *Advances in Nursing Science,* 9(1), 1–11.

Silva, M.C. and Rothbart, D. (1984). An analysis of changing trends in philosophies of science on nursing theory development and testing. *Advances in Nursing Science,* 6(2), 1–13.

Silva, M.C. and Sorrell, J.M. (1992). Testing of nursing theory: Critique and philosophical expansion. *Advances in Nursing Science,* 14(4), 12–23.

Smith, M.J. (1986). Human-environment process: A test of Rogers' principle of integrality. *Advances in Nursing Science,* 9(1), 21–28.

Walker, L.O. and Avant, K.C. (1995). *Strategies for theory construction in nursing* (3rd ed.). East Norwalk, CT: Appleton & Lange.

Wewers, M.E. and Lenz, E.R. (1987). Relapse among ex-smokers: An example of theory derivation. *Advances in Nursing Science,* 9(2), 44–53.

Wilson, J. (1969). *Thinking with concepts.* London: Cambridge University Press.

Woods, N.F. (1985a). Employment, family roles, and mental ill health in young married women. *Nursing Research,* 34(1), 4–10.

Woods, N.F. (1985b). Relationship of socialization and stress to perimenstrual symptoms, disability, and menstrual attitudes. *Nursing Research,* 34(3), 145–149.

Zetterberg, H.L. (1963). *On theory and verification in sociology* (Rev. ed.). Totowa, NJ: Bedminster Press.

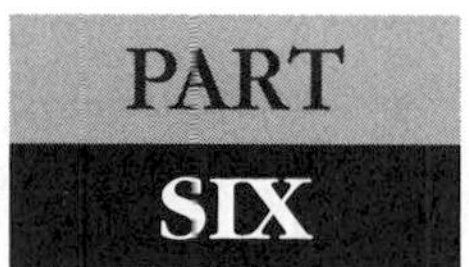

Our Pioneers: The Theorists and the Theories

Part Six is devoted to a discussion of nursing theories in relation to current nursing practice. This part emphasizes several themes introduced in other parts and develops them further by providing interpretive examples. The first theme is that nursing theories have evolved from a sociocultural context, were influenced by the educational and experiential background of the theorists, and cannot be understood or adequately analyzed without considering these influences. The second theme is that existing theories are not competitive but are complementary and may be used by the same person for different purposes or by different people for different purposes. The third theme is that theories can be viewed, interpreted, and used in many different ways and are not restricted to the purposes for which they were developed.

Theory users and their interpretations of theories are significant to the progress of the discipline. A final theme, not directly or explicitly presented in this part, but one that could be indirectly derived, is that progress in the discipline of nursing is measured by the development of theories, research, the theorists, the researchers, and the number of central problems that can be answered in existing theories.

Chapters 15 through 18 describe, analyze, critique, and provide examples of tests of nursing theories that were selected to represent some of the domain concepts. The model proposed in Chapter 14 is used to guide the presentation of each of the theories. The description, analysis, critique, and examples of tests presented here are preliminary and condensed. They are offered to assist you in embarking on your own critical analysis. The extensive bibliography offered in Chapter 21 is intended to support readers who may choose a more thorough analysis and critique of theories. I also encourage you to consider other domain concepts and other nursing theories. Although the theories are organized around domain concepts, the description is general and encompasses as much of the theorists' conceptualizations as possible.

CHAPTER 15

On Nursing Clients

The works of three theorists emerge as significant developments in the conceptualization of the nursing client. Central questions for these theorists are: Who is the nursing client? In what ways does a nursing client benefit from nursing care? What is the outcome of care? The three theorists are Dorothy Johnson, Sister Callista Roy (a mentoree and Johnson's student), and Betty Neuman. Johnson asserted in all her metatheory as well as theory publications that what differentiates nursing from medicine and other health sciences is its perspective of a nursing client as a behavioral system. To Roy, a client is an adaptive being with two subsystems for adapting—the regulator and cognator mechanisms—and four adaptive modes. The human being as represented by central structure, lines of defense and resistance becomes a client according to Neuman when threatened or attacked by environmental stressors. This chapter offers a description, an analysis, and a beginning critique of the three theorists' conceptualizations.

Dorothy Johnson

Theory Description

The early questions Dorothy Johnson addressed pertained to the knowledge base nurses needed for nursing care (Johnson, 1959a). Nursing care to her did not depend on medical care, nor was its goal recovery from illness or adoption of more desirable health practices. She labeled nursing's responsibilities that are related to medical care and better health "delegated medical care" and "health care," respectively (Johnson, 1961). Although nurses also performed functions related to "delegated medical care," the essence of nursing, its central mission, should lie in "nursing care," which Johnson considered ill defined with no delineated theoretical framework. When the latter is defined, when the specific goals are articulated, then we will be able to speak of a science of nursing (Johnson, 1959b).

Johnson's conceptualization of nursing, then, is based on the premise that nursing has a unique, independent contribution to health care that is distinct from its delegated dependent contributions (Johnson, 1964). All contributions delegated to and unique to patient care and cure are significant but, as professionals, nurses are obligated to articulate and communicate to the public their primary mission and their nursing goals, as well as their secondary mission that is delegated from medicine. The public is aware of the latter but less aware of the former. A client, to Johnson, behaves in an integrated, systematic, patterned, ordered, and predictable way. Behavior is goal oriented, and goals are an organizing framework for all behavior. Behavior is the sum total of biologic, social, cultural, and psychological behaviors. Nurses deal with the integrated responses of clients.

Johnson (1980) conceptualized a nursing client as a behavioral system, with behaviors of interest to nursing organized into seven subsystems of behavior (Table 15-1). Each one of the subsystems is analogous to the anatomy of a biologic subsystem. It identifies the components and the subcomponents by which we can identify the subsystem of behavior (Johnson, 1990).

First is the *drive* or the *goal* of the subsystem. Goals or drives are universal; however, the strength of the goal may differ and, in fact, may fluctuate in the same person from strong to weak. Goals have different meanings in different people or at different

Table 15-1 ***The Subsystems of Behavior—Johnson****

ACHIEVEMENT SUBSYSTEM

The function is mastery or control of either some parts of environment or of self in such areas as physical, creative, mechanical, social, and intellectual skills. These are measured against some acceptable yardstick.

AFFILIATIVE SUBSYSTEM

Inclusion into relations, intimacy, relating, bonding with the ultimate function of survival.

AGGRESSIVE SUBSYSTEM

Modes used to protect and preserve oneself from dangers, whether real or imaginary.

DEPENDENCE SUBSYSTEM

Used interchangeably with attachment; the ultimate function being approval, attention, or recognition and physical assistance through assistance from a repertoire of others.

ELIMINATIVE SUBSYSTEM

Difficult to differentiate from the biologic elimination system. It incorporates modes of behavior in the excretion of wastes, addresses when, how, why, and under what conditions a person externalizes what is internal and what needs to be expelled.

INGESTIVE SUBSYSTEM

Similar to digestive biologic system but incorporates when, why, how, and under what normative conditions the internalizing of external environment takes place. Its function is "appetitive satisfaction."

SEXUAL SUBSYSTEM

Recognizes strong similarity to biologic system but considers all other behaviors that are related to subsystem (eg, gender–role identity, courting, mating). The function is procreation and gratification.

** Based on Grubbs, J. (1980). An interpretation of the Johnson behavioral system model. In J. P. Riehl and C. Roy (Eds.), Conceptual models for nursing practice (2nd ed., pp. 217–254). New York: Appleton-Century-Crofts; and based on Johnson, D. E. (1980), The behavioral system model for nursing. In J. P. Riehl and C. Roy (Eds.), Conceptual models for nursing practice (2nd ed., pp. 207–216). New York: Appleton-Century-Crofts.*

times in the same person. Another parameter on which goals may differ is the object of the goal. For example, when observing the eating behavior of a Middle Eastern immigrant, an inference may be made that the goal of eating is to achieve appetite pleasure or to internalize an external environment (universal drive). The variety of the food and the total absorption into the act of eating (to the exclusion of external environment) may demonstrate the strength and the meaning of the eating behavior. The object is the type of food preferred by Middle Eastern immigrants—usually highly salty, high in protein, and free of pork and alcohol.

A second structural component is the *set*, which is the ordinary, regular, normal behavior a client uses to meet the goal of the subsystem. For example, pureed vegetable soup is a type of food normally eaten by Middle Eastern immigrants during an illness. Another example of set is a Middle Eastern immigrant's preference to have a room full of visitors at all times to meet his affiliative needs, which happens to be the usual way this particular person has of handling the stress of hospitalization. Therefore, expecting and maintaining a large group of family members at the bedside is a normal pattern of behavior for this particular person.

Choices represent to Johnson another component in the structure of a subsystem. Choices represent the available repertoire of options that a person has to meet particular goals. Choices are regulated by gender, age, cultural background, and socioeconomic status, among other variables. To meet the needs of procreation without a commitment to a partner—for example, through artificial insemination—is an option within the repertoire of some women and not of others, based on their perception of their own choices.

Finally, the goal, set, and choice are complemented by directly observing the *behavior* of the client. The behaviors that bring about desired goals and whether or not the normal patterns of behavior are appropriate under the circumstances of the health/illness situation are examples of observations and analyses that may be useful. Behaviors are also compared and contrasted with available options for the individual.

Each of the subsystems also has a *function* that is analogous to the physiology of biologic systems. The goal of the subsystem that is part of the structure is not entirely distinct from its function.

Subsystems, and indeed the client system, continue to grow, develop, and remain viable. Therefore, Johnson questioned what assistance subsystems may need to be able to do so, and her answer was "certain functional requirements" (1980, p. 212) that can be met by the individual or by others when the individual cannot meet such requirements. These functional requirements are:

1. Protection from unwanted, disturbing stimuli
2. Nurturance through giving input from environment (food, friendship, caring)
3. Stimulation by experiences, events, behavior that would "enhance growth and prevent stagnation" (Johnson, 1980, p. 212)

Subsystems continue to maintain themselves as long as both the internal and external environments are orderly, organized, and predictable and as long as each of the goals is met. When there is a disturbance in structure, in function, or even in the functional regimen (even though the structure and function may not have been affected), nursing care is indicated. Nursing has the goal of maintaining, restoring, or attaining a balance or stability in the behavioral subsystem or the system as a whole. Nursing acts as an "external regulatory force" to modify or change the structure or to provide ways in which subsystems fulfill the structure's functional requirement (Johnson, 1980, p. 214).

Johnson based her theory on a number of explicit and implicit assumptions (Table 15-2). The theory specifies that the behavior of the person who is ill is the object of nursing care. Therefore, nursing's specific contribution to patient welfare is fostering efficient and effective behavioral functioning in the patient during and following illness (Johnson, 1980, p. 207).

Nursing makes its contribution through identification of a behavioral subsystem or subsystems that are threatened or could potentially be threatened by illness or hospitalization. In Johnson's theory, the source of difficulty is clearly within the subsystem or within the functional requirements, whether or not manifested in structure, in function, or in the functional requirements. Johnson's assumptions are explicit and clear (Johnson, 1990). The theory provides useful definitions of person, health, nursing problem, and nursing therapeutics and no definitions for nursing process, interactions, or environment. Definitions are highly abstract; however, extensions offered by Auger (1976) and Holaday (1980) provide clear operationalization of definitions of person and

Table 15-2 ***Assumptions—Johnson***

EXPLICIT ASSUMPTIONS*

- Behavior is the sum total of physical, biologic, and social factors/behaviors.
- "The behavior of an individual evident at any given point in time is the product of the net aggregate of consequences of these factors over time and at that point in time."
- "When these regularities and constancies are disturbed, the integrity of the person is threatened and the functions served by such order are less than adequately fulfilled."
- A person is a system of behavior characterized by repetitive, regular, predictable, and goal-directed behaviors that always strive toward balance.
- There are different levels of balance and stabilization. Levels are different at different time periods.
- Balance is essential for effective and efficient functions of the individual (a minimum of energy expenditure, maximum satisfaction, and survival).
- Balance is developed and maintained within the subsystem or the system as a whole to maintain adaptation and environment.
- Changes in structure or function of a behavioral subsystem are related to dissatisfied drive, lack of functional requirements, or changes in environmental conditions.

IMPLICIT ASSUMPTIONS

- A person could be reduced to small components to be studied.
- A person as a system is the sum total of its parts (ie, subsystems).
- All behaviors can be observed through sensory data.

** This section is based on D. Johnson's class notes from the University of California, Los Angeles, 1970 and Johnson, 1968a.*

of nursing therapeutics. One of the potential problem areas in clarity is the use of some concepts with different meanings, one more acceptable and less esoteric than another (such as ingestion and elimination) that, when considered from a biologic standpoint, denote a different meaning (Tables 15-3 and 15-4).

The consequences that Johnson alluded to are adjustment and adaptation. An unintended consequence that was not discussed by Johnson is unwarranted dependence on others for meeting the needs of the subsystems. The theory does not address the potential consequences of such dependence.

Johnson did not clearly identify theoretical propositions in her published work, but she has discussed the implications of her theory for nursing research in a number of theory and research conferences. Her position has been that appropriate, cumulative research in nursing is only possible when we agree on the mission and goals of nursing (Johnson, 1974). Propositions in Johnson's theory are existence propositions. Existence propositions (Zetterberg, 1963) in this case lead to factor-isolating theories (Dickoff, James, and Wiedenbach, 1968) (Table 15-5).

Theory Analysis

The Theorist

Dorothy Johnson, a pediatric nurse by training, received her bachelor of science degree from Vanderbilt University School of Nursing in Nashville, Tennessee and a master of public health degree from Harvard University. She spent the balance of her nursing career as a professor of pediatrics at the University of California, Los Angeles (UCLA), where she influenced the lives and theoretical identities of many faculty members, administrators, and students. Her interest in sociology and psychology influenced the development of her theory.

Johnson worked with students in the master's program. Although some wrote master's theses and many went on the further education, the focus of the program for which she held a primary responsibility in pediatrics was on preparing clinical specialists in the program. Perhaps that may explain the paucity of research related to her theory.

Table 15-3 ***Concepts—Johnson***

Behavior	Structural	Nurturance
Subsystems of	Components	Internal Regulation
Behavior	Goal	External Regulation
Affilliative	Set	Restore
Ingestive	Choice	Maintain
Eliminative	Action	Attain
Aggressive	Function	Stability
Sexual	Functional Requirements	Instability
Dependence	Protection	
Achievement	Stimulation	

Table 15-4 **Definition of Domain Concepts—Johnson**

Nursing	An external regulatory force that acts to preserve the organization and integration of the patient's behavior at an optimal level under those conditions in which the behavior constitutes a threat to physical or social health or in which illness is found (Johnson, 1980, p. 214).
Goal of nursing	Restore, maintain or attain behavioral integrity, system stability, adjustment and adaptation, efficient and effective functioning of system (Johnson, 1980, p. 214).
Health	Efficient and effective functioning of system; behavioral system balance and stability.
Environment	Identified internal and external environments, but provided no specific definition.
Human being	A biopsychosocial being who is a behavioral system with seven subsystems of behavior.
Nursing client	A biopsychosocial being as a behavioral system threatened by loss of order, predictability, or stability due to illness or potential illness. "All patterned, repetitive, purposeful ways of behaving that characterize each man's life are considered to comprise his behavioral system." (Johnson, 1980, p. 209)
Nursing problem	Instability in the system or one of the subsystems due to functional or structural stress: a) inadequate drive satisfaction; b) inadequate fulfillment of the functional requirements; c) changes in environmental conditions (Grubbs, 1980, p. 224).
Nursing process	Not addressed.
Nurse–patient relations	Not addressed.
Nursing therapeutics	Regulate and control: a) providing protection, nurturance, or stimulation to subsystems; b) by external mechanisms restricting, defending, inhibiting, or facilitating (Johnson, 1961, 1980).
Focus	Responses of person to stress, the reduction of stress, and the support of natural defenses and adaptive processes (Johnson, 1961, p. 66).

Paradigmatic Origins

Johnson stated that her theory is a product of philosophical ideas, sound theory and research, her clinical experiences, and many years of thinking, discussing, and writing (Johnson, 1978). Her theory had several sources. First and foremost, her conception of a person as a system of behavior is analogous to the concept of a person as a biologic system, differentiated into a set of biologic systems, such as cardiovascular, skeletal, endocrine, digestive, and so on. Just as each biologic subsystem is differentiated by a structure demonstrated in anatomic dissection, a behavioral system has a structure when abstractly dissected. A structure has several components: a goal, a set, a choice, and behavior. Biologic subsystems have functions and so do behavioral subsystems. Physiology speaks to biologic subsystem functions. Both sets of subsystems have functional requirements.

Johnson's assumptions are congruent with general systems theory assumptions, and concepts consistently evolve from Johnson's systems assumptions. For example,

Table 15-5 **Potential Propositions—Johnson**

PERSON

1. Behavior is orderly, systematic, and organized around seven subsystems of behavior. Each subsystem of behavior is identifiable by structure, goal, set, choice, behavior by function, and by a number of functional requirements.
2. Internal regulatory mechanisms affect the structure, function, and functional requirements in the subsystem of behavior of the entire system.
3. Behavioral subsystem disorders are manifested in disturbances in structure, function, or functional requirements in each subsystem. Behavioral subsystem disorders are differentiated into insufficiency in one of the subsystems, dominance in one or more of the subsystems, or incompatibility between two or more of the subsystems.

ENVIRONMENT

1. External regulatory mechanisms affect each subsystem of behavior, and the entire system is demonstrated by structure function and the subsystem functional requirements.

HEALTH

1. Health, a behavioral system balance or stability, is manifested in the effective and efficient attainment of the goals and functions of each subsystem of behavior as judged by the nurse and mediated by the right of the patient.
2. Balance could be determined through manifestations of general harmony with and between the behavioral systems.

NURSING PROCESS

1. Johnson's theory does not yield any theoretical propositions related to the nursing process. Assessing and diagnosing, using Johnson's theory, brings about efficient and effective nursing care.

INTERACTIONS

1. Johnson's theory does not yield any theoretical propositions related to the nursing process except when we consider subsystem interactions.

NURSING THERAPEUTICS

1. Nursing is an external force that functions through control or modification of external regulatory mechanisms for the purpose of achieving balance and stability as demonstrated by efficient and effective functioning.
2. Nursing therapeutics are differentiated into nurturance, stimulation, and maintenance.
3. Nursing therapeutics deal with insufficiency, dominance, and incompatibility.

functioning of systems, interdependency of subsystems, balance in subsystems, regularity and constancy of behaviors, energy, boundaries, and disequilibrium are concepts defined by Bertalanffy (1968). Some concepts were used by Johnson with consistent meaning. Johnson considered integration, wholeness, organization, interaction, and integration of a human being as subsystems, all of which are derived from systems theory. The impact of her writings on nursing science in general and on theory in particular underwent a revival in the 1980s. More writing in theory in the 1980s demonstrated the profound impact of her 1950s renaissance theory ideas.

Johnson's theory is also based on a systems paradigm, as perceived from a sociological background. One sees the influence of Talcott Parsons (1951) on her writing in more than one way, but especially in her attempt to conceptualize all nursing as dealing with a person as a system of behavior. Parsons attempted to conceptualize one theory to encompass all sociology. He perceived the science for the Social System Analysis, the social system representing society as the focus of sociological explorations. Components of the structure of a social system—goal, set, choice, and behavior—are the same in Johnson's theory as in Parsons' theory.

Johnson relied on practice to provide the impetus for her theory, on sociology to provide the paradigm, and on psychology to support the validity of the derived concepts, such as Ainsworth's (1972) on affiliation and Feshback's (1970) on aggression. She acknowledges the profound influence of Nightingale on her thinking about nursing and on the development of her theory (Johnson, 1992).

Internal Dimensions

Johnson's theory embodies an analytical model of what a nursing client is and the problems resulting from this conceptualization. It is a theory developed to answer the questions: What is nursing? and When does a person become a nursing client? The answers focus on concepts, and it is a concatenated theory. It is based on a field system of relations focusing on the ill or potentially ill person. It revolves around a concept.

Johnson's theory has a constructive beginning that is a hypothetical conceptualization of a human being from a nursing perspective. It is based on a parallel conceptualization of a human being as a set of biologic subsystems. It is also analogous to the conceptualization of Parson's (1951) social system in terms of a structure, function, goals, set, choices, action, functional imperatives, and the goal of stability for the subsystems. Therefore, Johnson's is a deductive, hypothetical theory.

Although Johnson's goal was that her ideas would describe and explain all behaviors that are within the domain of nursing and of all action (therefore to be a macrotheory of nursing), it is useful microtheory of the client in nursing as a behavioral system. It is a middle-range theory addressing normal and abnormal patterns of behavior in the nursing client. It has a broad scope as it describes and explains a wide range of problems related to assessment of clients (all drives, needs, regulators affecting behavior).

It is interesting to note that, whereas Johnson advocates that nursing should develop knowledge of control (1968a), the phenomena that she addresses and develops are related to knowledge of order and somewhat to the beginnings of knowledge of disorder.

Theory Critique

Johnson's theory provides nursing with a sufficiently broad scope to include a number of diverse areas of nursing. However, the theory is limited to nursing's concern for the ill, hospitalized person and less congruent with nursing's orientation toward health (eg, Johnson, 1987).

Johnson offers the nursing practice a concept, broad in scope, of a person as a system of behavior; this concept helps in organizing assessment of normal patterns of behavior and deviations from normalcy of internal and external mechanisms that may influence subsystems. Although the theory includes concepts of nursing problems and nursing therapeutics, these concepts are highly abstract in Johnson's work. The extensions offered by Auger (1976) and somewhat by Grubbs (1980) provide an operationalization of definitions of a person and nursing therapeutics. Johnson's theory helps explain the component of a person's behavior that is of interest to nursing. Knowledge of order (normal patterns of behavior) and knowledge of disorder (abnormal patterns of behavior) are synthesized from social, behavioral, and natural sciences. The theory provides, in abstraction, broad guidelines to knowledge of control; the theory's complexity, however, stems from its high abstraction.

The nursing process used by many educational and nursing service institutions was not addressed in Johnson's theory because Johnson focused on a theory of human behavior responses to the stress of illness. Grubbs (1980) demonstrated how Johnson's client assessment theory could be used in conjunction with the nursing process.

The major utility of this theory lies in its framework for the assessment component of the nursing process. Auger and Dee (1983) used it as a guideline to develop a patient classification system. The system provided nursing and hospital administration with the capability to establish levels of staffing based on patients' needs. Clinicians used Johnson's theory as a basis for the development of a classification system that was helpful in providing patients in psychiatric units with purposeful care (Dee and Auger, 1983). The classification system could be used in other settings (Dee, 1986, 1990).

Several other analyses documented the utility of the theory in practice (Derdiarian, 1993a, 1993b). Holaday (1980) discussed the use of the theory in pediatrics for assessment and in conjunction with other theories for intervention. Small (1980) used the theory to interpret her research and as a framework for caring for visually impaired children. As a consequence of the theory, the authors found it helpful in providing a framework for diagnosis, in selecting interventions, and in evaluating outcomes. Rawls (1980) described and evaluated the utility of the theory in caring for patients with amputations. The theory's utility for nursing therapeutics is yet to be realized and adequately developed (Reynolds and Cormack, 1991).

Johnson's theory is focused on individual care, it is better suited for long-term care, and the complexity of the model requires a professional nurse with sound grounding in a number of sciences. It provides an effective guide for assessment and a frame for diagnosis and intervention. However, patterns of behavior that require the care of the nurse are yet to be identified, defined, and developed.

Johnson has profoundly influenced theoretical thinking since 1959, but sparse publication of her theory has limited the radius of her ideas. Johnson always maintained that nursing curricula should be guided with a well evaluated conceptualization of nursing (Johnson, 1989). Within that belief system, several curricula emanated from her theory. Most of the application work was done at the institution where Johnson taught—UCLA (implementation began about 1964). However, the mobility of her colleagues and students has helped in implementing her theory in educational programs at the University of Colorado (Hadley, 1970), the University of Hawaii, and Vanderbilt University.

The use of Johnson's theory in the United States was based on an operationalization of the theory into the UCLA curriculum and on the fact that Wu (1973) and Auger

(1976) developed and published their books, extending Johnson's ideas. The combination of these two books provided the beginning student with knowledge of order that replaced the old fundamentals of nursing. Those fundamentals were based on the medical model and were taught to beginning students. No published material is available to describe the painstaking efforts of the University of California School of Nursing faculty in translating Johnson's ideas into a curriculum—a curriculum that was later emulated with refinements in Hawaii and Colorado. In the 1980s, Harris (1986) chronicled the utilization of Johnson's theory as a framework for the curriculum at UCLA.

External Components

Johnson diligently identified the assumptions, defined most of the nursing domain concepts, and provided guidelines for utilization in conjunction with the nursing process. The assumptions and conceptualizations are congruent with current professional values regarding the uniqueness of nursing, its separateness, and its interdependence. Also, the view of stability is becoming accepted as a world view for nursing. However, the theory's focus on the individual and disorder is incongruent with nursing's claim to health maintenance and promotion and to nursing's interest in aggregates as seen in the concept of community health.

Johnson was one of first nursing scholars to identify the significance of congruence between nursing goals and societal expectations (Johnson, 1974, p. 376). She continued over the years to emphasize that the client and the public are the ultimate judges of the nursing mission. The theory grew from her conviction that improvement in care is the ultimate goal. The studies done by Grubbs (1980), Holaday (1981), and Small (1980) assume such congruence and speak to patients' satisfaction of care. However, as with all other theories, such congruence between public expectations and nurses' stated goals needs to be explored. Perhaps the public's interest in health and in health care commensurate to its cost is in the best interest of nurses and will augment nurses' views of their mission with the public's view of nursing's goals. Until then, it is safe to assume that a theorist who spoke vehemently for improved patient care and for the significance of the public view in shaping the nursing mission has translated those views into her theory.

Theory Testing

Johnson, in presenting her theory, invariably spoke of the significance of theory in guiding research (1968b). She admonished that research using her theory should focus on identifying and explaining "the behavioral system disorders which arise in connection with illness, and . . . develop the rationale for and means of management" (Johnson, 1968b, p. 6).

Damus (1980) explored the validity of theory in practice and collected observations related to behavioral system disorder in patients with posttransfusion hepatitis. Her study demonstrated a positive relationship between behavioral and physiologic disequilibrium and a relationship between nursing diagnosis and nursing intervention.

More important, this study lent support to the idea that, indeed, the "source of subsystem disorders can be identified and predicted" and also lent unequivocal support to the usefulness of the theory in nursing practice (Damus, 1980, p. 287).

Holaday's study of achievement in well and chronically ill children (1974, 1981) and Holaday and Turner-Henson's (1987) and Porter's (1972) work on stimulation of premature infants lend validity to notions of the subsystem, its utility, and isolation in patient care. Holaday completed two research studies related to the affiliative subsystem of behavior (1981, 1982) and the achievement subsystem (1974). In the first, the cry of the chronically ill infant received a different pattern of maternal response than the cry of the well infant. The set goal components of the subsystems provided the interpretation for the mother's responses to the cry. Derdiarian (1990a) provided further support to the utility of the theory as a framework for enhancing nurses' satisfaction. She also supported Johnson's assumptions about the interrelationships between the subsystems of behavior (Derdiarian, 1990b). The theory was also used as a framework to explain the attitudes of nurse administrators toward nurses who are impaired by alcohol and drug use (Lachicotte and Alexander, 1990). The theory was also used as a framework for a study about pain management of adult patients with cancer (Wilkie, 1990).

Five research tools were developed to measure perceived quality of nursing care and perceived behavioral changes of cancer patients, based on Johnson's theory. The first patient indicators of nursing care were developed to record "incidences of readily observable physiological complications acquired by institutionalized patients" and to measure quality of care (Majesky, Brester, and Nishio, 1978, p. 365). They were based on Johnson's assumption that the occurence of a complication is a manifestation of a person's "ability to cope with stresses on the behavioral systems" (p. 365). Therefore, to monitor behavioral changes, a nurse can derive the status of a person on a health/illness continuum. The 105 items of potential complications representing infection, immobility, and fluid imbalance were subjected to validity screening and reliability testing.

The second research tool, the Derdiarian behavioral system model, resulted in 193 items categorized to represent each subsystem of the behavior, which are useful for identifying perceived changes due to cancer (Derdiarian, 1983, 1984; Derdiarian and Forsythe, 1983). Derdiarian (1990a, 1991) demonstrated that the use of theory-driven assessment tools enhances satisfaction of nurses and patients and the quality of care. These attempts are useful beginnings of factor-isolating, categorizing, and providing empirical descriptions of some central concepts in the theory.

The third research tool was a projective test developed by Lovejoy (1983, 1985) to assess family functioning as perceived by children with leukemia. The fourth instrument was developed and validated by Dee (1986) as a classification instrument for psychiatric patients. The fifth was developed by Bruce, Hinds, Hudak, Mucha, Taylor, and Thompson (1980) to measure the quality of outcomes for patients with renal disease. Each of these tools has the potential for further support of theory and its utility.

These tools demonstrate the usefulness of the theory in the assessment of nursing problems. One of the requirements for subsystem survival is the provision of stimulation. To identify the needs of premature infants, Porter (1972) explored the relationship of sensory stimulation and growth and development of premature infants. Subsequently, others have provided evidence that indeed marked growth and development occurred when premature infants are stroked frequently and when infants are handled frequently.

Attributions of success to internal and external variables differentiated between chronically ill and normal children. The chronically ill children tended to attribute success and failure to outside variables and normal children tended to attribute the same to internal variables. Holaday (1974) interpreted the results to indicate disequilibrium in the achievement subsystem. Both studies lend more empirical clarity to two of Johnson's subsystems. She further built on her previous studies by considering chronically ill children's use of out-of-school time (Holaday and Turner-Henson, 1987). The dependency subsystem also received some investigative attention (Stamler and Palmer, 1971). These studies support the presence of subsystems conceptually and their relationship to other subsystems.

Other studies are based on psychiatric patients (Dee, 1986) or have developed and published a description of indicators in patient care that are central to nursing (Majesky, Brester and Nishio, 1978). The potential in these studies is tremendous because the researchers are attempting to delineate patient care outcomes based on nursing interventions.

Outcomes of behavioral system stability are still complex and highly abstract. Factor-isolating studies and exemplars are needed to delineate different states of stability. The theory's clarity is demonstrated in its view of the person and its lack of clarity is viewed in outcomes. Nursing service administrations have used the theory to develop nursing assessment forms for history, nursing admission, and discharge. The questions in the forms evolve from a behavior system framework that characterizes this theory (Dee, 1986; Dee and Auger, 1983).

Theories can be used as a framework for interpretation. A good example of this use is provided in the research of Holaday (1981, 1982, 1987), described previously. Holaday found that maternal responses to ill infants were characterized by quick response time and immediacy; mothers were in close vicinity of infants at all times; and the mother's interventions were multiple rather than singular. In other words, mothers tended to pick up the ill infant, rock, pat, and give a pacifier, as compared with just picking up the well infant. Mothers of the ill infants did not discriminate between different types of cries as well as did mothers of the well infants (eg, cries due to pain or restlessness). Holaday interpreted her results using Johnson's components of the behavioral subsystems theory, that is, set-goal, which was narrow in the case of the ill children. In other words, mothers of chronically ill children responded to every cry with no discrimination. With this theory-based interpretation, nursing implications according to Holaday (1981, 1987) were for helping mothers with their set-goal of the affiliative subsystem, that is, the subsystem that focuses on relationships.

Johnson's theory was used internationally as a framework to describe perceived rights for disclosure of information related to each subsystem of behavior. Two factors emerged to be significantly related to perceptions of rights for disclosure. These factors correspond to the achievement, ingestion, and elimination subsystems. The findings support these subsystems' functions of the need for mastering the environment through information and the need for incorporating information regarding patients' concerns (Naguib, 1988).

Sister Callista Roy

Theory Description

The central questions of Sister Callista Roy's theory are: Who is the focus of nursing care? and What is the target of nursing care?; and to a lesser extent, When is nursing care indicated? As with other current theories in nursing, the outcome of nursing care received limited consideration in Roy's descriptive theory.

Roy's first ideas appeared in 1964 in a graduate course paper written at UCLA. Roy published these ideas in 1970, and subsequently, different components of her framework crystallized during the 1970s, 1980s, and 1990s. Over the years, Roy identified the assumptions on which her theory is based (Table 15-6). More recently, versions of her theory incorporated humanistic assumptions regarding the dignity of human beings and the role of nurses in promoting integrity in life and death. Roy also made the client appear more visible in the care process, although this visibility is more philosophical in nature and less operationalized in practice.

Table 15-6 ***Assumptions—Roy***

EXPLICIT ASSUMPTIONS (ROY, 1989, AND ROY AND ANDREWS, 1991)

- The person is a biopsychosocial being.
- The person is in constant interaction with a changing environment.
- To cope with a changing world, the person uses both innate and acquired mechanisms, which are biologic, psychological, and social in origin.
- Health and illness are one inevitable dimension of the person's life.
- To respond positively to environmental changes, the person must adapt.
- The person's adaptation is a function of the stimulus he is exposed to and his adaptation level.
- The person's adaptation level is such that it comprises a zone indicating the range of stimulation that will lead to a positive response.
- The person has four modes of adaptation: physiologic needs, self-concept, role function, and interdependence (Roy, 1980, pp. 180–182).
- "Nursing accepts the humanistic approach of valuing other persons' opinions and viewpoints" (Roy, 1984, p. 36). Interpersonal relations are an integral part of nursing (Roy, 1984, p. 36).
- There is a dynamic objective for human existence with the ultimate goal of achieving dignity and integrity (Roy, 1984, p. 38).

IMPLICIT ASSUMPTIONS

- A person can be reduced to parts for study and care.
- Nursing is based on causality.
- Patients' values and opinions are to be considered and respected.
- A state of adaptation frees an individual's energy to respond to other stimuli (Roy, 1984, p. 38).

Roy's assumptions in general are in agreement with current views in nursing regarding adaptations, human beings, and nursing. Her implicit assumptions attest to the totality of the individual as manifested in behavior, active participation of individuals in life, and an individual's potential for self-actualization. New humanistic values have been identified in Roy's theory (1984, 1987, 1988a; Roy and Andrews, 1991). The principles of humanism are creative power, holism, subjectivity, purposefulness in life, interpersonal relations, and activity. Although others have tended to view the holistic nature of the theory (Mastal and Hammond, 1980), it was not until 1984 that Roy emphasized the holistic nature of a person and the humanistic care of nurses. In 1987 and 1988, these humanistic values were described. Roy and Corliss (1993) presented a set of revised assumptions for Roy's theory that included attention to holism, interdependence, central processes of systems, information feedback, and the complexity inherent in living systems. These assumptions reflected a general systems theory approach to viewing her theory and clarified the philosophical origins of Roy's theory.

According to Roy's theory, a person—a biopsychosocial being, an adaptive system, a human being—is in constant interaction with a changing environment; therefore, a person is continually changing and attempting to adapt. When he is not adapting positively and is therefore manifesting ineffective responses, he is of concern to nursing; however, once a person manifests effective behavior, he no longer needs nursing attention. A person uses both innate and acquired mechanisms to ready himself to adapt to his environment (Andrews and Roy, 1986). A person is also defined in terms of purposefulness of existence and as reflecting the context of the unity of purpose of humankind and the common good, as well as the value and meaning inherent in life (Roy, 1988a). In addition, Roy views the innate creative powers as essential to understanding the nature of a human being. In an adaptive person, "veritivity," that she uses to mean the truth of human nature, reflects activity, creativity, unity, purpose, and value (Roy, 1987).

A person is an adaptive system with two major internal central mechanisms used for adapting. These are the regulator and the cognator subsystems, which are viewed as innate or acquired coping mechanisms. These innate or acquired mechanisms are used to deal with a constantly changing environment (Roy, 1991; Roy and Andrews, 1991). The regulator mechanism works primarily through the autonomic nervous system to organize a reflex action that prepares the individual to respond and adapt to the environment. The major parts of the regulator subsystem are the neural, endocrine, and perception–psychomotor parts (Roy and McLeod, 1981). The regulator mechanism receives stimuli from the internal and external environments, both of which are basically chemical or neural, and receives all input into the central nervous system. Body responses observed by the nurse are effects of autonomic responses, responsiveness of endocrine glands, and the perception process. The latter is altered by cultural and social factors (external stimuli) and "must remain in short-term memory long enough for a psychomotor choice or response to be made" (Roy and McLeod, 1981). The bodily responses, brought about through chemical–neural–endocrine channels, are fed back as additional stimuli to the regulator system (Roy, 1984, pp. 28–36).

The second mechanism is the cognator subsystem, which identifies, stores, and relates stimuli so that a symbolic meaning can be attached to the behavior. The cognator mechanism is composed of several parts and corresponding processes: (1) perceptual/information processing manifested in the processes of selective attention, coding, and memory; (2) learning, manifested in imitation, reinforcement, and insight; (3) judgment, which involves the process of problem solving and decision making; and (4) emotion, which is manifested in defenses to seek relief and affective appraisal and attachment (Roy, 1988b; Roy and Andrews, 1991). These processes are influenced by internal and external stimuli and affect the psychomotor choice of response of orientation, approach, avoidance, flight, or hiding as demonstrated in the form of spoken or unspoken words. Failure in either the regulator or the cognator mechanisms results in maladaptation (Roy, 1984).

All *input* is channeled through the processes of the regulator and the cognator and produces responses through four effector modes: physiologic needs, self-concept, role function, and interdependence. The two subsystems are related to each other through perception and are related to each effector mode differently. Whereas the regulator is related predominantly to the physiologic mode,

> . . . since very little is known physiologically about the process of perception formation, memory, and choice of psychomotor responses, the other modes of self-concept, role function, and interdependence must relate to the meaning of a given perception for the individual human system. The meaning of the perception will, therefore, influence the body response (Roy and McLeod, 1981, p. 67)

On the other hand, the cognator subsystem is related to all adaptive modes. Processes such as selective attention, imitation, problem solving, and appraisal influence nutritional intake in the physiologic mode, role function, self-concept, and interdependence. Within each mode, all cognator processes could be manifested; for example, attachment, reinforcement, and memory are integral parts of role cues selected by a person. The physiologic mode is a result of the needs of individuals for physiologic integrity. This mode allows individuals to respond physically to their environment. There are five basic physiologic needs and four regulator processes in this mode. The physiologic needs are activity and rest, nutrition, elimination, oxygenation, and protection. The regulator processes are described as the senses, fluids, and electrolytes, neurologic functions, and endocrine functions.

The self-concept mode is related to the need for psychic integrity (Roy and Andrews, 1991). Self-concept is defined by a person through significant others, and it includes perceptions of the physical and personal selves. The physical self is manifested in body sensations (feelings and experience) and image (view of self). The components of the personal self are self-consistency (continuity of self), self-ideal (expectations), and the moral–ethical–spiritual self (values) (Andrews and Roy, 1986; Roy, 1987). Self-esteem is a component of self-concept and is defined as the extent to which individuals perceive their self-worth (Andrews, 1991).

The role function and interdependence mode is focused on the need for social integrity. Role is viewed in Roy's theory as a set of expectations of individuals toward each other. She classified roles as primary (based on age, sex, and development), secondary (acquired through relations with others and made permanent), and tertiary (activities that are more temporary) (Andrews and Roy, 1986). The interdependence between individuals is expressed in the ability to love, to respect, and to value, and to receive love and respect and to be valued.

Stimuli affecting modes and mechanisms are identifiable as focal stimuli (those that are immediate in an individual's life), residual stimuli (attitudes and previous experiences), and contextual stimuli (all other stimuli, eg, heat, aggravating a rash, or noise that is irritating to a person in pain).

In early writings, Roy and McLeod (1981) proposed that a theory of the person as an adaptive system (ie, regulator and cognator mechanisms) should be used in conjunction with the Roy adaptation model. This was later modified and synthesized so there was no differentiation between the model and the theory (Roy, 1984). A person is conceptualized as an adaptive system that includes input (stimuli and an adaptation level), control processes (the regulator and the cognator as coping mechanisms), effectors (four modes), and output (adaptive and ineffective responses) (Roy, 1984, p. 30) (Table 15-7).

Table 15-7 ***Concepts—Roy***

- Adaptation
  - Adaptation level
  - Adaptation zone
  - Adaptive response
- Client: An Adaptive System
  - Biologic
    - Anatomy
    - Physiology
  - Psychological
    - Perceiving
    - Learning
    - Acting
  - Social
    - Family
    - Community
    - Work group
    - Society
- Adaptive System
  - Cognator
  - Regulator
- Adaptive Stimuli
  - Focal
  - Contextual
  - Residual
- Physiologic Modes
  - Activity and rest
  - Nutrition
  - Elimination
  - Oxygenation
- Psychological Modes
  - Self-concept
    - Psychic integrity
    - Physical, personal, moral–ethical–spiritual self
    - Self-consistency
    - Self-ideal/self-expectancy
    - Learning
    - Inner cell of self-concept
    - Self-esteem
- Adaptive Modes
  - Regulator process
  - The senses
  - Neurologic function
  - Endocrine function
  - Fluid and electrolyte
- Role Function
  - Expressive
  - Instrumental
  - Primary role
  - Secondary role
  - Tertiary role
  - Role function
  - Position
  - Role performance
  - Role mastery
  - Social integrity
- Interdependence
  - Nurturing
  - Affectional adequacy
  - Significant other
  - Support systems
  - Receptive behaviors (love, respect, value)
  - Contributive behaviors (love, respect, value)

Later developments in Roy's theory have helped to clarify her view of a person. However, some concepts remain ambiguous and overlapping. Although concepts are mainly derived from other paradigms, the primitive ones (regulator and cognator) are not as precisely identified and defined. Concept boundaries are not clear. For example, effector modes and focal stimuli overlap (there is overlap in some effector modes, such as in interdependence role, self-concept, and role function). There is also overlap between adaptive modes and mechanisms, and there is lack of clarity in the definitions, as others have discussed (Mastal and Hammond, 1980). Environment and internal stimuli remain operationally undifferentiated (Tiedeman, 1983) (Table 15-8).

Roy and McLeod (1981), Roy and Roberts (1981), Roy and Andrews (1991), and Roy and Corliss (1993) have provided a useful systematic presentation of all possible links between variables resulting in a multitude of theoretical propositions. This is clearly a theory that lends itself to the development of propositions and hypotheses. The propositions provided by the theorist are theoretically sound, structurally adequate, systematic, and relational. The researcher's task is in operationalizing propositions for research projects. The propositions tend to focus on biologic events (physiologic response, intact neural pathways) rather than nursing phenomena. The propositions are linear and bivariate, but Roy is striving for nonlinear and multivariate relationships (Roy and Roberts, 1981, p. xiv).

Roy's theory has a high descriptive and explanatory power of the individual as an adaptive system, but the theory has limited predictive and prescriptive power. The descriptive and explanatory potential could be further enhanced with existence propositions. This is the task most needed for the further development and refinement of this theory. Although Roy has attempted to establish the theoretical validity of each coping system and effector mode, work now should proceed to establish their empirical validity.

Theory Analysis

The Theorist

After receiving a master of science degree in pediatric nursing, Sister Callista Roy, who was a pediatric nurse by training, studied sociology at UCLA, where she received her doctorate in 1976. The impetus of her theory was inspired by her having been the advisee and student of Dorothy Johnson. Her first manuscript, conceptualizing man as an adaptive system, was based on Helson's (1964) theory of adaptation level and was written for Johnson's graduate class on conceptual models in nursing. Later influenced by Ralph Turner, the sociologist, Roy derived her explication of self-concept and role function.

Forces in the development of her model have been her administrative position at Mount St. Mary's College (Los Angeles, CA), which allowed her to further develop theory in curricula and allowed her use of the expertise and support of faculty members who taught at that institution. Sister Callista Roy is an eloquent speaker and prolific writer, with a great deal of energy that has helped spread her ideas nationally and internationally. After completing a postdoctoral fellowship at the University of California,

Table 15-8 ***Definition of Domain Concepts—Roy***

When nursing is needed	The adaptive system of a person who is ill or has the potential of illness "when unusual stresses or weakened coping mechanisms make the person's usual attempts to cope ineffective."
Goal of nursing	To enhance the adaptation of the patient in the four modes to free energy to respond to other stimuli. Freed energy promotes healing abilities and wellness (Roy and Roberts, 1981). "To promote adaptation" (Roy, 1984, p. 36) and "to decrease ineffective responses" (Roy, 1984, pp. 37–38).
Health	A state of adaptation that is manifested in free energy to deal with other stimuli. A process of promoting integrity and wholeness (Roy, 1984, p. 39). A continuous process of being and becoming integrated (Roy and Gliss, 1993).
Environment	Internal and external stimuli. There are three classes of stimuli: the focal stimuli (immediately confronting a patient); contextual (all stimuli); residual (pertinent stimuli), but cannot validate effect on current situation. In other words, it is "all conditions, circumstances, and influences surrounding and affecting the development and behavior of persons and groups" (Roy, 1984, p. 39; Roy and Gliss, 1993).
Human being	Functions holistically (Roy, 1984, p. 36), highest possible fulfillment of human potential (Andrews and Roy, 1986).
Nursing client	A person, family, group, or community. Biopsychosocial adaptive systems with two processor subsystems that are mechanisms for adapting or coping—the regulator and the cognator. The system has four affectors of adaptation, or the adaptive modes: physiologic needs, self-concept, role function, and interdependence (Roy and Roberts, 1981, p. 43). A holistic, adaptive system (Roy, 1984, p. 36).
Nursing problem	The source of difficulty is coping activity that is inadequate to maintain integrity in the face of a need deficit or excess (Roy, 1980, p. 184).
Nursing process	A "particular format" used in nursing that uses the problem-solving approach. It comprises the six steps of assessment of behaviors, assessment of influencing factors, nursing diagnosis, goal setting, intervention, and evaluation (Roy, 1984, pp. 42–62; Andrews and Roy, 1991).
Nurse–patient relations	Acknowledged in 1984 as important, but not defined. Defined in 1987 through nursing process.
Nursing diagnosis	"Changes in internal or external environment can trigger need deficits or excesses. Within the appropriate adaptive mode, coping activation is stimulated. When the coping mechanism is ineffective in meeting the demand, ineffective behavior results" (Roy and Roberts, 1981, p. 47). "The behavior with its predominant stimulus" (Roy and Roberts, 1981, p. 47).
Nursing therapeutics	Traditional techniques such as comfort measures or health teaching, or entirely new activities that have not been discovered, all with the goal of promoting adaptation (Roy and Roberts, 1981, pp. 47–48).
Focus	On persons, groups, families, communities, or societies with ineffective behavior, and on manipulation of stimuli so that they would fall within the patient's zone of positive coping. Increase, modify, decrease internal or external stimuli. Traditional interventions such as providing comfort or health teaching, or new undiscovered interventions (Roy, 1984, p. 28).

San Francisco School of Nursing (where she was trained as a clinical scholar on a Robert Wood Johnson fellowship in 1985), she embarked on a new phase in her research/practice theory career. As a clinical scholar and while in the program, she has used her theory in a clinical neurology setting. During the 90s she also directed the doctoral program at Boston College.

Paradigmatic Origins

Roy's theory is a synthesis of concepts developed outside the domain of nursing and redefined within the context of nursing. Although Helson's adaptation level theory appears to be the impetus for the central concept in this theory—adaptation as a process—Roy clearly and admittedly was also influenced by her mentor and teacher, Dorothy Johnson. Johnson conceptualized a person as a behavioral system with seven subsystems, and Roy conceptualized a person as a system with two subsystems as coping mechanisms and four modes of coping. The similarities continue to encompass goals of nursing (homeostasis), focus (external regulatory mechanisms), the patients (maladaptive or potentially maladaptive people), and later, a person with ineffective behavior.

Roy's doctoral education in sociology and her work with Ralph Turner influenced her development of the role, interdependence, and self-concept (an interactionist approach) as effector modes.

> One's self-concept is defined by interaction with others. One to one interactions between individuals are characterized by the use of verbal and nonverbal symbolic communication. (Roy and Roberts, 1981, p. 205)

To be specific, Roy's theory evolved from a synthesis of concepts from the adaptation, systems, and interactional paradigms. Parallels exist between the list of concepts with the physiologic modes, Johnson's subsystems of behaviors, Henderson's activities of daily living, and unmet needs (eg, rest, elimination, circulation). Elements of systems theory influenced the development of the subsystems (Bertalanffy, 1968). Roy (1970; Roy and Corliss, 1993) acknowledges the influences of Levine (1966), Henderson (1960), Nightingale (1859/1995), and Chardin (1965) among other theorists and philosophers.

The development of Roy's theory progressed rather rapidly to meet curricular needs of Mount St. Mary's College. Therefore, some sense of urgency, and the backgrounds of existing faculty, may have contributed to some of the seemingly fragmented and overlapping concepts. The expediency may have created content to be used in a curriculum rather than content that would enhance the development of nursing knowledge through questioning and refinement. All these influences and forces have been acknowledged in later writings (Andrews and Roy, 1986). The shift to more clinical focus is apparent in the later writings of Roy (Roy and Andrews, 1991; Roy and Corliss, 1993) and is credited to her postdoctoral education.

Internal Dimensions

Roy's theory is a moderately abstract, logically deductive microtheory of the nursing client developed around descriptions of concepts; thus, it is a concatenated theory developed around adaptation and its modes. Roy uses a field approach with units of analysis in terms of other miniunits. The theory has a broad scope. It attempts to address a broad range of problem areas related to the client who has demonstrated ineffective responses to internal and external stimuli. The goal of the theory is to conceptualize the nursing client, in Roy's early writings, as four coping modes, and in later writing, as a system with two subsystems—the regulator and the cognator—and even later as input, two subsystems, four effector modes, and output (Roy, 1984). Roy and Roberts (1981) proposed the Roy theory as "a nursing practice theory . . . which is the knowledge of disorder" (p. 24), but in fact it provides a framework to organize knowledge that addresses modes and mechanisms of adaptation as well as ineffective behavior.

Theory Critique

Roy's theory evolved from mental imagery of what nursing is, who the nursing client is, and what the goal of nursing care is. It was deductively derived from other theoretical formulations but was not based on previous research findings, nor did it generate many published research findings (Roy, 1976, p. 691; Roy and McLeod, 1981). During 25 years of development of theory, Roy has clarified her own philosophical assumptions and discussed them (Roy, 1988a; Roy and Corliss, 1993). Some of her assumptions could be propositions and therefore could be tested. One example is the conceptualization of human beings with four coping modes. Furthermore, which behaviors are components of what mode of coping need also be subjected to evaluation. Roy acknowledges such directions in formulating propositions (Roy, 1980) (Table 15-9).

Roy is given a great deal of credit as a theorist who has systematically attempted to develop theoretical propositions to enhance the potential of research. Nevertheless, the propositions are based more on neurologic and biologic sciences. Some of these propositions tend to reduce the person to responding to chemical or neural stimuli through neural inputs (Roy and Roberts, 1981, pp. 62– 66). The perspective is demonstrated in attention to central concepts and attention to careful articulation of assumptions congruent with the nature of nursing. Clarity of the concepts could be enhanced by theoretical distinctiveness, operational definitions, valid empirical referents, and reliable data. Clarity of a theory in nursing could be enhanced by explicit relatedness between central concepts of the theory.

Table 15-9 ***Propositions—Roy***

- Nursing actions promote a person's adaptive responses.
- Nursing actions can decrease a person's ineffective adaptive responses.
- People interact with changing environment in an attempt to achieve adaptation and health.
- Nursing actions enhance the interaction of persons with environment.
- Enhanced interactions of persons with environment promote adaptation.

Many studies were conducted using Roy's theory; some were directed to exploring and further developing concepts that are not as central to the theory, such as perceptions of the nursing clients. However, perception of the patient was not a central concept of the early conceptualization of man. Nevertheless, the earliest research projects focused on perceived adaptation levels of the elderly client (Idle, 1978) and perceptions of decision making (Roy, 1977) rather than on empirically describing systems, effectors, or ineffective responses. When developing her theory later, perception emerged as a central concept that links the regulator and cognator mechanisms (Bunting, 1988). Others, such as Randall, Poush-Tedrow, and Van Landingham (1982) provided support for the centrality of perceptions. Roy acknowledged and supported the notion of client involvement in their care.

> According to this nursing model, the person is to be respected as an active participant in his care . . . The goal arrived at is one of mutual agreement between the nurse and patient. Intervention[s] are the options that the nurse provides for the patient. (Roy and Roberts, 1981, p. 47)

Roy's theory was used to develop research instruments, to describe responses to different health/illness concepts, and to evaluate interventions. Tools were developed to measure perceptions of adaptation levels (Idle, 1978), perceptions of powerlessness in decision making (Roy, 1979), health care outcomes for cancer patients (Lewis, Firsich, and Parsell, 1978, 1979), and regaining functional abilities after delivery (Tulman and Fawcett, 1988). Roy's theory was used as a framework to study the experiences and responses of clients to parental touch of preterm infants (Harrison, Leeper, and Yoon, 1990), spinal cord-injured women during pregnancy (Craig, 1990), of adult survivors of multiple traumas (Strohmyer, Noroian, Patterson, and Carlin, 1993), and spousal adaptation to mates' coronary artery bypass surgery (Artinian, 1991, 1992).

What the theory may lack in research utilization, it more than compensates for in practice, education, and administrative utility. The theory has synthesized theory with the process of clinical judgment adequately and has offered an excellent checklist for assessment of variables responsible for the problematic behavior (ie, focal, contextual, and residual stimuli) and the setting of priorities for action. Although there is no systematic evidence of effect of use of the theory on staff or educators, many personal testimonies across the country attest to a sense of direction and organization when the theory has been used. The theory offers less direction in prescribing.

In developing and testing an assessment tool based on Roy's theory, Wagner (1976) indicated the lack of boundaries between role function, interdependence, and self-concept modes, but demonstrated the theory's utility in various diverse practice settings. The theory was used in assessing and planning care for patients in surgical settings (Roy, 1971), in community settings (Hanchett, 1990; Schmitz, 1980), and in obstetric and pediatric settings, in short, in distributive and episodic settings (Wagner, 1976). The setting that created the most difficulty was the intensive care setting (Wagner, 1976). The theory has demonstrated its usefulness in assessing gerontology patients (Janelli, 1980; Farkas, 1981), young children (Galligan, 1979), cardiac patients (Gordon, 1974), patients with organic brain damage (Hamer, 1991), postpartum patients (Kehoe, 1981), and fathers whose mates undergo cesarean delivery (Fawcett, 1981a). It has been useful in neonatal care (Downey, 1974), in demonstrating depression and life satisfaction among a group of retired people (Hoch, 1987), and for acute psychiatric patients (Kurek-Ovshinsky, 1991).

In all these studies, the utility of a checklist to identify normal behavior and deviations from normal behavior was demonstrated, and the potential of the theory in identifying outcome criteria to be used for quality assurance was also demonstrated (Laros, 1977). At the same time, however, they demonstrated a lack of concept boundaries, a severe limitation of the theory's framework for understanding person–environment interactions. There are some thoughtful and useful directions for developing nursing therapeutics based on theory.

The circle of contagiousness of the theory in education is wide and extensive compared with other theories. Conferences were planned in the 1970s and 1980s for educators interested in using the theory as a framework for their curriculum. The annual conference planned by Mount St. Mary's College is another indication of the wide interest that continues for the theory (Wallace, 1993). For educational settings faced with the need for the development of a conceptual framework for curricula, the availability of a theory that has been operationalized at Mount St. Mary's College School of Nursing, including the textbooks and literature to use, made for enthusiastic adoption of the theory. Roy's theory has been used in 11 states (27 schools) and also in Canada and Switzerland (Fawcett, 1984). The theory has also been used in specialty curricula (Brower and Baker, 1976). The challenges inherent in operationalizing and implementing Roy's theory drive faculty to develop some innovative approaches to promote a more adaptive implementation (Morales-Mann and Logan, 1990).

Clinical setting administrators have also attempted a further operationalization of the theory in several settings. In each instance, it provided a framework for assessment of patient needs in each of the modes and a ready-made, usable classification system for the stimuli. Recording patient care needs was rendered more organized and simple, and there were indications of increased patient satisfaction and expanded professional practice (Laros, 1977; Mastal, Hammond, and Roberts, 1982). In a case study analysis Gless (1995) demonstrated the clinical utility of Roy's theory in supporting and promoting a quadriplegic patient's ability to copy with living in a long-term care facility.

All concepts related to the physiologic mode, or effectors, are concrete and are most directly related to observable data; data related to this mode tend to predominate the findings. Perhaps this is partially because concepts from the other three modes are generally abstract, less operationalized, and beset with unclear boundaries. The concepts are theoretically defined but lack both boundary validity and operational definition. Adaptation, the consequence of nursing care—a process and an end result—lacks both theoretical and operational definition and validity. Exemplars of adapted patients and patients with ineffective behavior (process and product) could help in beginning to develop theoretical definition.

Concepts are tautological, such as focal stimuli, which are also identified behaviors in each of the modes. The view of a person as an open interacting system and the view of input and output appear to be inconsistent, even though Roy, in her later writing, incorporated both input and output within her conceptualization of a person. On the whole, Roy used a field approach and logical method in the development of her theory, and she defined units in terms of other miniunits.

External Components of Theory

Society and other health care professionals would agree that nursing deals with the physiologic needs of the patient and the goal of adaptation in that mode, but there may be less agreement on the role of nursing in relation to other modes. Perhaps this is due to decreased clarity of those modes or the focus of the health care system on biologic and physiologic aspects of care. The systematic assessment potential that Roy's theory offers is congruent with the prevailing view of the need for an organized system in assessment and intervention and utility of the nursing process in patient care.

The simplicity of the theory and the available operationalized teaching-oriented literature enhanced its wide geographical spread but limited its more thoughtful and inquisitive use; coping mechanisms of cognator and regulator are limited in utility due to lack of clarity. The complexity of the propositions has hampered its operationalization for research. Educators and clinicians in search of a coherent way to present and discuss their care or teaching found the theory useful and provided more face validity to the concepts of the theory. Researchers, on the other hand, either ignored the theory or found the complexity of the propositions and their physiologic perspective cumbersome or unrepresentative of the nursing perspective, so they turned to other perspectives. For whatever reasons, creative energies centered around face validity studies rather than on construct, criterion validity, or relational research.

The strength of Roy's theory lies in its exemplary nature of theory development. The theory evolved from a belief that nursing has a unique contribution to patient care and that the recipient of care is an open adaptive system. After structurally identifying major components of theory, assumptions, and concepts, Roy developed the functional components (ie, utility in education, practice, and research). The she backtracked and systematically identified theory propositions. The theory is ready for some systematic research.

Theory Testing

Studies were conducted by Roy during her postdoctoral Robert Wood Johnson fellowship at the University of California, San Francisco, to determine cognitive processes in patients with head injury and to test different propositions of the theory (Roy and Andrews, 1991). The results provided detailed descriptions of patterns of information processing of patients over the course of their illness due to head injury. Results also supported the proposition that nursing interventions using Roy's theory tended to improve cognitive processing of these patients (Roy and Andrews, 1991). Others have used the theory to describe responses to chronic illness (Pollock, 1986), perceptions of stressors of children in an intensive care unit (Munn and Tichy, 1987), the needs of spouses of surgical patients (Silva, 1987), and the differences between recovery rates in the functional abilities of postpartum vaginal and cesarean delivery patients (Tulman and Fawcett, 1988).

The effects of interventions designed within an adaptation framework were evaluated in several studies. Examples are evaluation of effects of using a birth chair on mothers and infants (Cottrell and Shannahan, 1986, 1987) and of prenatal education on unplanned cesarean birthing (Fawcett and Henklein, 1987). Fawcett's (1981b) research in identifying the needs of parents facing cesarean section is an example of significant research offering support to Roy's modes of adaptation as a primary assessment framework. Levels of adaptation have been an elusive consequence but a most significant aid in understanding the nursing care process and its intended goals. The study of Lewis, Firsich, and Parsell (1979), geared toward developing an instrument to measure the adaptation level of chemotherapy patients, is a step in the right direction in the empirical definition of adaptation. Roy's studies reported in Roy and Andrews (1991) also support the effectiveness of interventions driven by Roy's theory in improving cognitive functioning of patients with head injury. Contributions of research findings synthesized by Pollock, Frederickson, Carson, Massey, and Roy (1994) provided guidelines for further testing of the theory and the rationale for collaboration of researchers who are using the same theory. Relationships between study variables and theory concepts need further analysis (see Tables 15-8 and 15-9).

Betty Neuman

Theory Description

The central questions for Betty Neuman are: How can nurses organize the vast knowledge needed to deal with complex human situations that require nursing care? and How do nursing clients interact, adjust to, and react to stress? Neuman considers her theory wellness oriented and a holistically focused conceptualization of client and nurse responses and actions (Neuman, 1989a). Neuman articulated a number of basic assumptions about client systems, environmental stressors, responses to stress, lines of resistance and defense health, energy, and wellness (Neuman, 1989a, p. 17–22). These explicit assumptions are described in Table 15-10. Central concepts of her theory are included in Table 15-11.

To Neuman, nurses deal with clients as a whole. Nursing clients are people who are anticipating stress or who are dealing with stress (Neuman and Young, 1972). Nurses focus their attention on responses that could be labeled stressful and these responses are then within the domain of nursing. The nurse diagnoses the level of stability, internal and external environment stressors, and the effect of stressors on a client's system stability. Levels of stability can be determined through the analyses of lines of defense, lines of resistance, basic structure energy resources or survival factors, and the five interacting, dynamic variables: physiologic, psychological, sociocultural, developmental, and spiritual (Neuman, 1989a). The spiritual aspects of Neuman's theory were absent in her earlier work (Neuman, 1982); they were added to other variables and developed in her

Table 15-10 ***Assumptions—Neuman****

1. Nursing clients are dynamic; they have both unique and universal characteristics and are in constant energy exchange with environments.
2. The relationship between client variables—physiologic, psychological, sociocultural, developmental, and spiritual—influence a client's protective mechanisms and determine a client's response.
3. Clients present normal range of responses to the environment that represent wellness and stability.
4. Stressors attack flexible lines of defense, then normal lines of defense.
5. Nurses' actions are focused on primary, secondary, and tertiary prevention.

* *These assumptions are based on Neuman (1995).*

1989 conceptualization of the composite client system. To Neuman, a client system is a whole system. A client is a physiologic, psychological, sociocultural, developmental, and spiritual being.

The client system, also referred to as the client, is defined in terms of a core structure and a series of concentric circles in addition to the five variables. The core structure includes basic survival factors that are universal and that characterize all species as well as all unique features of a particular client system. The basic universal survival factors are the innate and genetic factors and natural strengths and weaknesses of the system. Therefore, according to Neuman, this component of the universal core structure is where the innate factors that regulate temperatures, the genetic response patterns, and any innate strengths or weaknesses in all body organs are found. However, this core structure also contains unique aspects of a client system that characterize a person, such as cognitive abilities. A client's response patterns are determined and regulated by this core structure. Both universal and unique features of a client system are described by Neuman as normal temperature range, genetic structure, response pattern, organ strength and weakness, ego structure, and "knowns" or commonalities (1989a, pp. 27–29).

Table 15-11 ***Concepts—Neuman***

Variables	Environment
Physiologic	Internal
Psychological	External
Sociocultural	Created
Developmental	Health
Spiritual	Wellness
Flexible line of defense	Stability
Normal line of defense	Prevention
Lines of resistance	Primary
Basic structure/energy resources	Secondary
Stressors	Tertiary
Intrapersonal	Reconstitution
Interpersonal	Theory of optimum client system stability
Extrapersonal	Theory of prevention

A client system is also described through two lines of defenses, a flexible one and a normal one (Neuman, 1982). All environmental stressors first attempt to attack the flexible line of defense. It is visually represented in Neuman's diagrams as the outermost circle surrounding the basic core structure of energy sources; the line is depicted as broken to signify its flexible nature. It is a buffer to a client's normal line of defense, also known as the "client's normal or stable state." The function of this line of defense is to fight the invasions of stressors or to fight the reactions to stressors. Neuman (1989a) describes this line of defense as:

> . . . accordionlike (sic) in function. As it expands away from the normal defense line, greater protection is provided; as it draws closer, less protection is available. It is dynamic rather than stable and can be rapidly altered over a relatively short time period or in a situation like a state of emergency or a condition like undernutrition, sleeplessness, or dehydration. (pp. 28 and 29)

The function of the flexible line of defense as buffer to the normal line of defense is rendered ineffective by some stressors, singularly or in groups. The stressors will then attack the normal line of defense, and when that in turn becomes ineffective in warding off the effect of the stressor to penetrate the core structure or allowing reactions to stress to occur, then a response to stress will be manifested. Responses are described as instability or illness.

The normal line of defense is another component of the client system. It is vital in protecting the basic core structure and integrity of the system. "This line represents what the client has become, the state to which the client has evolved over time or the usual wellness level" (Neuman, 1989a, p. 30). Although not quite as flexible as the flexible line of defense, the normal line of defense still has the capability of expanding or contracting over time. It is depicted with a solid circle surrounding the next layer of the client system, which is the lines of resistance. This is where the system stability and integrity are manifested, and this is where the normal patterns of wellness levels for the client system are found. Its dynamic nature is apparent in its ability to remain stabilized in dealing with stressors.

Stressors singularly or in groups could continue to penetrate the client system, heading for its basic structure and energy resources. Before the stressor is allowed to influence the basic core of a client system, however, it has to penetrate what Neuman calls lines of resistance. These lines involuntarily activated are three broken concentric circles surrounding the core of a client system. As a stressor succeeds in penetrating the normal lines of defense, the lines of resistance are activated. "These resistance lines contain certain known and unknown internal factors that support the clients' basic structure and normal defense line, thus protecting system integrity" (Neuman, 1989a, p. 30).

Neuman provides the "mobilization of white blood cells" as an example of activation of a line of resistance. If lines of resistance succeed in warding off stressors, that is "reversing the reaction to stressors," then the client system reconstitutes its energy resources and basic structure (Neuman, 1989a, p. 31). If lines of resistance fail, then energy will be depleted. The degree of energy depletion goes from minimal to death.

Each one of these concentric circles has a major function. The flexible line of defense shields the normal line of defense; the normal line of defense is a buffer to each of the lines of resistance; and all these lines combine function to prohibit the stressor from invading the core structure of a human being. All the lines combined also protect the core structure from reacting to stress. Each defense and resistance line varies according to such variables as age and development (Neuman, 1995).

To Neuman, stressors are all environmental, and they have the potential for disrupting the stability of the client system (1989a, p. 50). Stressors attempt to penetrate the flexible and normal lines of defense, and the results are positive or negative responses. How a client system responds to stress is determined by the resistance demonstrated through lines of defense and resistance and by the dynamic relationship of five variable areas. The five variable areas are: physiologic, which describe bodily structure and function; psychological, which are related to mental processes and relationships; sociocultural, which relate to social and cultural functions; developmental, referring to life development processes; and spiritual, referring to the spiritual belief system. Neuman (1989a) maintained that the spiritual component has not been well developed in nursing.

To answer her central question about nursing, Neuman (1974, 1989a) demonstrated that a systems/stress theory of human beings would help nurses organize the vast knowledge amassed about human beings and their environments. An elaborate depiction of stressors and their penetrating abilities and of human beings and their natural and acquired resistance abilities emerged as a framework that nurses could use in describing their clients' problems and the territory for nursing intervention.

As outlined in Table 15-12, nurses also assess stressors in the environment. Environments are internal, external and created, and all may influence a client system in a circular fashion. Client system and environments relate reciprocally, and the outcome of this relationship is corrective or regulative for the client system. The internal environment is intrapersonal, the external environment includes the interpersonal and extrapersonal components, and the created environment is a composite of the intrapersonal, interpersonal, and extrapersonal components. Neuman described the internal and external environments in the following way:

> The internal environment consists of all forces or interactive influences internal to or contained solely within the boundaries of the defined client/client system. It correlates with the model intrapersonal factors or stressors. The external environment consists of all forces or interactive influences external to or existing outside the defined client/client system. It correlates with both the model's inter and extrapersonal factors or stressors. (Neuman, 1989a, p. 31)

The created environment is dynamic and is an interface that exists and connects the internal and external environments. Although the created environment may be created unconsciously by a client, it acts as a reserv oir for the existence or for the maintenance of the integrity of the client system. The expressions related to this environment are conscious or unconscious or both. The environment infiltrates all systems and all structures, it is purposeful, and it protects the functions of client/client systems.

> The insulating effect of the created-environment changes the response or possible response of the client to environmental stressors, for example, the use of denial or envy (psychological), physical rigidity or muscular constraint (physiological), life cycle continuation of survival patterns (developmental), required social space range (sociocultural), and sustaining hope (spiritual). (Neuman, 1989a, p. 32)

Table 15-12 ***Definition of Domain Concepts—Neuman***

Nursing	Is concerned with all and potential stressors. Deals with assessment of effect and potential effects of environmental stressors (Neuman, 1989a, p. 34).
Goal of nursing	To keep client's system stable. To assist clients to adjust, which is a requirement for optimum wellness level (1989a, p. 34). "Facilitate optimum wellness for the client through retention, attainment or maintenance of client system's stability" (1989a, p. 25).
Health	Health is wellness. It is a point on a continuum running from greatest negentropy to maximum entropy (1989a, p. 25). When all parts of a client are in harmony or in balance, and when all needs are met, optimal health is achieved. Health is also energy.
Human being	A physiologic, psychological, sociocultural, developmental, and spiritual being. Represented by central structure, lines of defense, and lines of resistance.
Nursing client	A human being who is threatened with, or who is attacked by, environmental stressors.
Environment	"All internal and external factors or influences surrounding the identified client or client system." Three types of environments were identified: internal, external, and created. The stressors are part of the environment. The internal environment is contained within the boundaries of the client system. The external environment contains forces outside a client system. The created environment denotes a client's unconscious mobilization of such structural components as energy factors, stability, and integrity (1989a, pp. 31–33, 1995).
Nursing problem	A whole client system threatened with or actually manifesting responses to stressors.
Nursing process	Neuman describes three central steps: nursing diagnoses, nursing goals, and outcomes (1989a, pp. 39–41).
Nurse–patient relations	Not discussed.
Nursing intervention	Prevention is the intervention identified by Neuman. There are three components in her intervention typology: primary, secondary, and tertiary. Reconstitution is part of tertiary prevention.

The created environment's goal is the unconscious stimulation of the client's health. It includes self-esteem, values, beliefs, and energy exchanges. Therefore, caregivers should explore ideas, beliefs, and fears as much as they explore symptoms and other causal factors. Finally, we should remember that energy is continuously flowing between client and environment. The caregiver's assessment and intervention is for the purpose of bringing optimal stability, which is the best possible state of wellness. Determining levels of wellness is accomplished through a consideration of client energy levels (Neuman, 1989a, p. 33). When more energy is expended than generated, the client system moves to entropy or illness. As more and more energy is needed to expend and less and less energy is being generated, death may result. Neuman defined entropy as "a process of energy depletion and disorganization, moving the system toward illness or possible death" (Neuman, 1989a, p. 48).

The goal of the caregiver is to maintain or to bring about the system's stability, a process Neuman calls *reconstitution.* Reconstitution brings the system a state of stability or wellness that is higher or lower than the previous state. Nursing actions are described in terms of prevention. Prevention is primary, secondary, and tertiary. Preventive aspects of care that occur before the stressors invade the client system are primary. Primary prevention identifies potential stressors and augments positive coping and function. When stressors attack the client system, nurses then mobilize and support internal and external responses, protect the core structure, facilitate treatment, and continue with any needed primary prevention. These actions are described by Neuman as secondary prevention (Neuman, 1989a, p. 21, 1989b, p. 56).

Neuman describes the development of a theory that evolved from her theory of nursing—the theory of optimal client system (Neuman and Koertvelyessy, 1986, cited in Neuman, 1989a, p. 46). Other theories could be developed as well. Neuman's theory has the potential for many theoretical propositions. A number of propositions are described in Table 15-13.

Theory Analysis

The Theorist

Betty Neuman, a community mental health nurse, received her bachelor's degree in nursing in 1957 and master's degree in nursing in 1966 from UCLA. She started her teaching job in 1966 (when we became office mates at UCLA) and was charged with coordinating the community mental health consultation clinical specialist program.

Although the UCLA faculty were busily operationalizing and implementing Johnson's theory at that time, Neuman was uninvolved in this process. She was concerned about the development of a framework to describe the consultation role of nurses, one that could help students describe and explain their actions and the rationale for their actions. The result of that concern was the development of her theory of a client who is in need of health care. Because the role of community mental health consultant is not necessarily exclusively a nursing role, this may explain why Neuman maintains in her writings that her theory is designed for use by any health professional.

Neuman has worked as a teacher, a consultant, and a writer and has maintained a small private practice as a licensed marriage and family counselor. She taught programs in stress reduction and in self-help for retarded children. Neuman received a doctorate from Ohio University in 1985. Currently, she lectures, writes, and consults, and she is a consultant for the Neuman Systems Model implementation trustee group (Neuman, 1989c, p. 453).

Table 15-13 ***Propositions—Neuman***

- Primary prevention prevents stressors from penetration of flexible line of defense.
- Primary prevention prevents stress responses.
- Secondary prevention enhances wellness and decreases stress.
- By supporting strengths of clients' systems and conserving their energy, nurses can increase level of wellness.

Paradigmatic Origins

Neuman's theory has several paradigmatic origins. One origin that is explicitly identified by Neuman is systems theory as conceptualized by Bertalanffy (1968). Neuman used Caplan's (1964) preventive functions, which she used in teaching the master's program in community mental health to define the levels of actions of nurses (Neuman, 1989c). Other origins identified by Neuman are Chardin's (1955) conceptualization of wholeness; Putts' (1972) application of systems theory in nursing; ideas about adaptation and environment (Neuman, 1989a, p. 12); Marxist ideas of synthesis of man and environment (Cornu, 1957); Gestalt psychology (Edelson, 1970), in which the interactions of people and their environments are described; and Selye's (1950) ideas about stress and bodily responses. Neuman relied heavily on these sources, which are all equally appropriate for use by mental health workers. It is the multiplicity of Neuman's sources that provides the breadth in her theory and its potential interdisciplinary nature.

Internal Dimensions

This is a highly abstract and a deductive theory constructed from hypothetical beginnings, and it was derived from a number of paradigms. The theory is hierarchical, evolving from a set of principles describing relationships between lines of defense, lines of resistance, basic structure, and energy resources. Neuman's is a field theory that explains the relationship of a client system to the environment, and it is a macrotheory that attempts to describe client system relationships with environment and nurse actions in any situation that requires nursing care. The theory has a broad scope; it provides a framework that describes components of the domain of nursing as a whole. It is also a macrotheory of the domain of nursing, and it explains the primary, secondary, and tertiary prevention needs of nursing clients and the nursing actions for each level of prevention.

Neuman's theory was constructed to provide her with a framework for teaching community mental health consultation in a graduate program. It was constructed through the synthesis of different theories that she believed are essential for use by community mental health consultants in their practice. Examples of such theories are systems theory, crisis theory, Gestalt theory, and stress and adaptation theory. Neuman's theory was also developed to identify nurse's actions and the focus of such actions. It provides a comprehensive description of nursing clients and a framework to describe nursing interventions. It describes knowledge of order; that is, it provides a descriptive account of the normal structure of client's systems and the patterns by which stress tends to attack human beings. The theory lacks a framework to identify, describe, and explain the different patterns of responses to stress.

Neuman's theory is logically developed, as demonstrated in her conceptualization of a client system as having several parts, with these parts interacting and relating to form a larger whole (Barnum, 1994). Interventions also have parts and levels. Primary, secondary, and tertiary prevention are identified, but it is not clear why other intervention actions are excluded, or, if included, where they should be within the conceptualization of interventions that she provides in the theory. Many nurses would question the rationale, the utility, and the assumptions in including all nursing interventions within a prevention framework. There are other critical questions of the theory. Neuman addresses antithetical and mutually exclusive concepts without addressing their complementarity and supplementarity. Examples are stability and dynamism, the conscious and unconscious environments, and holism and isolated responses (eg, psychological responses of denial). The relationship between these opposites and ways by which they are synthesized have not been addressed.

One of the strengths of this theory is Neuman's use of clear diagrams. These diagrams, used in all the descriptions of her theory, make the theory visually appealing; they enhance its clarity and provide nurses with opportunities to consider the logic and the interrelationships between the theory concepts.

Theory Critique

Neuman clearly identified some assumptions on which her theory is built (Fawcett, 1989). There are some implicit assumptions not well defined, such as valuing individuality of clients (Lancaster and Whall, 1989, p. 262). Although this is a theory with a potential to use families and communities as clients, Neuman does not identify assumptions related to such potential. Values inherent in nursing in relationship to the role of patients in maintaining and promoting health are not addressed.

The central concepts of her theory lack clarity. For example, health and wellness are used interchangeably and the relationship between health care as advocated by her theory and the World Health Organization's mandate for health for all by the year 2000 could be clearer (Haggart, 1993). Different meanings and interpretations are inherent in these diverse definitions. These potential variations, if acknowledged and addressed, could enhance the power of the theory.

Neuman (1989c) describes a wide circle of contagiousness for her theory that spans the United States and other countries. Use of her theory encompasses all program levels and a variety of nursing sources. Neuman details an impressive list of utilizers of her theory during the 1970s and 1980s (Neuman, 1989c, pp. 460–466). This extensive use prompted the development of slide shows, videotapes, and the Neuman Systems Model Trustee Group, Inc., which is charged with the task of seeing that her theory flourishes and continues to be used accurately.

The utility of Neuman's theory has been demonstrated in the diversity of its use (Campbell and Keller, 1989). Neuman (1989b) describes patient situations in which her theory could be used in suicide counseling, and Lillis and Cora (1989) provide an analysis of the use of Neuman's theory in a case study. Neuman's theory has been used in community health nursing settings (Beddome, 1989; Benedict and Sproles, 1982), as a framework for family assessment (Reed, 1989), as a guide for assessing and intervening in dysfunctional families (Herrick and Goodykoontz, 1989), for preventing abuse in the elderly (Delunas, 1990), in caring for patients in hospital settings (Brink, Neuman, and Wynn, 1992; Burke, Capers, O'Connell, Quinn, and Sinnott, 1989), as a framework for perinatal nursing (Dunn and Trepanier, 1989), for assessing renal patients (Breckenridge, 1989), in critical care (Bergstrom, 1992; Heffline, 1991), as a framework for patients recovering at home from myocardial infarction (Ross and Bourbonnais, 1985; Smith, 1989), in the care of patients positive for human immunodeficiency virus (Pierce and Hutton, 1992), and for nursing during the acute stage of spinal cord injury (Foote, Piazza, and Schultz, 1990; Hoeman and Winters, 1990; Sullivan, 1986).

Buchanan (1987) offers a modification of the theory for use with aggregates, families, and communities. She clarified and added an extension to each of the central theory concepts; however, the major additional contribution appears to be the collaborative decision-making process. These additions are congruent with Neuman's rationale for the development of her ideas, which is the development of a framework to be used by different members of the health care team. The extensions are also congruent with the theory assumptions. The theory's potential application to caring of people with different cultural heritages was discussed by Sohier (1989).

Neuman's theory is reported to have guided the development of curricula in Neuman's college (Mirenda, 1986), as well as being used as a framework for programs in transition from associate to baccalaureate programs (Lowry and Jopp, 1989; Sipple and Freese, 1989), as a framework for some specific students' experiences (Dale and Savala, 1990), and as a framework for cooperative (two-school) baccalaureate programs (Nelson, Hansen, and McCullagh, 1989). The faculty and administrators in most of these programs found Neuman's theory clear; it provided a holistic vision of nursing—a clear nursing perspective, and it provided an emphasis on client's perceptions—a useful framework for analysis of clients. One example of this evaluation is in Nelson, Hansen and McCullagh (1989).

Mrkonich, Hessian, and Miller (1989) describe using Neuman's theory as a framework for three accredited baccalaureate nursing programs that are situated in private, religious, and liberal arts colleges. The authors report that the theory's use was enhanced by its common language, which facilitated communication among health care professionals (p. 93). They also credit the theory for its potential to stimulate research and further development of theory (Mrkonich, Miller and Hessian, 1989). Mirenda (1986) described the Neuman college nursing process tool that was developed to be used by students in assessing nursing clients. The tool is reported to help students use Neuman's theory clinically.

Neuman's theory is used as a framework for demonstration of the process of concept development. The richness of the diagrammatic representation of the theory concepts and relationships has helped faculty members in one college devise visual representations to assist students to learn about conceptual models (Johnson, 1989).

There are many indications of the theory's international use. Examples of this are provided by Ross, Bourbonnais, and Carroll (1987) and Bourbonnais and Ross's (1985) descriptive accounts of the theory's utility for the fourth and final year of a baccalaureate program in Canada. Story and Ross (1986) demonstrated the theory's effective utility in the development and implementation of a framework for clinical learning experiences for nursing with families of the elderly at home. These authors also discussed the feasibility of using multiple nursing theories within the same curriculum to guide different learning experiences.

Similar examples of utility in curricula were provided by many others. These examples were collected by Neuman in a book of readings (Neuman, 1989a). This collection demonstrates the extensive utility of her theory for baccalaureate programs and associate degree programs as well as for a framework for multilevel planning.

The theory's utility in administrative practice has also been demonstrated. It was used as a framework for community health administration (Drew, Craig, and Beynon, 1989), and it was used as a framework for the reorganization of structure and function of the nursing department at Jefferson Davis Memorial Hospital (Hinton-Walker and Raborn, 1989). Kelley, Sanders, and Pierce (1989) describe the utility of the theory in guiding nurse administrators in their management and leadership roles in educational and practice settings. They also report the development of a tool for assessing and evaluating "conditions upon which the nurse administrators' goals are established and modified" (p. 129).

The Neuman Systems Management Tool, well described and illustrated, is tailored to provide administrators with a guide for actions and decisions within 3 minutes of use. No reports of validity or reliability of the tool were provided. Others report its use in the development of nursing care plans (Capers and Kelly, 1987) as well as in planning and implementation of the theory in nursing practice (Capers, O'Brien, Quinn, Kelly and Fenerty, 1985).

External Components of Theory

Neuman's theory is congruent with values about holism in nursing and the reciprocal relationship between environments and client systems. The theory is also highly useful for nurses who tend to speak in terms of prevention rather than treatment or intervention. The focus of the theory on involvement of clients and on assessment that includes defense and resistance is an acceptable nursing focus. The theory is particularly useful for nurses who believe that all health care professionals share the same goals and actions. In proposing the universality of assessment and intervention among the different health professionals, Neuman failed to identify the unique contributions of nurses to the health care team.

Theory Testing

Neuman's theory has generated limited research, but research projects driven by her theory have been increasing (Louis, 1995). One of the theory's propositions—that primary prevention inhibits the impact of the stress of surgery—was tested by Ziemer (1983). The study results failed to support the theoretical proposition. Although there is a potential for using the theory as a framework for research, the limited use of Neuman's theory in research raises many questions about its descriptive and explanatory powers. However, Harris, Hermiz, Meininger, and Steinkeler (1989) report increasing empirical use of Neuman's theory.

Louis and Koertvelyessy (1989) surveyed schools of nursing to determine the use of nursing models in curricula and research. The questionnaires contained specific information related to the use of Neuman's theory. The response rate of 38% was analyzed, and the results indicated that 92% of the responding schools used one of 26 nursing models in their graduate programs as a framework. The respondents identified 41 different models studied by graduate students. Neuman's was one of the most cited models. The authors of the survey report were able to identify 38 research studies that used Neuman's theory. They concluded that the studies were descriptive and that most of the concepts of Neuman's theory were studied, with the exception being the spiritual variable. The researchers used the theory as an outline of the phenomenon, as a framework for the methodology, and as a framework for interpretation and for implications. The report did not include information on the nature of the studies, the findings, or the implications of the findings on Neuman's theory or nursing practice. No citations were provided.

Despite the limitations of Neuman's theory in stimulating research, the utility of the theory in the clinical and educational spheres has been amply documented.

REFERENCES

Johnson

Ainsworth, M. (1972). Attachment and dependency: A comparison. In J. Gewirtz (Ed.), *Attachment and dependency.* Englewood Cliffs, NJ: Prentice-Hall.

Auger, J.A. (1976). *Behavioral systems and nursing.* Englewood Cliffs, NJ: Prentice-Hall.

Auger, J.A. and Dee, U. (1983, April). A patient classification system based on the behavioral system model of nursing: Part 1. *The Journal of Nursing Administration,* 13, 38–43.

Bertalanffy, L. von (1968). *General systems theory: Foundations, development, application.* New York: George Braziller.

Bruce, G.L., Hinds, P., Hudak, J., Mucha, A., Taylor, M.C., and Thompson, C.R. (1980). Implementation of ANA's quality assurance program for clients with end-stage renal disease. *Advances in Nursing Science,* 2(2), 79–95.

Damus, K. (1980). An application of the Johnson behavioral system model for nursing practice. In J.P. Riehl and C. Roy (Eds.), *Conceptual models for nursing practice* (2nd ed.). New York: Appleton-Century-Crofts.

Dee, V. (1986). Validation of a patient classification instrument for psychiatric patients based on the Johnson model for nursing. Unpublished doctoral dissertation. University of California, San Francisco.

Dee, V. (1990). Implementation of the Johnson model: One hospital's experience. In M.E. Parker (Ed.), *Nursing theories in practice* (pp. 33–44). New York: National League for Nursing.

Dee, U. and Auger, J.A. (1983). A patient classification system based on the behavioral system model of nursing: Part 2. *The Journal of Nursing Administration,* 13, 18–23.

Derdiarian, A. (1983). An instrument for theory and research development using the behavioral systems model for nursing: The cancer patient, Part I. *Nursing Research,* 32(4), 196–201.

Derdiarian, A. (1984). An investigation of the variables and boundaries of cancer nursing: A pioneering approach using Johnson's behavioral systems model for nursing. In *Proceedings of the 3rd International Conference on Cancer Nursing.* Melbourne, Australia: The Cancer Institute/Peter MacCallum Hospital and the Royal Melbourne Hospital.

Derdiarian, A.K. (1990a). Effects of using systematic assessment instruments on patient and nurse satisfaction with nursing care. *Oncology Nursing Forum, 17,* 95–101.

Derdiarian, A.K. (1990b). The relationships among the subsystems of Johnson's behavioral system model. *Image: Journal of Nursing Scholarship, 22,* 219–225.

Derdiarian, A.K. (1991). Effects of using a nursing model-based assessment instrument on quality of nursing care. *Nursing Administration Quarterly,* 15(3), 1-16.

Derdiarian, A.K. (1993a). Application of the Johnson behavioral system model in nursing practice. In M.E. Parker (Ed.), *Patterns of nursing theories in practice* (pp. 285–298). New York: National League for Nursing.

Derdiarian, A.K. (1993b). The Johnson behavioral system model: Perspectives for nursing practice. In M.E. Parker (Ed.), *Patterns of nursing theories in practice* (pp. 267–284). New York: National League for Nursing.

Derdiarian, A. and Forsythe, A.B. (1983). An instrument for theory and research development using the behavioral systems model for nursing: The cancer patient, Part II. *Nursing Research,* 32(4), 260–267.

Dickoff, J., James, P., and Wiedenbach, E. (1968). Theory in a practice discipline, Part 1. Practice oriented theory. *Nursing Research,* 17(5), 415–435.

Feshback, S. (1970). Aggression. In P. Mussen (Ed.), *Carmichael's manual of child psychology* (3rd ed.). New York: John Wiley & Sons.

Grubbs, J. (1980). An interpretation of the Johnson behavioral system model. In J.P. Riehl and C. Roy (Eds.), *Conceptual models for nursing practice* (2nd ed.). New York: Appleton-Century-Crofts.

Hadley, B.J. (1970, March). The utility of theoretical frameworks for curriculum development in nursing: The happening at Colorado. Paper presented at WICHEN General Session, Honolulu, Hawaii.

Harris, R.B. (1986). Introduction of a conceptual model into a fundamental baccalaureate course. *Journal of Nursing Education*, 25, 66–69.

Holaday, B. (1974). Achievement behavior in chronically ill children. *Nursing Research*, 23(1), 25–30.

Holaday, B. (1980). Implementing the Johnson model for nursing practice. In J.P. Riehl and C. Roy (Eds.), *Conceptual models for nursing practice* (2nd ed.). New York: Appleton-Century-Crofts.

Holaday, B. (1981). Maternal response to their chronically ill infants' attachment behavior of crying. *Nursing Research*, 30(6), 343–347.

Holaday, B. (1982). Maternal conceptual set development: Identifying patterns of maternal response to chronically ill infant crying. *Maternal Child Nursing Journal*, 11(1), 47–58.

Holaday, B. (1987). Patterns of interaction between mothers and their chronically ill infants. *Maternal Child Nursing Journal*, 16(1), 29–45.

Holaday, B. and Turner-Henson, A. (1987). Chronically ill school-age children's use of time. *Pediatric Nursing*, 13, 410–414.

Johnson, D.E. (1959a). A philosophy of nursing. *Nursing Outlook*, 7(4), 198–200.

Johnson, D.E. (1959b). The nature of a science of nursing. *Nursing Outlook*, 7(5), 291–294.

Johnson, D.E. (1961). The significance of nursing care. *American Journal of Nursing*, 61(11), 63–66.

Johnson, D.E. (1964, June). Is there an identifiable body of knowledge essential to the development of a generic professional nursing program? Paper presented at First Interuniversity Faculty Work Conference Nursing Council, NEBHE, Stowe, VT.

Johnson, D.E. (1968a). Theory in nursing: Borrowed or unique. *Nursing Research*, 17(3), 206–209.

Johnson, D.E. (1968b, April). One conceptual model of nursing. Paper presented at Vanderbilt University, Nashville, TN.

Johnson, D.E. (1974). Development of theory: A requisite for nursing as a primary health profession. *Nursing Research*, 23(5), 372–377.

Johnson, D.E. (1978). State of the art of theory development in nursing. In *Theory development: What, why, how?* New York: National League for Nursing.

Johnson, D.E. (1980). The behavioral system model for nursing. In J.P. Riehl and C. Roy (Eds.), *Conceptual models for nursing practice* (2nd ed.). New York: Appleton-Century-Crofts.

Johnson, D.E. (1987). Evaluating conceptual models for use in critical care nursing practice. *Dimensions of Critical Care Nursing*, 6(4), 195–197.

Johnson, D.E. (1989). Some thoughts on nursing. *Clinical Nurse Specialist*, 3(1), 1–4.

Johnson, D.E. (1990). The behavioral system model for nursing. In M.E. Parker (Ed.), *Nursing theories in practice* (pp. 23–32). New York: National League for Nursing.

Johnson, D.E. (1992). The origins of the behavioral system model. In F.N. Nightingale, *Notes on nursing: What it is, and what it is not* (Commemorative edition, pp. 23–27). Philadelphia: J.B. Lippincott.

Lachicotte, J.L., and Alexander, J.W. (1990). Management attitudes and nurse impairment. *Nursing Management*, 21, 102–104, 106, 108, 110.

Lovejoy, N. (1983). The leukemic child's perceptions of family behaviors. *Oncology Nursing Forum* 10(4): 20–25.

Lovejoy, N. (1985). Needs of vigil and nonvigil visitors in cancer research units. In *Fourth Cancer Nursing Research Conference Proceedings.* Honolulu: American Cancer Society.

Majesky, S.J., Brester, M.H., and Nishio, K.T. (1978). Development of a research tool: Patient indicators of nursing care. *Nursing Research*, 27(6), 365–371.

Naguib, H.H. (1988). *Physicians', nurses', and patients' perceptions of the surgical patients' educational rights.* Unpublished doctoral dissertation. University of Alexandria, United Republic of Egypt.

Parsons, T. (1951). *The social system.* New York: Free Press.

Porter, L. (1972). The impact of physical-physiological activity on infants' growth and development. *Nursing Research*, 21(3), 210–219.

Rawls, A.G. (1980). Evaluation of the Johnson behavioral model in clinical practice. *Image*, 12, 13–16.

Reynolds, W. and Cormack, D.F. (1991). An evaluation of the Johnson Behavioral System Model of Nursing. *Journal of Advanced Nursing*, 16(9), 1122–1130.

Small, B. (1980). Nursing visually impaired children with Johnson's model as a conceptual framework. In J.P. Riehl and C. Roy (Eds.), *Conceptual models for nursing practice* (2nd ed.). New York: Appleton-Century-Crofts.

Stamler, C. and Palmer, J.O. (1971). Dependency and repetitive visits to the nurse's office in elementary school children. *Nursing Research*, 20(3), 254–255.

Wilkie, D. (1990). Cancer pain management: State-of-the-art care. *Nursing Clinics of North America, 25*, 331–343.

Wu, R. (1973). *Behavior and illness.* Englewood Cliffs, NJ: Prentice-Hall.

Zetterberg, H.L. (1963). *On theory verification in sociology* (Rev. ed.). Totowa, NJ: Bedminster Press.

Roy

Andrews, H.A. (1991). Overview of the self-concept mode. In C. Roy and H.A. Andrews, *The Roy adaptation model: The definitive statement* (pp. 269–279). East Norwalk, CT: Appleton & Lange.

Andrews, H.A. and Roy, C. (1986). *Essentials of the Roy adaptation model.* Norwalk, CT: Appleton-Century-Crofts.

Artinian, N.T. (1991). Stress experience of spouses of patients having coronary artery bypass during hospitalization and 6 weeks after discharge. *Heart and Lung*, 20, 52–59.

Artinian, N.T. (1992). Spouse adaptation to mate's CABG surgery: 1 year follow-up. *American Journal of Critical Care*, 1(2), 36–42.

Bertalanffy, L. (1968). *General system theory.* New York: George Braziller.

Brower, H.T. and Baker, D.J. (1976). Using the adaptation model in a practitioner curriculum. *Nursing Outlook*, 24(11), 686–689.

Bunting, S.M. (1988). The concept of perception in selected nursing theories. *Nursing Science Quarterly*, 1(4), 168–174.

Chardin, P.T. (1965). *Hymn of the universe.* (S. Bartholomew, Trans.). New York: Harper & Row.

Cottrell, B. and Shannahan, M. (1986). Effect of the birth chair on duration of second stage labor and maternal outcome. *Nursing Research*, 35(6), 364–367.

Cottrell, B. and Shannahan, M. (1987). A comparison of fetal outcome in birth chair and delivery table births. *Research in Nursing and Health*, 10, 239–243.

Craig, D.I. (1990). The adaptation to pregnancy of spinal cord injured women. *Rehabilitation Nursing*, 15(1), 6–9.

Downey, C. (1974). Adaptation nursing applied to an obstetric patient. In J.P. Riehl and C. Roy (Eds.), *Conceptual models for nursing practice.* New York: Appleton-Century-Crofts.

Farkas, L. (1981). Adaptation problems with nursing home application for elderly persons: An application of the Roy adaptation nursing model. *Journal of Advanced Nursing*, 6, 363–368.

Fawcett, J. (1981a). Assessing and understanding the cesarean father. In C.F. Kehoe (Ed.), *The cesarean experience: Theoretical and clinical perspectives for nurses.* New York: Appleton-Century-Crofts.

Fawcett, J. (1981b). Needs of cesarean birth parents. *Journal of Obstetric, Gynecologic, and Neonatal Nursing*, 10, 371–376.

Fawcett, J. (1984). *Analysis and evaluation of conceptual models of nursing.* Philadelphia: F.A. Davis.

Fawcett, J. and Henklein, J. (1987). Antenatal education for cesarean birth: Extension of a field test. *Journal of Obstetric, Gynecologic, and Neonatal Nursing*, 16, 61–65.

Galligan, A.C. (1979). Using Roy's concept of adaptation to care for young children. *American Journal of Maternal Child Nursing*, 4(1), 24–28.

Gless, P.A. (1995). Applying the Roy adaptation model to the care of clients with quadriplegia. *Rehabilitation Nursing*, 20(1), 11–16.

Gordon, J. (1974). Nursing assessment and care plan for a cardiac patient. In J.P. Riehl and C. Roy (Eds.), *Conceptual models for nursing practice.* New York: Appleton-Century-Crofts.

Hamer, B.A. (1991). Music therapy: Harmony for change. *Journal of Psychosocial Nursing and Mental Health Services*, 29(12), 5–7.

Hanchett, E.S. (1990). Nursing models and community as client. *Nursing Science Quarterly*, 3, 67–72.

Harrison, L.L., Leeper, J.D., and Yoon, M. (1990). Effects of early parent touch on preterm infants' heart rates and arterial oxygen saturation levels. *Journal of Advanced Nursing*, 15, 877–885.

Helson, H. (1964). *Adaptation-level theory: An experimental and systematic approach to behavior.* New York: Harper & Row.

Henderson, V. (1960). *Basic principles of nursing care.* London: International Council of Nurses.

Hoch, C. (1987). Assessing delivery of nursing care. *Journal of Gerontological Nursing*, 13(1), 10–17.

Idle, B.A. (1978). SPAL: A tool for measuring self-perceived adaptation level appropriate for an elderly population. In E.E. Bauwens (Ed.), *Clinical nursing research: Its strategies and findings* (Monograph series No. 2). Indianapolis: Sigma Theta Tau.

Janelli, L.M. (1980). Utilizing Roy's adaptation model from a gerontological perspective. *Journal of Gerontological Nursing*, 6(3), 140–150.

Kehoe, C.F. (1981). Identifying the nursing needs of the postpartum cesarean mother. In C.F. Kehoe (Ed.), *The cesarean experience: Theoretical and clinical perspectives for nurses.* New York: Appleton-Century-Crofts.

Kurek-Ovshinsky, C. (1991). Group psychotherapy in an acute inpatient setting: Techniques that nourish self-esteem. *Issues in Mental Health Nursing*, 12, 81–88.

Laros, J. (1977). Deriving outcome criteria from a conceptual model. *Nursing Outlook*, 25, 333–336.

Levine, M.E. (1966). Adaptation and assessment: A rationale for nursing intervention. *American Journal of Nursing*, 66, 2450–2453.

Lewis, F., Firsich, S.C., and Parsell, S. (1978). Development of reliable measures of patient health outcomes related to quality nursing care for chemotherapy patients. In J.C. Krueger, A.H. Nelson, and M.O. Wolanin, *Nursing research: Development, collaboration, utilization.* Germantown, MD: Aspen.

Lewis, F.M., Firsich, S.C., and Parsell, S. (1979). Clinical tool development for adult chemotherapy patients: Process and content. *Cancer Nursing*, 2(2), 99–108.

Mastal, M.F. and Hammond, H. (1980). Analysis and expansion of the Roy adaptation model: A contribution to holistic nursing. *Advances in Nursing Science*, 2(4), 71–81.

Mastal, M.F., Hammond, H., and Roberts, M.P. (1982). Theory into hospital practice: A pilot implementation. *Journal of Nursing Administration*, 12(6), 9–15.

Morales-Mann, E.T. and Logan, M. (1990). Implementing the Roy model: Challenges for nurse educators. *Journal of Advanced Nursing*, 15, 142–147.

Munn, V.A. and Tichy, A.M. (1987). Nurses' perceptions of stressors in pediatric intensive care. *Journal of Pediatric Nursing*, 2, 405–411.

Nightingale, F. (1859). *Notes on nursing: What it is and what it is not.* London: Harrison. Reprinted 1995. Philadelphia: J.B. Lippincott.

Pollock, S.E. (1986). Human responses to chronic illness: Physiologic and psychological adaptation. *Nursing Research*, 35(2), 90–95.

Pollock, S.E., Frederickson, K., Carson, M.A., Massey, V.H., and Roy, C. (1994). Contributions to nursing science: Synthesis of findings from adaptation model research. *Scholarly Inquiry for Nursing Practice*, 8(4), 361–372.

Randall, B., Poush-Tedrow, M., and Van Landingham, U.J. (1982). *Adaptation nursing: The Roy conceptual model applied.* St. Louis: C.V. Mosby.

Roy, C. (1970). Adaptation: A conceptual framework for nursing. *Nursing Outlook, 18*(3), 42–45.

Roy, C. (1971). Adaptation: A basis for nursing practice. *Nursing Outlook*, 19(4), 254–257.

Roy, C. (1976). *Introduction to nursing: An adaptation model.* Englewood Cliffs, NJ: Prentice-Hall.

Roy, C. (1977). *Decision-making by the physically ill and adaptation during illness.* Unpublished doctoral dissertation, University of California, Los Angeles.

Roy, C. (1979). Relating nursing theory to education: A new era. *Nurse Educator*, 4(2), 16–21.

Roy, C. (1980). The Roy adaptation model. In J.P. Riehl and C. Roy (Eds.), *Conceptual models for nursing practice* (2nd ed.). New York: Appleton-Century-Crofts.

Roy, C. (1984). *Introduction to nursing: An adaptation model* (2nd ed.). Englewood Cliffs, NJ: Prentice-Hall.

Roy, C. (1987). Roy's adaptation model. In R.R. Parse, *Nursing science: Major paradigms, theories, and critiques* (pp. 35–45). Philadelphia: W.B. Saunders.

Roy, C. (1988a). An explication of the philosophical assumptions of the Roy adaptation model. *Nursing Science Quarterly*, 1(1), 26–34.

Roy, C. (1988b). Altered cognition: An information processing approach. In P.H. Mitchell, L.C. Hodges, M. Muwaswes. and C.A. Walleck (Eds.), *AANN's neuroscience nursing: Phenomenon and practice: Human responses to neurological health problems* (pp. 185–211). East Norwalk, CT: Appleton & Lange.

Roy, C. (1989). The Roy adaptation model. In J.P. Riehl-Sisca, *Conceptual models for nursing practice* (3rd ed., pp. 105–114). East Norwalk, CT: Appleton & Lange.

Roy, C. (1991). The Roy adaptation model in nursing research. In C. Roy and H.A. Andrews, *The Roy adaptation model: The definitive statement* (pp. 445–458). East Norwalk, CT: Appleton & Lange.

Roy, C. and Andrews, H.A. (1991). *The Roy adaptation model: The definitive statement.* East Norwalk, CT: Appleton & Lange.

Roy, C. and Corliss, C.P. (1993). *The Roy adaptation model: Theoretical update and knowledge for practice* (pp. 215–229). New York: National League for Nursing.

Roy, C. and McLeod, D. (1981). Theory of the person as an adaptive system. In C. Roy and S.L. Roberts, *Theory construction in nursing: An adaptation model* Englewood Cliffs, NJ: Prentice-Hall.

Roy, C. and Roberts, S.L. (1981). *Theory construction in nursing: An adaptation model.* Englewood Cliffs, NJ: Prentice-Hall.

Schmitz, M. (1980). The Roy adaptation model: Application in a community setting. In J.P. Riehl and C. Roy (Eds.), *Conceptual models for nursing practice* (2nd ed.). New York: Appleton-Century-Crofts.

Silva, M.C. (1987). Needs of spouses of surgical patients: A conceptualization within the Roy adaptation model. *Scholarly Inquiry for Nursing Practice: An International Journal*, 1, 29–44.

Strohmyer, L.L., Noroian, E.L., Patterson, L.M., and Carlin, B.P. (1993). Adaptation six months after multiple trauma: A pilot study. *Journal of Neuroscience Nursing*, 25, 30–37.

Tiedeman, M.E. (1983). The Roy adaptation model. In J.J. Fitzpatrick and A.L. Whall (Eds.), *Conceptual models of nursing: Analysis and application.* Bowie, MD: Robert J. Brady Company.

Tulman, L. and Fawcett, J. (1988). Return of functional ability after childbirth. *Nursing Research*, 37(2), 77–81.

Wagner, P. (1976). Testing the adaptation model in practice. *Nursing Outlook*, 24(11), 682–685.

Wallace, C.L. (1993). Resources for nursing theories in practice. In M.E. Parker (Ed.). *Patterns of nursing theories in practice* (pp. 301–311). New York: National League for Nursing.

Neuman

Barnum, B.J.S. (1994). *Nursing theory: Analysis, application, evaluation* (4th ed.). Philadelphia: J.B. Lippincott.

Beddome, G. (1989). Application of the Neuman systems model to the assessment of community-as-client. In B. Neuman, *The Neuman systems model* (2nd ed.). East Norwalk, CT: Appleton & Lange.

Benedict, M.B. and Sproles, J.B. (1982). Application of the Neuman model to public health nursing practice. In B. Neuman, *The Neuman systems model: Application to nursing education and practice.* Norwalk, CT: Appleton-Century-Crofts.

Bergstrom, D. (1992). Hypermetabolism in multisystem organ failure: A Neuman systems perspective. *Critical Care Nursing Quarterly*, 15(3), 63–70.

Bertalanffy, L. (1968). *General system theory.* New York: George Braziller.

Bourbonnais, F.F. and Ross, M.M. (1985). The Neuman systems model in nursing education: Course development and implementation. *Journal of Advanced Nursing*, 10(2), 117–123.

Breckenridge, D.M. (1989). Primary prevention as an intervention modality for the renal client. In B. Neuman, *The Neuman systems model* (2nd ed.). East Norwalk, CT: Appleton & Lange.

Brink, L.W., Neuman, B., and Wynn, J. (1992). Transport of the critically ill patient with upper airway obstruction. *Critical Care Clinics*, 8(3), 633–647.

Buchanan, B.F. (1987). Human environment interaction: A modification of the Neuman systems model for aggregates, families, and the community. *Public Health Nursing*, 4(1), 52–64.

Burke, Sr., M.E., Capers, C.F., O'Connell, R.K., Quinn, R.M., and Sinnott, M. (1989). Neuman-based nursing practice in a hospital setting. In B. Neuman, *The Neuman systems model* (2nd ed.). East Norwalk, CT: Appleton & Lange.

Campbell, V. and Keller, K.B. (1989). The Betty Neuman health care systems model: An analysis. In J.P. Riehl-Sisca, *Conceptual models for nursing practice* (2nd ed.). East Norwalk, CT: Appleton & Lange.

Capers, C.F. and Kelly, R. (1987). Neuman nursing process: A model of holistic care. *Holistic Nursing Practice*, 1(3), 19–26.

Capers, C.F., O'Brien, C., Quinn, R., Kelly, R., and Fenerty, A. (1985). The Neuman systems model in practice: Planning phase. *Journal of Nursing Administration*, 15(5), 29–39.

Caplan, G. (1964). *Principles of preventive psychiatry.* New York: Basic Books.

Chardin, P.T. (1955). *The phenomenon of man.* London: Collins.

Cornu, A. (1957). *The origins of Marxian thought.* Springfield, IL: Charles C. Thomas.

Dale, M.L. and Savala, S.M. (1990). A new approach to the senior practicum. *Nursing Connections*, 3(1), 45–51.

Delunas, L.R. (1990). Prevention of elder abuse: Betty Neuman health care systems approach. *Clinical Nurse Specialist*, 4(1), 54–58.

Drew, L.L., Craig, D.M., and Beynon, C.E. (1989). The Neuman systems model for community health administration and practice: Provinces of Manitoba and Ontario, Canada.

In B. Neuman, *The Neuman systems model* (2nd ed.). East Norwalk, CT: Appleton & Lange.

Dunn, S.I. and Trepanier, M. (1989). Applications of the Neuman systems model to perinatal nursing. In B. Neuman, *The Neuman systems model* (2nd ed.). East Norwalk, CT: Appleton & Lange.

Edelson, M. (1970). *Sociotherapy and psychotherapy*. Chicago: University of Chicago Press.

Fawcett, J. (1989). *Analysis and evaluation of conceptual models of nursing* (2nd ed.). Philadelphia: F.A. Davis.

Foote, A.W., Piazza, D., and Schultz, M. (1990). The Neuman systems model: Application to a patient with a cervical spinal cord injury. *Journal of Neuroscience Nursing*, 22, 302–306.

Haggart, M. (1993). A critical analysis of Neuman's systems model in relation to public health nursing. *Journal of Advanced Nursing*, 18, 1917–1922.

Harris, S.M., Hermiz, M.E., Meininger, M., and Steinkeler, S.E. (1989). Betty Neuman: Systems model. In A. Marriner-Tomey, *Nursing theorists and their work*. St. Louis: C.V. Mosby.

Heffline, M.S. (1991). A comparative study of pharmacological versus nursing interventions in the treatment of postanesthesia shivering. *Journal of Post Anesthesia Nursing*, 6(5), 311–320.

Herrick, C.A. and Goodykoontz, L. (1989). Neuman's systems model for nursing practice as a conceptual framework for a family assessment. *Journal of Child and Adolescent Psychiatric and Mental Health Nursing*, 2(2), 61–67.

Hinton-Walker, P. and Raborn, M. (1989). Application of the Neuman model in nursing administration and practice. In B. Henry, C. Arndt, M. Di Vicenti, and A. Marriner-Tomey, *Dimensions of nursing administration: Theory, research, education, practice*. Boston: Blackwell Scientific Publications.

Hoeman, S., and Winters, D.M. (1990). Theory based case management: High cervical spinal cord injury. *Home Health Care Nurse*, 8, 25–33.

Johnson, S.E. (1989). A picture is worth a thousand words: Helping students visualize a conceptual model. *Nurse Educator*, 14(3), 21–24.

Kelley, J.A., Sanders, N.F., and Pierce, J.D. (1989). A systems approach to the role of the nurse administrator in education and practice. In B. Neuman, *The Neuman systems model* (2nd ed.). East Norwalk, CT: Appleton & Lange.

Lancaster, D.R. and Whall, A.L. (1989). The Neuman systems model. In J.J. Fitzpatrick and A.L. Whall, *Conceptual models of nursing: Analysis and application* (2nd ed.). East Norwalk, CT: Appleton & Lange.

Lillis, P.P. and Cora, V.L. (1989). A case study analysis using the Neuman nursing process format: An abstract. In B. Neuman, *The Neuman systems model* (2nd ed.). East Norwalk, CT: Appleton & Lange.

Louis, M. (1995). The Neuman model in nursing research: An update. In Betty Neuman, *The Neuman systems model* (pp. 473–495). East Norwalk, CT: Appleton & Lange.

Louis, M. and Koertvelyessy, A. (1989). The Neuman model in nursing research. In B. Neuman, *The Neuman systems model* (2nd ed.). East Norwalk, CT: Appleton & Lange.

Lowry, L.W. and Jopp, M.C. (1989). An evaluation instrument for assessing an associate degree nursing curriculum based on the Neuman systems model. In J.P. Riehl-Sisca, *Conceptual models for nursing practice* (3rd ed.). East Norwalk, CT: Appleton & Lange.

Mirenda, R.M. (1986). The Neuman systems model: Description and application. In P. Winstead-Fry (Ed.), *Case studies in nursing theory*. New York: National League for Nursing.

Mrkonich, D.E., Hessian, M., and Miller M.W. (1989). A cooperative process in curriculum development using the Neuman health care systems model. In J.P. Riehl-Sisca, *Conceptual models for nursing practice* (3rd ed.). East Norwalk, CT: Appleton & Lange.

Mrkonich, D.E., Miller, M., and Hessian, M. (1989). Cooperative baccalaureate education: The Minnesota intercollegiate nursing consortium. In B. Neuman, *The Neuman systems model* (2nd ed.). East Norwalk, CT: Appleton & Lange.

Nelson, L.F., Hansen, M., and McCullagh, M. (1989). A new baccalaureate North Dakota-Minnesota nursing education consortium. In B. Neuman, *The Neuman systems model* (2nd ed.). East Norwalk, CT: Appleton & Lange.

Neuman, B. (1974). The Betty Neuman health-care systems model: A total person approach to patient problems. In J.P. Riehl and C. Roy, *Conceptual models for nursing practice*. New York: Appleton-Century-Crofts.

Neuman, B. (1982). *The Neuman systems model: Application to nursing education and practice*. Norwalk, CT: Appleton-Century-Crofts.

Neuman, B. (1989a). The Neuman systems model. In B. Neuman, *The Neuman systems model* (2nd ed.). East Norwalk, CT: Appleton & Lange.

Neuman, B. (1989b). The Neuman nursing process format: Family case study. In J.P. Riehl-Sisca, *Conceptual models for nursing practice* (3rd ed.). East Norwalk, CT: Appleton & Lange.

Neuman, B. (1989c). In conclusion—In transition. In B. Neuman, *The Neuman systems model* (2nd ed.). East Norwalk, CT: Appleton & Lange.

Neuman, B. (1995). *The Neuman systems model*. East Norwalk, CT: Appleton & Lange.

Neuman, B. and Young, R.J. (1972). A model for teaching total person approach to patient problems. *Nursing Research*, 21(3), 264–269.

Pierce, J.D., and Hutton, E. (1992). Applying the new concepts of the Neuman systems model. *Nursing Forum*, 27(1), 15–18.

Putt, A. (1972). Entropy, evolution and equifinality in nursing. In J. Smith (Ed.), *Five years of cooperation to improve curricula in western schools of nursing*. Boulder, CO: Western Interstate Commission for Higher Education.

Reed, K.S. (1989). Family theory related to the Neuman systems model. In B. Neuman, *The Neuman systems model* (2nd ed.). East Norwalk, CT: Appleton & Lange.

Ross, M.M. and Bourbonnais, F.F. (1985). The Betty Neuman systems model in nursing practice: A case study approach. *Journal of Advanced Nursing*, 10(3), 199–207.

Ross, M.M., Bourbonnais, F.F., and Carroll, G. (1987). Curricular design and the Betty Neuman systems model: A new approach to learning. *International Nursing Review*, 34(3), 75–79.

Selye, H. (1950). *The physiology and pathology of exposure to stress.* Montreal: ACTA.

Sipple, J.A. and Freese, B.T. (1989). Transition from technical to professional-level nursing education. In B. Neuman, *The Neuman systems model* (2nd ed.). East Norwalk, CT: Appleton & Lange.

Smith, M.C. (1989). Neuman's model in practice. *Nursing Science Quarterly*, 2(3), 116–117.

Sohier, R. (1989). Nursing care for the people of a small planet: Culture and the Neuman systems model. In B. Neuman, *The Neuman systems model* (2nd ed.). East Norwalk, CT: Appleton & Lange.

Story, E.L. and Ross, M.M. (1986). Family centered community health nursing and the Betty Neuman systems model. *Nursing Paper*, 18(2), 77–88.

Sullivan, J. (1986). Using Neuman's model in the acute phase of spinal cord injury. *Focus Critical Care*, 13(5), 34–41.

Ziemer, M.M. (1983). Effects of information on postsurgical coping. *Nursing Research*, 32(5), 282–287.

CHAPTER 16

On Human Being-Environment Interactions

When Martha Rogers asked the central question of her theory, What is the focus of nursing?, the answer was readily human being–environmental fields, "people and their world" (Rogers, 1992). Human beings and the environment are both unitary, irreducible, pandimensional, negentropic energy fields that are identifiable by pattern. Neither unitary human being nor unitary environment can be discussed, considered, or understood in isolation from the other. They are interrelated in an irreducible way. This fresh look at environment, unique to nursing and different from other theorists' views of environment, made it easy to consider Rogers as a significant force in our conceptual understanding not only of environment but of human being–environment relationships. Rogers' theory is described, analyzed, and critiqued in this chapter and classified as person–environment interactions. Rogers' science of unitary human beings also provides many insights about "environment" from a nursing perspective. Some tests of the theory proposition are also included. I also encourage you to look at Florence Nightingale's work for a conceptualization of environment as well as other theorists' conceptualizations of environment.

Martha Rogers

Theory Description

Rogers, a nurse leader and significant nursing theorist, specifically identified her theory, which she called the "science of unitary human beings," as a conceptual system of nursing intended to stimulate the development of nursing theories. Nursing theories, Rogers maintained, could only be developed as a result of nursing research that is completed within the conceptual system she conceived. In later work, Rogers relabeled her conceptualization as the science of unitary man (1980a), and then, even later, as a paradigm for nursing (Rogers, 1983a). She also changed the word "man" to "human beings" and "individuals." She proposed that the science of human beings is as applicable to groups as it is to individuals (Rogers, 1992). Groups may be a family, a social group, a community, a crowd, or any other combinations of individuals.

Examples of theories that may evolve from Rogers' paradigm are a "theory of accelerating evolution," a "theory for paranormal phenomena," and "rhythmical correlates of change" (1980a, 1987, 1992). Consistent with the premises of this book and based on the arguments developed in Chapter 8 on conceptual frameworks and theory, Rogers' conceptualization will be treated here as a theory. As has been done with each theory, the analysis and critique are provided to enhance understanding of the theory, to explain its role in the development of nursing's domain, and to encourage the further use, refinement, and development of the theory.

The central questions that Rogers attempted to answer are:

What is the focus of nursing?
Who is the nursing client?
What knowledge is needed to develop the science of nursing?

Rogers' conceptualization of nursing as a unique science is based on several explicit assumptions, presented in Table 16-1, and it encompasses several major concepts, presented in Table 16-2.

Most of Rogers' concepts are unique to her conceptualization. The concept of a unitary human being, with which Rogers' name has become synonymous, is a primitive concept. All other concepts are derived from a general systems theory (pattern, organization, negentropy), physics (electrodynamic), an evolutionary theory (life pro-

Table 16-1 ***Assumptions—Rogers***

EXPLICIT ASSUMPTIONS

- Nursing is concerned with the life process of a human being, which is irreversible, along a space–time continuum (Rogers, 1970, p. 59).
- The focus of the science of nursing is the unitary human being, his innovative wholeness, and his integral and continuous relationship with the environment. That relationship involves energy and matter exchange. Matter is energy (1970, pp. 47, 54).
- There is pattern and organization in the wholeness of the unitary human being, but causality cannot explain it (1970, pp. 53, 65).
- Conceptual systems are preludes to theories, and theories are tested in real life with a feedback to theories. The cycle is continuous, open, and changeable based on changes in knowledge (1970, pp. 83–88).
- Unitary human beings are characterized by the ability to use abstraction, imagery, language, thought, sensation, and emotion (1970, p. 73).
- Reality does not exist but appears to exist as expressed by human beings (1980, p. 333).
- Nursing is based on a humanistic and not a mechanistic model (1970, pp. 87, 138).
- Generalization can only occur from a study of the whole but not any of the parts in isolation.
- Human behavior demonstrates reason and feelings (1970).
- Unitary man possesses the ability to join in the process of change deliberately and with probability (1983b, p. 222, 1986).
- The human field and its environmental field are postulated to be coextensive with the universe (1983b, p. 222).

Table 16-2 ***Concepts—Rogers***

Unitary human being	Life process
Human field	Rhythmicity
Unitary environment	Self-regulation
Environment field	Negentropy
Energy field	Evolutionary emergence
Open	Unitary human processes
Pattern and organization	Helicy
Pandimensionality	Resonancy
Unidirectionality	Integrality
Sentience	Unpredictability
Thought	
Pattern	

cess, helicy), and adaptation theories (homeostasis, adaptation). Her concepts are abstract, general, conceptually defined, and documented, but they are limited in their operational referents, which may explain the slow use of the theory by nurses in general and nurses who are in practice in particular (Table 16-3).

To Rogers, a unitary human being is an irreducible, indivisible energy field in constant interaction with the environment, which is also an energy field and a unitary one. Energy fields are not reducible or indivisible nor are they the sum total of their parts, which may be physical, social, psychological, or biologic in nature. In fact, human beings and environments *do not have* energy fields; *they are* energy fields. They are open for exchange and extend to infinity. Energy fields are identifiable through dynamic–nonstatic wave patterns and organization that changes from "lower frequency, longer wave pattern to high frequency, shorter wave pattern" based on the principle of resonancy. Energy fields are pandimensional, transcend time and space, and therefore may have imaginary boundaries that are unique and changeable (Rogers, 1980a, 1983b, 1986, 1992). She considers fields as open "unifying concepts." Energy for her "signifies the dynamic nature of the field" (Rogers, 1992, p. 30). The four concepts that are basic to Rogers in her own last writings are energy fields, pattern, openness, and pandimensionality (Barrett, 1990a). Change is one of the basic tenets of her theory. Change is innovative, probabilistic, continuous, and relative. It furthers the differentiation of human and environmental fields from lower to higher diversity. Change is based on continuous interaction between a unitary human being's energy field and the environmental energy field. Human development was cited as a goal (Rogers, 1970) and rejected later (Malinski, 1986). The end point is not balance or equilibrium; rather, although there is no end point, there is a harmony that evolves and manifests in mutuality or integrality of person–environment–energy fields. These states of integrality, if we can call them states, are identified through patterns. Field pattern, which has been a central idea for Rogers since the beginnings of the formulation of her theory is:

> . . . an abstraction. It gives identity to the field. The nature of the pattern changes continuously. Each human field pattern is unique and is integral with its own unique environmental field pattern. (Rogers, 1986, p. 5)

Table 16-3 Definition of Domain Concepts—Rogers

Nursing	A learned profession, a science of unitary human beings, and the art of "imaginative and creative use of this knowledge in human service" (Rogers, 1980b, p. 122). It is concerned with living and dying. Fields of practice span the gamut of in and out of hospital, community, and the moon (Rogers, 1992).
Goal of nursing	To bring and promote symphonic interaction between a human being and his environment through participation in a process of change. This is done to "strengthen the coherence and integrity of the human field and to direct and redirect patterning of the human and environmental fields" (1970, p. 122). Maximum health potential (p. 86). "Meaningful life and meaningful transition from life to death" (1970, p. 125).
Health	Health and illness are not dichotomous but continuous, are part of the same continuum, and are an expression of the life process; they are socially defined. Health is "characteristics and behaviors emerging out of the mutual, simultaneous interaction of the human and environment fields" (1980b). One can extrapolate that Rogers' view of health could be the greater developmental coherence that evolves from human being–environment energy fields that are novel, emerging, and more diverse in pattern and organization. Health and illness are not differentiated, nor are there any norms of health (Madrid and Winstead-Fry, 1986)
Environment	"An irreducible, pandimensional, negentropic energy field, identified by pattern and manifesting characteristics different from those of the parts and encompassing all that is other than any given human field" (1983b, p. 222; modified in Rogers, 1992).
Human being	An irreducible, irreversible, pandimensional, negentropic energy field identified by pattern and manifesting characteristics that are different from those of the parts and which cannot be predicted from knowledge of the parts" (1983a, glossary). Unitary human being develops through three principles: helicy, resonancy, and integrality.
Nursing client	Human being–environment energy fields relationship (1970, p. 127).
Nursing problem	Not specifically addressed because Rogers believes labels of problems and illness are tentative and based on societal definition. Problems may denote changes in wave patterns and organization and in rhythmical correlates of change (1980a, pp. 334–335). Disharmony or lack of integrity in human being–environment energy fields.
Nursing process	Not specifically addressed. However, what Rogers says about scientific process applies here: "The subjective world of human feelings must be incorporated into so-called 'objective science' " (1970, p. 87).
Nurse–patient relations	Not addressed.
Nursing therapeutics	"Repatterning of man and environment for more effective fulfillment of life's capabilities" (1970, p. 127). Beliefs in innovative therapeutic modalities such as therapeutic touch (1985).
Focus	"Activities of daily living" must be considered within the context of the opportunities for human being–environment interchange that would stimulate the "flow of repatterning commensurate with the openness of nature" (1970, p. 123). Unitary human being in interaction with unitary environment. Human beings and environment are energy fields.

Rogers postulated three principles to describe the patterns of human being and environment interactions and change (Rogers, 1986). To understand the nature, direction, and power of change, one has to consider motion and changes in energy fields through these principles: resonancy, helicy, and integrality. *Resonancy* describes the direction of change from lower to higher wave patterns. The principle of *helicy* postulates that change manifested in increasing diversity and nonrepeating rhythmicity is continuous and unpredictable. *Integrality* describes the nature and the process of the mutuality between the human and energy fields. All three principles are characterized by their continuity and are manifested through patterns. Human and environmental fields are also characterized by their "pandimensionality," which replaced her earlier concepts of "four-dimensional" and "multi-dimensional" (Rogers 1992, p. 31). The change in this concept does not reflect a change in definitions, only a change in a label. Pandimensionality "is a way of perceiving reality," "it expresses the idea of a unitary whole," and it reinforces the nonlinearity and the lack of spatial and temporal characteristics (Rogers, 1992, p. 32). The changes that the human and environment fields experience are continuous; they emerge out of nonequilibrium and these changes are continuously accelerating.

Theory Analysis

The Theorist

It is difficult to think of the New York University nursing program without thinking of Martha Rogers. It is equally impossible to consider environment as a central concept in nursing without immediately thinking of Florence Nightingale and Martha Rogers. Both have left their imprints on nursing in more ways than one, but certainly on theoretical nursing and, more particularly, on the meaning of environment and its centrality to nursing.

Martha Rogers is one of the pioneers who envisioned a science of nursing in the late 1950s and early 1960s and advocated nursing having its own body of knowledge. She maintained that the science of nursing is unique and is not a synthesis of all sciences—it is more than that. Although synthesis may occur, the result is an integrated whole, as different from the parts as a unitary human being is different from the sum total of its parts. Martha Rogers began advocating that view in 1952.

Rogers received a diploma in nursing from Knoxville General Hospital School of Nursing, Knoxville, Tennessee, in 1936. She earned a bachelor of science degree from George Peabody College, Nashville, in 1937. From Teachers' College she received a master's degree in nursing in 1945, and she also received a master's degree in public health from Johns Hopkins University in 1952 (Rogers, 1983b). She worked as a public health nurse in rural Michigan and Connecticut and established the first visiting nurse service in Arizona (Hektor, 1989).

Rogers completed the requirements for her doctorate degree in science at Johns Hopkins one day in 1954, boarded a train and, one day later, was head of the nursing program at New York University. One of her first acts was to teach doctoral student seminars. She noted that the dissertation students in nursing were part and parcel of dissertation seminars in the education department. Rogers' belief in the uniqueness of nursing and its science prompted her to design a separate seminar for the nursing students. She quickly realized that the parameters of that unique knowledge had not been identified as yet. That became Rogers' mission in nursing (P. Winstead-Fry, personal communication, 1984).

As an advocate of diversity, Rogers demonstrated it in her personal life through her love of music and science fiction; in her writing, which incorporated philosophy, music, futurology, and physics; and the special talent with which she combined wit, humor, science, and art in speaking about nursing. Martha Rogers was one of the few scholars in nursing who will transcend her time and the profession. On a personal note, I invited Martha on behalf of the University of Alexandria in Egypt to give a keynote address for an international nursing conference. Her love for history, cultures, people, and life was evident in this last international trip before her death in 1994. I will always treasure having shared that trip with a great and courageous nurse scholar.

Paradigmatic Origins

Rogers developed her theory from a number of paradigms; concepts were synthesized into what is now a whole around unitary human being, unitary environment, energy fields, continuous interaction with the environment as an energy field, patterns, and change. Understanding of Rogers' theory is enhanced by the study of general systems theory (Rogers, 1985). The constant interaction between human beings and environment, the interrelationships of the energy field, and the openness of both to continuous exchange of matter and energy are based on Bertalanffy's (1968) definition of an open system. Although Rogers uses some of the terminology of systems theory, she denies the study of subsystems and isolated behavior as representing the whole of the unitary human being. Rogers also draws on the assumptions and concepts of the general systems theory in two other ways: the unitary human being as an organization of the whole, which is more than the sum of the parts, and the individuality and uniqueness of human beings as reflected in this pattern and organization and in their wholeness. Furthermore, Rogers uses the concept of negentropy—a general systems theory concept—to develop helicy, which is the "continuous innovative, probabilistic, increasing diversity of human and environmental field patterns characterized by nonrepeating rhythmicities" (Rogers, 1980a). Negentropy is a property of both the human being and his environment. Probabilism was later changed to unpredictability (Rogers, 1992).

Physics and electromagnetic theory provide some of the basic premises and concepts of Rogers' theory. The energy field of unitary human being and the environment are dynamic, are irreducible, are unbound, extend to infinity, and are identifiable by waves and patterns. Physicists provide the rationale for the existence of such energy fields and for understanding of resonancy as the "continuous change from lower frequency to higher frequency wave patterns" in human and environmental fields (Rogers, 1980b, p. 2).

The electrodynamic theory of life (Burr and Northrop, 1935) was used by Rogers as the link between physics and life processes in nursing. Rogers used the tenets of evolution theory to explain the increase in diversity, differentiation, complexity, and patterning in developing human and environmental behaviors. A unitary human being is always in the process of "becoming" rather than "being"; at any point, he is more than he has been because all his previous actions, experiences, interactions, and being are incorporated into his present being. A unitary human being is a homeodynamic being and is not homeostatic (Rogers, 1980c, 1992). The process is therefore evolutionary toward more complexity; and dynamic equilibrium, which characterizes adaptation theory, is not possible as a goal in life.

Rogers was influenced by the early Greek philosophers and modern theory and philosophy. Her writings drew on Burr and Northrop (1935), Chardin (1961), Polanyi (1958), and Lewin (1964), among others. In addition, she drew on her vast fiction reading, interest in classical music, and modern physics to describe her concept of nursing science. She was one of the few early thinkers in nursing who conceptualized nursing clients from a holistic perspective (Barnum, 1994).

Internal Dimensions

Rogers used the dialectic method of reasoning in developing her theory, due to the fact that higher level principles are subsumed under lower level concepts (Barnum, 1994). The theory is basically concatenated and has a hypothetical constructive beginning, evolving from synthesis of concepts from a number of fields, the core of which are a number of concepts that are central to nursing. These are unitary human being, unitary environment, energy field, open systems, patterns, pandimensionality, and human development. The relationships between concepts are still at a tentative stage.

Rogers' theory is a deductive theory that is monadic with several irreducible units, but it is macro in content and wide in scope as it purports to describe life processes that result from person–environment–energy fields interaction. The intent of the theory is to explain the continuous, evolving, but unpredictable patterns. It provides a framework to describe the life process of unitary human beings and could provide knowledge of order. The theory does not offer conceptual guidelines for knowledge of disorder or control. The concepts lead to description of patterns, rhythmicities, and symphonic harmony.

Theory Critique

The discipline of nursing deals with phenomena related to the life process of unitary human beings and their environments, which are expressed in health and illness. The discipline of nursing has science and art and nursing is a profession learned through education. The science of nursing is basic and it is the "organized body of abstract knowledge arrived at by scientific research and logical analysis" (Rogers, 1992, p. 28). The art of nursing, on the other hand, encompasses the innovative ways by which the science is used to enhance human beings' lives. "The aim of nursing is to assist people in achieving their maximum health potential . . . their maximum well-being within the capability of each person" (Rogers, 1970, pp. 86, 135). Rogers defined the goal of professional nursing as follows:

> Professional practice in nursing seeks to promote symphonic interaction between man and environment, to strengthen the conference and integrity of the human field,

> and to direct and redirect patterning of the human and environment fields for realization of maximum health potentials. (Rogers, 1970, p. 122)

She also proposed that the purpose of nursing "is to promote health and well being for all persons wherever they are" (Rogers, 1992, p. 28). A nurse using Rogers' theory works on mobilizing individual or family resources, heightening her integrity, and strengthening the human being–environment or family–environment relationships (Barrett, 1990a; Rogers, 1988).

The scope of Rogers' theory is broad and has the potential to encompass the phenomena of the domain of nursing. However, although it articulates the central phenomena, it does not define practice, nor does it attempt to do so. The theory appears too abstract; concepts—though defined theoretically—do not lend themselves readily to the practice arena or to measurable variables for research. Rogers never claimed her conceptualization to be a theory, and her thinking and ideas preceded all current attempts at theory building. This may be why she has not offered a systematic operationalization of her concepts for use in practice and research. Nevertheless, the notion of considering the individual as a whole and the focus of nursing on the human being–environment relationship is appealing to nursing and lends itself to a theory of human being–environment interaction.

Others have extended Rogers' theory and have postulated that the characteristics of a unitary human being could be related to needs and activities of daily living. Because unitary human beings can feel, exchange, be awake, move, choose, value, and relate, a group of nurses (theoreticians, clinicians, and researchers) have developed such a conception and delineated a number of nursing diagnoses according to these characteristics (Kim and Moritz, 1982) (Table 16-4).

Table 16-4 Characteristics of Unitary Human Being—Rogers

Factor I. Interaction	Factor II. Action
A. Exchanging	A. Valuing
1. Eating and drinking	1. Philosophical beliefs about health, human interactions, and spirituality
2. Eliminating	B. Choosing (human beings knowingly making choices—wise, unwise, or detrimental)
3. Breathing	1. Judgment and decision-making capacity regarding alternatives, consequences, commitments
4. Giving and receiving	C. Moving
B. Communicating	1. Mobility (rhythm and patterns)
1. Verbal	Factor III. Awareness
2. Nonverbal	A. Waking (sleep behavior, patterns, and quality
C. Relating	B. Feeling (as perceived and as manifested)
1. Spacing	C. Knowing (health knowledge, abstractions, motor skills)
2. Touching	
3. Eye contact	
4. Belonging	
5. Referencing	
6. Family response to patient illness	

Adapted from Lucy Field and Margaret Newman, Clinical application of the unitary man: Case study analysis. In Kim, M.J. and Moritz, D.A. (Eds.), (1982). Classification of nursing diagnosis: Proceedings of the third and fourth national conferences. New York: McGraw-Hill; copyright C.V. Mosby Co., St. Louis.

Diagnoses such as noncompliance (choosing), anxiety (feeling), respiratory dysfunction (exchanging), impairment of mobility (moving), spiritual concern (valuing), alternations in sleep/rest activity (waking), and alterations in patterns of sexuality (relating) have been defined in relation to a unitary human being (Kim and Moritz, 1982; Rossi and Krekeler, 1982, pp. 276–277).

Several writers have demonstrated some of the theory's utility in practice. Barrett (1990a) and Madrid and Winstead-Fry (1986) proposed a useful assessment framework derived from Rogers' focus on patterns. One component of this framework is living in the relative present, experiencing comfort with the past and present of the individual. Shared communication, a sense of rhythm (a flow in daily life), a connection to environment (a sense of place in a community), personal myth (a sense of self-identity), and system integrity (survival) are other components of the assessment framework. For each of the components, the authors offer a range of intervention options. Carboni (1995a) extended Rogers' ideas for practice and developed a theory of Rogerian nursing practice as an enfolding health as wholeness and harmony. In this theory, nurses and clients participate knowingly in patterning the human and environment fields and create health and wholeness.

Whelton (1979) synthesized Rogers' theory with nursing process theory in delivering care to patients with decreased cardiac input and impaired neurologic function. Others have demonstrated the theory's principles in therapeutic touch (Krieger, 1976) and in conceptualizing hyperactivity in children within the framework of synergism as being merely changes in a person's pattern of interaction with the environment (Blair, 1979). Rogers provided the potential for understanding aging and hyperactivity (1980a) by her theory. Minimal sleep needs of the hyperactive child are seen by Rogers as a response to increasing complexity and diversity of wave patterns and frequency of environmental fields; therefore, hyperactivity, if not viewed from unitary human being–environment interactions, tends to be labeled as a disease. Mason and Patterson (1990) used Rogers' theory to assess a problematic middle-aged man with 33 previous admissions to psychiatric hospitals; although they discussed some limitations such as their inability to use some holistic principles (such as touch), they concluded that the theory helped them break traditional practices and provided them with support to use visionary and innovative practices to help the patient.

Rogers' theory has inspired the development of assessment tools (Tettero, Jackson, and Wilson, 1993) and provided a framework to assess the perception and the meaning of passage of time and the need for diversional activities for the elderly (Biley, 1992).

Despite all these attempts at clinical operationalization and utilization, the general sentiment in practice, education, and administration remains the same: that this theory has application limitations. The potential is there in the theory, but the complex nature of its concepts and propositions, the esoteric concepts and level of abstraction, and the overlap between concepts due to lack of definition all render the use of Rogers' theory limited in practice. Not only is it difficult to operationalize and measure characteristics and actions of unitary human beings and energy fields to identify manifestations of patterns of energy fields, but one is also faced with the limitations of the existing English language in describing pandimensionality of a human being field and the influence of the tremendous acceleration of change on humanity (Rogers, 1980a). Rogers' approach, however, is more meaningful in the 1990s than it was in the previous three decades. It is more congruent with accelerating changes, fascination with outer space, acceptance of lack of predictability, and chaos theories.

External Components of Theory

A decade ago, Rogers' theory was an unknown; it was esoteric and not reflective of nursing. The changes in prevailing views of health, developments in physics, and the movement toward holism have facilitated nurses' acceptance to further explore her theory. The view that the discipline of nursing deals with unitary human beings who are in constant interaction with the environment has gained momentum and support particularly when it is equated erroneously with holism. There is indication that nursing practice is more positive about the potential of Rogers' theory (Garon, 1992; Rossi and Krekeler, 1982).

Each nurse–patient interaction is an interaction of energy fields that evolves into repatterning and reorganizing waves in the direction of increasing differentiation and diversity. Each encounter is unique; it moves forward and becomes more complex. Feelings, thoughts, experiences, and awareness of the nurse and patient and their environments blend together, each one emerging not totally the same as before. Repatterning is a new pattern evolving from a previous pattern that requires investigation into the "nature of field patterns and organization." These views are valued by nurses, consumers, and, indeed, more and more by other health professionals. Her work inspired many educators (Barrett, 1990b).

Theory Testing

Gill and Atwood (1981) attempted to use Rogers' theory as the basis for a study of wound healing in animals, but were legitimately criticized by Kim (1983) for reductionism, causality, and inappropriate use of the animal model. Others have successfully explained some of Rogers' propositions without resorting to reductionism or mechanistic approaches. For example, Rogers' proposition that unitary human beings/environments are dynamic fields of energy, always sending and receiving messages that change both the human and environment fields in complexity and diversity, has been tested and has received some support (Katz, 1971). Although Katz, a graduate of New York University, did not link her findings to Rogers' theory per se, her findings lend support to this proposition. Katz's experimental subjects, premature infants who were subjected to a patterned regimen of auditory stimulation from tape recordings of the maternal voice, achieved greater motor and tactile adaptive maturation.

Porter's (1972) findings support Katz's (1971) and Rogers' proposition that environmentally imposed motions speed up infant growth and development. Goldberg and Fitzpatrick (1980) hypothesized that movement therapy for institutionalized individuals, as a holistic nursing intervention derived from Rogerian theory, would improve psychological well-being as demonstrated in morale and in attitudes toward aging. The hypothesis was supported, lending further support to Rogers' theoretical propositions.

Heidt (1981), testing another intervention based on Rogerian premises, found that subjects who received nursing intervention through therapeutic touch had greater reduction in posttest anxiety scores than those who received it through casual or no touch.

Other studies reformulated and deduced a theorem regarding environmental disruption and sleep/wakefulness rhythms and tested it on a general population and a clinic population. More specifically, the theorem stated:

> Persons experiencing a deviation in the rhythmic relationship with their environment will manifest greater complexity and diversity in their sleep/wakefulness patterns than persons who are not experiencing a deviation in the rhythmic relationship with their environment. (Floyd, 1983, p. 43)

Although the findings demonstrated a significant difference in "increasing diversity" (total wakefulness time was greater for rotating shift workers than for nonrotating shift workers), there was minimal support for "increasing complexity" (rotating shift workers slept less than nonrotating shift workers). The study lends support to the theorem but raises some questions when the study used a clinical sample. Floyd's (1983) study represents an example of the potential innovation in testing Rogers' propositions and the significance of systematic study of propositions emanating from nursing theory.

Developmental stages and time orientation were the focuses of another study based on Rogerian theory that concluded that there is "support for the developmentally-based nature of specific dimensions of temporality" (Johnston, Fitzpatrick, and Donovan, 1982, p. 120). These studies, together with Newman's (1979, 1986) theory of health, are based on the interrelationships between time, space, consciousness, and movement and are fine extensions of Rogers' ideas.

Despite such progress, there are still major gaps in our methodology for unitary human beings/unitary environments and their energy fields (Butcher, 1993). Should such gaps in our present knowledge halt all research investigations using Rogers' theory? Is it possible to develop investigations accounting for all Rogers' premises and concepts with our present limited knowledge? The answer is "no" to both questions. As demonstrated previously, researchers who have been inspired by Rogers' theory and theoretical propositions have found innovative ways to test and support some theory propositions without adhering to or accounting for all assumptions and principles of the theory. For example, well-being in Goldberg and Fitzpatrick's (1980) study was measured in terms of psychological well-being rather than in terms of the greater developmental coherence that involves human being–environment energy fields, as Rogers would emphasize. There are indications of increasing congruency between her ideas and methods used for research, either because tools have been developed based on the theory assumptions such as the person–environment participation tool developed by Leddy (1995), or because creative processes of inquiry are proposed and developed (Carboni, 1995b). And as Winstead-Fry (personal communication, 1984) indicated, Rogers' students, colleagues, and others continue to work on developing congruent measures related to meditation, to measure development as defined by Rogers, and to engage in studies on creativity, differentiation, and parent/child interactions.

A valuable resource that contains comprehensive analyses of tests completed on Rogers' theory is edited by Malinski (1986). This compilation, in addition to a review of literature based on Rogers' theory, may indicate several conclusions about the theory, including:

- A world view is emerging in nursing that is congruent with Rogers' principles (Malinski, 1986).
- There are some universal questions about Rogers' world view (Meleis, 1988).
- Research work that uses Rogers' principles is increasing (Benonis, 1989; Quinn, 1989; Schodt, 1989).
- Existing methodological approaches are not entirely useful in investigating principles postulated in her theory (Moccia, 1985; Phillips, 1989; Smith, 1986, 1988), and therefore, "there is an essential need for methodological studies aimed at development, validation, and evaluation research tools and strategies for the unitary science framework" (Cowling, 1986, p. 74).
- There is a definite evaluation in the types of studies completed to test or further develop Rogers' principles (Clarke, 1986; Ference, 1986; Fitzpatrick, 1988).

Ference (1986) describes the mid-1960's studies, which are mainly doctoral dissertations, as studies of human development; in the 1970s the studies revolved around the principle of complementarity that was later relabeled integrality. Concurrently, several of Rogers' students studied body image in an attempt to explain human and environment fields. The variable of time dominated investigations in the mid-1970s, for example, Newman (1976, 1989) researched perception of time in relationship to gait tempo. According to Ference (1986, p. 38), "these studies helped future researchers to define the meaning of time in a space–time context."

According to Ference (1986), other studies during that period focused on locus of control, field independence, and differentiation. Several instruments unique to Rogers' theory have been developed. Two have been reported. These are the Human Field Motion Test (Ference, 1986) and the Human Field Power Test (Barrett, 1986).

Barrett (1990c) developed a measure of power as knowing participation in change. This measure has been used in many studies. For example, Caroselli (1995) demonstrated that among female nurse executives a weak relationship exists between power and feminism as measured by the "power as knowing participation in change" instrument. Observable manifestations of human patterning that Rogers (1986) describes as correlates were examined by Yarcheski and Mahon (1991) in a study comparing early, middle, and late adolescent boys and girls. The authors selected perceived field motion, human field rhythms, creativity, sentience, perception of time, and waking and sleeping periods. The findings, though not supporting the relationships proposed in Rogers' theory, suggest that age may be related to the correlates. This, according to the researchers, suggests some linearity that may have been deleted prematurely from Rogers' theory. Other researchers attempted to define and test the proposal of increasing frequency patterning in explaining the healing processes involved in recovery (Schneider, 1995) and patterns of perceived field motion and health status (Yarcheski and Mahon, 1995).

Smith (1995) compared patterns of power and spirituality in people who have survived polio and those who never had polio. Polio survivors show similar power and more spirituality than participants who did not have polio. This finding suggests that patterns of human field change were related to surviving polio. The study suggests that nurses' awareness of spirituality as a human potential may drive more attention to enhancing the different potentials of patients and they could facilitate the patients' ability to connect with other aspects of their energy fields. The investigators used Rogers' theory to drive the research questions and propose continuity to develop spirituality with this theory.

Another significant test of any theory is the extent to which it has stimulated theoretical published discourse. Rogers' theory inspired the development of other theories, such as Newman's theory of health (Newman, 1986). Others, particularly graduate students from Wayne State University, Case Western Reserve University, the University of Rochester, and New York University are engaged in researching propositions derived from Rogers' theory. Rogers' theory has been operationalized for educational settings. The curriculum of nursing at New York University is not the only one based on Rogers' theory. It has been used to develop curricula at Duquesne, College of Mount St. Vincent, and Fairleigh Dickinson University (P. Winstead-Fry, personal communication, 1984).

Rogers' theory is complex, is somewhat tautological (she acknowledges an overlap between concepts), and has an aura of coherent truth but with the reality of a challenge in operationalization. Although difficult for the American practitioner, it is understandable in the international arena. Its view of humanity and environment and the lack of separation between mind and body is congruent with the Eastern view, and it is expected that its circle of contagiousness will increase more rapidly than ever anticipated in the decade ahead. It is congruent with professional values in nursing and with the emerging perceptions of humanity.

REFERENCES

Barnum, B.J.S. (1994). *Nursing theory: Analysis, application, and evaluation* (4th ed.). Philadelphia: J.B. Lippincott.

Barrett, E.A. (1986). Investigation of the principle of helicy: The relationship of human field motion and power. In V.M. Malinski (Ed.), *Explorations on Martha Rogers' science of unitary human beings* (pp. 173–187). Norwalk, CT: Appleton-Century-Crofts.

Barrett, E.A. (1990a). Visions of Rogers' science-based nursing. In E.A. Barrett (Ed.), *Visions of Rogers' science-based nursing* (pp. 31–44). New York: National League for Nursing.

Barrett, E.A. (1990b). The continuing revolution of Rogers' science-based nursing education. In E.A. Barrett (Ed.), *Visions of Rogers' science-based nursing* (pp. 303–317). New York: National League for Nursing.

Barrett, E.A. (1990c). A measure of power as knowing participation in change. In O.L. Strickland and C.F. Waltz (Eds.), *Measurement in nursing outcomes* (pp. 159–175). New York: Springer.

Benonis, B.C. (1989). The lived experience of recovering from addiction: A phenomenological study. *Nursing Science Quarterly*, 2(1), 37–43.

Bertalanffy, L. von (1968). *General systems theory: Foundations, development, application.* New York: George Braziller.

Biley, F.C. (1992). The perception of time as a factor in Rogers' science of unitary human beings: A literature review. *Journal of Advanced Nursing*, 17(9), 1141–1145.

Blair, C. (1979). Hyperactivity in children: Viewed within the framework of synergistic man. *Nursing Forum*, 18, 293–303.

Burr, H.S. and Northrop, F.S.C. (1935). The electro-dynamic theory of life. *The Quarterly Review of Biology*, 10, 322–333.

Butcher, H.K. (1993). Kaleidoscoping in life's turbulence: From Seurat's art to Rogers' nursing science. In M.E. Parker (Ed.), *Patterns of nursing theories in practice* (pp. 183–198). New York: National League for Nursing.

Carboni, J.T. (1995a). Enfolding health-as-wholeness-and-harmony: A theory of Rogerian nursing practice. *Nursing Science Quarterly*, 8(2), 71–78.

Carboni, J.T. (1995b). The Rogerian process of inquiry. *Nursing Science Quarterly*, 8(1), 22–37.

Caroselli, C. (1995). Power and feminism: A nursing perspective. *Nursing Science Quarterly*, 8(3), 115–119.

Chardin, T. (1961). *The phenomenon of man.* New York: Harper Torchbooks.

Clarke, P.N. (1986). Theoretical and measurement issues in the study of field phenomena. *Advances in Nursing Science*, 9(1), 29–39.

Cowling, W.R. (1986). The science of unitary human beings: Theoretical issues, methodological challenges, and research realities. In V. Malinski (Ed.), *Explorations on Martha Rogers' science of unitary human beings.* Norwalk, CT: Appleton-Century-Crofts.

Ference, H. (1986). The re onship of time experience, creativity traits, differenti n, and human field motion. In V. Malinski (Ed.), E rations on Martha Rogers' science of unitary hu beings. Norwalk, CT: Appleton-Century-Crofts.

Fitzpatrick, J. (198 eory based on Rogers' conceptual model. *Journal ontological Nursing*, 14(9), 14–16.

Floyd, J.A. (198 earch using Rogers' conceptual system: Develo of a testable theorem. *Advances in Nursing Sc* 2), 37–48.

Garon, M. (ontributions of Martha Rogers to the develop nursing knowledge. *Nursing Outlook*, 40(2),

Gill, B.P wood, J.R. (1981). Reciprocity and helicy use TT and wound healing. *Nursing Research*, 30(

and Fitzpatrick, J.J. (1980). Movement ther aged. *Nursing Research*, 29(6), 339–346.

Go 1). Effect of therapeutic touch on anxiety level ized patients. *Nursing Research* 30(1), 32–37.

K. (1989). Martha E. Rogers: A life history. *Nursing Science Quarterly*, 2(2), 63–73.

R.L., Fitzpatrick, J.J., and Donovan, M.J. (1982). opmental stage: Relationship to temporal dimen- [Abstract]. *Nursing Research*, 31(2), 120.

(1971). Auditory stimulation and developmental avior of the premature infant. *Nursing Research*, 20(3), –201.

, H.S. (1983). Use of Rogers' conceptual system in esearch: Comments. *Nursing Research*, 32(2), 89–91.

n, M.J. and Moritz, D.A. (Eds.). (1982). *Classification of nursing diagnosis: Proceedings of the third and fourth national conference.* New York: McGraw-Hill.

Krieger, D. (1976). Healing by the laying on of hands as a facilitator of bioenergetic change: The response of in vivo human hemoglobin. *International Journal of Psychoenergetic Systems*, 1, 121–129.

Leddy, S.K. (1995). Measuring mutual process: Development and psychometric testing of the Person-Environment Participation Scale. *Visions: The Journal of Rogerian Nursing Science*, 3(1), 20–31.

Lewin, K. (1964). *Field theory in the social sciences.* New York: Harper Torchbooks.

Madrid, M. and Winstead-Fry, P. (1986). Rogers' conceptual model. In P. Winstead-Fry (Ed.), *Case studies in nursing theory.* New York: National League for Nursing.

Malinski, V. (1986). *Explorations on Martha Rogers' science of unitary human beings.* Norwalk, CT: Appleton-Century-Crofts.

Mason, T. and Patterson, R. (1990). A critical review of the use of Rogers' model within a special hospital: A single case study. *Journal of Advanced Nursing*, 15(2), 130–141.

Meleis, A.I. (1988). Book reviews (Malinski, V.M. [1986] *Explorations on Martha Rogers' science of unitary human beings*). *Research in Nursing and Health*, 11, 59–63.

Moccia, P. (1985). A further investigation of dialectical thinking as a means of understanding systems-in-development: Relevance to Rogers' principles [Commentary]. *Advances in Nursing Science*, 7(4), 33–38.

Newman, M.A. (1976). Movement, tempo, and the experience of time. *Nursing Research*, 25(4), 273–279.

Newman, M.A. (1979). *Theory development in nursing.* Philadelphia: F.A. Davis.

Newman, M.A. (1986). *Health as expanding consciousness.* St. Louis: C.V. Mosby.

Newman, M.A. (1989). The spirit of nursing. *Holistic Nursing Practice*, 3(3), 1–6.

Phillips, J.R. (1989). Science of unitary human being: Changing research perspective. *Nursing Science Quarterly*. 2(2), 57–60.

Polanyi, M. (1958). *Personal knowledge.* Chicago: University of Chicago Press.

Porter, L.S. (1972). The impact of physical-physiological activity on infant growth and development. *Nursing Research*, 21(3), 210–219.

Quinn, J.F. (1989). Therapeutic touch as energy exchange: Replication and extension. *Nursing Science Quarterly*, 2(2), 74–78.

Rogers, M.E. (1970). *An introduction to the theoretical basis of nursing.* Philadelphia: F.A. Davis.

Rogers, M.E. (1980a). Nursing: A science of unitary man. In J.P. Riehl and C. Roy (Eds.), *Conceptual models for nursing practice* (2nd ed.). New York: Appleton-Century-Crofts.

Rogers, M.E. (1980b). The science of unitary man [Audiotapes]. New York: Media for Nursing.

Rogers, M.E. (1980c, December). Science of unitary man: A paradigm for nursing. Paper presented at the International Congress on Applied Systems Research and Cybernetics, Acapulco, Mexico.

Rogers, M.E. (1983a). Science of unitary human being: A paradigm for nursing. In I.W. Clements and F.B. Roberts (Eds.), *Family health: A theoretical approach to nursing care.* New York: John Wiley & Sons.

Rogers, M.E. (1983b, June). Nursing science: A science of unitary human beings. Paper presented at the First National Rogerian Conference, New York University.

Rogers, M.E. (1985). A paradigm for nursing. In R. Wood and J. Kekahbah (Eds.), *Examining the cultural implications of Martha E. Rogers' science of unitary human beings.* Lecampton, KS: Wood-Kekahbah Associates.

Rogers, M.E. (1986). Science of unitary human beings. In V. Malinski (Ed.), *Explorations on Martha Rogers' science of unitary human beings.* Norwalk, CT: Appleton-Century-Crofts.

Rogers, M.E. (1987). Rogers' science of unitary human beings. In R.R. Parse (Ed.), *Nursing science: Major paradigms, theories, and critiques.* Philadelphia: W.B. Saunders.

Rogers, M.E. (1988). Nursing science and art: A perspective. *Nursing Science Quarterly*, 1(3), 99–102.

Rogers, M.E. (1992). Nursing science and the space age. *Nursing Science Quarterly*, 5(1), 27–34.

Rossi, L. and Krekeler, K. (1982). Small-group reactions to the theoretical framework "unitary man" (1980). In M.J. Kim and D.A. Moritz (Eds.). *Classification of nursing diagnosis: Proceedings of the third and fourth national conference.* New York: McGraw-Hill.

Schneider, P.E. (1995). Focusing awareness: The process of extraordinary healing from a Rogerian perspective. *Visions: The Journal of Rogerian Nursing Science*, 3(1), 32–43.

Schodt, C.M. (1989). Parental-fetal attachment and couvade: A study of patterns of human-environment integrality. *Nursing Science Quarterly*, 2(2), 88–97.

Smith, D.W. (1995). Power and spirituality in polio survivors: A study based on Rogers' science. *Nursing Science Quarterly*, 8(3), 133–139.

Smith, M.J. (1986). Human-environment process: A test of Rogers' principle of integrality. *Advances in Nursing Science*, 9(1), 21–28.

Smith, M.J. (1988). Testing propositions derived from Rogers' conceptual system. *Nursing Science Quarterly*, 1(2), 60–67.

Tettero, I., Jackson, S. and Wilson, S. (1993). Theory to practice: Developing a Rogerian-based assessment tool. *Journal of Advanced Nursing*, 18(5), [illegible]–782.

Whelton, B.J. (1979). An operationalization of M. Rogers' theory throughout the nursing process. *International Journal of Nursing Studies*, 16, 7–20.

Yarcheski, A. and Mahon, N.E. (1991). An empirical test of Rogers' original and revised theory of correlates in adolescents. *Research in Nursing and Health*, 14, 447–455.

Yarcheski, A. and Mahon, N.E. (1995). Rogers' pattern manifestations and health in adolescents. *Western Journal of Nursing Research*, 17(4), 383–397.

CHAPTER 17

On Interactions

Several nurse theorists addressed nursing as a process of interaction. Some, such as Ida Orlando, developed the focus of the nursing process in nursing. I selected the following theorists to represent the central domain concepts related to interaction: Imogene King, Ida Orlando (Pelletier), Josephine G. Paterson and Loretta T. Zderad, Joyce Travelbee, and Ernestine Wiedenbach. The theories of Orlando, Travelbee, and Wiedenbach may also be used as the frameworks to describe and explain significant questions related to the nursing process.

Imogene King—A Theory of Goal Attainment

Theory Description

King's theory evolved in the mid-1960s, when she was raising questions about the role of theory in nursing practice and how nurses make decisions in their daily practice. King was also attempting to describe the essence of nursing and the interactional patterns and goals that govern the nurse–patient relationship. Like other nurse theorists of her generation, she asked questions as an attempt to explain what nursing is (King, 1990a). The development of her convictions and conceptualization progressed from recommending that nursing could be provided through a framework that contains a synthesis of ideas (a frame of reference that she entitled, in 1971, "Toward a Theory for Nursing") to the development of a theory that prompted the title to shift to "A Theory for Nursing" in 1981. In a curious way, the difference between the first tentative title and the second is analogous to nursing's tentativeness about theory in the 1970s and the determination to theorize in the 1980s. The difference between King's two books can be found in the last chapter of the second book, where she articulated her theory "for" nursing. Her theory is that nursing is a process that is interactional in nature; these interactions lead to transactions resulting in goal attainment (King, 1990a, 1992a).

At the beginning of the 1990s, King also entitled her work, "general systems framework" as well as "theory of goal attainment" (King, 1992a, 1992b, 1996a, 1996b). King provided nursing with four sets of concepts as part of her conceptual framework for nursing (King, 1988a). These concepts are central to the field of nursing and provide the basis on which she developed a theory of goal attainment, beginning with an assumption that nurses as human beings interact with patients as human beings, and both are open systems who also interact with the environment. Therefore, the personal systems (nurse and patient) interact with each other in an interpersonal system and with the environment that she called the social system (society). The relationships between these systems led to the development of the theory of goal attainment, with a distinct set of concepts, some of which were derived from the conceptual framework. Other theories may evolve from the conceptual framework. To understand the theory fully, it should be read in conjunction with the conceptual framework.

The theory deals with the central questions of interaction between nurses and clients (King, 1996b). King considered questions related to the nature of the process of interaction that lead to the achievement of goals and the significance of mutual goal setting in achieving nursing care goals. The theory evolved from several explicit assumptions (Table 17-1). These assumptions are congruent with contemporary and future-oriented views that nursing holds and aspires to maintain. They speak to the significance of patient involvement in the care as well as in the decision-making process, the importance of collaboration, and the humanity of the nurse–patient encounter.

It is important to note, too, that King's assumptions encompass the nurse's perceptions, goals, needs, and values, and not only the patients' and these are expected to influence the interaction process and, indeed, the outcomes. Although King designated the nurse as a central concept in nursing theory, she did not go as far as Paterson and Zderad in focusing on the significance of the consideration of the continuous growth of the nurse in every interaction. The theory assumptions explicitly address the rationality of human beings and proceed to develop consistent concepts related to

Table 17-1 ***Assumptions—King***

EXPLICIT ASSUMPTIONS

- The central focus of nursing is the interaction of human beings and environment, with the goal being health for human beings (King, 1982, p. 143).
- Individuals are social, sentient, rational, reacting, perceiving, controlling, purposeful, action-oriented, and time-oriented beings (King, 1981, p. 143).
- The interaction process is influenced by perceptions, goals, needs, and values of both the client and the nurse (1981, 92).
- Human beings as patients have rights to obtain information, to participate in decisions that may influence their life, health, and community services, and to accept or reject care (1981).
- It is the responsibility of health care members to inform individuals of all aspects of health care to help them in making "informed decisions" (1981).
- Incongruities may exist between the goals of health caregivers and recipients. Persons have the right to either accept or reject any aspect of health care (1981, pp. 143–144).

IMPLICIT ASSUMPTIONS

- Patients want to participate actively in the care process.
- Patients are conscious, active, and cognitively capable to participate in decision making (Austin and Champion, 1983, p. 56).

clients who can perceive, interpret, and solve problems. Austin and Champion (1983) argued that, as such, the theory is not useful to some situations in nursing (eg, when patients are comatose or psychotic).

There are inconsistencies in the different lists of concepts provided by King (Table 17-2). In one instance, she listed human being, environment, health, and society as the abstract concepts. She also identified personal, interpersonal, and social systems as the major concepts (1981, p. 142). She defined interaction, perception, communication, transaction, role, stress, growth and development, time, and space as they represent the theory of goal attainment. Although King clarified the relationship between the latter set of concepts in the interpersonal system, it is not clear how these "major concepts in the theory" relate to human beings, environment, health, and society (King, 1988a). Perception appears to be a central concept in her theory (Bunting, 1988).

King offered, in the conceptual framework, almost every concept that nurses may have historically used in nursing care (see Table 17-2). It is not entirely clear how the goal attainment theory evolved from the myriad concepts that appear in the conceptual

Table 17-2 ***Concepts: A Conceptual Framework for Nursing—King***

PERSONAL SYSTEMS	
Perception	Growth and development
Self	Time
Body image	Space
INTERPERSONAL SYSTEMS	
Role	Transactions
Human interaction	Stress
Communication	Coping
SOCIAL SYSTEMS	
Organization	Decision making
Power, authority, status	Control
Goal attainment	
CONCEPTS: A THEORY OF GOAL ATTAINMENT	
Interaction	Time
Perception	Space
Communication	Goal attainment
Transaction	Effective nursing care
Role	Appropriate information
Stress	Satisfaction
Growth and development	
CONCEPTS: A THEORY OF ADMINISTRATION	
Organization	Decision making
Power	Perception
Authority	Communication
Status	Interaction
Role	Transaction
Control	

framework. In the goal attainment theory, she restricted concepts to the interaction system, central to the nursing act. Most of her concepts are derived except for goal attainment, health transaction, effective nursing, appropriate information, and satisfaction. Although the derived concepts are defined conceptually and have the potential for operational definition, they have not been delineated as central concepts, nor were they defined theoretically or operationally. However, the theory purports to have, as a goal, nurse–patient interactions.

Other concepts not defined are satisfaction and effective nursing care, and although these are seemingly central to patient outcomes, they are neither conceptually nor operationally defined. To attain goals, appropriate information should be given; what is "appropriate," what is considered "information," and who decides what is appropriate or information are only a few of the questions that point out the lack of theoretical definitions and lack of boundaries between concepts (Table 17-3), and incongruence between assumptions, concepts, and statements (Uys, 1987).

Incompleteness and inconsistency are evident in how King views health. Health is defined in terms of ability to function in a social role, but as Magan (1987) indicated, ways by which the levels and quality of that functioning could be assessed are not described. Explication of health terms of morbidity and mortality data and accidents is more congruent with a disease orientation than a role-functioning orientation. King's views of health and illness are also problematic. As Magan puts it:

> The difficulty with a consistent understanding of health in King's framework is further complicated by her assertion that health and disease do not constitute polarities, while she also maintained that illness is an interference or disturbance in health. (Magan, 1987, p. 119)

The inconsistencies in King's definition of health are manifest in viewing health and illness as nonpolar and not dichotomies and illness as an interference or disturbance, and at the same time viewing health in terms of a dynamic life experience.

King offers strategies to measure health (King, 1988b) and examples of how her theory can be tested through a set of propositions that link perceptions, transactions, goal attainment, satisfaction, and effective nursing care. Propositions are relative and tend to be deterministic (Zetterberg, 1963). They are based on a cause-and-effect approach and are designed for prediction, not description. Propositions link some of the defined concepts (transactions, interactions, role performance), but they also link the undefined concepts.

Theory Analysis

The Theorist

Imogene King is well known for more than her theory; she is one of the pioneers who promoted a theoretical base for nursing (King 1964, 1975, 1976). She is, like a number of other theorists, a graduate (EdD, 1961) of Teachers College of Columbia University. In 1945, she had graduated from St. John's Hospital School of Nursing in St. Louis and received a bachelor's degree in nursing education in 1948 and a master of science in nursing in 1957. She completed a postdoctoral study in systems research, advanced statistics, research design, and computers (King, 1986a).

Table 17-3 Definition of Domain Concepts—King

Nursing	"A process of human interaction between nurse and client whereby each perceives the other in the situation and, through communication, they set goals, explore means, and agree on means to achieve goals" (King, 1981, p. 144), "and their actions indicate movement toward goal achievement" (1987, p. 113). "A process of action, reaction, interaction and transaction" (1971, p. 89 and 1981, p. 2). Nursing services are called on when individuals cannot function in their roles.
Goal of nursing	"To help individuals to maintain their health so they can function in their roles" (1981, p. 3). "To help individuals to attain and restore health or die in dignity" (1981, p. 13). The goal of nursing is then to maintain, restore, and promote health (92).
Health	"A dynamic life experience of a human being, which implies continuous adjustment to stressors in the internal and external environment through optimum use of one's resources to achieve maximum potential for daily living" (1981, p. 5 and 1983, p. 186). Ability to function in social role. Process of growth and development (King, 1990b, 1992).
Environment	The internal environment of human beings transforms energy to enable them to adjust to continuous external environmental changes (1981, p. 5). The external environment is the formal and informal organization. "A social system is defined as an organized boundary system of social roles, behaviors, and practices developed to maintain values and the mechanisms to regulate practice and rules" (1981, p. 115). The nurse is part of the patient's environment.
Human being	Rational, sentient, social being, perceiving, thinking, feeling, able to choose between alternative actions, able to set goals, to select means toward goals, to make decisions, and to have a symbolic way of communicating thoughts, actions, customs, and beliefs. Is time-oriented and reacting. Reactions are based on perceptions, expectations, and needs (1981, p. 19).
Nursing client	A unique, total, open system with perception, self, body image, time, space, growth, and development throughout the life span and with experiences of changes in structure and function of body influencing perception of self (1981, pp. 19–20). Person as open system exhibits permeable boundaries permitting an exchange of matter, energy, and information (1981, p. 69). A person who cannot perform daily activities and cannot carry the responsibilities of their roles (1976).
Nursing problem	Inability to meet needs for daily living (1981, p. 5). Inability to function in their roles (1981, p. 3). The central problem is nonmutual goal setting and lack of agreement on goals and means leading to unattained goals (1981, p. 144). "Felt needs" as perceived by patient or real needs as perceived by nurse (1968, p. 29).
Nursing process	A focal concept in King's theory. The goal of nursing is to help patients attain their goals. The mechanism for that is the nursing process. Through this process, nurses interact purposefully with clients (1981, p. 176). The purpose is information sharing, setting of mutual goals, participation in decisions about goals and means, implementing plans and evaluations.
Nurse–patient relations	"A process of perception and communication between person and environment and between person and person, represented by verbal and nonverbal behaviors that are goal-oriented" (1981, p. 145). Variables affecting interactions are knowledge, needs, goals, past experiences, and perceptions of nurse and patient. The interaction process also includes reaction and transaction (1981, p. 145).
Nursing therapeutics	Transactions: informing, sharing, setting of mutual goals, participation in decisions about goals and means (1981, p. 176). Goal-oriented nursing record (1983, pp. 183–186).

A clinician, an administrator, but primarily an educator, King is currently enjoying retirement after having been a professor at the College of Nursing, University of South Florida at Tampa. She has been dean of the School of Nursing at Ohio State University, Columbus, and professor of nursing at Loyola University in Chicago. Besides being an author, she is an effective speaker whose joy in presenting and describing her theory are readily apparent to her audiences.

Paradigmatic Origins

King used the language of system theory in the introduction of her ideas. Fawcett classified her as a system theorist (1995, p. 117); she classifies her ideas as emerging from systems theory (King 1990a), and George classified her as an adaptation theorist (1980, p. 186). Her conceptual framework evolves from all paradigms that have been used in nursing, for example, the developmental paradigm (growth and development), systems (structural–functional view of role, open systems, social systems, energy), adaptation (continuous adjustment to stressors), psychoanalytical (self), and stress (energy response to environment). The theory of goal attainment derives a great deal from symbolic interactionism, and what King offers helps in understanding the nursing process and the process of interaction, and therefore prompts a classification of her theory as an interactionist theory.

Although King personally stated that she never used the symbolic interactionist school of thought (Fawcett, 1989, p. 116), the influence of interactionism is marked. Several indications of parallelism between King's theory and symbolic interactionism are the descriptions of a person as a social being, actor, and reactor, who is constantly structuring and restructuring his perception of the world, thereby communicating through symbols. Nurse–patient interactions occur with the perpetual repertoire of both. Present meaning of any situation and perceptions of time of both nurse and patient are significant to the interaction (King, 1981, p. 148). In addition, King's use of roles (though more congruent with a structural–functional approach) and the personal element perception and interpretation are also indications of an interactionist approach. King recognized that a functionalist view of role is related to the study of social systems, but . . .

> [t]he interactionist view of role is basic to understanding individuals in organizations when role is thought of as a relationship with another person or group of individuals, it is related to interpersonal systems. . . . The interactionist view relates to social interaction. (1981, p. 90)

Therefore, the entire focus of theory and the central question around process, interaction, and goal attainment make it more congruent with a symbolic interactionist approach. King herself asserts that systems theory represents the philosophical basis of her theory (King, 1990a). However, whether or not the refinement of the theory may be more enhanced if the backdrop is interaction rather than the inconsistent and mixed use of both system and interaction paradigms, is a question that continues to beg an answer (Burney, 1992). Finally, both the paradigmatic origin and the theory suffer from the limitation of viewing a person as a social being rather than a biopsychosocial being.

Internal Dimensions

The microtheory of goal attainment was developed from a field approach around concepts rather than propositions and is therefore concatenated in structure. It is a mental image, with a constructive beginning deduced from a conceptual framework whose concepts were also deduced from other paradigms. Its scope is limited to the process of interaction, focusing on perceptions of clients for the purpose of goal attainment. It deals with interactions of one nurse with one patient. Despite the fact that King extensively discusses the social system, her theory evolving from the interpersonal system is limited to nurse–patient interactions, as it ought to be. She later expanded it to incorporate the family and their perceptions (King, 1983a, 1983b, 1990b).

The microtheory of goal attainment purports to predict processes inherent in goal attainment and provides descriptions of the concepts and properties of the interpersonal system. The theory would be classified as providing a description of the nursing process; it mainly explains how and when to use transactions to achieve mutually agreed-on goals. It is a single-domain theory with an average abstraction. King developed her theory using a logical method of development. The parts of the interactional system (interaction, transaction) lead to goal attainment.

Theory Critique

Examples of the utility of King's theory for practice, research, education, and administration are numerous in the literature. Theory development progressed from a conceptual framework variety of unrelated concepts to a theory of nursing in the interpersonal system. King herself completed one research project and operationalized the theory for practice. Propositions emanating from the theory are presented in Table 17-4.

Table 17-4 ***Propositions—King***

1. If perceptual accuracy is present in nurse–patient interactions, transactions will occur.
2. If nurse and patient transact, goals will be attained.
3. If goals are attained, satisfactions will occur.
4. If goals are attained, effective nursing will occur.
5. If transactions are made in nurse–patient interactions, growth and development will be enhanced.
6. If role expectation and role performance, as perceived by nurse and patients, are congruent, transactions will occur.
7. If role conflict is experienced by nurse or patient or both, stress in nurse–patient interactions will occur.
8. If nurses with special knowledge and skills communicate appropriate information to patients, mutual goal setting and goal attainment will occur.
9. Knowledge of oneself will bring about a helping relationship with patients.
10. Accurate perceptions of time and space in nurse–patient interactions lead to transactions.

From King, I. M. (1981). A theory for nursing: Systems, concepts, process (p. 149). New York: John Wiley & Sons, and King, I. M. (1986a). King's theory of goal attainment. In P. Winstead-Fry (Ed.), Case studies in nursing theory. New York: National League for Nursing.

King's theory is parsimonious, with distinct concepts and limited relationships, but teleological because interaction is defined by interaction and transaction (King, 1981, p. 145). Goal attainment appears to be a process of transaction toward effective nursing care and is a product that is equated with effective nursing care and satisfaction (King, 1981, pp. 147 and 153).

Considering that interaction has emerged as one of the central concepts in nursing, King's contribution is substantial to nursing knowledge (King, 1987b). The theory's clarity is enhanced when considered as a theory to describe and answer questions related to nurse–patient interactions for the purpose of setting goals. The nursing care process has been conceived as a process involving assessment, diagnosis, intervention, and evaluation (King, 1986a). The process depends on two significant clinical tools: observation and interaction.

King offers the nursing profession a description of the properties of interaction and one of its goals—attainment of mutually agreed-on goals. King also offers a unique variation of the nursing process. The goal-oriented nursing record (GONR), developed as a tool analogous to the problem-oriented medical record developed by Weed (1969), includes both "process and outcomes in nursing situations" and a record of the goals, the means to achieve those agreed-on goals, and the process used to achieve them. It consists of five components: a data base, a problem list, a goal list, a plan, and progress notes (King, 1981, pp. 164–165).

The GONR is similar to the nursing process used by other theorists, but it offers a more dynamic dimension that addresses the process and not only the goals. GONR has the potential of offering organized nursing care, and it could facilitate nursing audits, enhance abilities in making nursing diagnoses, increase focus on patients' participation, and validate perceptions of patients during the process (King, 1981, p. 172). King expanded her theory to incorporate the family as a client in 1983 (Gonot, 1983, 1986).

The numerous examples of use of King's theory in clinical practice (Smith, 1988) include:

- An elderly patient with a cerebral vascular accident (King, 1983a)
- A patient with renal disease (King, 1984)
- Caring for families (King, 1983b)
- A problem-solving tool to facilitate the development of a healthy work environment and to decrease the incidence of diseases of the computer age such as carpal tunnel syndrome (Norgan, Ettipio, and Lasome, 1995)
- Providing community health nursing care (Asay and Ossler, 1984; Sowell and Lowenstein, 1994)
- Providing psychiatric care (Gonot, 1983)
- Caring for comatose patients (King, 1986a)
- Caring for adults with diabetes (Husband, 1988)
- As a framework for managed care (Hampton, 1994)

The theory was extended for testing under King's guidelines in Japan, Sweden, and the United States (Frey, Rooke, Sieloff, Messmer, and Kameoka, 1995) providing a forward-looking approach to collaboration, which is a hallmark for knowledge development in the future (Meleis, 1985). Woods (1994) used the theory to demonstrate how mutual identification and achievement of goals were facilitated between nurses and a group of elderly people with chronic health problems. The theory has been used with attention to new evolving concepts such as quality of care (Sowell and Lowenstein, 1994) and quality of life (King, 1994). The theory has been used to develop a framework for neonatal care that is built less on medical models and medicalization and more on a process of interaction between parents and nurses (Norris and Hoyer, 1993). Such examples of the theory–practice link support its utility and potential in transcending the boundaries of time, geography, and specializations; they also demonstrate that the theory has been used innovatively and with a trend-setting approach.

Despite these examples of the clinical utility of the theory, it appears to be more useful for assessing active, autonomous, collaborative, and individual (fewer examples of group or aggregate utility) relationships with nurses. It is more useful for long-term nurse–patient relationships to evaluate "satisfaction, goal attainment, and effective nursing care." The utility of GONR for care of infants, children, comatose patients, some psychiatric patients, dementia patients, or some mentally retarded patients is still in question (Austin and Champion, 1983; Barnum, 1994). King's theory is also limited in use to only some health care settings.

> The theory would have limited application in settings where clients are unable to interact competently. In addition, it is not clear how the theory could be utilized with groups. Utilizing transactions with groups of individuals who had different goals is not addressed by King. (Austin and Champion, 1983, p. 60)

There are a number of other limitations to clinical utility. The theory does not give explicit guidelines for assessment, diagnosis, or intervention. The theoretical boundaries to help a practitioner in assessing problems and potential problems and in deciding on clinical therapeutics are not identified. It analyzes problems but does not offer guidelines for interventions. The specificity to other nursing phenomena is lacking. Interaction is a process in all helping relationships; its uniqueness to nursing stems from its relationship to other phenomena. This is lacking in King's theory. Carter and Dufour (1994) disagree with these criticisms and develop compelling arguments for the theory's flexibility and utility.

Nursing administration could use the theory in developing a recording system for nursing care plans with refinement and modifications related to patient care outcomes. King promised that, if nurses use goal attainment theory and GONR to enhance accurate documentation and recording of goals identified and attained in interactions, effective nursing care could be measured (King, 1981, p. 155, 1989, pp. 42–45). King discussed the development of a theory of administration following the same principles used in developing a theory of goal attainment. King believed that when such theory is communicated in the literature, it will be useful for both nursing science administration and nursing education administration. Elberson (1989) presented a description of the utility of King's theory in nursing administration, and Byrne-Coker and Schreiber (1990) provided an analysis of effective use of the theory as a framework for nursing practice in an agency.

King's theory is amenable to use in nursing education as a basis for learning, one significant phase and component of the nursing process. Evidence suggests that the theory provides both a conceptual framework for curricula (Daubenmire and King, 1973; King, 1978, 1996c) and is used to guide a curriculum in continuing education (Brown and Lee, 1980). King provided guidelines for implementation of her theory in an educational setting (1968, p. 30), and in 1986, she published a book on curriculum development in which she carefully demonstrated how her theory could be used as a framework for curricula (King, 1986b). She also summarized the potential utility of theory in curricula (Gulitz and King, 1988; King, 1988a). King's theory has been used as a conceptual framework for a baccalaureate program at Ohio State University School of Nursing in Columbus (Daubenmire and King, 1973; King 1986b) and in models for improved patient care (Rooke, 1995). Other schools also used her theory or components of it as a framework (Fawcett, 1995).

Diagrams depicting relationships between central concepts of the theory, central concepts in nursing, and major propositions would have enhanced the clarity of the theory and would have pointed out the gaps in linkages.

External Components of Theory

The theory is congruent with values and beliefs about nursing, humanity, autonomy, patient advocacy, self-reliance, and planning that are espoused by Western societies, especially the United States, pertaining to the conscious, self-directed patient. The focus of the theory on mutual goal setting and attainment, on interacting with individuals, and on helping individuals become healthy enough to function in roles is congruent with Western philosophy and mores of pragmatism and usefulness of adult members of society. Many other societies that consider patients helpless, that espouse the sick role as abandonment of social roles and responsibilities, and that support the rights of patients to be sheltered from prognosis and health care goals (such as some Middle Eastern cultures) would consider this theory culturally limited (Meleis and Jones, 1983). Patients in these societies prefer to relinquish all decisions and goal setting to the expertise of the health care professionals.

Theory Testing

King outlined hypotheses for testing her theoretical propositions (King, 1987a) and proposed future studies to test these hypotheses (King, 1986a; Uys, 1987). Fawcett (1995) reports that in February 1988 a conference held at the University of South Florida College of Nursing focused on research designed to test King's theory. As Fawcett indicates, this is a reflection of a growing body of knowledge related to King. King also developed a criterion-referenced instrument designed to assess physical and behavioral functional abilities, goal setting with clients, and goal attainment (King, 1986a).

Several studies testing various properties derived from King's theory are reported in the literature. Brower (1981) described nurses' attitudes toward the elderly; Rosendahl and Ross (1982) described the relationship between attending behaviors on mental status; and Frey (1989) described the development and initial testing of parent support, child support, family health, and child health in families with insulin-dependent diabetes mellitus. Frey used King's theory as the basis for defining concepts, selecting indicators, and developing propositions for testing. The finding lends support to the relationship between interaction and health as proposed by King. The researcher questions the availability of appropriate instruments to use in testing King's theory (Frey, 1989, p. 146). There are also indications of the international utility of King's theory in research (Rooke and Norberg, 1988). The theory was used to describe awareness and perceptions of prostate and testicular cancers and an intervention to enhance such awareness (Martin, 1990). It was tested in terms of its cultural relevance by Frey, Rooke, Sieloff, Messmer, and Kameoka (1995) and Rooda (1992). The theory was used as a framework for testing postoperative recovery and satisfaction of patients (Hanucharurnkui and Vinya-nguag, 1991).

King also tested her theory and reported the results in her 1981 book. The study was designed to answer three questions:

1. What elements in nurse–patient interactions lead to transactions?
2. What are the relationships between the elements in the interactions that lead to transactions?
3. What are the essential variables in nurse–patient interactions that result in transactions? (King, 1981, p. 151)

The results of this descriptive study supported the components of the interpersonal system and lent construct validity. The study limitations are numerous, but the study could be considered a pilot for further research. The study was based on data generated by nonparticipant observations of verbal and nonverbal behaviors of nurses and patients. The sample consisted of 17 cases. The results of this descriptive study support the components of the interpersonal system and provide construct validity. Specifically, King's study indicated that interaction was verbal and nonverbal and that nurse–patient interactions lead to transactions and identification of problems, concerns, or disturbances in the patient's environment. Variables that helped in the achievement of goals were "accurate perceptions of nurse and patient, adequate communication, and mutual goal setting" (King, 1981, p. 155). Despite several limitations of the study (sample size, biases of the researchers, limited analysis) it is a pilot study that indicates the potential testability of the theory (King, 1996b).

Ida Orlando

Theory Description

In the mid to late 1950s, the Yale School of Nursing shifted from undergraduate to graduate education and integrated psychiatric concepts into the entire curriculum. Orlando's theory grew out of processes inherent in these curricular changes and out of dissatisfaction with the possibility that nursing care was being prompted by organizational rules rather than by attention to patients' needs. Orlando's theory is based on the central questions: What prompts nursing actions? What are the properties of dynamic nurse–patient relationships that may lead to effective care?

When Orlando began formulating her conceptualization of nursing, the answer to the first question was that nurses were prompted in their actions by physician's prescriptions, organizational needs, and personal repertoire of experiences rather than by patient needs—in other words, for reasons other than the patients' immediate experiences and immediate needs (1961, p. 60). This answer did not satisfy Orlando and may have initiated the ideas for the development of her theory. When Orlando revisited the terms she used in her theory and the goal of the theory she redefined it as a "nursing process theory" instead of a theory of "effective nursing care" (Orlando, 1990).

The focus of Orlando's theory is on identifying and clarifying the nurse–patient interpersonal process during health and illness situations. To her, basically, nurses' reactions or responses to patients may be automatic, "disciplined professional," (1972) or "deliberative" (1961, 1990). In each situation, the reaction is based on observation of the patient's verbal or nonverbal behavior and is influenced by perceptions, thoughts, and feelings related to the patient's action that prompted the nurse's reaction, or vice versa. The automatic response is guided by "secretiveness," during which neither the meaning of the behavior nor the perceptions of the nurse or the patient are validated. The "disciplined professional response" is guided by "explicitness" of perceptions, of thoughts, and of feelings, indicating that the patient's needs are validated and ambivalence and distress are explored. The disciplined professional response also indicates the nurse has validated the effectiveness of nurses' actions in helping the patient.

The nursing disciplined process requires the following conditions:

- What the nurse says to the individual in the contact must match (be consistent with) any or all of the items contained in the immediate reaction.
- What the nurse does nonverbally must be verbally expressed, and the expression must match one or all of the items contained in the immediate reaction.
- The nurse must clearly communicate to the individual that the item being expressed belongs to herself.
- The nurse must ask the individual about the item expressed to obtain correction or verification from that same individual (1972, pp. 29–30).

On the other hand, not all interactions are based on a nursing process discipline. Nurses may give automatic nursing care, exemplified in routine care (Orlando, 1961, 1972). Automatic nursing care does not encompass perception, thoughts, and feelings. These deal less with finding out and meeting the patients' needs for help. There are two types of automatic responses. One is stimulated by the patients' needs and, insofar as nurses respond to needs that patients cannot take care of by themselves, automatic response is expected to be effective. This is deliberative, automatic response. The other automatic responses are those that result from reasons other than the patients' immediate needs for help. Automatic responses neither acknowledge nor consider patients' perceptions and thoughts of the problem.

A nurse's professional identity is exemplified by her offering disciplined professional actions that are stimulated by knowledge of patient needs and that are validated by patient responses. These actions involve a continuous process of reflection as the nurse attempts to explore the meaning of the behavior of the patient. The nurse perceives the behavior and its meaning, shares these perceptions, and explores and validates the meanings of these perceptions with the patient. By sharing, exploring, and validating perceptions, misinterpretations are minimized. Modeling for interpretation and validation would enhance further use of this process and would enhance understanding of our own and others' reactions and actions (Schmieding, 1987).

When nurses provide these actions, the result is a patient who experiences improvement in behavior, who has needs met, who feels comfortable, who has a sense of adequacy, and who does not manifest helplessness or distress. Nurses deal with "immediate needs" in "immediate experiences" of a patient in an illness situation by engaging in "immediate exploration" of the patient's perceptions, thoughts, and feelings (Orlando, 1961, p. 65). If nurses provide effective nursing care, they will see immediate behavioral changes for the better, they will see increased ability and adequacy in better care of self, and eventually, they will see an increased sense of well-being. Need "is situationally defined as a requirement of the patient that, if supplied, relieves or diminishes his immediate distress or improves his immediate sense of adequacy or well-being" (Orlando, 1961, p. 5). Orlando based her conceptualization of nursing as dynamic interaction on several implicit assumptions (Table 17-5). It is also based on acknowledgment of feelings and emotions.

There are three problems with the assumptions. First, it is not clear how Orlando derived her assumptions; no documentation exists. Second, the nature of some of her

Table 17-5 ***Assumptions—Orlando***

IMPLICIT ASSUMPTIONS

- When patients cannot cope with their needs without help, they become distressed with feelings of helplessness (Orlando 1961, p. 11).
- Nursing, in its professional character, does not add to the distress of the patient (1961, p. 9).
- Patients are unique and individual in their responses (1961, p. 59).
- Nursing offers mothering and nursing analogous to an adult mothering and nurturing of a child (1961, p. 4).
- Nursing deals with people, environment, and health.
- Patients need help in communicating needs; they are uncomfortable and ambivalent about dependency needs (1961, p. 24).
- Human beings (nurses and patients) are able to be "secretive" or explicit about their needs, perceptions, thoughts, and feelings (1972, p. 26).
- The nurse–patient situation is dynamic; actions and reactions are influenced by both nurse and patient (1961).
- Human beings attach meanings to situations and actions that are not apparent to others.
- Patient entry into nursing care is through medicine (1961, p. 5).
- The patient cannot state the "nature and meaning of his distress for his need without the n[illegible] help or without her first having established a helpful relationship with him" (1961, p. 2[illegible]
- "Any observation shared and explored with the patient is immediately useful in ascerta[illegible] and meeting his need or finding out that he is not in need at that time" (1961, p. 36).
- Nurses are concerned with needs that patients cannot meet on their own (1961, p. 5)

assumptions limits nursing to administering only to patients who are under the care of medicine and who cannot meet their own needs comfortably. Neither of these assumptions is acceptable in nursing today; nurses may care for patients who are not under medical care and may help to more effectively meet the needs of patients who are able to meet their own needs. Third, the ratio of assumptions to propositions is high, necessitating too many conditions for the number of propositions and placing a severe limitation on the exploratory power of the theory. Fourth, there appears to be a mechanistic and reductionist view of human beings that is implicit in her theory (Sellers, 1991). However, Orlando was one of the early thinkers in nursing who proposed that patients have their own meanings and interpretations of situations, and therefore, nurses must validate their inferences and analyses with patients before drawing conclusions on patients' experiences or needs (Forchuk, 1991; Orlando, 1961).

Orlando's theory contains more primitive concepts that are unique to her theory (deliberative, automatic, disciplined professional, dynamic nurse–patient relationship) than derived concepts that have been discussed in other theories (needs, helplessness, environment), which give the theory its own unique focus and enhance its contribution to nursing theory (Table 17-6). Many of the central concepts are not defined (environment, health) or, when defined (eg, interaction), they are nonvariables (Hage, 1972) (Table 17-7). Because the concepts evolved from her conceptual image of nursing's potential reality, they have empirical references and therefore have the potential to be operationalized (Andrews, 1983).

Properties of action and reaction are well explicated, but outcomes are not defined—such as improvement, distress, need for help, helplessness—making it difficult not only to ascertain conceptually the need for help but also to ascertain the consequences of either automatic or deliberate nursing actions. The most significant variable—effective nursing care—is equated with either the disciplined professional process or lack of helplessness, distress, and even, at times, meeting the needs of patients, making the theory both tautological and teleological.

Table 17-6 ***Concepts—Orlando***

Need for help	Reaction
Distress	Perception
Immediate	Thought
Need	Feeling
Experience	Actions
Exploration	Secret
Behavioral changes	Automatic response
Sense of adequacy	Explicit
Helplessness	Personal response
Situational conflict	Improvement
Nursing process discipline	Reactions
Deliberative nursing process	Explicit
Disciplined professional response	Secret

Table 17-7 Definition of Domain Concepts—Orlando

Nursing	"Is responsive to individuals who suffer or anticipate a sense of helplessness." "Process of care in an immediate experience . . . for avoiding, relieving, diminishing, or curing the individual's sense of helplessness" (Orlando, 1972, p. 13). "Finding out and meeting the patient's immediate need for help" (1972, p. 20).
oal of nursing	Increased sense of well-being; increase in ability, adequacy in better care of self and improvement in patient's behavior (1961).
lth	Sense of adequacy or well-being Fulfilled needs. Sense of comfort (1961, p. 9, 1969)
nment	Not defined directly but implicitly in the immediate context for a patient (Orlando, 1972).
eing	Developmental beings with needs; individuals have their own subjective perceptions and feelings that may not be observable directly.
ent	Patients who are under medical care and who cannot deal with their needs or who cannot carry out medical treatment alone.
lem	Distress due to unmet needs due to "physical limitations," "adverse reactions to the setting," or "experiences which prevent the patient from communicating his needs (1961, p. 11).
	Ineffective nursing activities: acting in a way not helpful to patient or not achieving professional purpose (1961, p. 72).
	Ineffective patient behavior such as being uncooperative, unreasonable, demanding, or commanding behaviors that prevent the nurse from carrying out her care of maintaining a satisfactory relationship with the patient.
	The interaction of "1) the behavior of the patient, 2) the reaction of the nurse, and 3) the nursing actions which are assigned for the patient's benefit" (1961, p. 36). Process by which a nurse acts (1972, p. 29).
s	Central in theory and not differentiated from nursing therapeutics or nursing process.
	Direct function: "1) Initiates a process of helping the patient express the specific meaning of his behavior in order to ascertain his distress and 2) helps the patient explore the distress in order to ascertain the help he requires so that his distress may be relieved." Indirect function: Calling for the help of others (1961, p. 29)
	Whatever help the patient may require for his need to be met" (ie, for his physical and mental comfort to be assured as far as possible while he is undergoing ome form of medical treatment or supervision [1961, p. 5]).
	matic or deliberative instructing, suggesting, directing, explaining, informing, uesting, questioning, making decisions for the patient, handling the body of patient, administering medications or treatments or changing the patient's ediate environment. Automatic activities: 1) routines of patient care such as g food, evening care, 2) routines to protect the interests and safety of t, such as locking doors, adjusting side rails, 3) routine practices of orga- n, such as signatures for consent forms, and releases (1961, p. 84).
	activities redefined in 1972: 1) perception by five senses, 2) automatic , 3) automatic feelings, 4) action (p. 25).
	and professional activities: automatic activities plus matching of verbal rbal responses, validation of perceptions, matching of thoughts and h action (1972, pp. 25–32).

Theory Analysis

The Theorist

Ida Jean Orlando Pelletier was an associate professor and the director of the graduate program in mental health and psychiatric nursing (1958–1961) at Yale University School of Nursing when her 1961 book was published. The book was a product of a 1954–1959 National Institute of Mental Health grant to integrate mental health concepts in nursing programs (Crane, 1980). Her second book, in 1972, was a result of another supported research project (by the National Institute of Mental Health, Public Health Service) and a general research grant. She was, at that time, a clinical nurse consultant at McLean Hospital, Belmont, Massachusetts (1962–1972).

Orlando has held numerous other positions, including consultant to nursing service administration and nursing education to schools, to health departments, and to the many students who called her from across the United States. She was appointed consultant to the New England Board of Higher Education and the board of the Harvar[illegible] Community Health Plan. Orlando's most recent position was director of nursing at th[illegible] Tri-City Unit of Metropolitan State Hospital in Waltham, Massachusetts.

According to Schmieding (1986), Orlando's 1961 book has been translated into fi[illegible] languages. Orlando worked closely with and was influenced by Wiedenbach; she, in tu[illegible] influenced Travelbee's theoretical notions of nursing. Her book was reissued with n[illegible] introductions by the National League for Nursing (1990); this republication of her w[illegible] acknowledges the significance of her contributions and the timelessness of her idea[illegible]

Paradigmatic Origins

Although Orlando's theory evolved from extant practice through the analysis of [illegible] 2000 nurse–patient interactions to discern what is good and bad practice, Orl[illegible] writing appears to be influenced by Peplau's (1952/1991) focus on interperson[illegible] tionships in nursing. Peplau defined nursing in terms of relationships betwee[illegible] son in need of help and the nurse who is able to recognize such a need. Defini[illegible] Orlando and Peplau have some common properties and, considering that Pepla[illegible] were published in 1952 and Orlando began to formulate hers in 1954 (Yale re[illegible] grant for the purpose of developing an integrated program and, later, a faculty [illegible] development grant that facilitated testing some of Orlando's theoretical prop[illegible] one can make an assumption of Peplau's influence on Orlando. Peplau ackn[illegible] the influence of Harry Stack Sullivan on the development of her ideas; the[illegible] may deduce that Orlando's theory has also used some of Sullivan's co[illegible] assumptions (dynamic relations, inadequate communication).

Perceptions, meaning, and evaluation of meaning are central concept[illegible] ory and are also central to symbolic interactionism. Considering that Orl[illegible] method of research that grew out of the Chicago school of symbolic inte[illegible] the 1950s, understanding her theory could be enhanced by studying the [illegible] and major concepts of symbolic interactionism. Orlando used field metho[illegible] it became a world view in research.

Schmieding (1987) suggested that by studying established theories in other disciplines, nursing theories could be better clarified and developed. She therefore proposed to analyze Orlando's theory by using John Dewey's theory of inquiry. She described the similarities and the differences between Orlando's and Dewey's organizing principles around the meaning of experience, habit, and functions in acting and reacting. She demonstrated that Orlando used experiences, the meaning of experience, and the immediacy of nurse–patient situations as the basis for her theory and that these same principles are central to Dewey's theory. Orlando herself did not acknowledge the paradigmatic origins of her theory and no references appeared in her original writings.

Internal Dimensions

Orlando analyzed some 2000 nurse–patient interactions to identify the properties, dimensions, and goals of interaction. The theory that evolved inductively from these analyses focused on the nature and dynamics of nurse–patient interactions. All statements in the theory relate to interactions therefore, it is a concatenated theory. She used a field approach in developing the theory. Orlando's background in psychiatric nursing (her academic objectives were to identify psychiatric content that should be integrated in nursing curricula) has most probably influenced the focus of the theory on describing the psychosocial aspects of the nurse–patient interactions.

As a single-domain theory that is also a microtheory of nurse–patient interactions, it is limited to immediate exploration and responses to a given situation. The nurse is an integral part of this theory; nurses' perceptions, thoughts, and feelings affect their actions and the patients' reactions. The entire theory is built on nurse–patient encounters; therefore, using Barnum's (1994) classification method of theory development, Orlando used a mixture of operational and problematic methods—more of the former than of the latter.

Orlando identified a number of problems (helplessness, distress) and what nurses should do to handle these problems. The concepts in the problems are not operationally defined, and this limits the development of research hypotheses. Orlando's theory is focused on the delivery of nursing care through a disciplined nursing process. However, her focus is on how to deliver care and not on what care to give. Therefore, her theory provided an early attempt to conceptualize knowledge of process. It is a nursing process theory of medium- to low-level abstraction, leaning more toward the low-level abstraction. This analysis of theory was confirmed by Orlando in introducing her book for republication in (1990). She described her theory as a "nursing process theory."

Theory Critique

The early 1960s marked a milestone shift in the way the nursing perspective was viewed. The interaction theorists, epitomized by Orlando, marked a shift in the perspective of nursing from phenomena dealing with nurses, functions of nurses, and needs of patients to a focus on the process of interaction and the potential consequences for the patient. Orlando's theory—with its major proposition a deliberative nursing process, or the nursing process discipline, as it was relabeled in 1972—and then relabeled nursing process theory in 1990—is a more effective process for identifying patient needs and evaluating patient care. Providing effective care was the focus of many research projects and provided the framework for numerous Yale studies and published research (Diers, 1970).

Systematic explorations of relationships between each of the concepts in the theory and patient outcomes is possible when patient outcomes (improvement, met needs) are articulated, defined, and operationalized. Explorations could also focus on the effect of the "nursing process discipline" on the assessment process and on implementation of other clinical therapeutics (Orlando, 1972, p.4). Examples of potential propositions are presented in Table 17-8.

Although Orlando considered the theory to be a theoretical framework for the practice of professional nursing (Orlando, 1972, p. 1), the theory is more congruent in guiding nurse–patient interactions for the purpose of assessing needs and in providing the nursing therapeutics deemed necessary to patient care. The process is in fact considered a universal process of interactions between patients and all health professionals (Marriner-Tomey, Mills, and Sauter, 1989). What may make it more unique to nursing is the addition of such dimensions as space (hospital) and length of encounters (number of hours nurses interact with patients).

The theory has several limitations, among them the seeming focus on ill people in hospitals, and the focus on individuals—particularly those who are aware and conscious—on immediate time and situations, on short-term rather than long-term care and planning, and on the virtual absence of reference group or family members. Other limitations are the lack of definition of environment, health, patient outcomes, physiologic aspects of needs, and nonvariable nature of the central concepts of the theory (eg, improvement, immediacy, effectiveness). When we consider the theory goals to be limited only to describing the nurse–patient interaction process for assessment of needs and for evaluation of care, then its limitations diminish.

Nurses have used focused interactions and deliberative processes, whether they have been aware of it or not; even when they have been aware of this use, whether they credit Orlando or not remains debatable. Concepts and linkage from the theory, such as validation of observation and nurse–patient discussion of feelings, thoughts,

Table 17-8 ***Propositions—Orlando***

- There will be greater improvement in patient behavior and more effective nursing care when nurses use the disciplined professional response than when they use automatic personal response.
- The nursing situation includes perceptions, thoughts, feelings, and actions.
- When a nurse assesses a patient's immediate needs, immediate experiences, and immediate resultant behaviors, nursing care is more effective in decreasing distress and helplessness and increasing comfort.
- When nurse–patient dynamics and an "explicit" relationship are established, the patient is able to communicate his needs more clearly.
- Effective nursing interactions and processes enhance patients' comfort and decrease their stress.

perceptions, and reactions, are used in psychiatric settings as well as in many other settings. Further use would be enhanced by refinements, extensions, and proposition testing.

Orlando's theory evolved from the need for curricular changes, and it is therefore logical that her first test of ideas occurred in an educational setting (Yale University). The first book (1961) identified teaching and learning strategies and some of the content that could be used in teaching students how to use the deliberative nursing process.

In her second book (1972), Orlando relayed the results of a training program over a 3-month period. The training was for 28 staff nurses (as opposed to students in an educational system) in the use of the nursing process discipline. The purpose was to change their responsiveness from one that was "personal and automatic" to one that was "disciplined and professional" (Orlando, 1972, p. 4). Outcome variables were observed in nurses, and the study results indicated effective use of nursing process discipline in nurse–patient encounters by nurses who were in the training program (Orlando, 1972).

Although there are limited indications of the use of Orlando's theory in practice, educational, or administrative settings, the concepts permeate our educational and practice settings. Schmieding (1986) provides the most comprehensive use of Orlando's theory in nursing practice and nursing administration. Sheafor (1991) provides an analysis that supports the need to incorporate the deliberative Orlando approach in graduate programs. Each situation presented focused on problematic situations either with patients, nurses, physicians, or other colleagues. Nurses' immediate responses and deliberate process responses are then described illustrating Orlando's propositions. In each one of the vignettes offered, the deliberative process clarified assumptions, cleared misconceptions, checked judgmental thoughts, and enhanced expressions and interpretations.

External Components of Theory

The theory represents a shift from a view of nursing that was task oriented and function oriented, with goals that stemmed from organizational needs and with therapeutics that were offered and that were based on physicians' prescriptions to nursing as an interaction process. Values of nursing shifted because of, or as a product of, interaction theories. Theses theories proposed that nursing is a process, patients are the focus, patients should be consulted in their own care, and patients should be spared the distress and discomfort associated with misconceptions, misinterpretations, and noninvolvement in their own care. Patients' behaviors and participation in interpreting meaning and validating perceptions should be significant factors in nurses' reactions. Although the patient was still viewed as helpless and the deliberative process appeared to be always initiated by the nurse, many of the assumptions of the theory are congruent with social and professional values of the 1980s and 1990s.

The theory is culturally bound. Patients in other parts of the world and from other cultures may not want to participate in identifying their needs, nor do they feel free to engage in interpretations of meanings. They may prefer to rely on their significant others and the health care professionals to do that for them. They may misinterpret the continuous validation proposed in this theory as lack of knowledge, lack of expertise, or lack of accountability in the care process (Lipson and Meleis, 1983). The uniqueness of individuals assumed by the theory could counteract automatic responses of nurses because even a nursing process discipline or deliberative nursing process could turn into an automatic response if the nurse forgets the basic assumptions guiding the theory.

Theory Testing

The theory evolved from Orlando's observations of nurse–patient interactions. Although the findings were not reported in a research report, her 1961 book is based on that research. The research was done in various patient settings to explore the effect of the deliberative process, which includes perceptions, thoughts, and feelings of the patient and the nurse regarding patients' needs and the care given. Validation of perceptions, thoughts, and feelings is essential for enhancing the congruence between patients' needs and the care given. Results indicate unique nursing process is more effective than other approaches in dealing with pain (Barron, 1966; Bochnak, 1963), in reducing stress (Mertz, 1962), in understanding patients' needs (Cameron, 1963), in decreasing postoperative vomiting (Dumas and Leonard, 1963), in relieving distress experienced by patients during the process of admission to a hospital (Elms and Leonard, 1966), on the outcome of implicit and explicit verbal acceptance of a nursing procedure as well as on the degree of effectiveness of enemas and progress in labor (Tryon, 1963), and on the effectiveness of the enema, with the indicators being higher retention rate, more fecal return, and higher ratio of fluid intake and return (Tryon and Leonard, 1964).

A number of studies focused on explicating the properties and components of nurse–patient interactions (Diers, 1966; Gowan and Morris, 1964; Pienschke, 1973; Rhymes, 1964; Wolfer and Visintainer, 1975). Others explored the relationship between the nurses' social approval of patients and postoperative recovery behavior as an outcome, finding a significant but weak inverse relationship between physical status (self-report) and social desirability (Eisler, Wolfer, and Diers, 1972). These authors question the process and intent of validating experiences with patients (central to Orlando and Wiedenbach), suspecting that some patients may respond to validation on the basis of social expectation rather than "the patient's inner experience" (Eisler, Wolfer and Diers, 1972, p. 524).

A significant central concept in Orlando's theory—perceptions—was used as a framework to describe needs of grieving spouses. A study of the grieving spouses' perceptions of their own needs before and after the death event revealed high reliability in ability to identify needs and a consistency in the identified needs (Hampe, 1975). However, when identified needs were compared with met needs, a discrepancy became apparent. Implicitly, if the nurses had asked the grieving spouses to identify their own needs, perhaps the nurses would have more systematically and effectively planned to meet each of those needs. A deliberative interaction process can elicit perceptions of needs even when patients cannot communicate their needs (Gowan and Morris, 1964). When nurses used the previously identified needs of grieving spouses as specific targets in their nursing interventions, grieving spouses experienced more met needs (Dracup and Breu, 1978). In this latter study, the greater satisfaction in nursing care was attributed to the systematic approach in need identification.

Another study that supports Orlando's differentiation between presenting problems as perceived by nurses and those as perceived and validated by patients was by Gilliss (1976), who demonstrated that fewer patients suffering from sleeplessness required sleep medication in an experimental group in which Orlando's deliberative process was implemented. In this group, patients' specific needs were identified, defined, validated, and met.

Orlando's theory was used as a framework to research nursing administration. Schmieding (1988, 1990a, 1990b, 1990c) demonstrated that nursing administrators did not explore the reaction of their staff to problematic situations; the majority of them use an approach to handling problematic situations that did not involve the staff or they would tell the nurses what to do rather than solicit from nurses their thoughts or action plans. Using Schmieding's application of Orlando, Sheafor (1991) provided recommendations on how to enhance productivity in hospitals.

The processes of interaction, action, and decision making in nursing administration are similar to these processes involved in nurse–patient interactions. Schmieding (1983) systematically explored the nature of interaction, decision making, and action processes in problematic situations in nursing administration and discovered that Orlando's theory could provide the needed nursing focus in nursing service administration. An instrument was developed to describe the action process of different members of nursing service personnel (Schmieding, 1987). Orlando's theory was also used in describing the responses of nursing students to distressed patients (Haggerty, 1987).

The findings lend support to consideration of the interaction process in achieving effective patient and nursing care outcomes. However, numerous methodological issues are related to need identification and increasing patterns of interaction in the nursing process discipline. One such problem is the paucity of research tools to identify patient needs. Williamson (1978), in attempting to identify patient needs, questioned the existence of mutually exclusive variables such as physical and emotional needs and the contextuality of needs and socioeconomic cultural variables.

Josephine Paterson and Loretta Zderad

Theory Description

Paterson and Zderad (1988) addressed two central questions: How do nurses and patients interact? How can nurses develop the knowledge base for the act of nursing? The humanistic practice nursing theory proposes that the nurse and the patient are significant components in the nurse–patient situation. The act of caring increases the humanness of both. They both approach the situation with experiences that influence the encounter. Nurses, therefore, should consider such encounters as existential experiences and should describe them from a phenomenological perspective. The sum total of all these experiences will enhance the development of the science of nursing.

In selecting existentialism and phenomenology as context and method for the development of nursing knowledge, Paterson and Zderad operate from several premises. The progress of nursing as a human science is hampered by the mechanistic, deterministic, cause-and-effect methods that have dominated it; in other words, they rejected the received view, the logical positivism view of theory development (Paterson, 1971, p. 143). Paterson and Zderad were a decade ahead of the literature in nursing that later advocated such a move. They have also developed their ideas on the premise that the experiences of nurses in practice supply the impetus for any useful theory for nurses. However, they also warned us that preconceived notions influence what is significant and determinately affect the development of knowledge.

Nursing is a lived dialogue that incorporates an intersubjective transaction in which a nurse and a patient meet, relate, and are totally present in the experience in an existential way that includes intimacy and mutuality (Paterson and Zderad, 1970–1971). Nursing brings a person together with a nurse because of the call of that person for help and the response of the nurse. The encounter is influenced by all other human beings in the patient's and nurse's lives and by other things, whether ordinary objects (such as utensils, clothes, furniture) or special objects (such as life-sustaining equipment). The dialogue during these encounters occurs in a time frame as experienced by both partners. When there is synchroneity in timing, the intersubjective dialogue is enhanced. Dialogue occurs in a certain space that is objective, the physical setting, or subjective, personal space.

Paterson and Zderad's theory is based on a number of implicit assumptions (Table 17-9). The theory has the potential for highly abstract propositions related to nurse–

Table 17-9 ***Assumptions—Paterson and Zderad***

IMPLICIT ASSUMPTIONS

- Nursing involves two human beings who are willing to enter into an existential relationship with each other.
- Nurses and patients as human beings are unique and total biopsychosocial beings with the potential for becoming through choice and intersubjectivity.
- The present experiences are more than the sum total of the past, present, and the future, and are influenced by the past, present, and future. In their totality they are less than the future.
- Every encounter with another human being is an open and profound one, with a great deal of intimacy that deeply and humanistically influences members in the encounter.
- Human beings are free and are expected to be involved in their own care and in decisions involving them.
- All nursing acts influence the quality of a person's living and dying.
- Nurses and patients coexist; they are independent and interdependent.
- A nurse has to "accept and believe in the chaos of existence as lived and experienced by each man despite the shadows he casts, interpreted as poise, control, order, and joy" (Paterson and Zderad, 1988, p. 56).
- Human beings have an innate force that moves them to know their angular views and other's angular views of the world (Paterson and Zderad, 1976; Zderad, 1969).

From Paterson J.G. and Zderad, L.T. (1976). Humanistic nursing. New York: John Wiley & Sons; Zderad, L.T (1969). Empathetic nursing: Realization of a human capacity. Nursing Clinics of North America, 4, 655–662; and Paterson, J.G. and Zderad, L.T. (1988). Humanistic Nursing. NLN Publication, March (41–2218).

patient interactions (Table 17-10). The level of abstraction does not render propositions ready for testing. Concepts of the theory are well delineated (Table 17-11); however, some conceptual definitions are not complete in the theory (I/thou, I/it, we, all at once), and others provide useful conceptual definitions such as empathy (Zderad, 1969) and nursology (Paterson, 1971). The theorists did not offer operational definitions. Central nursing phenomena, such as environment or well-being, are not defined nor are central concepts of the theory, such as nurturance, comfort, empathy, and clinical process. Derived concepts, such as the nursing dialogue as meeting, relating, and presence are more comprehensively defined than any of the primitive concepts (Table 17-12).

Theory Analysis

The Theorists

Josephine G. Paterson, DNE, and Loretta T. Zderad, PhD, are nurse researchers at the Veterans Administration Hospital in Northport, New York. Paterson (diploma from Lenox Hill Hospital, BSNE from St. Johns University, MPH from Johns Hopkins University) received her DNS from the Boston University School of Nursing. Zderad (diploma from St. Bernard's Hospital, BSNE from Loyola University, MSNE from Catholic University) received her PhD from Georgetown University. Their interest in public health and psychiatric nursing, respectively, is complementary and well represented in their theory. Their ideas evolved in 1960 while collaboratively teaching graduate students. After completing their respective doctorates, they developed a course on humanistic nursing at the Veterans Administration Hospital in 1972. In the process of teaching the course, their theory evolved. Their 1976 collaborative book is a result of their teaching and observing clinicians in practice. Their book was republished by National League for Nursing in 1988, an indication of the contemporary nature of their ideas.

Paradigmatic Origins

It is easy to determine the paradigmatic origins of Paterson and Zderad's theory. The origins are explicitly identified as being existential philosophy for theory development

Table 17-10 Propositions—Paterson and Zderad

- Nursing's existential involvement in patient care is manifested in the active presence of the whole nurse in time and space as viewed by the patient.
- Nursing's goal of more well-being is enhanced by both nurse and patient as they experience the process of making responsible choices.
- Because nursing is involved with human beings, its phenomena are a person needing help and a person helping in his own situation.
- Intimacy and mutuality in relationships enhance more well-being.

Table 17-11 ***Concepts—Paterson and Zderad***

Between	Becoming
Nurturing	I/Thou
Comfort	I/it
Being and doing	We
Lived dialogue	All at once
Nurturing	Well-being
Intersubjective transaction	More-being
Meeting	Choices
Relating	Authenticity with one's self
Presence	Intellectual awareness
Intimacy	Community
Mutuality	Concepts for research
Call and response	Authenticity with self
Other human beings	Nursology
Things	
Time	
Synchronicity	
Space	

and phenomenology for research. Existentialism considers a person as a unique being and the sum of all undertakings. It does not purport to find out the "why" of human experience, but just describes the "is" of it. It views human existence as inexplicable and emphasizes the freedom of human choice and responsibility for one's acts. Existential philosophy projects that a person exists but lacks a fixed nature and is always in a state of becoming.

Phenomenology is the study of all aspects of a phenomenon in all its richness, in all its dimensions, in its entirety—without attempting to separate the human experiences of any partners in the study (Kant, 1953, pp. 80–90). The focus is on the here and now. Nursing deals with more than that; therefore, any limitations in the theory are limitations of the paradigmatic origins.

Paterson and Zderad relied heavily on such existentialist philosophers as Teilhard de Chardin, Martin Buber, Gabriel Marcel, and Frederick Nietzsche to develop their theory of nursing, and they also relied on such phenomenologists as James Agee. Both existentialism and phenomenology are compatible paradigms and allow the humanistic nursing theory to evolve. Barnum identified several advantages in the use of these paradigms to develop the nursing domain. A person could be considered in totality, experience could be viewed as a whole, and knowledge for nursing could be viewed as more than the sum total of diverse views from a variety of disciplines. Indeed, these paradigmatic origins give nursing its *raison d'etre* (Barnum, 1994, p. 275). Existential nursing furthers a better understanding of the environment of one's self. To use the accepting nature of existentialism is antithetical to the advocacy needed to make changes in intolerable and oppressive situations that are mitigated by illness or by other social or political conditions. Existential nursing may provide the rationale for accepting an unhealthy and noneffective status quo.

Table 17-12 ***Definition of Domain Concepts—Paterson and Zderad***

Nursing	A human discipline involving one human being helping another in an interhuman and intersubjective transaction "containing all the human potentials and limitations of each unique participant" (Paterson and Zderad, 1988, p. 3). Incorporates all human responses of a person needing another. "The ability to struggle with other man through peak experiences related to health and suffering in which the participants in the nursing situation are and become in accordance with their human potential" (1988, p. 7).
Goals of nursing	1. Humanistic nursing itself is a goal. 2. Help patients and self to develop their human potential and to come toward, through choice and intersubjectivity, well-being or more well-being. To help patients and self to increase possibility of making responsible choices (1988, p. 14–17).
Health	More than absence of disease: equated with more well-being, as much as humanly possible (1988, p. 12).
Environment	Objective world as manifested in "other human beings" and things. The subjective meaning of the people and things. Refers to nurses' and patient's environment (1988, pp. 31–33, 37).
Human being	A unique and "incarnate being always becoming in relation with men and things in a world of time and space" (1988, p. 18). Has the capacity to reflect, value, experience to become more. One who asks for help and one who gives help.
Nursing client	Both nurse and patient are the nursing clients (incarnate men), who are unique, when they "meet in a goal-directed (nurturing well-being and more well-being) intersubjective transaction (being with and doing with) occurring in time and space (as measured and as lived by patient and nurse)" (1988, p. 21).
Nursing problem	Seeming discomfort that prompts a call for help. "A person with perceived needs related to the health/illness quality of living" (1988, p. 18).
Nursing process	"Deliberate, responsible, conscious, aware, nonjudgmental existence of the nurse in the nursing situation, followed by disciplined, authentic reflection and description" (1988, pp. 7–8). Based on awareness on the part of the nurse, continuous assessment (p. 16), and developing the human potential of the patient for responsible choosing between alternatives.
Nurse–patient relations	The human dialogue is the essence of nursing, interaction is nursing. Nurse–patient experience is an intersubjective transaction with empathy.
Nursing therapeutics	A human dialogue involves being and doing, nurturing, well-being or more well-being, and comforting. Existential involvement that is an active presence besides the doing, to provide nurturing and comfort and involves experiencing, reflecting, and conceptualizing (1988, p. 12–23). Nurses offer alternatives and support responsible choosing, share self, knowledge, and experience.
Focus of nursing	On the person's unique being and becoming (1988, p. 19).

Internal Dimensions

The purpose of the theory is to describe humanistic nursing and its components and the human method of *nursology*; the study of nursing aimed toward the development of nursing theory. Paterson and Zderad used a method to develop theory, and the theory is the method. They aimed to develop a theory, using methodology and proposing research, congruent with the nature of nursing as a human science (Kleiman, 1986). The theory evolved deductively from a philosophical view—existentialism—but they used a phenomenological approach to inductively develop a theoretical conception of nursing. Because most of the concepts are derived from existentialism, one can deduce that the theory is more deductive than inductive.

This is a highly abstract theory developed around an interest in exploring interaction as a concept. The theory focuses on properties of the human encounter—the human situation that exists between nurses and patients; therefore, it is classified as a microtheory, with more derived than primitive concepts. Its scope is narrow, describing one aspect of nursing therapeutics or the nursing process—interaction—and one aspect of interaction—human encounter. Therefore, it is a single-domain theory. It deals with knowledge of process: How do people interact, particularly when one needs help and one is willing to give help?

Paterson and Zderad use a dialogue form for describing the "nursing dialogue." Therefore, McKeon (as cited in Stevens, 1984, p. 51) would consider their approach to theory development a dialectical one. They present a whole, explaining the whole (humanistic nursing) through the parts (the various concepts) and the parts through the whole. The uniqueness of this theory lies in the lack of boundaries between the experience of the authors as nurses, theoreticians, methodologists, and writers. Concepts in the theory describe all that, and all experiences describe concepts.

Theory Critique

The theorists, in proposing their humanistic theory of nursing, have also proposed a methodology congruent with the assumptions of the theory to develop nursing knowledge (Paterson, 1971). They use the logic of phenomenological methodology and call it *phenomenological nursology*. The method is aimed at the reality as experienced by the nurse and the patient subjectively and objectively. They propose the method for research and nursing practice. Existentialism is the context of nursing, and concepts are used to develop theory. Phenomenology is the process for clinical nursing and for research in nursing. Phenomenological nursology evolved from nursing practice and is usable for nursing research.

The theorists proposed five phases of phenomenological nursology (Paterson, 1971, pp. 144–146):

1. "Preparation of the nurse knower for coming to know." This could be accomplished by total immersion in selected and related literary work. Immersion includes reflecting, contemplating, and discussing.
2. "Nurse knowing of the other intuitively" by seeing the world through the eyes of the subject or the patient, becoming an insider rather than an outsider.

3. "Nurse knowing the other scientifically" by replaying the subjective experiences, reflecting on them, and transcribing the amalgamated view. The nurse considers relationships and analyzes, synthesizes, and then conceptualizes.
4. "Nurse complementarity synthesizing known others" by comparing and contrasting the differences of like nursing situations to arrive at an expanded view.
5. "Succession within the nurse from the many to the paradoxical one," evolving from the multiple realities to an inclusive conception of the whole that incorporates the multiplicities and contradictions.

This is a method to find truths related to everyday practice in nursing or as evolving out of nursing research.

The theory depicts a way of life, an attitude toward humanity, a goal of actualization worth striving for on all levels of personal and professional lives. However, it is limited in the form of guidelines for nursing practice. The only indication of the use of this theory in practice has been offered by Paterson and Zderad as occurring in the Veterans Administration Hospital in Northport, New York.

The theory is a philosophy and a methodology that purports to improve not only quality of care but also the quality of life for the nurse, the teacher, and the administrator. Objective criteria to measure outcomes are antithetical to the theory and the methodology proposed. Therefore, the subjective/objective assessment of each individual nurse is expected and accepted; there are no valid or reliable criteria to measure concepts nor are they warranted within the philosophical view that guides the theory.

This is a tautological theory; the process of humanistic nursing is described by the goal of humanistic nursing, and the complexity of the phenomenon it addresses stems from abstractness and lack of boundaries between its concepts. It appears to focus on the nurse rather than on the patient as becoming and actualizing in the course of nursing care. Barnum (1994, pp. 104–109) asked if what we need is really a holistic nurse, in which case the proper subject matter of existential nursing theory would appropriately be the nurse rather than the patient. If that is one of the focuses of nursing, and Donaldson would agree (1983), then Paterson and Zderad have offered a theory that appropriately describes one of the nursing phenomena.

External Components of Theory

The theory may be incongruent with some prevailing values of practice that address outcome over process, but it is congruent with values surrounding research and knowledge development in nursing that emerged in the mid-1980s in the United States. Humanistic theory proposes understanding of human beings and their experiences as they exist rather than how they ought to be or rather than changing them. The goals of humanistic nursing of understanding, supporting, and maintaining may be in direct conflict with other professional values and goals, such as intervention goals for changes in pain responses or for alleviation of suffering.

As illustrated by Barnum (1994, pp. 222–225), it is a common existential position that suffering brings about a state of heightened self-awareness, thereby creating an openness to authentic experience that the patient might not otherwise experience and express. Suffering creates a state in which the person is brought face to face with his own being. Most nurses, however, seek to remove (alleviate) suffering. It might be difficult for a nurse who is adhering to this theory to justify nursing acts that remove a patient from the authentic experience of suffering. Neither Travelbee nor Paterson and Zderad would advocate the removal of suffering. Nursing to them is to help the patients articulate their perceptions of the situation and the meaning of the suffering and to grow through this suffering.

According to this theory, a nurse–patient encounter involves an open human dialogue that incorporates a high degree of intimacy to enhance understanding of the subjective world of the patient (Barnum, 1994, pp. 215–226). How many such meetings can a nurse be involved in, in the course of her working day, and is there potential for emotional drainage leading to burnout? Do all patients seek and approve of such genuine encounters? Paterson and Zderad would argue that the higher levels of experience gleaned from each encounter indicate rejuvenation rather than burnout.

The theory is congruent with that segment of society that espouses subjectivity and being, but patients may want to experience and evolve their being in genuine encounters within their own circle rather than with the nursing staff.

When, in 1960, Paterson and Zderad were developing the seeds of their theory, they may or may not have anticipated the supportive literature of the 1980s that advocated phenomenology as the methodology most compatible with nursing. The 1980s witnessed an emerging world view in nursing, denouncing the empirical positivist view (see Chaps. 4 and 5) and supporting a phenomenological view (Menke, 1978; Munhall, 1982; Oiler, 1982). Paterson and Zderad advocated respecting nursing experiences as sources of knowledge and, indeed, of wisdom, providing nursing with nonmechanistic and nonpositivistic strategies for theory development and research (Paterson, 1978; Zderad, 1978). Nursing would do well to adopt their views.

Theory Testing

Although no research is reported specifically using Paterson and Zderad's method, numerous research findings have used grounded theory, modified phenomenological approaches, and qualitative approaches to nursing research. Researchers have used these concepts interchangeably to describe methodologies depicting part of each (Stern, 1980; Wilson, 1977). Paterson and Zderad have used the approach to articulate concepts of empathy (Zderad, 1968, 1969, 1970), and comfort (Paterson and Zderad, 1976), but these reports appear to be clinical insights as a prelude to systematic research findings. These reports inspired others to explore the same or similar concepts (Kolcaba and Kolcaba, 1991).

Research to explore these theory propositions has potential after the concepts have been operationalized. For example, the concepts of authenticity, the "between," more well-being, and all-at-once are abstract and lack definition to render them researchable. The potential of the theory to generate research is exemplified in the use of the self (the nurse) and different patterns of presence in the patient's "time-space spheres."

Joyce Travelbee

Theory Description

Nursing to Travelbee is an interpersonal process between two human beings, one of whom needs assistance because of an illness and the other who is able to give such assistance. The goal of the assistance is to help a human being cope with an illness situation, learn from the experience, find meaning in the experience, and grow from the experience. For a nurse to be able to achieve that goal, she also has to find meaning in each encounter. Because illness is suffering and pain, the role of the nurse is to deal with suffering and pain. If the nurse experienced personal suffering, she would be far better able to understand the patient's suffering. Nurses should not shy away from becoming involved with their patients because it is through such involvement that empathy, sympathy, and, eventually, rapport are established.

The central questions that Travelbee's theory answers are: How do nurse–patient, human-to-human relationships get established? For what purpose? Travelbee further asked: What is it that enables some individuals to cope with stress over a prolonged period of time? (J. Travelbee, personal communication, 1970) In attempting to answer these questions, Travelbee theorized that suffering is a common life experience that every person encounters at some point, that particularly occurs around illness, and that is divided into phases.

Human relationships help people cope with suffering, and Travelbee conceptualized relationships as progressing in stages, beginning with the phase of original encounter and evolving to the phase of rapport. A person's attitude toward suffering ultimately determines how effectively he copes with illness. The nurse's role is focused on helping patients find different meanings for suffering, meanings that are of particular importance to them.

Travelbee provides us with an exhaustive conceptualization of sympathy, rapport, and suffering as fine examples of a factor-isolating theory. Suffering is defined as

> . . . a feeling of displeasure that ranges from simple transitory mental, physical, or spiritual discomfort to extreme anguish and to those phases beyond anguish; namely, the malignant phase of despair, the feeling of "not caring," and the terminal phase of apathetic indifference. (Travelbee, 1966, p. 70)

It is an experience that is variable in its intensity, duration, and depth. Beyond the beginning feelings of suffering, and when suffering becomes extremely intense physically, mentally, and spiritually, suffering progresses to the malignant phase in which a person experiences anger, helplessness, and bitterness. If suffering persists, a person ceases to complain or express feelings related to anger and helplessness and instead displays apathetic indifference.

Although reactions to suffering are individualistic, there are some common responses. These are "nonacceptance, blaming self or others, bafflement, anger, self-pity, depression, anguish" during a "why me?" stage (Travelbee, 1966, p. 88). Or human beings may respond to suffering through no protest or even with an affirmative reaction, thereby accepting the suffering. Acceptance may occur because of personal philosophy, perception of the nature of humanity, or religious convictions. Pain and suffering are related. "To suffer is to be immersed in a black ocean of pain" (Travelbee, 1966, p. 89).

To deal with pain and suffering, a nurse has to establish nurse–patient interactions by getting to know the patient, by becoming involved, by ascertaining needs, and by fulfilling the purpose of nursing, which is to alleviate suffering and to help people find meaning in a situation. Communication is the key tool for the nurse. Nurses use various clinical therapeutics to keep channels of communication open, such as validating perceptions, reflecting by self or with patient, and using open-ended comments to solicit more information. Nurses can deliberately prevent communication breakdown by perceiving patients as human beings, recognizing levels of meaning when communicating, listening with reflection, and avoiding cliches, automatic responses, and undue interruptions (Travelbee, 1966, pp. 91–117).

Communication is the vehicle through which nurse–patient relationships are established. Such a relationship is defined as "an experience or series of experiences between a nurse and a patient . . . [or] a family member . . . in need of the service of the nurse." The relationship has two characteristics: it is a "mutually significant meaningful experience" and, through it, the nursing needs of the individual (or family member) are met (Travelbee, 1966, p. 125). Nurses and patients go through several stages to achieve the goal of established nurse–patient relationships. Each stage has certain tasks, and healthy development of the relationship is accomplished by mastering each task. The stages are:

1. **Phase of the original encounter:** Emotional knowledge colors impressions and perceptions of both nurse and patient during initial encounters. The task is "to break the bond of categorization in order to perceive the human being in the patient" and vice versa (Travelbee, 1966, p. 133).
2. **Phase of emerging identities:** Both nurse and patient begin to transcend their respective roles and perceive uniqueness in each other. Tasks include separating oneself and one's experiences from others and avoiding "using oneself as a yardstick" by which to evaluate others. Barriers to such tasks may be due to role envy, lack of interest in others, inability to transcend the self, or refusal to initiate emotional investment.
3. **Phase of empathy:** This phase involves sharing another's psychological state but standing apart and not sharing feelings. It is characterized "by the ability to predict the behavior of another" (Travelbee, 1966, p. 143).
4. **Phase of sympathy:** Sharing, feeling, and experiencing what others are feeling and experiencing is accomplished. This phase demonstrates emotional involvement and discredits objectivity as dehumanizing. The task of the nurse is to translate sympathy into helpful nursing actions (Travelbee, 1964).
5. **Phase of rapport:** All previous phases culminate into rapport, defined as all those experiences, thoughts, feelings, and attitudes that both nurse and patient

undergo and are able to perceive, share, and communicate (Travelbee, 1963, 1966, pp. 133–162).

When relationships are established, the nurse can help patients to accept and find meaning in their experiences or to accept their humanness through either circuitous or indirect methods (avoiding direct confrontation by using parables or by the nurse opening herself and sharing similar personal experiences) or direct methods (asking pertinent questions or logically explaining the situation). Establishment of rapport in nurse–patient relationships and finding meaning in suffering eventually lead to the development of hope in patients (Travelbee, 1971).

Travelbee based her theory on numerous assumptions that are interspersed throughout her book. These assumptions are presented in Table 17-13. Travelbee's assumptions are explicit and congruent with selected concepts and theory propositions. The concepts are abstract and have face validity, but the boundaries are not clear or operationally defined (What is hope and how can it be measured?) (Table 17-14). Travelbee is consistent in her views of humanity, uniqueness, existential

Table 17-13 Assumptions—Travelbee

- The nurse–patient relationship is the essence of the purpose of nursing (Travelbee, 1966, p. 13).
- Human beings are rational, social, and unique beings and are more different than alike (1966, p. 29).
- All human beings undergo certain experiences and will search for meaning in them during the process of living. These experiences could be considered as coherent wholes and could be understood (eg, illness, anxiety, joy, harm). Therefore, likeness and similarities between human beings are in the nature of their experiences (1966, p. 30).
- Labels tend to evoke stereotypical categories. Nurses should remember that patients are human beings who differ from other human beings only in "requesting the assistance of other human beings believed capable of helping them solve health problems" (1966, p. 34).
- Relationships are established when both partners perceive each other's uniqueness. Then, such human relationships transcend roles and are true, meaningful, and effective relationships based on perceptions of uniqueness (1966, p. 36).
- Nurse–patient relationships are based on perceiving the patient as an illness or nursing as a task. Illness is only understood in the context of perceptions of the patient and the nurse.
- Illness, suffering, and pain experiences could be self-actualizing if individuals find meaning in them.
- Human beings are motivated to search for and understand the meaning of all life experiences.
- Illness and suffering are not only physical encounters for human beings, they are emotional and spiritual encounters as well (1966, p. 69).
- Nurse–patient interaction, when purposeful, fulfills the goals of nursing (1966, p. 93).
- "Communication is a process that can enable the nurse to establish a nurse–patient relationship and thereby fulfill the purpose of nursing—namely to assist individuals and families, to prevent and cope with the experience of illness and suffering and, if necessary, to assist them to find meaning in these experiences" (1966, p. 94).
- Nurses are expected to ascertain the meaning of exchanged messages.

Table 17-14 ***Concepts—Travelbee***

Perception	Finding meaning in illness and suffering
Pain	Circuitous
Suffering	Parable approach
Communication	Veiled
Therapeutic self	Personal experience
Hope	Direct
Self-actualization	Questioning
Transcend self	Explanation
Therapeutic self	Transitory discomfort
Nurse–patient relationship/human to human relationship	Anguish
Phase of original encounter	Malignant despair
Phase of emerging identities	Not caring
Phase of empathy	Apathetic indifference
Phase of sympathy	Love
Phase of rapport	

encounters, and nursing. The theorist's definitions of health, nursing, relationships, nursing problems, and nursing therapeutics are conceptually clear, with the integrity of the assumptions preserved throughout the definitions (Table 17-15). Rapport is a phase toward the nurse–patient relationship; the phases overlap. Further operationalization will help determine which behaviors belong in which phase of the process of establishing nurse–patient relationships. Travelbee often relied on dictionary definitions. Research relating to different concepts was not cited. The theory lends itself to numerous propositions that are central to the practice of nursing. Examples are offered in Table 17-16.

Theory Analysis

The Theorist

The late Joyce Travelbee was a faculty member at several schools of nursing. She worked as an assistant professor in the Department of Nursing, Louisiana State University, New Orleans, then as an instructor in psychiatric and mental health nursing in the Department of Nursing Education at New York University, then as a professor at the University of Mississippi School of Nursing in Jackson, and finally at Hotel Dieu School of Nursing in New Orleans. She received a diploma in nursing from Charity Hospital, New Orleans, a bachelor of science from Louisiana State University, and graduated Yale with a master of science in nursing. She acknowledged Ida Orlando's influence on her work.

Table 17-15 ***Definition of Domain Concepts—Travelbee***

Nursing	An interpersonal process and service vitally concerned with change and influence of others. An interpersonal process whereby the professional nurse practitioner assists an individual or family to prevent or cope with the experience of illness and suffering and, if necessary, to assist the individual or family to find meaning in these experiences (Travelbee, 1966, pp. 5–6).
Goal of nursing	To assist an individual or family to prevent or cope with the experience or illness and suffering and, if necessary, to assist the individual or family to find meaning in these experiences (1966, pp. 10–12, 20), with the ultimate goal being the presence of hope (1971).
Health	World Health Organization (WHO) definition: "Health is a state of complete physical, mental, and social well-being and not merely the absence of disease or infirmity. The enjoyment of the highest attainable standard of health is one of the fundamental rights of every human being without distinction of race, religion, political, economic, or social condition" (1966, p. 7).
Environment	Not defined.
Human being	A unique thinking, biologic, and social organism, an irreplaceable individual who is unlike any other person, who is influenced by heredity, environment, culture, and experiences. Always in the process of becoming and capable of choosing (1966, pp. 26–34). Understanding of a human being is through his perception of himself.
Nursing client	A patient is a human being who requests assistance from another human being who he believes is capable of helping and will help in solving his health problems.
Nursing problem	Communication breakdown and distortion: "1. Failure to perceive patient as a human being 2. Failure to recognize levels of meaning in communication 3. Failure to listen, using value statements without reflection 4. Cliches and automatic responses 5. Failure to interrupt" (1966, pp. 106–117)
Nursing process	Process to ascertain needs, validate inferences, decide who should meet needs, plan a course of action, and validate. "Disciplined intellectual approach," a logical method of approaching nursing problems, using knowledge and understanding of concepts from all other sciences and nursing in caring for patients (1966, p. 15).
Nurse–patient relations	An experience between an individual in need of the services of a nurse, and a nurse for the purpose of meeting the needs of the individual.
Nursing therapeutics	Therapeutic use of self (nurse). Disciplined intellectual approach to patient problems. Everything the nurse does for and with the patient is designed to help the individual or family in coping with or bearing the stress of illness and suffering in the event the individual or family encounters these experiences (1966, p. 8). Help patients find meaning in their experiences (1966, p. 10). Methods to find meaning are: 1) Circuitous (indirect) method, which includes (a) parable method (tell analogous story), (b) veiled problem approach (use indefinite pronouns), or (c) personal experience approach (shared experience); 2) Direct method, which includes questioning in jest and explaining (1966, pp. 16–19, 173–179). "Communication techniques: Use of open-ended comments or questions Use of reflecting technique Use of sharing perceptions Deliberate use of cliches" (1966, pp. 106–110).

Table 17-16 ***Propositions—Travelbee***

- To know and understand perceptions of time and life experiences increases the nurse's abilities to meet the needs of patients.
- "The nurse's perception of patients is a major factor in determining the quality and quantity of nursing care she will render each patient" (Travelbee, 1966, p. 34).
- If nurses perceive patients as illnesses, tasks, or sets of stereotype characteristics, their focus in care in (institutional) rather than person-centered (1966, p. 36–41).
- As patients become a "chore and a task, the nurse withdraws and directs her energy toward meeting institutional needs" and patients experience anger, irritability, tension, restlessness, sadness, depression, hopelessness, apathy, and transient somatic symptoms (1966, pp. 38–40).
- An individual's socioeconomic status affects the level of dehumanization a person is subjected to.
- "The quality of nursing care given any patient is determined by the nurses' beliefs about illness, suffering, and death" (1966, p. 55).
- "The spiritual values of the nurse or her philosophical beliefs about illness and suffering will determine the extent to which she will be able to help patients find meaning (or no meaning) in these situations" (1966, p. 55).
- Nurses are able to empathize with patients who are similar to themselves (1966, p. 142).
- Experience of illness affects, to a varying degree, all those associated with the patient, and subsequently affects the patient's perception of the experience (1966, p. 66).
- There is a direct relationship between caring and suffering; the more a person cares and is attached to an object or a person, the more the person suffers when that object or person is lost (1966, p. 72).
- Responses to pain are influenced by cultural background of the person, philosophical premises, spirituality, level of anxiety, and responses of others to the person in pain (1966, p. 81).
- What are the properties of hope, determinants of hope and hopelessness (1971)?
- There is a direct relationship between the extent to which the individual's need for cognitive clarity and security are met and the individual's anxiety level (1971, p. 190).

Paradigmatic Origins

Travelbee based her theoretical formulations on existentialist philosophy from which she drew many of the theory assumptions. A developmental approach is somewhat demonstrated in her writing as she used the concepts of stages of development of the nurse–patient relationship, stages of suffering, tasks to be mastered, constant change and development, and the becoming nature (Chin, 1974), after going through each of the stages. The continuous sense of becoming is both a developmental and an existential concept.

The incongruence perhaps lies in assumptions of developmental theory of an orderly progression and the lack of orderliness inherent in the existentialist philosophy. Despite this shortcoming, Travelbee has effectively and usefully synthesized assumptions and concepts of both developmental theory and existential philosophy by depicting the complexity of humanity through significant milestones (Sarlore, 1966). Her conception of empathy could be clearer if cast within the framework of role theory, particularly role taking.

Travelbee herself credited Victor Frankel (1963) (with whom she corresponded and met) and Rollo May (1953) with the influence on her theories.

Internal Dimensions

Travelbee's theory is a hierarchical theory developed around the concepts of nurse–patient relationship, suffering, and pain to explore the relationship among them. It is both a concatenated theory, isolating and conceptualizing the central theory concepts, and a hierarchical one, as it interprets the relationship among these variables. Travelbee used the field approach in developing her theory, as is demonstrated in conceptualizing rapport in terms of other phases leading to and incorporating rapport. It is a descriptive and prescriptive microtheory that is also considered a single-domain theory.

The theory addresses one of the major concepts in nursing—interaction—but is limited to interaction surrounding illness. The theory focuses on the components of illness of concern to nursing: suffering and pain. It adds mainly to knowledge of process in nursing and provides significant existence propositions (nurse–patient interactions proceed through phases) and relational propositions (rapport increases patient's acceptance of illness).

Travelbee uses an operational method to develop highly abstract relationships. She incorporates the nurses' perceptions and acceptance with components of the nursing problem areas and nursing therapeutics. The nurse perceives, understands, and assigns meaning to behavior and is therefore part of the theory. The nurse's communication is one of the nursing problems, and the self could be used as the intervention through empathy and sympathy.

An operational method of theory development allows choices between alternate theories and actions. An example can be seen in the alternative that Travelbee provides to dealing with suffering through using the direct method of confronting the patient with his suffering or the indirect method of sharing one's own experiences. Operational methods tend to be more acceptable to nurses because of their preferences for well identified choices.

The theory's explanatory power is low (higher ratio of assumptions to explicitly stated propositions) and is limited to knowledge of disorder (suffering) and knowledge of process (relationships).

Travelbee used a deductive approach to develop her theory (Duffey and Muhlenkamp, 1974). Although she explicitly stated the sources that influenced the theory deductively (existentialist philosophy), the inductive approach is more assumed than explicit. It is assumed that she observed nurse–patient relationships in acute and suffering incidents. Such observations are not an integral part of her theory, and it is not clear whether she developed her theory based on extant or ought-to-be practice. One can deduce that it was the former rather than the latter.

Theory Critique

The theory is teleological. The process of establishing relationships is achieved after several stages in nurse–patient encounters, including rapport; however, rapport is the nurse–patient interaction. It is both goal and process; it is both process and product. The theory is tautological and parsimonious; assumptions and relationships could be presented without the numerous repetitions; and more attention needs to be given to the propositions. Finding meaning is analogous to coping but leads to coping, and vice versa.

The complexity of the theory is demonstrated in the abstractness of the concepts, limited operational definitions, and potential multiplicity of relationships. Therefore, its use in research, practice, education, and administration appears to be limited.

Although many of the central concepts in Travelbee's theory are derived from other theories (empathy, sympathy), she does not appear to have developed her propositions using findings of other research. Some of Travelbee's ideas are common practice in nursing. The nursing process as we have come to teach it and use it involves several of the steps outlined by Travelbee. Observations are carried out to validate the needs of patients, to validate inferences made, to make decisions about personally taking action or not, and to then plan a course of action; then, the action is evaluated. The patient is the final authority.

Doona (1979), in preparing a second edition of an earlier Travelbee book (1969), used Travelbee's intervention theory as a guideline for the field of psychiatric nursing. Beyond this publication, no published evidence was found that directly develops, implements, or refines Travelbee's ideas. The theory has the potential for use in practice within the limitations of its scope and its microtheory nature, both of which refer only to individual patients who are ill and suffering, who are conscious, who are willing to invest in the development of rapport, and who participate in finding meaning in and making decisions about their care.

Cook (1989) demonstrated the utility of the theory in assessing suffering of nurses due to job distress at the height of the nursing shortage that forced their hospital to adopt a new system of patient care. The theory was used to define the nature and degree of suffering, the nature of each phase in the development of meaningful interactions between members of a group of nurses who met regularly to deal with their job stress. The rapport described by Travelbee was achieved prior to planning interventions. The intervention plan based on Travelbee (1971) included alleviating suffering, redefining the situation, and finding meaning in their experiences through disciplined and intellectual approaches and the use of the self (Cook, 1989, p. 205). The process of rapport development and the interventions helped the group members to feel less victimized and to gain control over their professional lives. The result was improved self-esteem, better problem solving, a more supportive environment, and rediscovery that a new system is providing them with greater autonomy and more challenging roles.

No other published material uses Travelbee's theory in education or administration, despite favorable review of her 1966 book (Sloane, 1966; Wolff, 1966). Travelbee indicated that the University of Mississippi School of Nursing in Jackson was beginning to modify its curriculum to use her theory (personal communication, 1970). However, the limited scope of the theory restricts its utility for all aspects of nursing.

External Components of Theory

The focus of the theory on the uniqueness and dignity of the human being, on humanity, on autonomy, and on acceptance of others' values makes the assumptions of the theory congruent with Western values. The more recent emphasis on the role of hope—

the ultimate goal of finding meaning in suffering—in healing and recovery tends to give more theoretical credence to Travelbee's propositions pertaining to the meaning of an illness and attitudes toward suffering. However, illness is viewed by society as an aberration, an abnormality, or a condition to be avoided and eliminated. This value is antithetical to Travelbee's basic assumption that illness is a part of life, and finding meaning in illness and suffering is a growing experience. Therefore, professional values could clash with the theory values (used here as an assumption). Many patients could consider the assumption of shared nurse–patient relationships to find meaning problematic and may even go as far as questioning the cost effectiveness of such emphasis on relationships. The lack of a biologic view of the patient and the limited positivistic orientation of the theory undoubtedly limit the utility and the acceptance of the theory by nurses.

Relationships are significant in the helping fields; they are an integral part of assessment for care, and they are focal in delivering care. Travelbee articulated for nursing how such relationships are formed and for what purpose. Hers is a theory to describe one of the central domain concepts in nursing.

Theory Testing

Central relationships in Travelbee's theory—nurse–patient relationship's effect on suffering and coping—have not been researched. However, the concept of empathy has been the center of numerous research studies. Various tools have been developed to measure degrees of empathy (Barrett-Leonard, 1962; Cartwright and Lerner, 1963; Truax and Carkhuff, 1967). Most of the studies of the 1960s and 1970s concluded that existing tools lacked construct and predictive validity and that their reliability was low (Chinsky and Rappaport, 1970; Kurtz and Grummon, 1972).

Other studies using Travelbee's theory explore differences between perceptions of high and low empathizers in effective communication (Stetler, 1977) and properties of interaction surrounding pain (McBride, 1967). Results have been inconclusive. Freihofer and Felton (1976) explored the nature of nursing actions perceived to offer support, comfort, and ease the suffering of a terminally ill patient and significant others of terminally ill patients. More descriptive studies of this type will lend data to explore the construct validity of nurses' actions and options for suffering patients.

Ernestine Wiedenbach

Theory Description

Ernestine Wiedenbach developed a concept of nursing that was congruent with the prevailing ideas at Yale in the late 1950s and early 1960s and that shifted nursing focus from the medical model to a patient model. In her early work (1963), she attempted to develop a concept that encompassed all nursing; this evolved into a prescriptive theory. The theory addresses the central question: How do nurses help patients meet their needs? Help, to Wiedenbach, is an integral part of nursing, and it is all actions that enable individuals to overcome whatever hampers their ability to function.

Needs and functions that dominated nursing at the time continue to do so with an added dimension. Needs can only be ascertained if the nurse validates her perceptions, feelings, and thoughts with those of the patient. Therefore, nurses' actions should abide by the following parameters: actions should be mutually understood and agreed on with full knowledge of implications, and they should be either patient directed or nurse directed or both. When they are nurse directed, they must be deliberate and based on patient needs. To Wiedenbach, nurses develop a helping prescription with the reality of the situation (physical, physiologic, psychological, emotional, and spiritual) by exploring nurses' philosophies of nursing (central purpose and assessment of the situation). Throughout a continuous process of observation and validation, nurses' observations are focused on determining inconsistencies (deviations from normal) and perseverances in making the patients realize their needs. Nurses make plans for action to "minister help needed." The plan has to be validated by patients before implementation. Nurses use themselves, the patients, or others who are appropriate as therapeutic agents.

Wiedenbach (1970a) identified several assumptions that guided her theory, and there are other implicit assumptions (Table 17-17). There are some inconsistencies in the assumptions, such as uniqueness and orderliness, self-directed and dependent, but on the whole, Wiedenbach made a deliberate effort to identify the philosophical premises on which she developed her theory. A student of her theory may be confused with the numerous premises appearing at different points throughout her work. Inconsistencies also exist in using principles, philosophy, and assumptions interchangeably, when, at times, any one of these also were used to mean propositions.

Assumptions and concepts are congruent (Table 17-18). Concepts in the theory are mostly derived (needs, interaction, perception), and because Orlando, Wiedenbach, Dickoff, and James all worked together closely in developing their ideas, despite some of their perceptions of differences (Wiedenbach, 1970b), it is not easy to discern which concepts are primitive and which are derived. All these theories are extensions of each other; although Wiedenbach developed the concept of validation, validation is an integral part of Orlando's nursing process discipline. For Wiedenbach, one of nursing's goals is to promote comfort; for Orlando, it is to alleviate distress. Wiedenbach focused on perceptions of people in need of help and Orlando focused on perceptions as a significant concept in interaction. Concepts in general are not operationally defined, perhaps by design, because whether a patient is comfortable or not depends on the patient's perception and the meaning he attributes to the event and situation (Table 17-19).

The major concepts in this theory tend to be concrete and nonvariable (comfort, validation, need for help). The definitions are contextual, and this has the advantage of allowing variable definitions (comfort is in the eye of the beholder), but it also decreases utility in practice and research. Health and environment are not defined; a nursing client is defined in terms of hospital care and is contingent on awareness of needs. Relationships between concepts in Wiedenbach's early and later writing are not always clear (ie, prescription, validation). The explanatory power of the theory is hampered by a lack of clarity.

Table 17-17 ***Assumptions—Wiedenbach***

EXPLICIT ASSUMPTIONS

- "Each human being is endowed with a unique potential to develop within himself the resources that enable him to maintain and sustain himself" (Wiedenbach, 1970b, p. 1058).
- "The human being basically strives toward self-direction and relative independence and desires not only to make best use of his capabilities and potentialities, but desires to fulfill his responsibilities as well" (1970b, p. 1058).
- "The human being needs stimulation in order to make best use of his capabilities and realize his self-worth" (1970b, p. 1058).
- Whatever the individual does represents his best judgment at the moment of doing it" (1970b, p. 1058).
- "The helping art of clinical nursing is a deliberate blending of thoughts, feelings, and overt actions" (1964, p. 11).
- "There are three more basic premises in nursing: "reverence for the gift of life," "respect for dignity, worth, autonomy, and individuality of each human being," and "resolution to act dynamically in relation to one's beliefs" (1964, p. 16).
- Characteristics of professionalism: clarity of purpose, mastery of skills and knowledge, sustaining purposeful working relationships with others, interest in advancing knowledge and dedication to furthering the goal of mankind" (Dickoff, James, and Wiedenbach, 1968).

IMPLICIT ASSUMPTIONS

- Patients are dependent beings normally willing to utilize help (Wiedenbach, 1970b, p. 1060).
- Patients can use their sensitivities to frustrate health caregivers and "thwart their efforts to obtain the results they desire" (1970b, p. 1060).
- Individuals like to live an orderly life, and life is an orderly process.
- Factors such as physical, physiologic, psychological, and spiritual influence the nursing situation.
- Individuals want and have the resources to be healthy, comfortable, and capable (1964).
- Professional nursing respects dignity, worth, autonomy, and individuality of each human being.

The theory lacks propositions and linkages between concepts, but one can derive propositions related to the process of assessment and intervention. The principles of help are amenable to the development of existence propositions and, subsequently, relational propositions (Table 17-20).

Theory Analysis

The Theorist

Ernestine Wiedenbach holds a bachelor of arts degree from Wellesley College, Wellesley, Massachusetts, and a diploma in nursing from Johns Hopkins School of Nursing, Baltimore. She received her master's degree in public health nursing from Teachers College, Columbia University. She practiced as a nurse midwife. At the time of theory development, she was an associate professor of maternity nursing at the School of Nursing,

Table 17-18 **Concepts—Wiedenbach**

Need for help	Ministeration
Help	Realities
Inconsistency/consistency	Central purpose
Purposeful perseverance	Prescription
Self-extension	Skills
Preconception	Procedural
Interpretation	Communication
Actions	
Rational	
Reactionary	
Deliberate	

Yale University (she began working there around 1952) (Bennet and Foster, 1980). She worked closely with two philosophers, Patricia James and James Dickoff, who were teaching a course in philosophy for nurses. She also worked closely with Ida Orlando. Currently, Wiedenbach is retired and an associate professor emeritus.

Paradigmatic Origins

Basically, Wiedenbach's view of a human being and her view of a nurse are functional. She views patients in terms of their capabilities to function and carry out their responsibilities. Wiedenbach was influenced by Ida Orlando, James Dickoff, and Patricia James (and perhaps the reverse is also true). Such influence is seen in her explication of nurses' actions and reactions and the focus on interpretation and validation of perceptions, feelings, thoughts, and actions. Therefore, it would be useful for the reader to also review the discussion of paradigmatic origins found under Orlando.

Some of Wiedenbach's assumptions and concepts regarding the motivation of human beings and nurses' impulsive responses appear at times to reflect conditions or stimulus–response types of actions and reactions (Wiedenbach, 1968). Careful analysis of the theory may identify developmental themes or parallel themes with a psychoanalytical orientation, such as internal needs, frustrations, and motivations. However, the meaning of the situation or the event as perceived and expressed by an individual demonstrates a departure from psychoanalytical concepts to a phenomenological approach. These are speculations on paradigmatic origins. One origin is clear and documented; the theory evolved out of 40 years of clinical and teaching experiences (Wiedenbach, 1964, p. vii, 1968, 1969), and later developments supported the process nature of the theory (Wiedenbach and Falls, 1978).

Internal Dimensions

Wiedenbach's theory was developed around the need for help and validation of such need through patient perceptions and is therefore a concatenated theory that lends itself first and foremost to existence propositions. It is an inductive theory evolving from observations of clinical practice and patients' needs for help after many years of prac-

Table 17-19 ***Definition of Domain Concepts—Wiedenbach***

Nursing	A helping art with knowledge and theories. A goal-directed and deliberate blending of thoughts, feelings, perceptions, and actions to understand the patient and his condition, situation, and needs, to enhance his capability, improve his care, prevent recurrence of problem, and deal with anxiety, disability, or distress (Wiedenbach, 1964).
Goal of nursing	"To facilitate the efforts of the individual to overcome the obstacles which currently interfere (or maybe later interfere [1970b, p. 1058]) with his ability to respond capably to demands made of him by his condition, environment, situation, and time" (1963, p. 55). "To meet the need the individual is experiencing as a need for help" (1963, p. 55).
Health	Not defined.
Environment	Conglomerate of objects, policies, setting, atmosphere, time, human beings, happenings past, current, or anticipated that are dynamic, unpredictable, exhilarating, baffling, and disruptive (1970, p. 1061).
Human being	Possesses self-direction and relative independence, makes best use of capabilities, fulfills responsibilities, has resources to maintain self; in other words, is a functioning being (1964).
Nursing client	A person who is under care of some member of health care personnel, who is in a vulnerable position, with a perceived need for help.
Nursing problem	Inability or impaired ability of an individual to cope with situational demands due to interferences (1963, p. 56). Discomfort.
Nursing process	Deliberative, to identify need for help and interferences with ability to cope. Through observation, understanding, and clarification of the meaning of cues, determination of causes of discomfort (through inspection, palpation, temperature, etc.) and determination of whether or not patient is able to meet his own needs. Ministration of help needed and, the last step in the process, validation that help given was indeed help needed (1963, p. 56–57).
Nurse–patient relations	The deliberate use of nurses' perceptions, thoughts, feelings, and actions.
Nursing therapeutics	Deliberate action that is either nurse directed, patient directed, or mutually understood and agreed on (1970b, p. 1059). (These are the nurse's options and the choice is hers.) It is designed to deal with a person who is in need of help by "any measure or action required and desired by the individual that has the potential for restoring or extending his ability to cope with the demands implicit in his situation" (1963, p. 56). Help, which is any measure or action that enables the individual to overcome whatever interferes with his ability to function capably in relation to his situation (1963, p. 56). Giving advice, information, referral, ministering or applying a comfort measure. Deliberate actions are mutually understood and agreed on, patient directed, and nurse directed. Communication is an important tool. Helping is based on three principles: inconsistency or consistency, purposeful perseverance, and self-extension (1970b).
Focus of nursing	Goal-directed activities focused on identifying "the patient's perception of his condition" and his need for help (1963, p. 55).

Table 17-20 ***Propositions—Wiedenbach****

- When nurses observe inconsistencies in patients' actions, they use their perseverance in identifying the need for help and in offering help.
- Exploration and validation of nurses' and patients' perceptions, thoughts, and feelings increase the effectiveness of help offered to patients in need of help.
- Deliberate nursing action is an overt act consisting of several components: the need for help, validation, and ministration of help.
- Congruent nurse and patient perceptions of the need for help and evaluation of help enhance effective care and decrease discomfort.
- Mutually understood and agreed-on nursing actions will have a positive effect on the patient.
- Help give to individuals in need of help is categorized as: identification of variance from normal (principle of inconsistency/consistency); identification of an individual's need for help (principle of purposeful perseverance); utilizing self or others for help, advice, information, referral, or comfort (principle of self-extension).

** Propositions delineated under Orlando could also be propositions derived from this theory.*

tice in the maternal and child nursing subspecialty. It is a microtheory explicating a component of the interaction process focused on validating perceptions, thoughts, and feelings before a deliberate action is planned. It is a theory with narrow scope—the deliberative nurse–patient interactive process in a clinical situation to identify needs and verify actions. It addresses one component of one of the central concepts in nursing: nurse–patient interaction. It deals with knowledge of process, describing a component of the process inherent in assessing and providing care.

Wiedenbach used a field approach in identifying dimensions of interaction and validation and used a combination of operational and problem approaches to theory development. She focused her conceptualization around problems of discomfort and the need for help and around the function of the nurse in observing, assessing, and exploring and validating feelings, thoughts, and fears. She used persuasion and personal beliefs to drive the concepts home to nurses.

Perhaps because of the concreteness of the theory, the circle of contagiousness of ideas was wide and reached diverse geographical locations and settings. Although nurses may not articulate the concepts and linkages emanating from Wiedenbach, the central ideas of her theory are used widely. Her's is a good example of theory with tautology, lack of parsimoniousness in presenting ideas (presented in philosophical dialogue), and teleology (identifying the need for help is both a process and an outcome). The ratio of assumptions to existing propositions decreases its current power of explanation.

Theory Critique

The patient's perspective has become an integral part of the lexicon of nursing since the 1980s. Whether these concepts infiltrated nursing thought as a result of Orlando and Wiedenbach can only be determined through extensive analysis of nursing literature and through comparison of writings the decades prior to 1960 and the decades following the publications of Orlando, Wiedenbach, Travelbee, Paterson, Zderad, and other interactionist theorists. An analysis of networking of ideas and people and the development of conceptual genealogical trees may enable us to ascertain the influence of the different theorists on the development of nursing knowledge.

It is apparent that the circle of contagiousness for research was limited to research in or surrounding Yale, but the circle of contagiousness for practice was much wider and engulfed the United States and foreign countries. Concepts such as patient-centered care, perceptions, validation, and exploration of thoughts, feelings, and actions are used in many practice settings. The theory gives guidelines for implementing the nursing process and has stimulated many attempts at conceptualizing the interaction process, but it is limited in its power for prescription (Rickleman, 1971). The scope of the theory remains limited to individuals who are conscious in a hospital setting, who are basically motivated to participate in their own care, who are inconsistent (in a state of disharmony with their surroundings, situation, or expectations) (Wiedenbach, 1965), and who are able to perceive their need for help Patients who are consistent (do not deviate from normalcy), who are noncompliant, and who do not perceive a need for help are not nursing clients. Therefore, its use in practice is limited.

Administration literature in nursing may be considered an extension of Wiedenbach's theory; however, deliberate action perceptual clarification, and validation could be claimed by any effective and efficient organizational theory.

External Components of Theory

The external components of Wiedenbach's theory are the same as those for Orlando's theory.

Theory Testing

As with Orlando's theory and perhaps in combination with it, numerous research studies were launched to test the what and how of a deliberative process and validation of interaction in assessing and intervening with patients in need of help. A review of the research and publications based on Wiedenbach's theory revealed two findings: first, both Orlando and Wiedenbach are cited in most research related to concepts of either theory, and second, Wiedenbach's ideas are still appearing in the literature as researchers continue to test propositions emanating from theory.

One type of research using Wiedenbach's theory focused more on the prescriptive propositions of effect of deliberate nursing process (validation) on several patient outcomes. Such research was hospital oriented (preoperative preparation, admission procedures, obstetric preparation, and patients in need of pain relief). (See discussion under Orlando.) Experimental groups usually received care that included identification of patient's needs focused on verbal and nonverbal behavior (Shields, 1978), nurses' perceptions compared and contrasted with patients' perceptions, and actions to provide help to restore the patient's functional ability based on a continuous process of validation.

On the other hand, nonexperimental care given to the control group was personal, automatic, technique oriented, organizationally focused, and more authoritarian or friendly, but not deliberate and goal oriented. Patient outcomes generally were significantly better in the first than in the second group. Outcomes considered included physiologic measures, such as emesis during postoperative or postdelivery recovery, and degree of change in heart and respiration. Other outcomes were psychological and included subjective patient reports of alleviation of distress (Elms and Leonard, 1966; Leonard, Skipper and Woolridge, 1967; Wolfer and Visintainer, 1975).

Other research was related to the exploration of an implicit assumption that the client is truthful in validating the nurse's perception of his condition. Eisler, Wolfer, and Diers (1972) found that a slight correlation existed between social approval needs of patients (but not the patients' inner experience) and their reports of physical well-being, thereby casting doubt on previously unchallenged assumptions that validation indeed gets at patients' true perceptions of the situation.

Numerous other research reports could be related to the theory, providing further validation or invalidation of its concepts. For example, Larson (1977) found that a client's socioeconomic status and social desirability of the diagnosis affected the nurse's perceptions of the patient's characteristics. The "should" advice in Wiedenbach's theory is therefore expanded to include the "realities" of the nurse–patient situation. There is no indication that Wiedenbach made any substantial changes in her conceptualization based on the results of these research studies. A set of propositions for using change as an outcome variable is presented in Table 17-20.

REFERENCES

King

Asay, M.K. and Ossler, C.C. (Eds.). (1984). *Conceptual models of nursing. Applications in community health nursing.* Proceedings of the Eighth Annual Community Health Nursing Conference. Chapel Hill, NC: Department of Public Health Nursing, School of Public Health, University of North Carolina.

Austin, J.K. and Champion, V.L. (1983). King's theory for nursing: Explication and evaluation. In P. Chinn (Ed.), *Advances in nursing theory development.* Germantown, MD: Aspen.

Barnum, B.J.S. (1994). *Nursing theory: Analysis, application, and evaluation* (4th ed.). Philadelphia: J.B. Lippincott.

Brower, H.T. (1981). Social organization and nurses' attitudes toward older persons. *Journal of Gerontological Nursing,* 7, 293–298.

Brown, S.T. and Lee, B.T. (1980). Imogene King's conceptual framework: A proposed model for continuing nursing education. *Journal of Advanced Nursing,* 5(5), 467–473.

Bunting, S. (1988). The concept of perception in selected nursing theories. *Nursing Science Quarterly,* 1(4), 168–174.

Burney, M.A. (1992). King and Neuman: In search of the nursing paradigm. *Journal of Advanced Nursing,* 17, 601–603.

Byrne-Coker, E. and Schreiber, R. (1990). King at the bedside. *Canadian Nurse,* 86(11), 24–26.

Carter, K.F. and Dufour, L.T. (1994). King's theory: A critique of the critiques. *Nursing Science Quarterly,* 7(3), 128–133.

Daubenmire, M.J. and King, I.M. (1973). Nursing process models: A systems approach. *Nursing Outlook,* 2(8), 512–517.

Elberson, K. (1989). Applying King's model to nursing administration. In B. Henry, C. Arndt, M. Di Vincenti, and A. Marriner-Tomey (Eds.), *Dimensions of nursing administration.* London: Blackwell Scientific Publications.

Fawcett, J. (1989). *Analysis and evaluation of conceptual models of nursing* (2nd ed.). Philadelphia: F.A. Davis.

Fawcett, J. (1995). *Analysis and evaluation of conceptual models of nursing* (3rd ed.). Philadelphia: F.A. Davis.

Frey, M. (1989). Social support and health: A theoretical formulation derived from King's conceptual framework. *Nursing Science Quarterly,* 2(3), 138–148.

Frey, M.A., Rooke, L., Sieloff, C., Messmer, P.R., and Kameoka, T. (1995). King's framework theory in Japan, Sweden, and the United States. *Image: Journal of Nursing Scholarship,* 27, 127–130.

George, J.B. (1980). Imogene King. In The Nursing Theories Conference Group, *Nursing theories: The base for professional nursing practice.* Englewood Cliffs, NJ: Prentice-Hall.

Gonot, P.J. (1983). Imogene M. King: A theory for nursing. In J.J. Fitzpatrick and A.L. Whall (Eds.), *Conceptual mod-*

els of nursing: Analysis and application. Bowie, MD: Brady.

Gonot, P.J. (1986). Family therapy as derived from King's conceptual model. In A.L. Whall (Ed.), *Family therapy for nursing: Four approaches.* Norwalk, CT: Appleton-Century-Crofts.

Gulitz, E.A. and King, I.M. (1988). King's general systems model: Application to curriculum development. *Nursing Science Quarterly,* 1(3), 128–132.

Hampton, D.C. (1994). King's theory of goal attainment as a framework for managed care implementation in a hospital setting. *Nursing Science Quarterly,* 7(4), 170–173.

Hanucharurnkui, S. and Vinya-nguag, P. (1991). Effects of promoting patients' participation in self-care on postoperative recovery and satisfaction with care. *Nursing Science Quarterly,* 4(1), 14–20.

Husband, A. (1988). Application of King's theory of nursing to the care of the adult with diabetes. *Journal of Advanced Nursing,* 13, 484–488.

King, I.M. (1964). Nursing theory: Problems and prospects. *Nursing Science,* 2, 394–403.

King, I.M. (1968). A conceptual frame of reference for nursing. *Nursing Research,* 17(1), 27–31.

King, I.M. (1971). *Toward a theory for nursing.* New York: John Wiley & Sons.

King, I.M. (1975). A process for developing concepts for nursing through research. In P.J. Verhonick (Ed.), *Nursing Research* (Vol. 1). Boston: Little, Brown.

King, I.M. (1976). The health care system: Nursing intervention subsystem. In W.H. Werley, A. Zuzich, M. Zajkowski, A.D. Zagornik (Eds.), *Health research: The systems approach* (pp. 51–60). New York: Springer-Verlag.

King, I.M. (1978). USA: Loyola University of Chicago, School of Nursing. *Journal of Advanced Nursing,* 3, 390.

King, I.M. (1981). *A theory for nursing: Systems, concepts, process.* New York: John Wiley & Sons.

King, I.M. (1983a). The family coping with a medical illness. Analysis and application of King's theory of goal attainment. In I.W. Clements and F.B. Roberts (Eds.), *Family health: A theoretical approach to nursing.* New York: John Wiley & Sons.

King, I.M. (1983b). King's theory of nursing. In I.W. Clements and F.B. Roberts (Eds.), *Family health: A theoretical approach to nursing.* New York: John Wiley & Sons.

King, I.M. (1984). Effectiveness of nursing care: Use of a goal oriented nursing record in end stage renal disease. *American Association of Nephrology Nurses and Technicians Journal,* 11(2), 11–17, 60.

King, I.M. (1986a). King's theory of goal attainment. In P. Winstead-Fry (Ed.), *Case studies in nursing theory* (Chap. 7). New York: National League for Nursing.

King, I.M. (1986b). *Curriculum and instruction in nursing.* Norwalk, CT: Appleton-Century-Crofts.

King, I.M. (1987a). King's theory of goal attainment. In R. Parse (Ed.), *Nursing science: Major paradigms, theories, and critiques.* Philadelphia: W.B. Saunders.

King, I.M. (1987b). Translating research into practice. *Journal of Neuroscience Nursing,* 19(1), 44–48.

King, I.M. (1988a). Concepts: Essential elements of theories. *Nursing Science Quarterly,* 1(1), 22–25.

King, I.M. (1988b). Measuring health goal attainment in patients. In C.F. Waltz and O. Strickland (Eds.), *Measurement of nursing outcomes: Measuring client outcomes.* New York: Springer.

King, I.M. (1989). King's systems framework for nursing administration. In B. Henry, C. Arndt, M. Di Vincenti, and A. Marriner-Tomey (Eds.), *Dimensions of nursing administration.* London: Blackwell Scientific Publications.

King, I.M. (1990a). King's conceptual framework and theory of goal attainment. In M.E. Parker (Ed.), *Nursing theories in practice* (pp. 73–84). New York: National League for Nursing.

King, I.M. (1990b). Health as the goal for nursing. *Nursing Science Quarterly,* 3(3), 123–128.

King, I.M. (1992a). Window on general systems framework and theory of goal attainment. In M. O'Toole (Ed.), *Miller Keane encyclopedia and dictionary of medicine, nursing, and allied health* (p. 604). Philadelphia: W.B. Saunders

King, I.M. (1992b). King's theory of goal attainment. *Nursing Science Quarterly,* 5, 19–26.

King, I.M. (1994). Quality of life and goal attainment. *Nursing Science Quarterly,* 7(1), 29–32.

King, I.M. (1996a). A systems framwork for nursing. In M.A. Frey & C.L. Sieloff (Eds.). *Advancing King's systems framework and theory of nursing* (pp. 14–22). Los Angeles: Sage.

King, I.M. (1996b). The theory of goal attainment. In M.A. Frey & C.L. Sieloff (Eds.), *Advancing King's systems framework and theory of nursing* (pp. 23–32). Los Angeles: Sage.

King, I.M. (1996c). The theory of goal attainment in research and practice. *Nursing Science Quarterly,* 9(2), 61–66.

Magan, S. (1987). A critique of King's theory. In R. Parse (Ed.), *Nursing science: Major paradigms, theories, and critiques.* Philadelphia: W.B. Saunders.

Martin, J.P. (1990). Male cancer awareness: Impact of an employee education program. *Oncology Nursing Forum,* 17, 59–64.

Meleis, A.I. (1985). International nursing for knowledge development. *Nursing Outlook,* 33(3), 144–147.

Meleis, A.I. and Jones, A. (1983). Ethical crises and cultural differences. *Western Journal of Medicine,* 138(6), 889–893.

Norgan, G.H., Ettipio, A.M., and Lasome, C.E.M. (1995). A program plan addressing carpal tunnel syndrome: The utility of King's goal attainment theory. *American Association of Occupational Health Nursing,* 43, 407–411.

Norris, D.M. and Hoyer, P.J. (1993). Dynamism in practice: Parenting within King's framework. *Nursing Science Quarterly,* 6(2), 79–85.

Rooda, L.A. (1992). The development of a conceptual model for multicultural nursing. *Journal of Holistic Nursing,* 10(4), 337–347.

Rooke, L. (1995). Focusing on King's theory and systems framework in education by using an experiential learning model: A challenge to improve the quality of nursing care. In M.A. Frey and C. Sieloff (Eds.), *Advancing King's framework and theory for nursing* (pp. 278–293). Newbury Park, CA: Sage.

Rooke, L. and Norberg, A. (1988). Problematic and meaningful situations in nursing interpreted by concepts from King's nursing theory and four additional concepts. *Scandinavian Journal of Caring Sciences,* 2(2), 80–87.

Rosendahl, P.B. and Ross, V. (1982). Does your behavior affect your patient's response? *Journal of Gerontological Nursing*, 8, 572–575.

Smith, M.C. (1988). King's theory in practice. *Nursing Science Quarterly*, 1(4), 145–146.

Sowell, R.L. and Lowenstein, A. (1994). King's theory as a framework for quality: Linking theory to practice. *Nursing Connections*, 7(2), 19–31,

Uys, L.R. (1987). Foundational studies in nursing. *Journal of Advanced Nursing*, 12(3), 275–280.

Weed, L.L. (1969). *Medical records, medical education, and patient care.* Cleveland: Case Western Reserve University Press.

Woods, E.C. (1994). King's theory in practice with elders. *Nursing Science Quarterly*, 7(2), 65–69.

Zetterberg, H.L. (1963). *On theory and verification in sociology* (Rev. ed.). Totowa, NJ: Bedminster Press.

Orlando

Andrews, C.M. (1983). Ida Orlando's model for nursing. In J. Fitzpatrick and A. Whall (Eds.), *Conceptual models of nursing: Analysis and application.* Bowie, MD: Robert J. Brady Company.

Barnum, B.J.S. (1994). *Nursing theory: Analysis, application, and evaluation* (4th ed.). Philadelphia: J.B. Lippincott.

Barron, M.A. (1966). The effects varied nursing approaches have on patients' complaints of pain [Abstract]. *Nursing Research*, 15(1), 90–91.

Bochnak, M.A. (1963). The effect of an automatic and deliberative process of nursing activity on the relief of patients' pain: A clinical experiment. *Nursing Research*, 12(3), 191–192.

Cameron, J. (1963). An exploratory study of the verbal responses of the nurse–patient interactions. *Nursing Research*, 12(3), 192.

Crane, M.D. (1980). Ida Jean Orlando: In Nursing Theories Conference Group, *Nursing theories: The base for professional nursing practice.* Englewood Cliffs, NJ: Prentice-Hall.

Diers, D.K. (1966). The nurse orientation system: A method for analyzing the nurse–patient interactions [Abstract]. *Nursing Research*, 15(1), 91.

Diers, D. (1970). Faculty research development at Yale. *Nursing Research*, 19(1), 64–71.

Dracup, K.A. and Breu, C.S. (1978). Using nursing research findings to meet the needs of grieving spouses. *Nursing Research*, 27(4), 212.

Dumas, R.G. and Leonard, R.C. (1963). The effect of nursing on the incidence of postoperative vomiting. *Nursing Research*, 12(1), 12–15.

Eisler, J., Wolfer, J., and Diers, D. (1972). Relationship between the need for social approval and postoperative recovery and welfare. *Nursing Research*, 21(5), 520–525.

Elms, R.R. and Leonard, R.C. (1966). The effects of nursing approaches during admission. *Nursing Research*, 15(1), 39–48.

Forchuk, C. (1991). A comparison of the works of Peplau and Orlando. *Archives of Psychiatric Nursing*, 5, 38–45.

Gilliss, L. (1976). Sleeplessness: Can you help? *The Canadian Nurse*, 72(7), 32–34.

Gowan, N.I. and Morris, M. (1964). Nurses' responses to expressed patient needs. *Nursing Research*, 13(1), 68–71.

Hage, J. (1972). *Techniques and problems of theory construction in sociology.* New York: John Wiley & Sons.

Haggerty, L.A. (1987). An analysis of senior nursing students' immediate responses to distressed patients. *Journal of Advanced Nursing*, 12, 451–461.

Hampe, S.O. (1975). Needs of grieving spouses in a hospital setting. *Nursing Research*, 24(2), 113.

Lipson, J. and Meleis, A.I. (1983). Issues in health care of Middle-Eastern patients. *The Western Journal of Medicine*, 139, 854–861.

Marriner-Tomey, A., Mills, D., and Sauter, M. (1989). Ida Jean Orlando (Pelletier): Nursing process theory. In A. Marriner-Tomey (Ed.), *Nursing theorists and their work.* St. Louis: C.V. Mosby.

Mertz, H. (1962). Nurse actions that reduce stress in patients. In *Emergency intervention by the nurse* (Monograph 1, pp. 10–14). New York: American Nurses Association.

Orlando, I.J. (1961). *The dynamic nurse–patient relationship.* New York: G.P. Putnam's Sons.

Orlando, I.J. (1972). *The discipline and teaching of nursing process.* New York: G.P. Putnam's Sons.

Orlando, I.J. (1990). Preface to the NLN edition. In I.J. Orlando, *The dynamic nurse patient relationship: Function, process, and principles* (pp. vii–viii). New York: National League for Nursing.

Peplau, H.E. (1991). *Interpersonal relations in nursing: A conceptual frame of reference for psychodynamic nursing.* New York: Springer. (Original work published 1952).

Pienschke, D. (1973). Guardedness or openness on the cancer unit. *Nursing Research*, 22(6), 484–490.

Rhymes, J. (1964). A description of nurse–patient interaction in effective nursing activity. *Nursing Research*, 13(4), 365.

Schmieding, N.J. (1983). An analysis of Orlando's theory based on Kuhn's theory of science In P.L. Chinn (Ed.), *Advances in nursing theory development.* Rockville, MD: Aspen Systems.

Schmieding, N.J. (1986). Orlando's theory. In P. Winstead-Fry (Ed.), *Case studies in nursing theory.* New York: National League for Nursing.

Schmieding, N.J. (1987). Problematic situations in nursing: Analysis of Orlando's theory based on Dewey's theory of inquiry. *Journal of Advanced Nursing*, 12, 431–440.

Schmieding, N.J. (1988). Action process of nurse administrators to problematic situations based on Orlando's theory. *Journal of Advanced Nursing*, 13, 99–7.

Schmieding, N.J. (1990a). Do head nurses include staff nurses in problem-solving? *Nursing Management*, 21(3), 58–60,

Schmieding, N.J. (1990b). A model for assessing nurse administrators' actions. *Western Journal of Nursing Research*, 12(3), 293–306.

Schmieding, N.J. (1990c). An integrative nursing theoretical framework. *Journal of Advanced Nursing*, 15(4), 463–467.

Sellers, S.C. (1991). A philosophical analysis of conceptual models of nursing. *Dissertation Abstracts International*, 52, 1937B. (University Microfilms No. AAC91-26248)

Sheafor, Marian (1991). Productive work groups in complex hospital units: Proposed contributions of the nurse-executive. *Journal of Nursing Administration*, 21(5), 25–30.

Tryon, P.A. (1963). An experiment of the effect of patients' participation in planning the administration of a nursing procedure. *Nursing Research*, 12(4), 262–265.

Tryon, P.A. and Leonard, R.C. (1964). The effect of patients' participation on the outcome of a nursing procedure. *Nursing Forum*, 3(2), 79–89.

Williamson, Y. (1978). Methodologic dilemmas in tapping the concept of patient needs. *Nursing Research*, 27(3), 172.

Wolfer, J.A. and Visintainer, M.A. (1975). Pediatric surgical patients' and parents' stress responses and adjustment. *Nursing Research*, 24(4), 244–255.

Paterson and Zderad

Barnum, B.J.S. (1994). *Nursing theory: Analysis, application, and evaluation* (4th ed.). Philadelphia: J.B. Lippincott.

Donaldson, S.K. (1983). Let us not abandon the humanities. *Nursing Outlook*, 31(1), 40–43.

Kant, I. (1953). Prolegomena to any future metaphysics (P.G. Lucas, Trans.). Manchester, England: University of Manchester Press.

Kleiman, S. (1986). Humanistic nursing: The phenomenological theory of Paterson and Zderad. In P. Winstead-Fry (Ed.), *Case studies in nursing theory*. New York: National League for Nursing.

Kolcaba, K.Y. and Kolcaba, R.J. (1991). An analysis of the concept of comfort. *Journal of Advanced Nursing*, 16(11), 1301–1310.

Menke, E.M. (1978). Theory development: A challenge for nursing. In N.L. Chaska (Ed.), *The nursing profession: Views through the mist*. New York: McGraw-Hill.

Munhall, P.L. (1982). Nursing philosophy and nursing research: In apposition or opposition? *Nursing Research*, 31(3), 776–786.

Oiler, C. (1982). The phenomenological approach in nursing research. *Nursing Research*, 31(3), 178–181.

Paterson, J.G. (1971). From a philosophy of clinical nursing to a method of nursology. *Nursing Research*, 20(2), 143–146.

Paterson, J.G. (1978) The tortuous way toward nursing theory. In *Theory development: What, why, how?* (NLN Publication No. 15–1708, pp. 49–65.) New York: National League for Nursing.

Paterson, J.G. and Zderad, L.T. (1970–1971). All together through complementary syntheses are the worlds of the many. *Image: Journal of Nursing Scholarship*, 4(3), 13–16.

Paterson, J.G. and Zderad, L.T. (1976). *Humanistic nursing*. New York: John Wiley & Sons.

Paterson, J.G. and Zderad, L.T. (1988). *Humanistic nursing* (2nd ed.). New York: National League of Nursing.

Stern, P.N. (1980). Grounded theory methodology: Its uses and processes. *Image*, 12, 20–23.

Stevens, B.J.S. (1984). *Nursing theory: Analysis, application, and evaluation* (2nd ed.). Boston: Little, Brown.

Wilson, H.S. (1977). Limiting intrusion: Social control of outsiders in a healing community. *Nursing Research*, 26(2), 103–111.

Zderad, L.T. (1968). A concept of empathy. Doctoral dissertation, Georgetown University.

Zderad, L.T. (1969). Empathetic nursing: Realization of a human capacity. *Nursing Clinics of North America*, 4, 655–662.

Zderad, L.T. (1970). Empathy: From cliche to construct. *Proceedings of the Third Nursing Theory Conference*. Lawrence, KS: University of Kansas Medical Center Department of Nursing.

Zderad, L.T. (1978). From here and now to theory: Reflections on "how." In *Theory development: What, why, how?* (NLN Publication No. 15–1708, pp. 35–48.) New York: National League for Nursing.

Travelbee

Barrett-Leonard, G.T. (1962) Dimensions of therapist responses as causal factors in therapeutic change. *Psychological Monographs*, 76(43, Whole No. 562).

Cartwright, R.D. and Lerner, B. (1963). Empathy, need to change, and improvement with psychotherapy. *Journal of Consulting Psychology*, 27, 138–144.

Chin, R. (1974). The utility of system models and developmental models for practitioners. In J. Riehl and C. Roy (Eds.), *Conceptual models in nursing practice*. New York: Appleton-Century-Crofts.

Chinsky, J.M. and Rappaport, J. (1970). Brief critique of the meaning and reliability of "accurate empathy" ratings. *Psychological Bulletin*, 73, 379–382.

Cook, L. (1989). Nurses in crisis: A support group based on Travelbee's nursing theory. *Nursing and health care*, 10(4), 203–205.

Doona, M.E. (1979). *Travelbee's intervention in psychiatric nursing* (2nd ed.). Philadelphia: F.A. Davis.

Duffey, M. and Muhlenkamp, A.F. (1974). A framework for theory analysis. *Nursing Outlook*, 22(9), 570–574.

Frankel, V. (1963). *Man's search for meaning: An introduction to logotherapy*. New York: Washington Square Press.

Freihofer, P. and Felton, G. (1976). Nursing behaviors in bereavement: An exploratory study. *Nursing Research*, 25(5), 332–337.

Kurtz, R.E. and Grummon, D.L. (1972). Different approaches to the measurement of therapist empathy and their relationship to therapy outcomes. *Journal of Consulting and Clinical Psychology*, 30, 106–115.

May, R. (1953). *Man's search for himself*. New York: W.W. Norton.

McBride, M.A. (1967). Nursing approach, pain, and relief: An exploratory experiment. *Nursing Research*, 16(4), 337–341.

Sartore, J.P. (1966). Existentialism. In W.V. Spanos (Ed.), *A casebook on existentialism*. New York: Thomas V. Crowell.

Sloane, A. (1966). Review of "Interpersonal aspects of nursing" by J. Travelbee. *American Journal of Nursing*, 66(6), 77.

Stetler, C. (1977). Relationship of perceived empathy of nurses' communication. *Nursing Research*, 26(6), 432–438.

Travelbee, J. (1963). What do we mean by rapport? *American Journal of Nursing*, 63(2), 70–72.

Travelbee, J. (1964). What's wrong with sympathy? *American Journal of Nursing*, 64(1), 68–71.

Travelbee, J. (1966). *Interpersonal aspects of nursing.* Philadelphia: F.A. Davis.

Travelbee, J. (1969). *Intervention in psychiatric nursing.* Philadelphia: F.A. Davis.

Travelbee, J. (1971). *Interpersonal aspects of nursing* (2nd ed.). Philadelphia: F.A. Davis.

Truax, C. and Carkhuff, R.R. (1967). *Toward effective counseling and psychotherapy.* Chicago: Aldine.

Wolff, I.S. (1966). Review of "Interpersonal aspects of nursing" by J. Travelbee. *American Journal of Nursing*, 66(7), 1504–1506.

Wiedenbach

Bennett, A.M. and Foster, P.C. (1980). Ernestine Wiedenbach. In The Nursing Theories Conference Group, *Nursing theories: The base for professional nursing practice.* Englewood Cliffs, NJ: Prentice-Hall.

Eisler, J., Wolfer, J.A., and Diers, D. (1972). Relationship between the need for social approval and postoperative recovery welfare. *Nursing Research*, 21(5), 520–525.

Elms, R.R. and Leonard, R.C. (1966). Effects of nursing approaches during admission. *Nursing Research*, 15(1), 37–48.

Larson, P.A. (1977). Nurse perception of client illness. *Nursing Research*, 26(6), 416–421.

Leonard, R.C., Skipper, J.K., and Woolridge, P.J. (1967). Small sample field experiments for evaluating patient care. *Health Services Research*, 2(1), 47–50.

Rickleman, B.L. (1971). Bio-psycho-social linguistics: A conceptual approach to nurse–patient interaction. *Nursing Research*, 20(5), 398–403.

Shields, D. (1978). Nursing care in labor and patient satisfaction. A descriptive study. *Journal of Advances in Nursing*, 3, 535–550.

Wiedenbach, E. (1963). The helping art of nursing. *American Journal of Nursing*, 63(11), 54–57.

Wiedenbach, E. (1964). *Clinical nursing· A helping art.* New York: Springer-Verlag.

Wiedenbach, E. (1965). Family nurse practitioner for maternal and child care. *Nursing Outlook*, 13, 50–52.

Wiedenbach, E. (1968). Nurse's role in family planning: A conceptual base for practice. *Nursing Clinics of North America*, 3(2), 355–365.

Wiedenbach, E. (1969). *Meeting the realities in clinical teaching.* New York: Springer-Verlag.

Wiedenbach, E. (1970a). Comment on beliefs and values: Basis for curriculum design. *Nursing Research*, 19(5), 427.

Wiedenbach, E. (1970b). Nurses' wisdom in nursing theory. *American Journal of Nursing*, 70(5), 1057–1062.

Wiedenbach, E. and Falls, C.E. (1978). *Communication: Key to effective nursing.* New York: Tiresias Press.

Wolfer, J. and Visintainer, M. (1975). Pediatric surgical patients' and parents' stress responses and adjustment. *Nursing Research*, 24(4), 244–255.

CHAPTER 18

On Nursing Therapeutics

The nursing activities and actions that are deliberately designed for caring for patients, potential patients, or people at risk (or families or communities) are grouped under nursing therapeutics. Theorists have described and discussed nursing therapeutics with various degrees of emphasis. Two images emerge when the concept "nursing therapeutics" is considered. One is Levine's proposed actions for conservation of energy and the second is Orem's proposed strategies to enhance self-care. Others may be delineated from the writings of different theorists (see Chap. 11, Tables 11-6, 11-12, and 11-18). Levine's and Orem's theories are evaluated in this chapter.

Myra Levine

Theory Description

The central questions that Levine addressed are:

What are the ways in which nursing care is delivered?
What are the goals of nursing actions?
Why are nursing actions provided?

To answer these questions, Levine conceptualized the methods of nursing as conservation of patient resources, as alteration of environment to fit the resources, and as an extension of the patient's perceptual system until his own system is healed. These questions address nursing therapeutics and, to a lesser degree, a perspective on health. The central idea in her theory is well manifested and exemplified in the label she chose for her theory, that is, energy conservation: a universal concept (Levine, 1990).

The impetus for Levine's conceptualization of nursing appears to be her attempt to separate the domains of medicine and nursing. Her first published work focused on proposing "trophicognosis" as a new label for nursing assessment and "plan of action to substitute the concept of nursing diagnosis" (Levine, 1966a, p. 57). Her rationale for the proposal was her desire to differentiate between diagnoses that have the connotation of medical diagnosis and disease orientation; the medical diagnosis tends to address and highlight the overlap between medicine and nursing rather than highlight the differences.

Trophicognosis is defined as "a nursing care judgment arrived at by the scientific method" (Levine, 1966a, p. 57). It denotes the knowledge of the art of nursing and is analogous to diagnosis and prognosis for the art of medicine. Labeling nursing assessment as a nursing diagnosis is only giving medical diagnosis a new label, but when trophicognosis is used, it emphasizes nursing care judgment based on the process of scientific method. Levine offered, then, a useful beginning for the use of the nursing process. Although the new label was not used in nursing, Levine's attempts in 1965 (published in 1966a) supported what other theorists had begun doing: delineating nursing's focus and differentiating between nursing and medicine. However, Levine later admonished nurses to simplify their language and not to invent language that confuses other health care providers (1989a).

Levine then put her energy into conceptualizing a human being as an adaptive being, in constant interaction with the environment, whose behaviors are integrated wholes in response to internal and external environmental stimuli. Nurses are interested in integrated responses of whole patients to noxious stimuli, particularly when the individual is not able to adapt behavior to environmental demands. Nursing is expected to create an atmosphere (therefore environment was beginning to emerge here as a central phenomenon in nursing) to encourage healing and to promote adaptation (1966b). Although this is classified as a theory that focused on nursing therapeutics, and some have used it as a framework for diagnosis and intervention (Taylor, 1989), Levine provided a detailed description of environment. She described environment dimensions as internal and external. Responses of human beings emanate from the internal environment. Both the internal and external environments influence each other, and the internal environment is constantly challenged to meet the external environment's demands. Throughout these challenges and changes, the body maintains its integrity through some control mechanisms that lead to autoregulation of the internal environment (Levine, 1973).

The external environment is perceptual, operational, and conceptual. The *perceptual environment* is that component "which an individual responds to with sense organs" (Levine, 1973, p. 12). The *operational environment* includes all that affects an individual physically, such as microorganisms and pollutants. The *conceptual environment* includes symbols, values, culture, language, thinking, and personal styles, among others (Levine, 1973; 1989b). The interaction between the internal and the external environments is where a person's adaptation resides; it is where the fit between person and environment occurs (Levine, 1989b).

Levine (1973) identified nine models to guide assessment (the relationship between each major theory concept and every model is not entirely explicit):

1. Vital signs
2. Body movement and positioning
3. Ministration of personal hygiene needs
4. Pressure gradient systems in nursing intervention (fluids)
5. Nursing determinants in provision for nutritional needs
6. Pressure gradient system in nursing (gases)
7. Local application of heat and cold

8. Administration of medication
9. Establishing an aseptic environment

Assessment would include organismic and environmental systems. The first allows for description of all physiologic and biologic adaptive integrative systems, such as response to fear (fight or flight), response to inflammation, and response to stress. The other systems of response are to the environment, which is more than one's immediate surroundings (Levine, 1969). It is the perceptual environment "depending on the ability of a person to receive sensory stimuli via his sense organs," the operational environment, including all those physical entities that do not need to be recorded by senses (radiation, microorganisms), and the conceptual environment "determined by the dependence of human beings on the symbolic exchange of language and ideas." It also includes cultural determinants (Levine, 1971a, p. 262).

> The environment is not always 'user-friendly.' Successful engagement with the environment depends upon the individual's repertoire—that store of adaptations which is either built into the genes or achieved through life experience. While there are redundant or back-up systems that offer options when the initial response is insufficient, health and safety are products of a competent conservation process. The goal of conservation is health. (Levine, 1990, p. 193)

The "holistic nursing challenge" is to nurse whole patients at the interface of organism and environment to promote adaptation. Adaptation could be accomplished through energy conservation. Conservation of energy is important to the disease process and begins with regulation of metabolism in response to noxious forces that have instigated the disease process. It does not only mean limitation of activity, it also means "proper disbursement of energy expense, allowing for activity within the range of the individual's capability, safety, and comfort" (Levine, 1971a, p. 259). Conservation of structural integrity is accomplished through tasks that support the physiologic and anatomic positioning. Conservation of integrity is related to environmental processes. It includes conservation of personal integrity through preservation of sense of worth and integrity and conservation of social integrity through the recognition of cultural, ethnic, religious, and family relationships (Levine, 1967).

Levine defines health through the definitions of integrity and wholeness. She defines integrity as

> having the freedom to choose; to move without constraint, as slowly or as swiftly as desired, and to exercise decisions in all matters—trivial and otherwise—without apology, indebtedness, or guilt. Integrity is the experience of life, the sensations of the body and its limbs, the sensory recording of every place and time on the mind and in the spirit. (Levine, 1990, p. 93)

Maintenance of system integrity depends on perceptual systems (basic orienting, visual, auditory, hepatic, and taste and smell). When perceptual systems are deficient, the organismic responses are altered, and the nurse uses her perceptual system in an attempt to maintain wholeness in the individual. This is how healing can proceed (Levine, 1969).

Levine's conceptualization is based on numerous implicit and explicit assumptions that were dispersed throughout her writings between 1966 and 1989. They are presented in Table 18-1. Basic to her theory are her beliefs in wholeness of patients (not

Table 18-1 ***Assumptions—Levine***

IMPLICIT ASSUMPTIONS

- The nurse creates an environment in which healing could occur (Levine, 1966a).
- A human being is more than the sum of parts.
- Human beings respond in a predictable way (1966a).
- Human beings are unique in their responses (1966a).
- Human beings know and appraise objects, conditions, and situations (1973).
- Human beings sense, reflect, reason, and understand (1973).
- Human beings' actions are self-determined even when emotional (1973).
- Human beings are capable of prolonging reflection through such strategies as raising questions or redirecting attention.
- Human beings make decisions through prioritizing courses of actions.
- Human beings must be aware and able to contemplate objects, conditions, and situations in order to act purposively.
- Human beings are agents who act deliberately to attain goals (1973, pp. 12–13).
- Adaptive changes involve the whole individual (1967).
- A human being has unity in his response to the environment. He responds in an integrated way (1966a).
- Every person possesses a unique adaptive ability based on one's life experience, which creates a unique message (1967).
- There is an order and continuity to life (1966a).
- Change is not random.
- A human being (as a whole) responds organismically in an everchanging manner (1967).
- A theory of nursing must recognize the importance of detail of care for a single patient within an empiric framework that successfully describes the requirements of all patients (1966a).
- A human being is a social animal.
- A human being is in constant interaction with an everchanging society.
- Change is inevitable in life (1973, p. 10).
- Nursing meets existing and emerging demands of self-care and dependent care (1985).
- Nursing is associated with conditions of regulation of exercise or development of capabilities of providing care (1973).

clients, because clients come from a Latin root that means a follower) (Levine, 1989c, p. 126), although client does not exactly mean a follower. The derivation of client is from Latin *clinare*, to bend or incline and *cliens*, one who has someone to lean on, which comes from Greek *klinein*, to lean, which has its roots in Sanskrit *srayate*, he leans on (*Webster's Third New International Dictionary*, 1986). Patients are partners in the care process and nurses should help in developing a trusting dialogue.

All major concepts are derived from other paradigms except for the concepts of trophicognosis and conservation, which are primitive to this theory (Table 18-2). Both are theoretically defined; the first was also operationally defined, but because of its esoteric nature, nurses preferred "nursing diagnosis" over trophicognosis. The derived concepts are not operationally defined and have unclear boundaries. Concepts such as

Table 18-2 Concepts—Levine

Wholeness	Intervention
Holism	Supportive
Noxious stimuli	Therapeutic
Organismic responses	Perceptual systems
Fight or flight	Basic orienting
Inflammatory responses	Visual
Stress	Auditory
Perceptual awareness	Hepatic
Homeostasis	Taste, smell
Homeorhesis	Environment
Adaptation	Perceptual
Equilibrium	Operational
Environmental exchange	Conceptual
Orderly synchronization = Health	Perceptual systems
Desynchronization = Disease	Basic orienting
Conservation	Anatomical
Energy	Visual
Integrity	Dynamic exchange
Structural	Trophicognosis
Personal	
Social	

wholeness, social well-being, integrity, and adaptation are used interchangeably and are not well differentiated (Table 18-3).

Levine's theory offers existence propositions that are based on conceptualizing assessment of levels of responses, internal and external environments, and focus of nursing as conservation of energy and integrity through therapy or support. It offers concepts that appear on the surface to be linked together; however, relationships between each set of these concepts are not clear (eg, well-being and adaptation, conservation and responses). Therefore, as it stands now, this is a theory with existence propositions and no relational ones. Levine's propositions are summarized in Table 18-4.

Although Levine described the conservation principles in what may be construed as assumptions, her principles could formulate the major propositions. She proposed that the goal and the process of nursing action is the conservation of energy, the goal of conservation is health, and health is to be whole with integrity (Levine, 1990). Such propositions are supported by assumptions emanating from other paradigms about the significance of energy and integrity for a human being.

Levine in a personal communication (cited in Fawcett, 1989, p. 157) provided further support for the classification of her theory as a theory for nursing therapeutics. She proposed a theory she called "therapeutic intervention" in which she described seven areas of therapeutic interventions that are still in the process of being developed. These are therapeutic regimens to support the healing process of the body, to substitute for failure of autoregulation, to focus on restoring integrity and well-being of individuals, to promote comfort and human concern, to decrease the threat of disease, to create functional changes, and to correct metabolic imbalances.

Table 18-3 ***Definition of Domain Concepts—Levine***

Nursing	Has a unique body of knowledge and is a human interaction. Its goal is to conserve energies and integrities through changes in the environment.
Goal of nursing	Restoration of individual's wholeness, integrity, well-being, and independent activity. Conservation of energy, social, personal, and structural (Levine, 1967). When necessary, maintenance of appropriate balance between patient abilities, involvement in the care, and nurses' actions. Maintenance and individuality.
Health	"Health and illness are patterns of adaptive change" (1966b, p. 2452). Is equated with successful adaptation; in fact, one criterion of successful adaptation is the attainment of social well-being (1966b, p. 2452). Health as integrity means being in control of one's life and having the freedom to choose (Levine, 1990).
Environment	Is both internal and external. It is a setting, a background, and the dynamic exchange that involves both the individual organism and the setting and background. Environment is perceptual, operational, and conceptual. Perceptual environment is based on a person's sense organs' interpretation. Operational environment includes the things that affect an individual physically, such as virus, and the conceptual environment evolves out of an individual's cultural patterns, values, and spirituality and is mediated by symbols of language and thought (1969, p. 94; 1973, p. 12).
Person	An everchanging organism who is in constant interaction with his environment and who is constantly striving to maintain his integrity. Responses of a human being are a unified whole.
Nursing client	A total, whole person, a system of systems, in a state of dyssynchronization and in need of assistance to conserve energy, structural, personal, and social integrity (1969; 1973). An ill client maintains his integrity through four levels of physiologically predetermined protective responses. These are fear, inflammatory process, stress, and perceptual awareness as mediated through sense organs.
Nursing problem	The internal or external environment as it threatens the total integrity of a whole person. Organism responses to threat coexist in a single individual: (1) Response to fear by fight or flight, an instantaneous reaction, a most primitive reaction; (2) Inflammatory response, a second-level response, a response of entire resources of an individual, a systematized energy directed as exclusion and removal of intruding irritant or pathogen; (3) Response to stress produces defensive response in the form of changes that are nonspecific in a human being. Structural changes and gradual loss of adaptation energy occurs, until exhaustion is reached; (4) Sensory response producing perceptual awareness, the information and experience in life are only meaningful when perceived in an integrated whole by the individual. All are energy exchange transmissions from individual to environment and back. The result is a physiological or behavioral activity.
Nursing process	Assessment, diagnosis, and intervention, using steps of the scientific method, with great emphasis on observation as a central tool (1973, pp. 23–29).

(continued)

Table 18-3 ***Definition of Domain Concepts—Levine*** *(Continued)*

Nurse-patient relations	"Depend on perceptual system of both persons" (1969, p. 97). The nursing process and action are for conservation.
Nursing therapeutics	The nurse acts in a therapeutic way when the intervention changes the course of adaptation toward a renewed social well-being. The nurse acts in a supportive way when the intervention maintains or fails to maintain the status quo and when there is no alteration in the course of adaptation (1966a; 1967). Focus is on creating an atmosphere where healing could occur; therefore, the target is the environment. Based on appreciation of the patient's responses. To conserve patient's resources, alter the environment to fit the resources and act as the patient's perceptual system when his own is impaired.
Adaptation	The process of change whereby the individual retains his integrity, his wholeness within the realities of his environment (1969, p. 95).
Focus of nursing	Organism responses that are singular but integrated, maintenance of wholeness. Nurse–patient interaction.
Consequences	Adaptation process of change within which an individual maintains his integrity and his wholeness.
Illness	Dyssynchronization with outer events Loss of a portion of well-being Loss of wholeness; "Health and illness are patterns of adaptive response (Levine, 1966b, p. 2452)."

Theory Analysis

The Theorist

Myra Levine is a graduate of the Cook County diploma program, and she has a non-nursing bachelor's degree from the University of Chicago, and a master of science in nursing from Wayne State University, Detroit. She took postgraduate courses at the University of Chicago (Artigue, Foli, Johnson, Marriner-Tomey, Poat, Poppa, Woeste, and Zoretich, 1994). She is currently retired and a professor emeritus in the medical-surgical nursing graduate program at the University of Illinois, Chicago, where she taught and collaborated in teaching the theory seminars. Her writings evolved while she was a predoctoral and postgraduate student at the University of Chicago. She has an extensive clinical (private duty nurse, staff nurse), administrative (director of nursing), and teaching background (preclinical instructor in Cook County; a faculty member at

Table 18-4 ***Propositions—Levine***

Awareness of an environment influenced behavior at all times.
Conservation of patients' energy is a consequence of nursing intervention.
Components of nursing interventions are conservation of individual patient's structural integrity, personal integrity, and social integrity.
Nurses are participants in every patient's environment and influence patient's adaptation.

Loyola University, at Rush University, and at the University of Illinois) (Esposito and Leonard, 1980).

Paradigmatic Origins

In introducing holism in the mid-1960s, Levine was critical of the scientific approach that advocated experimentation, deductive thinking, and analysis of experiences that only led to more mechanistic and dualistic approaches to patient care. The ultimate result was compartmentalization of human beings. She recommended an inductive approach that evolved from experience and clinical practice and incorporated the wisdom of the person. To her, there was a paradox between holism and humanism on the one hand and dualism and scientific thought on the other. Despite these admonitions, Levine used a deductive approach to develop her theory and recommended the scientific method for collecting data about nursing care.

Levine's clinical background in medical-surgical nursing and the close association of this background with medical, biologic, and pathophysiologic sciences influenced the development of her theory. The theory draws on concepts and assumptions from systems theory (Bertalanffy, 1968), adaptation theories (Cannon, 1939; Dubos, 1966; Selye, 1956), developmental theory (surprisingly, Erik Erikson [1968] was cited for the definition of wholeness, totality, and system [Levine, 1969, p. 94]), existentialism (Buber, 1967; Tillich, 1961), and nursing theorists (Abdellah and Levine, 1986; Nightingale, 1969; Rogers, 1961).

Levine also drew her ideas from several concepts that, in her view, had a major impact on nursing. These are the natural healing concept, the germ theory, theory of multiple factors, and the unified theory of health and disease. Although she promoted the scientific method for nursing in both the development of nursing science (Levine, 1966b) and in the development of nursing process (Levine, 1966a), she encouraged us to consider life processes holistically by transcending the duality of mind and body. She also warned against the apparent dissociation between environment and individual as evidenced in the nature/nurture arguments. Cause-and-effect mechanistic views are dehumanizing and antiholistic. Organism responses, purposeful life, integrative approach, and adaptation are concepts that guided her view of nursing. She advocated a return to nursing as it used to be.

> Nursing has always been characterized by an intensely humanistic purpose, an expression at once of the selfless giving, selfish rewards that accompany human interaction. (Levine, 1971a, p. 263)
>
> It is, after all, in the role of patient advocate that the nurse has historically fulfilled her responsibility to bring compassion, protection, and commitment to the bedside. (Levine, 1971b, p. 43)

Internal Dimensions

Levine's is a concatenated theory developed around concepts of adaptation, conservation, responses, and environment and therefore has an appropriate set of existence propositions. It is a microtheory with limited scope, addressing conservation of energy and integrity. It evolved deductively out of hypothetical beginnings, a view of what nursing ought to be. It is a descriptive theory that attempts to describe strategies of nursing care and of the nursing client. It addresses mainly phenomena of disorder, fight or flight, stress responses, inflammation responses, and perceptual awareness responses.

Levine used a problematic method approach in her theory (Barnum, 1994, pp. 29). Responses of people are holistic but are differentiated into four different problems; conservation is offered separately in four different types. Whereas a person is not reduced to components, responses are limited to four problematic responses. Nurses' actions are limited to conservation. It could be argued, therefore, that there is a certain element of reductionism in Levine's theory.

Theory Critique

Levine developed her notions in the mid-1960s when nurses were struggling with increasing mechanization, when they were beset with fragmentation caused by specialization, and when they were trying to differentiate between different types of nursing and also between nursing and medicine. She began by differentiating between medical and nursing judgment, by offering trophicognosis to replace nursing diagnosis. She saw the process of clinical judgment—the nursing process—as a means of focusing on nursing issues in patient care. Holism and humanism, person–environment interactions, are abstract concepts attached to the nursing act and not clearly defined, but Levine was among the first to redraw our attention to them. The essence of the nursing act is conservation. It is what all human beings strive for and, when not able to adapt to noxious stimuli, the nurse becomes their conservator.

Fortunately, or unfortunately, the theory drew heavily from pathophysiology and was therefore perceived as a theory oriented to acute care of ill individuals. However, Hirschfeld (1976) discussed the cognitively impaired older adult and demonstrated how Levine's four principles of conservation could be applied to give direction to nursing interventions when impairments are present. This appears to be the only published indication of Levine's utility in the practice arena, and it does provide support for the notion that the theory can be used clinically.

Levine's use of holism, humanism, and integrative approaches to understanding response and in nursing care is abstract and in need of operational referents. There is inconsistency in how they are used, which may arise from the view of human beings through a pathophysiologic approach and reduction of responses to those responses that are biologically bound. The inclusion of perceptual awareness amidst the focus on biologic responses to fear, stress, and inflammation almost seems an additive thought and not an integrative one. The major concepts of the theory adaptation and energy are not well defined.

The complexity of the theory is perhaps due to the lack of clarity and disconnectedness of its concepts. It is a teleological theory, adding to the lack of clarity of the boundaries of the concepts (Levine, 1971a, p. 258). Conservation is a goal and an intervention process in different parts of the theory, but organismic and environmental responses overlap when Levine discusses perceptual awareness. In later work she defined the goal of conservation as health and health as integrity (Levine, 1990). It could be argued that three responses—fear, stress, and inflammation—are simply syndromes in response to stress as defined by Selye. Complete definitions and development of propositions connecting responses, environment, and conservation would render this theory testable.

Other functional limitations in the theory may have deterred others from using it. Holistic nursing appears to be limited to integrating social and personal aspects of care in acute care individuals who are dependent on the health care professional. It does not lend itself readily without extensive interpretation to long-term care and care of families or communities. However, Cox (1991) provides a compelling example of how the theory was translated for use in long-term care. The theory offers guidelines for assessment of responses and environment and guidelines for goals of nursing therapeutics, but it is limited in conceptualizing the means by which the nurse can achieve these goals. The theory does not lend itself readily to preventive and health promotion care, but the potential for extensions exists. However, the theory has been used effectively as a framework to guide community nursing services for the homeless in Philadelphia (Pond, 1990).

Some have used the theory in curricula development for educational settings (Grindley and Paradowski, 1991; Hall, 1979; Riehl, 1980). Others have used it in administration settings as a framework for identification of outcome criteria for nursing care of patients on a neurology unit (Taylor, 1974). Taylor's account of her use also substantiates the utility of the theory for the use of the nursing process in assessment and diagnosis.

The circle of contagiousness of the theory is limited. The use of theory for research, education, and administration has suffered from the problematic approach in articulating the theory, the lack of interpretation of holistic and total human being, the limited operationalization of integrative responses, the overlap between concepts (eg, personal and social integrity), and, most of all, the lack of propositions. That is not to say that the potential is not there; it only means that the existing literature by Levine focuses on assumptions, concepts, and definitions. Each of the conservation principles lends itself to existence propositions and each of the nine descriptive models can generate research questions.

External Components of Theory

The theory is congruent with general professional and societal views of health and patient care. Levine espoused holistic care before holism became an accepted lexicon in both nursing and societal language. The total individual has a parallel in Rogers' unitary human being (Rogers, 1970). Two other of Levine's ideas are widely accepted now in nursing thought: the focus of nursing on life processes and the significance of the environment (Donaldson and Crowley, 1978; Flaskerud and Halloran, 1980).

To use an individual's natural resources, to conserve energy and to preserve the integrity of the individual are values of the future. Their social significance would make the theory appealing to the general public, but the challenge remains. How do we achieve these goals of nursing care? What are the outcome criteria by which we nurses know when we have and when we have not achieved these goals? Are they or are they not cost effective in prevention and intervention?

While nursing was attempting to devise ways to measure energy and study unitary human beings and the meaning of healing, Levine demonstrated inconsistencies in ideas and displayed impatience with the lack of use of scientific data in studying therapeutic touch. In response to an article by Krieger, she wrote a scathing letter to the editor, admonishing nurses to stick to science in developing nursing (Levine, 1979). In this letter she warned:

> The professional implications of nurses engaging in "healing" based on the spurious notion that "excesses of energy" in the human body can be transmitted to the "ill person who can be thought of as being in less than an optimal energy state" are frightening. The science is spurious, as is the explanation that this "appears to be done physiologically by a kind of electron transfer resonance." (p. 1379)

Levine charges that this type of thinking will take nursing on to a "hocus pocus" "faith healing" path and that nursing cannot afford to indulge in this kind of "charlatanism" (p. 1380).

Levine is an advocate of theoretical formulations that are based on coherence, but calls for corroboration of truth in nursing. She offered nursing in the mid-1960s a forward view of environment, holistic nursing, the total person, potential significance of perceptual apparatus in nursing, and nursing action as conservation.

Theory Testing

One research study tested a proposition that could be viewed as an extension of Levine's theory. The proposition states that mediation of stimuli through the perceptual system of the nurse could be enhanced if the nurse and the patient share the same subjective time. To explore this proposition, which is closely related to Levine's notion of hepatic perceptual system (which mediates touch, thought, muscles, joints, and skeletal system), Tompkins (1980) explored the effect of restricted mobility on perceived duration. She found that "decreased perceived duration . . . may be a mechanism for preserving system integrity in those whose mobility is restricted" (p. 333). This is the only published study that has tested the relationship between system integrity and perceptual systems.

Hirschfeld (1976) applied Levine's theory to the care of the cognitively impaired elderly patients and found the theory useful in determining priorities. Newport (1984) used Levine's theory as a framework for a study designed to contrast temperatures of newborns who were put in warmers with those who were placed in a skin-to-skin contact with mothers. Other research could evolve from the propositions described earlier in Table 18-4.

Dorothea Orem

Theory Description

Orem's theory has been one of the most discussed and used theories in nursing. The impetus of Orem's ideas, as is the case for a number of other theorists, was to define content for nursing curricula. The seeds of her theory were first published in 1959 in a guide for developing a curriculum for practical nurses (Orem, 1959). As a member of a curriculum subcommittee at Catholic University (1965–1968), Orem recognized that work needed to continue in developing a conceptualization of nursing. Five of the subcommittee members continued to work with another six colleagues for about a decade (1968–1979) to formalize a theory of the process of nursing. In the process, Orem published the first formal articulation of her ideas (1971), and the group articulated the process of nursing theory development and identified universal elements in nursing that are congruent with Orem (Nursing Development Conference Group, 1973, 1979). The second edition of her book appeared in 1980, when she refined and extended the theory that appeared in the first edition (Orem, 1980).

Orem proposed three theories that are interrelated and have come to be considered as one by many of the utilizers. Central to all three theories is that people function and maintain life, health, and well-being by caring for themselves. The first theory, "self-care deficits," is the most comprehensive and is the core of her ideas. It is a conceptual image of the recipients of care as people who are incapable of continuous self-care or independent care due to health-related or health-derived limitations (Orem, 1985, p. 34). The second theory, "theory of self-care," is based on the central idea that a relationship exists between deliberate self-care actions and the development and functioning of individuals and groups. The third theory, "theory of nursing system(s)," describes therapeutic self-care requisites and the actions or systems involved in self-care within the context of their contractual and interpersonal relations in human beings with self-care deficits (Orem and Taylor, 1986, p. 44). All three theories together become a general theory of nursing that she entitled the self-care deficit theory of nursing (Orem, 1995). The relationship between the three theories is described in the following way: "the theory of nursing systems subsumes the theory of self-care deficit, which subsumes the theory of self-care" (Orem, 1991, p. 66). She describes each of the theories in terms of some "postulated entities," which are: persons in space–time matrices; properties of persons; properties of relationships, motion, or change; and product. These entities differentiate among the three theories (Orem, 1991, p. 68).

The focus of the three theories is on *self-care*, defined as "the practice of activities that individuals initiate and perform on their own behalf in maintaining life, health, and well-being" (Orem, 1985, p. 84). Self-care is not limited to a person providing care for himself; it includes care offered by others on behalf of the person. Care may be offered by members of the family or outsiders until a person is able to perform self-care. Self-care is purposeful and contributes to human structural integrity, functioning, and development (Orem, 1985, p. 86). The purposes to be attained are universal, developmental, and health-deviation self-care requisites (Table 18-5).

The three types of self-care requisites are universal, developmental, and health deviation. The universal self-care requisites are found in all human beings and are associated with their life processes and their general well-being. Developmental requisites are related to the different stages that human beings undergo, such as adolescence and pregnancy, among other stages in the life cycle. The third set of requisites result from or are attached to deviations in structural or functional aspects of human beings (Orem, 1991, p. 125). Orem operationalizes each one of these requisites. The focus of nursing is on the identification of self-care requisites, the designing of meth-

Table 18-5 ***Self-Care Requisites—Orem***

UNIVERSAL SELF-CARE REQUISITES

- The maintenance of a sufficient intake of air
- The maintenance of a sufficient intake of water
- The maintenance of a sufficient intake of food
- The provision of care associated with elimination processes and excrements
- The maintenance of a balance between activity and rest
- The maintenance of a balance between solitude and social interaction
- The prevention of hazards to human life, human functioning, and human well-being
- The promotion of human functioning and development within social groups in accord with human potential, known human limitations, and the human desire to be normal (Orem, 1985, pp. 90–91)

DEVELOPMENTAL SELF-CARE REQUISITES

- The bringing about and maintenance of living conditions that support life processes and promote the processes of development; that is, human progress toward higher levels of the organization of human structures and toward maturation
- Provision of care either to prevent the occurrence of deleterious effects of conditions that can affect human development or so as to mitigate or overcome these effects from various conditions (1985, p. 96)

HEALTH-DEVIATION SELF-CARE REQUISITES

- Seeking and securing appropriate medical assistance in the event of exposure to specific physical or biologic agents or environmental conditions associated with human pathologic events and states, or when there is evidence of genetic, physiologic, or psychological conditions known to produce or be associated with human pathology
- Being aware of and attending to the effects and results of pathologic conditions and states
- Effectively carrying out medically prescribed diagnostic, therapeutic, and rehabilitative measures directed to the prevention of specific types of pathology, to the pathology itself, to the resolution of human integrated functioning, to the correction of deformities or abnormalities, or to compensation for disabilities
- Being aware of and attending to or regulating the discomforting or deleterious effects of medical care measures performed or prescribed by the physician
- Modifying the self-concept (and self-image) in accepting oneself as being in a particular state of health and in need of specific forms of health care
- Learning to live with the effects of pathologic conditions and states and the effects of medical diagnostic and treatment measures in a life-style that promotes continued personal development (1985, pp. 99–100)

ods and actions to meet the requisites, and "the totality of the demands for self-care action" (Orem, 1985, p. 88).

The totality of self-care actions to be performed for some duration to meet human self-care requisites by using valid methods and related sets of operations or actions is termed the *therapeutic self-care demand* (1985, p. 88). Therapeutic self-care demand is based on deliberate action (Orem, 1991, p. 135). "Deliberate actions of persons are based on their judgments about what is appropriate under existent conditions or circumstances" (Orem, 1991, p. 79). Nurses use "compound actions" meaning that their actions need to be coordinated, performed simultaneously, or related. The agent who performs the action must have "sensory knowledge" and an "awareness" of the situation; the agent "reflects" on that knowledge and "makes decisions." Actions are performed in phases (Orem, 1991, pp. 79–86).

The provider of self-care, whether self or other, is considered a *self-care agent.* It is an entity to be described in terms of development and operability, which is influenced by such variables as genetics, cultural or experiential backgrounds, and in terms of adequacy. The latter could be evaluated by considering self-care capabilities and self-care demand (Orem, 1987).

Nursing care is therapeutic self-care designed to supplement self-care requisites in the absence of capabilities to do so. Nursing actions, called "the theory of nursing systems," are:

- **Wholly compensatory**: The nurse is expected to accomplish all the patient's therapeutic self-care or to compensate for the patient's inability to engage in self-care, or when the patient needs continuous guidance in self-care.
- **Partly compensatory**: Both nurse and patient engage in meeting self-care needs.
- **Supportive educative system**: The system requires assistance in decision making, behavior control, and acquisition of knowledge and skills. Under this system, patients are able to perform self-care with assistance (Orem, 1985, pp. 152–156).

Orem's theory is based on explicit and implicit premises (Orem, 1983, 1987) (Table 18-6) that "do not express a singular belief in a clear way at either the philosophical or more general level of discourse" (Smith, 1987, p. 93).

Orem provides nursing with a number of primitive concepts that are defined theoretically and operationally, the esoteric nature of the terminology being one of the

Table 18-6 ***Assumptions-Orem***

EXPLICIT ASSUMPTIONS

- Nursing is a deliberate, purposeful helping service performed by nurses for the sake of others over a period of time.
- Persons (human agency) are capable and willing to perform self-care for self or for dependent members of the family.
- Self-care is part of life that is necessary for health, human development, and well-being.
- Education and culture influence individuals.
- Self-care is learned through human interaction and communication.
- Self-care includes deliberate and systematic actions performed to meet known needs for care (Orem, 1980, pp. 34–38).
- "Human agency is exercised in discovering, developing and transmitting to others ways and means to identify needs for and make inputs to self and others" (1987, p. 73).

IMPLICIT ASSUMPTIONS

- People should be self-reliant and responsible for their own care needs as well as for others in the family who are not able to care for themselves.
- People are individuals with entities that are distinct from others and from their environment.

obstacles that may have influenced the initial slow use of the theory in practice (Anna, Christensen, Hohn, Ord, and Wells, 1978). The theory includes both abstract (health, self-care agency) and concrete (universal self-care needs) variables (Table 18-7).

When concepts are defined, their relationships are not entirely clear as, for example, with health and self-care or illness and self-care deficit. The primitiveness, the overlap, and the undefined boundaries between concepts create multiple interpretations, particularly for those who are new to operationalizing the theory. The self-care agency is an example of an undefined concept or a primitive concept with multiple meanings. When should an agent be identified? What is the extent of self-care performed by an agent to make it self-care by self or by others? How do you determine the agent? By whose perception? (Anna, Christensen, Hohn, Ord, and Wells, 1978; Smith, 1979). These are examples of what an adequate theoretical and operational definition could do to decrease ambiguity and enhance clarity. Some of the variables are nonvariables (eg, self-care), thereby limiting their propositional power (Table 18-8).

Orem offers propositions that are summarized in Table 18-9. Propositions developed by Orem (1985) correspond to her three proposed theories and their central ideas. Propositions have progressed from existence propositions, attesting to the stage of development of the theory to relational and predictive propositions (Orem, 1995). Despite the complexity of the construct of self-care, Orem's theory has become part of the lexicon of health care and is beginning to be adopted by patients and health care professionals alike.

Theory Analysis

The Theorist

Dorothea Orem earned her diploma and bachelor of science in the 1930s and master of science in 1945 from the Catholic University of America, Washington, DC and honorary doctorates in 1976 from Georgetown University, Washington, DC, and in 1980 from Incarnate Word College, San Antonio, Texas. She has established a private consulting company, Orem and Shields, Inc., in Chevy Chase, Maryland, perhaps to accommodate the diverse practice arenas that are using her theory and that need her assis-

Table 18-7 ***Concepts—Orem***

Self-care	Self-care requisites
Deficits	Universal self-care
Capabilities	Developmental self-care
Demands	Health-deviation self-care
Dependent care	Therapeutic self-care demands
Dependent care deficit	Self-care agency
Nursing systems	Dependent care agency
Wholly compensatory	Theory of self-care
Partly compensatory	Theory of self-care deficits
Supportive educative	Theory of nursing systems

Table 18-8 **Definition of Domain Concepts—Orem**

Nursing	Nursing is art, a helping service, and a technology (Orem, 1985, pp. 144–146). Actions deliberately selected and performed by nurses to help individuals or groups under their care to maintain or change conditions in themselves or their environments (p. 5). Encompasses the patient's perspective of health condition, the physician's perspective, and the nursing perspective. Universal, developmental, and health deviation self-care requisites.
Goal of nursing	To render the patient or members of his family capable of meeting the patient's self-care needs (1985, p. 54). "1. To maintain a state of health; 2. To regain normal or near normal state of health in the event of disease or injury; 3. To stabilize, control, or minimize the effects of chronic poor health or disability" (1980, p. 124).
Health	"Health and healthy are terms used to describe living things . . . [it is when] they are structurally and functionally whole or sound . . . wholeness or integrity . . . includes that which makes a person human, . . . operating in conjunction with physiological and psychophysiological mechanisms and a material structure (biologic life) and in relation to and interacting with other human beings (interpersonal and social life)" (1980, pp. 118–119). "A state of being whole and sound" (1985, p. 176). Well-being is a perception of contentment, happiness and pleasure, by spiritual experiences and through a sense of personalization (1985, p. 179).
Environment	Environment components are environmental factors, environmental elements, environmental conditions, and developmental environment (1985, pp. 140–141). Limited view of environment to its usefulness as a helping method. Therefore defined under Nursing Therapeutics. Though environment is mentioned in a diagram (1985, p. 85) and in the definition of nursing, (1985, p. 53), it is not defined.
Human being	Has the capacity to reflect, symbolize, and use symbols (1985, p. 174). Conceptualized as a total being with universal, developmental needs and capable of continuous self-care (1985). A unity that can function biologically, symbolically, and socially (1985, p. 175).
Nursing client	A human being who has "health-related or health-derived limitations that render him incapable of continuous self-care or dependent care or limitations that result in ineffective or incomplete care" (1985, pp. 34–35). A person who is deficient in universal, developmental, or health-related self-care requisites. . . . A human being is the focus of nursing only when a self-care requisite exceeds self-care capabilities (1985, p. 35).
Nursing problem	Deficits in universal, developmental, and health-derived or health-related conditions.
Nursing process	A system to determine (1) why a person is under care, (2) a plan for care, (3) the implementation of care.
Nurse–patient relations	Not defined.
Nursing therapeutics	Deliberate, systematic, and purposeful action. Total compensatory, partly compensatory, or educative supportive care in universal, developmental, and health-deviation self-care deficits, using several helping methods; acting or doing for others, guiding, supporting, providing a developmental environment, teaching (1985, pp. 88–90).
Focus	"The special concern of nursing is the individual's need for self-care action and the provision and management of it on a continuous basis in order to sustain life and health, recover from disease or injury, and cope with their effects" (1985, p. 54). Dependency or incapacities due to health/illness situation (1983, p. 208).

Table 18-9 ***Propositions—Orem***

PERSON AND NURSING CLIENT

- Human beings have capabilities to provide their own self-care or care for dependents to meet universal, developmental, and health-deviation self-care requisites. These capabilities are learned and recalled.
- Self-care abilities are influenced by age, developmental state, experiences, sociocultural background as well as other variables.
- Self-care deficits are to balance between self-care demands and self-care capabilities and an indication of a state of social dependency.
- Self-care or dependent care is mediated by age, developmental stage, life experience, sociocultural orientation, health, and available resources.

NURSING THERAPEUTICS

- Therapeutic self-care includes actions of nurses, patients, and others that regulate self-care capabilities and meet self-care needs.
- Nurses assess the abilities of patients to meet their self-care needs and their potential for refraining from performing their self-care.
- Nurses engage in selecting valid and reliable processes or technologies or actions for meeting self-care demands.
- Components of therapeutic self-care are wholly compensatory, partly compensatory, and supportive–educative.

Based on Orem (1985) and Orem and Taylor (1986).

tance. She has been involved in nursing practice, nursing service, and nursing education at different levels of education (practical, diploma, baccalaureate, and graduate). She taught at two schools of nursing: the Catholic University of America and the Medical College of Virginia, Richmond (Foster and Janssens, 1980).

The impetus of Orem's theory was an attempt to conceptualize a curriculum for a diploma program by isolating and specifying nursing actions. She continued her theory development activities as a member of two overlapping crucial groups, the Nursing Model Committee of the Catholic University nursing faculty and the Nursing Development Conference Group.

Paradigmatic Origins

Orem's theory has been classified as a systems theory by Riehl and Roy (1980), as an interaction model by Riehl-Sisca (1989), and as developmental by Fawcett (1989). Orem used concepts from these three paradigms that may lead to the conclusion that the theory evolved from them. Her definition of health as a state of wholeness, her conception of the integrity of the person, and the use of systems of nursing all evolved from systems theory. These, however, are isolated concepts, more like terms, not derived conceptually or defined in terms of the original paradigm. A system model implies a feedback mechanism between nurse and patient, and such bidirectional movement is not congruent with this theory in which the nurse—patient relationship is predicated by the one-way transfer of agency (Melnyk, 1983, p. 173).

Similarly, Orem views a person with self-care deficits as socially dependent; the capability to engage in self-care and to meet universal self-care needs appears to characterize a more integrated development. These are concepts reflecting a developmental view of humanity, yet their lack of centrality in the theory, lack of definition, and absence of developmental stages and deliberate progression to more complex entities deny the theory a developmental origin. In fact, classifying the theory as either a system or a developmental theory would highlight gaps in defining concepts and propositions central to the two paradigms but tangential to Orem's theory.

The paradigmatic origin of the theory is more appropriately the needs theory of Henderson (1966) or the functional theory of Abdellah, Beland, Martin, and Matheney (1961). Henderson (1966, pp. 16–17) identified 14 needs. Universal self-care needs are similar to the needs identified by Henderson, although the uniqueness of Orem's theory lies more in the expectation of that person's capability to engage in his own self-care. Health-deviation requisites are an extension and not a refinement of Henderson's concept of nursing. Orem offers a fine example of the process inherent in theory development based on other theories in which new concepts evolve and others are derived. It is an example to be emulated as nurses refine and extend other theories.

Internal Dimensions

Orem's theories are interrelated and centered around self-care. Their level of development and interrelationship suggest that they are concepts and part of one theory, a nursing therapeutic theory of self-care. Orem's theory of self-care is a descriptive theory developed around an attempt to clarify the components of care offered by nurses and a conceptualization of the nursing client. It is a deductive theory with a hypothetical constructive beginning (Orem, 1985, 1991). Orem herself credits her own practice and reflections on others' practice for her theory's beginnings, making it an inductive theory. It is a concatenated theory with more potential for existence propositions to describe the properties of the various concepts and to delineate the elements of such complex constructs as the exercise of self-care. It uses a field approach to theory construction. The units are understood in terms of other miniunits.

The theory is focused on and limited to dealing with individual self-care deficits rather than with the biopsychological being. It deals essentially with one of the domain concepts—clinical therapeutics—and offers one modality for care—the development of self-care abilities. It focuses on actions and deals with knowledge of control. It is a theory developed using an operational method; alternative methods of action are dependent on the nurse's discrimination and decision about the needs and the action (Barnum, 1994, pp. 143–144). It is the agent's perspective that decides on alternative action. All actions are deliberate.

Theory Critique

Orem's theory has been operationalized and used in research, practice, and administration. It lends itself to research for a number of reasons. Orem herself has developed propositions linking the theory concepts and addressing at least two of the central con-

Orem also continues to revise and refine her theory. However, the the- therapeutic theory and appeals to the "relevance to nursing criteria" used more to guide practice than research. It is about practice and for used to guide evaluation, it has lent itself to evaluation of the clinical theory (Backscheider, 1974).

ory demonstrates a great, but limited, utility for nursing practice; it provides that has usage potential in parts, but is limited to only a component of e. Despite this limitation, there are several reasons for the rather speedy of the theory by nursing practice. The language of the theory extends con- anced by Henderson, Abdellah and, to some extent, Nightingale. Nurses, ifting from a medical model, have used a needs and functional approach to care; therefore, the shift becomes more gentle and gradual, both of which are to Orem's theory. Orem also delineated the technical and professional aspects sing practice in both the Nursing Development Conference publications (1973, and in her first book (Orem, 1971).

Orem's theory also incorporates the medical perspective rather than rejects it (John- n, 1983) and purports to build nursing practice on it. Furthermore, it uses medical ence language, with which most nurses are familiar and many prefer. The theory is eveloped around the ill person and conveys the centrality of individual and institu- ional care, perhaps the most appealing feature for the majority of nurses who care for the sick. Orem extended the use of the theory to the care of families (Orem, 1983). It also appeals to those who wish to model Kinlein (1977) who "hung her own shingle" when she went into private practice. It is perhaps due to all these reasons, and the operational method in theory development, that we see more documentation in the literature of the utility of this theory for practice than is true of other theories.

The wide appeal of theory in practice is demonstrated in using the theory to care for chronically ill patients, particularly the diabetic patient (Allison, 1973; Backscheider, 1971, 1974: Fitzgerald, 1980), in caring for amyotrophic lateral sclerosis patients (Taylor, 1988), in psychiatry (Buckwalter and Kerfoot, 1982; Caley, Dirksen, Engalla and Hennrich, 1980; Underwood, 1980), in critical and acute care settings (Mullin, 1980; Noone, 1995), in preoperative and postoperative care (Bromley, 1980; Campuzano, 1982; Dropkin, 1981), in hospice care (Murphy, 1981; Walborn, 1980), and with adolescents (Michael and Sewall, 1980; Norris, 1991) and adult and geriatric patients (Anna, Christensen, Hohn, Ord, and Wells, 1978). The theory was used to individualize care for cancer patients (Morse and Werner, 1988), for patients with end stage renal disease (Greenfield and Pace, 1985), and for patients with drug problems (Compton, 1989). The theory was also used for caring for gerontologic patients in community health nursing settings (Clark, 1986). The theory also has institutional utility (Bonamy, Schultz, Graham, and Hampton, 1995) and the potential for use as a framework for community health care (Taylor and McLaughlin, 1991).

Limitations of the theory to practice are demonstrated in the analysis of the definitions and the central propositions in the theory. It appears that the theory is illness oriented, both acute and chronic, with no indication of its use in wellness settings. Although some extended its use to the care of patients other than adults (Michael and Sewall, 1980; Norris, 1991), the theory itself addresses adults more than any other group (Melnyk, 1983). It presumes a list of needs that evolve out of a pathophysiologic or medical focus, explaining its utility to hospital care. It establisi a sick person and a nurse and not enough of a relationship be a nurse. It also provides limited utility for nurses who care for achieve their maximum level of independence (Easton, 1993). Th is questionable in light of its complexity, but the diversity of its ut in a variety of subspecialties. It provides nurses with collegial visibil and once nurses acquire the language of the theory through staff d grams, they tend to use it (McLaughlin 1993; Walker, 1993).

Nurse administrators have found the theory amenable to implementa ber of institutions and a greater number of chief nurses (16 of 24) of Depart erans' Affairs medical centers reported using either Orem's theory or a com Orem with other theorists (Bonamy, Schultz, Graham, and Hampton, 199 (1989) herself proposed a framework for nursing administration. Miller (198 lenged nursing administrators to create a climate to enhance the use of theory, alt she did not give much guidance or exemplars for implementation on a large involving nursing administrators. She offered a model for nursing practice based Orem's theory, demonstrating its utility for care in acute illness, convalescence, an restored health. The model was based more on a developmental, health/illness continuum than on Orem's theory. Others have described the utility of the theory as "a guide for the nursing activities within a hospital nursing service" (Coleman, 1980, p. 323), in organizing nursing care in independent practice (Backscheider, 1974), in psychiatric units (Underwood, 1980), particularly, in nurse-run clinics (Allison, 1973), in five pilot units at the Toronto General Hospital (Reid, Allen, Gauthier, and Campbell, 1989), and in a Veterans' Administration Medical Center (Bonamy, Schultz, Graham, and Hampton, 1995). It was also used effectively as a framework for a hospital-based utilization review process (Harrison-Raines, 1993).

The theory evolved from interest in curricula for diploma and baccalaureate programs and the need to differentiate between technical and professional education. Therefore, its utility to nursing education is enhanced by the theorist's interest. The curriculum subcommittee of the School of Nursing, Georgetown University, of which Orem, Backscheider, and Kinlein were members, developed a curriculum based on ideas of theory (or theory ideas evolved out of curriculum). Not surprisingly, the theory has been used as a conceptual framework in associate degree programs (Fenner, 1979). The framework is also used in the schools of nursing at the University of Southern Mississippi in Hattiesburg and the University of Missouri at Columbia (Fawcett, 1989, pp. 236–237).

The theory's circle of contagiousness in research, education, and administration is limited, but it has the widest circle of all theories in practice.

External Components of Theory

Orem's theory is congruent with the era of nursing practice that prevailed and focused on the ill and the institutionalized. As we shift focus to the well individuals and to the community, extensions and refinements will need to be made. The focus on health deficits due to illness creating self-care deficits will need to be supplemented with focus

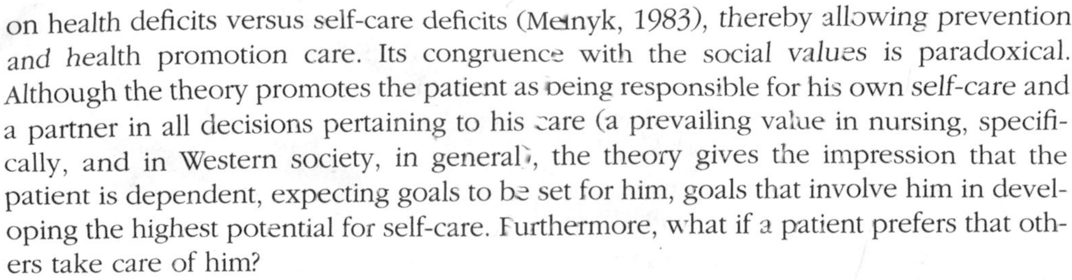
on health deficits versus self-care deficits (Melnyk, 1983), thereby allowing prevention and health promotion care. Its congruence with the social values is paradoxical. Although the theory promotes the patient as being responsible for his own self-care and a partner in all decisions pertaining to his care (a prevailing value in nursing, specifically, and in Western society, in general), the theory gives the impression that the patient is dependent, expecting goals to be set for him, goals that involve him in developing the highest potential for self-care. Furthermore, what if a patient prefers that others take care of him?

The theory seemingly needs adaptation for use with other cultures; for example, values of patients in Japan include group care and the inseparability of the environment and the individual. On the other hand, it is usable in some societies where, although hospital patients are not expected to be self-care agents, family members are expected to and actually do become the self-care agents, as in many Middle Eastern countries. The nurse's role in these countries is to educate and support family members who assume the care. When these patients come to the United States alone, without their families or other self-care agents, they are unreceptive to nurses' attempts to promote self-care skills.

Orem's proposed theory may indeed make a substantial and valued difference in the lives of people whose self-care abilities are curtailed due to acute or chronic conditions, but it may not make the same difference in enhancing prevention and promoting health and well-being.

Theory Testing

Orem's theory has been used as the basis for the development of research instruments to assist researchers in using the theory (Clinton, Denyes, Goodwin, and Koto, 1977; Denyes, 1982; Kearney and Fleischer, 1979; Kuriansky, Gurland, Fleiss, and Cowan, 1976). Kearney and Fleischer (1979) described the development of a valid and reliable instrument to measure the exercise of self-care agency (McBride, 1987). The instrument can be used to measure the level of involvement of patients in self-care, and eventually measurements could be developed to determine outcomes of the increase in patients' abilities of self-care. Hanson and Bickel (1985) and Weaver (1987) developed, described, and critiqued an instrument to measure patients' perceptions of self-care agency. A self-care practice questionnaire was developed and tested by Moore (1995) for the special purpose of measuring the self-care practice of children and adolescents. The Danger Assessment Instrument (Campbell, 1986) was developed to measure the danger level of homicide for battered women. Along the same lines, the Performance Test of Activities of Daily Living (PADL) is another tool developed to measure the self-care agency (Kuriansky, Gurland, Fleiss, and Cowan, 1976).

The focus of these studies lends support to the need for a process of operationalizing complex theory constructs and for the development of valid and reliable instruments based on these constructs. These studies represent effective steps in the further testing of central theory propositions that now exist, but with the potential for relational ones. The lack of clarity of concepts and tautology in ideas may have limited applications, but they have prompted the present line of investigation.

Fawcett reported that there are numerous unpublished ongoing or completed studies that have been presented in the annual conferences based on theory that are held at Georgetown University School of Nursing and Wichita (Kansas) State University. Fawcett also reported on dissertations that used Orem as a theoretical framework for the research (Fawcett, 1989, p. 233).

Several descriptive studies focused on self-care practices. Allan (1988) examined the use and interpretation of health information in the practice of self-care activities of women as related to their weight. She found that women in her study were more concerned about their self-image than risk factors, and she was able to describe the self-care activities that they used to protect that image in the face of the reality of failure to maintain their weight. Miller (1982) used the theory to identify categories of self-care needs for diabetic patients, and Storm and Baumgartner (1987) illustrated through a research case study method the use of self-care theory in the successful discharge of ventilator-dependent patients. Kubricht (1984) described self-care needs of radiation patients, and Sandman, Norberg, Adolfsson, Axelsson, and Hedly (1986) described Alzheimer-type dementia patients and nurses' needs and actions. Maunz and Woods (1988) described self-care actions by women. The theory was used to assess the perceived demands or changes in universal and self-care activities, and the degree of perceived difficulty in attempting to meet these demands among English and Spanish-speaking women with human immunodeficiency virus infection. For these women, the universal self-care tasks with the highest burden were caring for their children, engaging in physical activity, and attempting to fulfill the demands of their work responsibilities (Anastasio, McMahan, Daniels, Nicholas, and Paul-Simon, 1993). Infant birth weight was significantly and directly related to self-care agency and prenatal care actions (Hart, 1995).

Other studies tested relationships between propositions. One example is Denyes (1988) who provided partial support for the relationship between self-care agency and self-care in determining health outcomes. Hartley (1988) tested the relationship between nursing system and self-care behavior by examining the congruence between teaching strategies and learning styles of women and their effect on accuracy and frequency of performance of breast self-examination. The study demonstrated that self-care agency could evolve through the recall of observations or actions of others: "Knowledge of self-care breast self-examination developed through the use of supportive-educative nursing system, a system through which efficient and effective learning occurred" (Hartley, 1988, p. 166). Hart (1995) provided support for the significant relationship between basic prenatal care actions and self-care agency, which, in turn, was directly related to infants' birth weight.

Other tests of interventions lend further support to the utility of Orem's theories. The relationship between self-care as a nursing therapeutic and nursing outcome was examined in a number of studies. For example, Toth (1980) examined the relationship of a structured transfer preparation on patients' anxiety; Watkins (1995) tested patients' comprehension of discharge instructions based on Orem; Rothlis (1984) explored the effect of self-help groups on perceptions of hopelessness and helplessness; and Moore (1987) described the effects of various learning strategies on the development of autonomy and self-care agency among school-aged children. Using Orem as a framework, it was demonstrated that patients tended to accept responsibility for self-infusion at home, which increased their independence and sense of freedom (Gardulf, Bjorvell, Andersen, Bjorkander, Ericson, Froland, Gustafson, Hammarstrom, Nystrom, Soeberg, and Smith, 1995). Dashiff (1988) reviewed research and clinical literature in psychiatric nursing that is based on Orem's self-care deficit theory. She compared the contributions of this literature to the development of theory for use in psychiatric nursing with other nursing specialties and concluded that psychiatric nurses are using Orem's theory; however, there were limited indications of research productivity. Hanucharurnkui and Vinya-nguag (1991) tested the use of Orem's and King's theories on expediting the rate of recovery from surgery and increasing satisfaction with adult patients undergoing surgery. Interventions derived from Orem's and King's theories were related to less pain sensation and distress, using fewer analgesics, more ambulation, and higher satisfaction of patients than those who did not receive the theory-driven care. The theory was also used as a framework for a community-based intervention study in a smoking cessation program, with results pointing to the need for "tailored" self-care strategies (Williams, Shuster, Merwin, and Williams, 1994).

An indirect effect of focusing on a nursing theory was reported by Denyes, O'Connor, Oakley, and Ferguson (1989). A collaborative research project was initiated between nursing service and nursing education, focusing on contraceptive nursing care and self-care of women using primary care facilities. The results of the research—that women are their own self-care agents—gave impetus "for revising the clinic's family planning standards so that they would more fully operationalize the concepts" (Denyes, O'Connor, Oakley, and Ferguson, 1989, p. 144).

Theory-driven research is most effective and productive when a program of research is established versus a single study approach. Williams and Ramos (1993) demonstrated this in a series of four studies based on Orem's theory to describe the self-care needs of people with symptomatic mitral valve prolapse. The approach resulted in more focused questions that built on each other, which contributed to building systematic knowledge about the experience of patients suffering from this disease. The phases of the research included a review of medical records, analysis of health perception and body image, and a survey of cardiovascular nurses; and it led to the construction and validation of a research instrument.

As with all other theories, Orem's could be used more broadly as a schematic to analyze the focus of research conducted in nursing and to set a direction for future research in nursing (Smith, 1979). On the whole, although the potential is there, the theory is used more as a guide for practice, with few having used it to evaluate the outcome of care (Chang, 1980; Roberts, 1982). In general, theory testing has been problematic, due to the different levels of its utilization in research (Silva, 1986). Research driven by Orem's theory, published 1986–1991, was evaluated by Spearman, Duldt, and Brown (1993). They concluded that 32% of the studies used Orem's theory minimally, and 55% used it insufficiently, that is, the researchers used the theory superficially as a framework but the theory was not used in the discussion of the results. Only 13% of the studies used the theory adequately. Among these are studies that tested propositions relevant to health and health promotion among adolescent diabetics (Frey and Fox, 1990), and relevance of the effects of computer-assisted instruction on avoidance of dust in adult asthmatics (Huss, Salerno, and Huss, 1991).

REFERENCES

Levine

Abdellah, F.G. and Levine, E. (1986). *Better patient care through nursing research* (3rd ed.). New York: Macmillan.

Artigue, G.S., Foli, K.J., Johnson, T., Marriner-Tomey, A., Poat, M.C., Poppa, L.D., Woeste, R., and Zoretich, S.T. (1994). Myra Levine: Four conservation principles. In A. Marriner-Tomey (Ed.). *Nursing theorists and their work* (4th ed., pp. 199–210). St. Louis: C.V. Mosby.

Barnum, B.J.S. (1994). *Nursing theory: Analysis, application, and evaluation* (4th ed.). Philadelphia: J.B. Lippincott.

Bertalanffy, L. (1968). *General system theory.* New York: George Braziller.

Buber, M. (1967). *Between man and man.* New York: Macmillan.

Cannon, W.B. (1939). *The wisdom of the body.* New York: W.W. Norton.

Cox, R.A., Sr. (1991). A tradition of caring: Use of Levine's model in long-term care. In K.M. Schaefer and J.B. Pond (Eds.), *Levine's conservation model: A framework for nursing practice* (pp. 179–197). Philadelphia: F.A. Davis.

Donaldson, S.K. and Crowley, D.M. (1978). The discipline of nursing. *Nursing Outlook,* 26(2), 113–120.

Dubos, R. (1966). *Man adapting.* New Haven, CT: Yale University Press.

Erikson, E. (1968). *Identity, youth and crisis.* New York: W.W. Norton.

Esposito, C.H. and Leonard, M.K. (1980). Myra Estrin Levine: In The Nursing Conference Group, *Nursing theories: The base for professional practice.* Englewood Cliffs, NJ: Prentice-Hall.

Fawcett, J. (1989). *Analysis and evaluation of conceptual models of nursing* (2nd ed.). Philadelphia: F.A. Davis.

Flaskerud, J.H. and Halloran, E.J. (1980). Areas of agreement in nursing theory development. *Advances in Nursing Science,* 3(1), 1–7.

Grindley, J. and Paradowski M. (1991). Developing an undergraduate program using Levine's model. In K.M. Schaefer and J.B. Pond (Eds.), *Levine's conservation model: A framework for nursing practice* (pp. 199–208). Philadelphia: F.A. Davis.

Hall, K.V. (1979). Current trends in the use of conceptual frameworks in nursing education. *Journal of Nursing Education,* 18(4), 26–29.

Hirschfeld, M.J. (1976). The cognitively impaired older adult. *American Journal of Nursing,* 76(12), 1981–1984.

Levine, M.E. (1966a). Trophicognosis: An alternative to nursing diagnosis. In *Exploring progress in medical-surgical nursing practice.* New York: American Nurses Association.

Levine, M.E. (1966b). Adaptation and assessment: A rationale for nursing intervention. *American Journal of Nursing,* 66(11), 2450–2453.

Levine, M.E. (1967). The four conservation principles of nursing. *Nursing Forum,* 6(1), 45–59.

Levine, M.E. (1969). The pursuit of wholeness. *American Journal of Nursing,* 69(1), 93–98.

Levine, M.E. (1971a). Holistic nursing. *Nursing Clinics of North America,* 6(2), 253–264.

Levine, M.E. (1971b, June). Time has come to speak of health care. *AORN Journal,* 13, 37–43.

Levine, M.E. (1973). *Introduction to clinical nursing* (2nd ed.). Philadelphia: F.A. Davis.

Levine, M.E. (1979). The science is spurious [letter to the editor]. *American Journal of Nursing,* 79(8), 1379–1383.

Levine, M.E. (1989a). The ethics of nursing rhetoric. *Image: Journal of Nursing Scholarship,* 21(1), 4–6.

Levine, M.E. (1989b). The four conservation principles: Twenty years later. In J.P. Riehl (Ed.), *Conceptional models for nursing practice* (3rd ed.). East Norwalk, CT: Appleton & Lange.

Levine, M.E. (1989c). Ethical issues in cancer care: Beyond dilemma. *Seminars in Oncology Nursing,* 5(2), 124–128.

Levine, M.E. (1990). Conservation and integrity. In M.E. Parker (Ed.), *Nursing theories in practice* (pp. 189–202. New York: National League for Nursing.

Newport, M.A. (1984). Conserving thermal energy and social integrity in the newborn. *Western Journal of Nursing Research,* 6, 176–197.

Nightingale, F. (1969). *Notes on nursing. What it is and what it is not.* New York: Dover Publications.

Pond, J.B. (1990). Application of Levine's conservation model to nursing the homeless community. In M.E. Parker (Ed.), *Nursing theories in practice* (pp. 203–216). New York: National League for Nursing.

Riehl, J.P. (1980). Nursing models in current use. In J.P. Riehl and C. Roy (Eds.), *Conceptual models for nursing practice* (2nd ed.). New York: Appleton-Century-Crofts.

Rogers, C.R. (1961). *On becoming a person.* Boston: Houghton-Mifflin.

Rogers, M.E. (1970). *An introduction to the theoretical basis of nursing.* Philadelphia: F.A. Davis.

Selye, H. (1956). *The stress of life.* New York: McGraw-Hill.

Taylor, J.W. (1974). Measuring the outcomes of nursing care. *Nursing Clinics of North America,* 9(2), 337–348.

Taylor, J.W. (1989). Levine's conservation principles: Using the model for nursing diagnosis in a neurological setting. In J. Riehl-Sisca (Ed.), *Conceptual models for nursing practice* (3rd ed.). East Norwalk, CT: Appleton & Lange.

Tillich, P. (1961). The meaning of health. *Perspectives in Biology and Medicine,* 5, 92–100.

Tompkins, E.S. (1980). Effect of restricted mobility and dominance on perceived duration. *Nursing Research,* 29(6), 333–338.

Webster's Third New International Dictionary. (1986). Springfield, MA: Merriam-Webster.

Orem

Abdellah, G.F., Beland, I.L., Martin, A., and Matheney, R.V. (1961). *Patient-centered approaches to nursing.* New York: Macmillan.

Allan, J.D. (1988). Knowing what to weigh: Woman self-care activities related to weight. *Advances in Nursing Science,* 11(1), 47–60.

Allison, S.E. (1973). A framework for nursing action in a nurse-conducted diabetic management clinic. *Journal of Nursing Administration,* 3(4), 53–60.

Anastasio, C., McMahan, T., Daniels, A., Nicholas, P.K., and Paul-Simon, A. (1995). Self care burden in women with human immunodeficiency virus. *Journal of the Association of Nurses in AIDS Care,* 6(3), 31–42.

Anna, D.J., Christensen, D.G., Hohn, S.A., Ord, L., and Wells, S.R. (1978). Implementing Orem's conceptual framework. *Journal of Nursing Administration,* 8(11), 8–11.

Backscheider, J.E. (1971). The use of self as the essence of clinical supervision in ambulatory patient care. *Nursing Clinics of North America,* 6(4), 785–794.

Backscheider, J.E. (1974). Self-care requirements, self-care capabilities, and nursing systems in the diabetic nurse management clinic. *American Journal of Public Health,* 64(12), 1138–1146.

Barnum, B.J.S. (1994). *Nursing theory: Analysis, application, and evaluation.* Philadelphia: J.B. Lippincott.

Bennett, J.G. (1980). Forward to the Symposium on the Self-care Concept in Nursing. *Nursing Clinics of North America,* 15(1), 129–130.

Bonamy, C., Schultz, P., Graham, K., and Hampton, M. (1995). The use of theory-based nursing practice in the Department of Veterans' Affairs Medical Centers. *Journal of Nursing Staff Development,* 11(1), 27–30.

Bromley, B. (1980). Applying Orem's self-care theory in enterostomal therapy. *American Journal of Nursing,* 80(2), 245–249.

Buckwalter, K.C. and Kerfoot, K.M. (1982). Teaching patients self-care: A critical aspect of psychiatric discharge planning. *Journal of Psychiatric Nursing and Mental Health Services,* 20(5), 15–20.

Caley, J.M., Dirksen, M., Engalla, M., and Hennrich, M. (1980). The Orem self-care nursing model. In J.P. Riehl and C. Roy (Eds.), *Conceptual models for nursing practice* (2nd ed.). New York: Appleton-Century-Crofts.

Campbell, J.C. (1986). Nursing assessment for risk of homicide with battered women. *Advances in Nursing Science,* 8(4), 36–51.

Campuzano, M. (1982, April/May). Self-care following coronary artery bypass surgery. *Focus,* 55–56.

Chang, B.L. (1980). Evaluation of health care professionals in facilitating self-care: Review of the literature and a conceptual model. *Advances in Nursing Science,* 3(1), 43–58.

Clark, M.D. (1986). Application of Orem's theory of self-care: A case study. *Journal of Community Health Nursing,* 3(3), 127–135.

Clinton, J.F., Denyes, M.J., Goodwin, J.O., and Koto, E.M. (1977). Developing criterion measures of nursing care: Case study of a process. *Journal of Nursing Administration,* 7(7), 41–45.

Coleman, L.J. (1980). Orem's self-care concept of nursing. In J.P. Riehl and C. Roy (Eds.), *Conceptual models for nursing practice* (2nd ed.). New York: Appleton-Century-Crofts.

Compton, P. (1989). Drug abuse, a self-care deficit. *Journal of Psychosocial Nursing,* 27(3), 22–26.

Dashiff, C.J. (1988). Theory development in psychiatric-mental health nursing: An analysis of Orem's theory. *Archives of Psychiatric Nursing,* 2(6), 366–372.

Denyes, M.J. (1982). Measurement of self-care agency in adolescents [Abstract]. *Nursing Research,* 31(1), 63.

Denyes, M.J., O'Connor, N.A., Oakley, D., and Ferguson, S. (1989). Integrating nursing theory, practice and research through collaborative research. *Journal of Advanced Nursing,* 14, 141–145.

Dropkin, M.J. (1981, April). Development of a self-care teaching program for postoperative head and neck patients. *Cancer Nursing,* 103–106.

Easton, K.L. (1993). Defining the concept of self-care. *Rehabilitation Nursing,* 18(6), 384–387.

Fawcett, J. (1989). *Analysis and evaluation of conceptual models of nursing* (2nd ed.). Philadelphia: F.A. Davis.

Fawcett, J. (1995). *Analysis and evaluation of conceptual models of nursing* (3rd ed.). Philadelphia: F.A. Davis.

Fenner, K. (1979). Developing a conceptual framework. *Nursing Outlook,* 27, 122–126.

Fitzgerald, S. (1980). Utilizing Orem's self-care nursing model in designing an educational program for the diabetic. *Topics in Clinical Nursing,* 2(2), 57–65.

Foster, P.C. and Janssens, N.P. (1980). Dorothea E. Orem. In The Nursing Theories Conference Group (Eds.), *Nursing theories: The base for professional nursing practice.* Englewood Cliffs, NJ: Prentice-Hall.

Frey, M.A. and Fox, M.A. (1990). Assessing and teaching self-care to youths with diabetes mellitus. *Pediatric Nursing,* 16, 597–800.

Gardulf, A., Bjorvell, H., Andersen, V., Bjorkander, J., Ericson, D., Froland, S.S., Gustafson, R., Hammarstrom, L., Nystrom, T., Soeberg, B., and Smith, C.I.E. (1995). Lifelong treatment with gammaglobulin for primary antibody deficiencies: The patients' experiences of subcutaneous self-infusions and home therapy. *Journal of Advanced Nursing,* 21(5), 917–927.

Greenfield, E. and Pace, J. (1985). Orem's self-care theory of nursing: Practical application to the end stage renal disease (ESRD) patient. *Journal of Nephrology Nursing,* 2(4), 187–193.

Hanson, B.R. and Bickel, L. (1985). Development and testing of the questionnaire on perception of self-care agency. In J. Riehl-Sisca, *The science and art of self-care.* Norwalk, CT: Appleton-Century-Crofts.

Hanucharurnkui, S. and Vinya-nguag, P. (1991). Effects of promoting patients' participation in self-care on post-operative recovery and satisfaction with care. *Nursing Science Quarterly,* 4(1), 14–20.

Hart, M.A. (1995). Orem's self-care deficit theory: Research with pregnant women. *Nursing Science Quarterly,* 8(3), 120–126.

Hartley, L.A. (1988). Congruence between teaching and learning self-care: A pilot study. *Nursing Science Quarterly,* 1(4), 161–167.

Harrison-Raines, K. (1993). Nursing and self-care theory applied to utilization review: Concepts and cases. *American Journal of Medical Quality,* 8(4), 197–199.

Henderson, V. (1966). *The nature of nursing.* New York: Macmillan.

Huss, K., Salerno, M., and Huss, R.W. (1991). Computer-assisted reinforcement of instruction: Effects on adherence in adult atopic asthmatics. *Research in Nursing and Health,* 14(4), 259–267.

Johnston, R.L. (1983). Orem self-care model of nursing. In J. Fitzpatrick and A. Whall (Eds.), *Conceptual models of nursing: Analysis and application*. Bowie, MD: Robert J. Brady Company.

Kearney, B.Y. and Fleischer, B.J. (1979). Development of an instrument to measure exercise of self-care agency. *Research in Nursing and Health*, 2(1), 25–34.

Kinlein, M.L. (1977). Self-care concept. *American Journal of Nursing*, 77, 598–601.

Kubricht, D. (1984). Therapeutic self-care demands expressed by outpatients receiving external radiation therapy. *Cancer Nursing*, 7, 43–52.

Kuriansky, J., Gurland, B., Fleiss, J., and Cowan, D. (1976). The assessment of self-care capacity in geriatric psychiatric patients by objective and subjective methods. *Journal of Clinical Psychology*, 32, 95–102.

Maunz, E.R. and Woods, N.F. (1988). Self-care practices among young adult women: Influence of symptoms, employment, and sex-role orientation. *Health Care for Women International*, 9, 29–41.

McBride, S. (1987). Validation of an instrument to measure exercise of self-care agency. *Research in Nursing and Health*, 10, 311–316.

McLaughlin, K. (1993). Implementing self-care deficit nursing theory: A process of staff development. In M.E. Parker (Ed.), *Patterns of nursing theories in practice* (pp. 241–251). New York: National League for Nursing.

Melnyk, K.A.M. (1983). The process of theory analysis: An examination of the nursing theory of Dorothea E. Orem. *Nursing Research*, 32(3), 170–174.

Michael, M.M. and Sewall, K.S. (1980). Use of the adolescent peer group to increase the self-care agency of adolescent alcohol abusers. *Nursing Clinics of North America*, 15, 157–176.

Miller, J.F. (1980). The dynamic focus of nursing: A challenge to nursing administration. *The Journal of Nursing Administration*, 10(1), 13–18.

Miller, J.F. (1982). Categories of self-care needs of ambulatory patients with diabetes. *Journal of Advanced Nursing*, 7, 25–31.

Moore, J.B. (1987). Effects of assertion training and first aid instruction on children's autonomy and self-care agency. *Research in Nursing and Health*, 10, 101–109.

Moore, J.B. (1995). Measuring self-care practice of children and adolescents: Instrument development. *Maternal-child Nursing Journal*, 23(3), 101–108.

Morse, W. and Werner, J.S. (1988). Individualization of patient care using Orem's theory. *Cancer Nursing*, 11(3), 195–202.

Mullin, V.I. (1980). Implementing the self-care concept in the acute care setting. *Nursing Clinics of North America*, 15(4), 177–190.

Murphy, P.P. (1981). A hospice model and self-care theory. *Oncology Nursing Forum*, 8(2), 19–21.

Noone, J. (1995). Acute pancreatitis: An Orem approach to nursing assessment and care. *Critical Care Nurse*, 15(4), 27–35.

Norris, M.K. (1991). Applying Orem's theory to the long-term care of adolescent transplant recipients. *American Nephrology Nurses' Association Journal*, 18(1), 45–47, 53.

Nursing Development Conference Group. (1973). *Concept formalization in nursing: process and product.* Boston: Little, Brown.

Nursing Development Conference Group. (1979). *Concept formalization in nursing: process and product* (2nd ed.). Boston: Little, Brown.

Orem, D.E. (1959). *Guides for developing curricula for the education of practical nurses.* Washington, DC: U.S. Department of Health, Education, & Welfare, Office of Education.

Orem, D.E. (1971). *Nursing: Concepts of practice.* New York: McGraw-Hill.

Orem, D.E. (1980). *Nursing concepts of practice* (2nd ed.). New York: McGraw Hill.

Orem, D.E. (1983). The self-care deficit theory of nursing: A general theory. In I.W. Clements and F.B. Roberts (Eds.), *Family health: A theoretical approach to nursing care.* New York: John Wiley & Sons.

Orem, D.E. (1985). *Nursing: Concepts of practice* (3rd ed.). New York: McGraw-Hill.

Orem, D.E. (1987). Orem's general theory of nursing. In R. Parse, *Nursing science: Major paradigms, theories, and critiques.* Philadelphia: W.B. Saunders.

Orem, D.E. (1989). Theories and hypotheses for nursing administration. In B. Henry, M. Di Vincenti, C. Arndt, and A. Marriner (Eds.), *Dimensions of nursing administration. Theory, research, education, and practice.* Boston: Blackwell Scientific Publications.

Orem, D.E. (1991). *Nursing: concepts of practice* (4th ed.). St. Louis: C.V. Mosby.

Orem, D.E. (1995). *Nursing: Concepts of practice* (5th ed.). St. Louis: C.V. Mosby.

Orem, D.E. and Taylor, S.G. (1986). Orem's general theory of nursing. In P. Winstead-Fry (Ed.), *Case studies in nursing theory.* New York: National League for Nursing.

Reid, B., Allen, A., Gauthier, T., and Campbell, H. (1989). Solving the Orem mystery: An educational strategy. *Journal of Continuing Education in Nursing*, 20(3), 8–11.

Riehl, J.P. and Roy, C. (Eds.). (1980). *Conceptual models for nursing practice* (2nd ed.). New York: Appleton-Century-Crofts.

Riehl-Sisca, J.P. (1989). *Conceptual models for nursing practice* East Norwalk, CT: Appleton & Lange.

Roberts, C.S. (1982). Identifying the real patient problems. *Nursing Clinics of North America*, 17(3), 481–489.

Rothlis, J. (1984). The effect of a self-help group on feelings of hopelessness and helplessness. *Western Journal of Nursing Research*, 6, 157–173.

Sandman, P.O., Norberg, A., Adolfsson, R., Axelsson, K., and Hedly, V. (1986). Morning care of patients with Alzheimer-type dementia. A theoretical model based on direct observations. *Journal of Advanced Nursing*, 11, 369–378.

Silva, M.C. (1986). Research testing nursing theory: State of the art. *Advances in Nursing Science*, 9(1), 1–11.

Smith, M.C. (1979). Proposed metaparadigm for nursing research and theory development. *Image*, 11(3), 75–79.

Smith, M.C. (1987). A critique of Orem's theory. In R.R. Parse, *Nursing science. Major paradigms, theories, and critiques.* Philadelphia: W.B. Saunders.

Spearman, S.A., Duldt, B.W. [illegible] Brown, S. (1993). Research testing theory: A selecti[illegible]view of Orem's self-care theory, 1986–1991. *Jo*[illegible]*of Advanced Nursing*, 18, 1626–1631.

Storm, D.S. and Ba[illegible]er, R.G. (1987). Achieving self-care in the ven[illegible]pendent patient: A critical analysis of a case [illegible] *[illegible]national Journal of Nursing Studies*, 24, 95–[illegible]

Taylor, S.G [illegible]rsing theory and nursing process: [illegible]ractice. *Nursing Science Quarterly*, [illegible]

[illegible]aughlin, K. (1991). Orem's general theory [illegible] Orem's [illegible]nd community nursing. *Nursing Science* [illegible] 1(3), [illegible]3–160.

Taylo[illegible] Effect of structured preparation for trans-[illegible] anxiety on leaving coronary care unit. *Nurs-*[illegible], 29(1), 28–34.

[illegible].R. (1980). Facilitating self-care. In P. Pothier [illegible] *[illegible]chiatric nursing*. Boston: Little, Brown.

Walborn, K.A. (1980). A nursing model for hospice: Primary and self-care. *Nursing Clinics of North America*, 15(1), 205–217.

Walker, D.M. (1993). A nursing administration perspective on use of Orem's self-care deficit nursing theory. In M.E. Parker (Ed.), *Patterns of nursing theories in practice* (pp. 252–264). New York: National League for Nursing.

Watkins, G. R. (1995). Patient comprehension of gastroenterology (GI) educational materials. *Gastroenterology Nursing*, 18(4), 123–127.

Weaver, M.T. (1987). Perceived self-care agency: A LISREL, factor analysis of Bickel and Hanson's questionnaire. *Nursing Research*, 36, 381–387.

Williams S. and Ramos, M.C. (1993). Mitral valve prolapse and its effects: A program of inquiry within Orem's self-care deficit theory of nursing. *Journal of Advanced Nursing*, 18, 242–251.

Williams, S., Shuster, G.F., III, Merwin, E., and Williams, B. (1994). A community-based smoking cessation program: Self-care behaviors and success. *Public Health Nursing*, 11(5), 291–299.

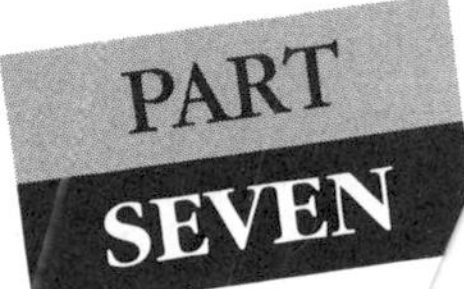

Our Theoretical Future (A Holograph of Past and Present)

Part Seven views the future of theoretical nursing as it is evolving from its past and present. It considers future challenges, stages, and milestones as they relate to the stages and milestones articulated and discussed in Part One. Further progress is explored under some of the premises also presented in Part One. The view presented in this part is not linear but holographic, that is to say, it sees past, present, and future through the same lenses and at the same instant it projects the future by seeing the past. The view is not static either but is limited to forces that exist at the turn of the 21st century. As new paradigms gain support within the discipline (paradigms that combine the empiricism of the West with the mysticism of the East) and as new trends influence nurses and their clients as human beings, the future may take different shapes and different forms.

This part closes with a short summary of salient future recommendations representing the perspective taken in this book.

CHAPTER 19

Theoretical Thinking and Practical Wisdom: Challenges for the Future

The task of developing theoretical frameworks that reflect clinical practice and better inform practice and drive the research in the discipline is not complete yet, nor will it ever be finished in dynamic and responsive disciplines (Meleis, 1992a). Theory as the link between research findings and practice utilization is dynamic, changing, and constantly evolving. Clinicians need and use theory to inform their practice. What helps clinicians is not *only* that patients' uncertainty about diagnosis and prognosis may be positively and directly related to slow progress in wound healing. It is also knowing that uncertainty in patients who have a life-style based on planning and certainty or who function better with a sense of control in their environment tend to have different recovery patterns than others who have had a life with more uncertainty. The first is a research hypothesis; the second is a theoretical proposition.

Theory is also the link between fragmented research and a coherent research program. How patients experience symptoms and interpret them, and the strategies they use to care for their symptoms in particular, and their health in general, is a theoretical question that may drive a number of research studies with populations who have experiences with different symptoms. The results of these studies add knowledge to self-care theories, provide support to develop new theories, and may refine existing theories on managing a number of illness experiences such as pain and shortness of breath, among other symptoms.

Theory provides the contextual interpretation of research findings and the framework to connect the different experiences nurses encounter. A theory on transition and health may alert nurses to use knowledge related to facilitating admission transition to inform their caring for patients undergoing other transitions. These experiences may, in turn, modify some of the theoretical interpretations regarding the admission transition. Theories allow the more complex interrelationships to be considered and, therefore, responses could be viewed more within a context of antecedents, consequences, as well as patterns, rather than isolated relationships, events, or responses.

Although theory has been instrumental in the general progress of the discipline of nursing, the most cogent and significant contributions that the nursing theorists have made is the promotion of theoretical thinking. Theoretical thinking is characterized by the ability to use frameworks to promote understanding, as well as the ability to be skeptical about the frameworks and their utility in exploring any, all, or part of health–illness situations. It is the ability to connect seemingly discrete, unconnected thoughts, observations, or facts and to see a coherent whole. It is abstract thinking that is grounded in exemplars from practice. A theoretical thinker is a reflective thinker who suspends the "fragmentedness" to allow exploring, explaining, and reinterpreting of wholes. A critical thinker is someone who is able to explore and describe patterns and not only discrete facts, and who engages in individual ontological dialogues, as well as similar dialogues with others. A theoretical thinker is a critical thinker with a goal of discerning patterns, connecting ideas, and developing explanatory models, to ask and answer the whats, why nots, and what ifs. A critical thinker is one who is inquisitive, truth seeking, systematic, and analytical (Dewey, 1982; Facione, Facione, and Sanchez, 1994). A theoretical thinker would not allow procedures and rules alone to drive his or her focus or explorations; rather he or she would use them only as tools that must be considered, revisited, and revised. Theoretical thinking includes critical consideration of the discipline's central phenomena and questions. Theories are dynamic and always changing and as Levine (1995) admonished, they "are not written in stone."

A theoretical thinker would question whichever prevailing models have governed his or her nursing care. An example of a model that has been critically analyzed is the biomedical model. The biomedical model as a framework for health care has been challenged because of its limited effectiveness (Engel, 1977) and challenged by nurses as inappropriate for the mission of nursing (Allan and Hall, 1988; Shaver, 1985). Others have described the differences in perspectives between nursing and other health fields and the uniqueness of the nursing perspective despite its dependent and interdependent functions (Visintainer, 1986).

Nursing theorists have demonstrated theoretical thinking and are among those nurses who not only challenged the biomedical model, but who also proactively conceptualized different aspects of the territory of nursing. Their conceptualizations provided the bases for identifying nursing perspectives and for defining our nursing domain. It is because of their pioneering work that members of the discipline continue to discuss the theoretical bases of practice and pose and answer theoretically driven questions. This theoretical thinking must continue to be promoted in nursing education, administration, and research.

This concluding chapter has three purposes. Its first purpose is to discuss the challenges that may shape theoretical nursing in the future. Its second purpose is to identify the next stages and milestones in the development and progress of theoretical nursing. Its third purpose is to provide the reader with some recommendations and guidelines related to the continuous progress of theoretical nursing. The ultimate purpose of this chapter is to maintain an open and ongoing dialogue about theoretical nursing.

Challenges

Theories developed in the future will reflect a close connection with clinical practice. Clinical practice is shaped by societies and, therefore, changes in society and in the health care system are driving the changes in clinical practice in nursing. Clinical practice, in turn, will influence the nature of theories that are developed in the discipline. To stimulate you to identify social trends that you think may influence the types of theories developed, I selected a few to share with you. These, I believe, are a few vital trends that will be reflected in the kinds of theories that nurses will develop (Meleis, 1996).

The Nature of Practice

The nature of nursing practice is profoundly influenced by the sociocultural and political events in any society. Major changes have occurred in the health care system during the 1990s that will continue to influence the types of theories that nurses may develop as well as the utility of these theories. The movements to primary health care and managed care increase the potential of maintaining a primary caregiver, but also decrease the amount of time that nurses spend with patients. Theories of the late 1990s that provided guidelines for developing trust and strong interpersonal ties with patients, the role of the self in the healing processes, and the extensive assessment and monitoring that nurses were able to perform during long hospitalizations or repeated visits will be limited. Models to promote patient–nurse relationships within the constraints dictated by time and more economically driven health care encounters will be developed. Therefore, the nature of relationships needs to be redefined, and ways by which such relationships may be established need to be reconsidered.

Most of the theories that have been developed have started from the premise that the nursing client is a hospitalized person. Over the years, patients have moved out of hospitals earlier, and whenever possible they are cared for on an outpatient basis. Although public health nurses have always given care to patients in communities and in their homes, the practice of public health nursing is undergoing drastic changes simultaneously, and patients are also going home with more acute conditions and with a need for monitoring of their critical needs with time limitations and budgetary constraints.

The nature of practice is also changing in a third major way. International mandates (World Health Organization, 1978) for better health care have advocated community-based primary health care as the practice of choice to ensure better health care for people and better access to health care. Community-based health care requires the development of models for care that are more complex and contextual and created with clients' involvement.

The nature of practice is also being influenced by the changing roles of the advanced nursing practice clinicians and may require rethinking theories needed for their practice (Davies and Hughes, 1995). An additional example is the increasing number of generalists and primary health care providers in medicine and the changes in their educational preparation and training. Another is the increasing number of care assistants and physician's assistants.

The Nature of Clients

Who the clients are and how they tend to define and interpret their patient status will drive theoretical nursing of the future. Clients have become more informed over the years and have become vocal about what they need from their health care providers.

Clients are embedded in multidimensional and dynamic contexts that are constantly changing (Reed, 1995). Theories that have defined clients as passive recipients of care or as human beings who are waiting for information and those that assumed that the nurse's role is to ensure compliance are no longer congruent with how clients define themselves (Allen, 1987). Clients come to the health care system either with their consciousness raised about their rights for information, for care, and for participation in decision making, or if they do not come with such expectations, the caring encounter may then include opportunities for consciousness raising. In either case, theories for the future must be developed to reflect the changing assumptions about clients and their levels of awareness and consciousness and must also provide some strategies by which consciousness may be raised within the value and belief systems of the clients.

Nurses deal with much more diversity in clients than has been the case historically; diversity in clients with regard to gender, race, ethnicity, or religion has always been, to a certain extent, a hallmark of health care practice; however, at the turn of the century, diversity has taken on another meaning and more significance because it comes with more questioning about the melting pot model of integration. Clients assert their identities, whether that identity is related to ethnic background or to sexual orientation. Clients are saying, "We like who we are, we do not want to assume or pretend otherwise, and we want to be respected and treated with sensitivity and with competence that includes our value systems and beliefs." This assertion requires different assumptions and different propositions that must be reflected in theories of the future.

Many world events are increasing transitions of people between countries and within countries through immigration and emigration. These transitions profoundly influence the health care and health outcomes of populations. There is also an increased population of the elderly in the world, and this brings with it a corresponding increase in health care needs. The elderly require different types of expertise from nurses. Nurses are also needed to help individuals live with and cope with long-term illnesses. Who the clients are, how they respond to their situation, how society has defined them, and how they define and redefine themselves are questions that can be answered only within sociocultural, economic, and political contexts. Attention to these questions and their answers could increase the power of theories to explain responses to health care.

The Nature of the Environment

Clients' environments and nurses' environments are undergoing tremendous changes that will then drive theory development in different ways. A plausible scenario is the expansion of the environment to include outer space, with all the changes in the nature of care that will need to become more congruent with the changing environment. Other changes in environment are related to levels of risks in the environment, such as increasing pollution, decreasing protection offered by the ozone layer, increasing aggression and decreasing safety, and increasing globalization. Each one of these will influence and drive the nature of theories in different ways and will require models that address the nature of healthy environments and strategies by which a healthy environment may be created and supported. Theories of the future will also have to address global issues, as well as strategies to provide care that evolve from an international perspective (Kleffel, 1996).

There have been many natural disasters (earthquakes and floods) and human-made disasters (wars; nuclear plant explosions like the one in Chernobyl, Ukraine, in 1986; and bombings) that not only require the immediate involvement of nurses, but require long-term attention while people are coping with the aftermath of these events. These situations drive the need for even more informed theories about environments and the different meanings of environments. For example, the earthquake in Kobe, Japan in 1995 and the Loma Prieta earthquake near San Francisco in 1989 prompt a reflection on nursing and ways by which nursing could contribute to the health care of people who have experienced such devastating events. The questions that these events raise for nurses are:

Who are the target populations?

Who gets marginalized during the disaster and during the long healing processes?

What processes do people go through as they begin to heal from the effects of the experience?

What strategies do nurses use to create a healing environment and to enhance people's well-being in the process of transition toward healing?

What are the milestones and critical periods in the long recovery process that nurses need to be aware of?

These are some of the questions that will drive the theories that will be developed to inform nursing practice.

The Nature of Analysis

A tendency to develop taxonomies characterized disciplinary analyses during the last decade of this century. Two types of taxonomies were developed—nursing diagnosis and nursing intervention. The work on defining and identifying nursing diagnosis began in nursing in 1950 (Gordon, 1979; McManus, 1950) and in the 1980s on nursing intervention in Iowa (Iowa Intervention Project, 1993, 1995). The taxonomic definitions were seriously considered after the pioneering efforts of Gebbie and Lavin, who initiated the first national conference on classification of nursing diagnosis in St. Louis in 1971 (Gebbie and Lavin, 1975). The results of seven such conferences have been the identification of 50 to 70 labels for nursing diagnosis and an increasing number of research projects in which the authors designed studies to validate nursing diagnosis and other studies to identify nursing diagnosis in diverse groups (Gordon, 1985; Kim, 1989). The result also has been an acceptance of nursing diagnosis as a significant step in clinical judgment and as a concept with great utility in nursing practice, as evidenced in the number of clinical writings about the concept, its appearance on agendas for nursing conferences, and its inclusion in the definition of nursing (American Nurses Association, 1995). Taxonomies will continue to shape the nature of knowledge developed. To project into the future, let's step back into the past to analyze how nursing diagnosis and theory were connected. There are two ways to consider the relationship between nursing theory and nursing diagnosis: first, one can consider how nursing theory has influenced the development of nursing diagnosis; and second, one can consider how nursing diagnosis has contributed to the development of nursing theory.

The impetus for the development of nursing diagnosis has some theoretical characteristics when viewed from the perspective of identifying and defining labels for judgments that nurses make in their daily practice. As Kritek (1978) indicated, these judgments about assessments are examples of factor-isolating theories, which were defined by Dickoff, James, and Wiedenbach in 1968. This type of theory specifies, describes, defines, and classifies concepts.

The process of identifying what nurses assess and what judgments they make is also characterized by some features that later nursing philosophers and theorists advocated. Nurses were asked to look at their own practice, to trust their assessments, to uncover their judgments, and to collaborate in a long process of specifying, defining, and identifying. The processes that organizers of the nursing diagnosis conferences, the attendees, and all others who participated in the nursing diagnosis movement have used are processes of theoretical thinking geared toward the goal of the theoretical development of the discipline.

Nursing diagnoses or nursing interventions, however, did not emerge from a coherent philosophical approach or from a theoretically defined domain. Although they represent the realities of those nurses who participated in developing the taxonomies and the classifications, they do not represent the majority of nurses who have been caring for clients and for communities for years and whose levels of expertise range from the novice to the expert, nor could they do that. Assumptions held by nurses and shared assumptions of the domain have not been adequately, carefully, or systematically discussed, nor have they reflected on the nursing diagnosis and intervention literature. Therefore, to summarize comments on ways by which nursing theory has influenced nursing diagnosis and interventions, I would say that the quest for theoretical development of the discipline may have guided the *process* of attempting to classify labels used in judging the condition of nursing clients and nurses' actions, but it did not guide the *content* of these labels. The content of the classification categories was predicated on diverse values, assumptions, and visions of the mission of nursing that remain to be identified and defined; they were also predicated on a problem orientation to care rather than an asset approach to care. A theoretical approach based on assets, health maintenance, and health promotion is a more congruent approach to the mission of nursing. This approach continues to be limited in the current framework for nursing diagnosis and intervention.

Attempts at relating existing nursing theories to the accepted diagnoses and interventions and to the development of useful, coherent, and supported nursing theories that may create new diagnoses and interventions should be of interest to theory students. One approach to theory development may be more useful than the other; however, with the level of enthusiasm in the classification of nursing diagnosis and nursing intervention movements, I propose that we carefully chart mechanisms to ensure that the former approach (accepted diagnoses and interventions) should not overshadow the latter (the development of theory leading to new diagnoses and interventions).

A second way by which the relationship between nursing theory and nursing diagnosis and intervention could be considered is to analyze the contributions of the classification systems to the development of nursing theory. I will focus here on the nursing diagnoses as an example. Similar analysis could be applied to nursing interventions.

There are at least three consequences of the nursing diagnosis movement to theoretical nursing.

First, nursing diagnosis created a theoretical discourse in the literature that is useful in analyzing philosophical bases and values and potentially useful in the further development and progress of theoretical nursing. Examples are the Shamansky and Yanni (1983) and Kritek (1985) debates about assumptions regarding the development of nursing diagnosis, the role of nursing diagnosis in knowledge development in the discipline, and the implicit limitations of the concept of nursing diagnosis. Other examples are the analysis of implicit values inherent in nursing diagnosis and in the dependent and independent roles of nurses (Jacoby, 1985; Kim, 1985; Kritek, 1979).

Second, the publication and use of nursing diagnoses have prompted a reevaluation of some of the labels and their meanings, a theoretical process that is defined as concept classification (Dennison and Keeling, 1989; Jenny, 1987).

Third, the nursing diagnosis movement has stimulated nursing researchers to initiate studies to identify nursing diagnoses and to validate existing ones (Gordon, 1985; Kim, 1989). A next step beyond the analysis of research findings is the initiation of further dialogue to interpret the theoretical and philosophical implications of these findings.

A taxonomy of nursing diagnoses and nursing interventions does not represent a theory; it is just a classification system Each of the diagnostic labels and each of the intervention's labels represent a concept that may be a building block for a potential nursing theory related to that concept, if and when the concept is defined within a context of assumptions, values, nursing mission, and other concepts representing the domain of nursing; and when it is related to health and well-being as the goals of nursing. Two types of theories could be developed: descriptive/explanatory and prescriptive theories. The nursing diagnosis label of "comfort (alterations in)," for example, is only meaningful within a theory that describes comfort and its relationship to the health of clients as viewed from the perspective of the domain of nursing, with its focus on person–environment interaction and responses to health and illness. It is also useful when they are based on some well defined and shared ontological beliefs and dialogues about the epistemology used to arrive at the classification systems that are well formed and informed.

The Nature of Technology and Information

Theories of the future will be profoundly influenced by the nature of technological development and by how technology is used in practice, research, teaching, and administration. We are moving steadfastly into an era where there will be client-centered information systems, organized data sets, where many aspects of people's lives will be dominated by computers, and increasing availability of health care information to the public will be disseminated through network systems. Our challenge is to address ways by which theoretical frameworks and informatics will interface, especially while nurses continue to adopt pluralistic philosophies in defining, connecting, and using data for nursing practice, research, and policy development. Although there is equal concern in selecting one theory or classification system prematurely to guide these processes, the risks may be higher in not settling on one shared framework. The challenge is to resolve these conflicts and to settle on a framework or frameworks that will facilitate exchanges and drive a more common and congruent set of outcomes. The challenge to face in the future is in the development of processes to integrate the development of informatic and theoretical nursing and to guide and develop informatics within the mission, the goals, and theories that reflect the discipline and the goals of health care (Hays, Norris, Martin, and Androwich, 1994).

Because of increased use of technology, insurance-driven policies related to hospitalization and discharge, and increasing costs of hospitalization worldwide, patients tend to leave hospitals earlier and continue their recovery and rehabilitation transition at home. The transition to recovery is somewhat more protracted, and patients need expert and competent care at home. These trends will drive the development of theories to reflect a new set of emerging care needs for patients.

Theoretical Nursing and Theory Development

These challenges will shape the future of theoretical nursing which, in turn, will influence the types of theories nurses develop as well as nursing education and administration.

The development of theories in the future must avoid what Bradshaw (1995) warns against—ignoring the nursing tradition of practical tasks and techniques of physical care and focusing only on a psychosocial approach to patient care and knowledge development. She proposes that nurses engaged in the development of knowledge must consider rediscovering theories that hold together the personal, the relational, the scientific, and technological aspects of patient care. The significance of theories in answering the pressing questions in nursing will depend on the extent to which these theories reflect the history and practice of nursing and the extent to which they include the principles outlined below.

A Global View

One of the principles that could empower nurses is to participate in the development of cross-national knowledge that benefits from participation of colleagues from different parts of the world. Although certain aspects of nursing interventions are culturally contexted, the phenomena themselves transcend cultures and societies. Comforting patients, helping wounds heal, feeding the elderly, increasing mobility and activity, rehydrating populations, preserving the integrity of clients, promoting health, developing healthy environments, promoting rest, supporting sleep, intubating, monitoring, managing symptoms, and decreasing pain are examples of phenomena that nurses deal with around the globe.

Covering the various dimensions about the nature of phenomena through international work creates knowledge that is more culturally sensitive and empowers nurses to influence policy changes related to health care. Sharing and reciprocating findings about phenomena increases nurses' repertoires of therapeutics that would, in turn, enhance their effectiveness in caring for diverse populations. The principle of a global view and worldliness could ensure that nurses' efforts in knowledge development become more cumulative and more culturally sensitive. Culturally sensitive theories help nurses become more culturally competent in a world that is constantly in transition and in a world in which patients tend to reflect diversity. This principle mandates thinking internationally in every aspect of our work and in the theories that we attempt to develop.

Marginalization

Dr. Hiroshi Nakajima, the Director General of the World Health Organization, warned us that history will judge the 20th century as the "era when human development faltered and gave rise to a wave of poverty" (Nakajima, 1995, p. 25). Growing inequality in the world and within countries is in his words, "a matter of life and death." There is an urgent need to develop knowledge about marginalization and about responses to marginalization on the quality of health care delivered to and received by marginalized people. Several components of marginalization are pertinent to nursing. The definition of marginalization highlights the effects of being in stigmatized jobs, being from another culture, having a sexual preference different from the prevailing norms, or for not having some of the more mainstream characteristics that represent those who are at the center of communities; rather, they are at the peripheries of communities. The elderly who live alone, or who have memory loss, are marginalized. People who fall between the cracks are marginalized, for example, in earthquakes, they are the rescue workers, they are the bystanders, they are the ones who may not be direct victims, but nevertheless, they experience the traumas and their well-being is profoundly influenced (Taylor and Frazer, 1982). When people are marginalized, they are stripped of their voice, stripped of their power, and stripped of their rights to resources. Marginalized people tend to be reflective about their own situation and develop their own symbols and language that marginalize them more. Having unique symbols, language, dress code, and place to meet further marginalizes them. Having delayed reactions may marginalize people. Although they may not represent another culture—the language, their responses, and their reactions reflect their own lexicon and their own symbols. This lexicon and the symbolism in it may not be well understood by others and they become even more pushed to the periphery and less powerful. Marginalized people tend to be more sensitive to the needs of others, know more about nonmarginalized people, and to be less demanding of other people, but the reverse is not always true (Hall, Stevens, and Meleis, 1994). Theories of the future must address the situation of marginalized clients in the health care system and reflect health and illness responses within a context of marginalization.

Situation-Specific Theories

A third principle is that of specificity. It may seem paradoxical to speak of global views and worldliness and at the same time of specificity as principles to guide the progress in theory development. Although the nature and goals of these two guiding principles are different, they are complementary rather than mutually exclusive. Whereas worldliness requires attention to what nurses tend to diagnose and practice in different countries, specificity calls for the development of theories that are more situation specific. Theories developed with the principle of specificity require a focus on describing, explaining, or predicting a phenomenon within a specific descriptive and explanatory context. These are also theories that focus on uncovering voices, identifying patterns, and interpreting themes. These theories are contextualized and represent many truths about similar situations with different populations. They help illuminate the experiences of populations, as well as the situation for nurses. Situation-specific theories respect mind–body wholeness, environment–person connections; they allow for multiplicity of truth, for tentativeness of interpretation, and for complexity of contexts. Situation-specific theories are generally used to formulate questions and answer questions within a context. They help in explaining situations that are limited in scope and in focus. An example of such theories is symptom-specific theory versus a theory of symptom management or a theory of unpleasant symptoms. Another example is a theory identity and health versus African-American identity and the psychotherapeutic environment (Brown, 1996; Lenz, Suppe, Gift, Pugh, and Milligan, 1995; Meleis, Isenberg, Koerner, Lacey, and Stern, 1995; University of California, San Francisco, School of Nursing Symptom Management Faculty Group, 1994).

Theoretical Nursing and Nursing Education

Theoretical nursing includes a discourse about the structure of nursing knowledge, the philosophical bases of nursing science, theory development, the history of nursing knowledge, and nursing theories. Aspects of these components have been included in doctoral nursing programs in the United States (Jacobs-Kramer and Huether, 1988) and internationally. A more limited version has been included in master programs with more emphasis on presentations and critique of existing nursing theories (Jacobson, 1987). Although nursing theories have been used as frameworks for nursing curricula in undergraduate programs during the 1970s and 1980s, only a limited number have included opportunities to discuss theoretical nursing and approaches to theory development (Jacobs-Kramer and Huether, 1988; Meleis and Price, 1988).

Theoretical thinking, the pride a member of a discipline has in the theoretical threads in one's discipline, a belief in the self as a proactive developer of knowledge, and an identity that incorporates the ability to structure nursing knowledge are values essential for quality care and for the continuous development of the discipline. The seeds for such values could and should be planted in students as early as possible in nursing education. It is not enough to promote these values in doctoral programs, or in master's programs; they should be planted as early as the first year of nurses' educations (Rafferty, Allcock, and Lathlean, 1996). Introducing theoretical nursing to students at the undergraduate level is not too early (Batra, 1987). Therefore, if nursing expects to have a significant impact on health care through development and use of theory, content related to the purpose, generation, and use of theory must be introduced into the curricula much earlier than it currently is (Jacobs-Kramer and Huether, 1988, p. 376).

In introducing such content, educators may reflect on the place for such content in curricula. When content related to theory and knowledge development is introduced as a separate component of a nursing curriculum, students and faculty experience difficulties in relating this content to other curricular components. Although this practice may have been necessary in the decades when the primacy of theoretical nursing was still debated, faculty members and students may now be ready to integrate that content with clinical and research components of the curriculum. To capture students' attention, to sensitize them to the significance of theory in their practice or research, and to demystify theory, teaching of theory must come out of its closet and it must be innovative and integrated (Karmels, 1993). When faculty are skeptical about theoretical nursing, they cannot persuade students of its importance (Levine, 1995).

Theoretical nursing provides nursing curricula with a perspective that is uniquely nursing's; it provides nursing students with frameworks that help them define their values, concepts in their work, significant problems in their fields, and approaches to structuring and developing knowledge. More importantly, a theoretical nursing perspective promotes the primacy of discovering, developing, and structuring nursing knowledge.

The relationship between theory and nursing curricula is similar to the relationship that research had to nursing curricula. Educators asked whether or not research courses should be in the curriculum, at what level they should be introduced, and what should be included (Wilson, 1985). The questions related to theory, theoretical nursing, and philosophy are no longer whether theory should be a component of nursing programs, or at what level it should be introduced; rather the questions educators will grapple with during the next decade are what aspects of theory should be introduced at every educational level and what are the most effective and meaningful ways by which they should be included.

Theoretical Nursing and Nursing Administration

> Nursing administrators can directly influence efforts to generate nursing's knowledge by providing access to a virtually untapped theory building resource—the non-university service setting. (DeGroot, Ferketich, and Larson, 1987, p. 38)

This sentiment of the close connection between nursing administration and nursing knowledge and of the potential of nursing theory construction by or as promoted by nursing administrators was expressed repeatedly in the late 1980s (an example is the volume edited by Henry, Arndt, Di Vincenti, and Marriner-Tomey, 1989). Until the late 1980s, there was a limited dialogue about the relationship of nursing theory and nursing administration (Christmyer, Catanzariti, Langford, and Reiz, 1988). Some addressed the shortcomings of that limited dialogue, indicating that specialty nursing cannot afford to be distanced from mainstream nursing by claiming that nursing theories do not represent them (Dashiff, 1988).

Viewing nursing administration from a domain perspective and investigating theoretical and clinical questions from that perspective could lead to a more coherent approach to structuring knowledge that is as useful to clinicians as it may be to administrators. Theories for the future must address the innovative relationship between practice, information, computer usage, skills acquisition, and clinical judgments (Anderson,

Dobal, and Blessing, 1992). Theoretical aspects of the domain of nursing may provide clinicians and administrators with a unifying framework that could further contribute to the development of coherent theories to guide nursing care (Jennings and Meleis, 1988; Meleis and Jennings, 1989).

New Stages . . . New Milestones

Stages

In Chapter 3, the development of theoretical nursing was described in terms of six stages. These were:

Stage of Practice
Stage of Education and Administration
Stage of Research
Stage of Nursing Theory
Stage of Philosophy
Stage of Integration

In Chapter 10, nursing was described as a scholarly discipline. The next stages in the development of nursing knowledge are projected as the reaching out/public stage.

The Reaching Out/Public Stage

This stage is defined as going beyond the confines of the discipline and beyond the usual mainstream nursing clients. Reaching out includes but is not limited to reaching out to develop theories that are useful in understanding and caring for clients from different socioeconomic and cultural backgrounds. It also includes having a voice and marketing nursing discoveries, ideas, and goals to members of other disciplines and the public.

Characteristics of this stage are a focus on the development of phenomena that reflect the situation and the experiences of minorities and vulnerable, underserved, and underrepresented populations. Theories developed during this stage allow for understanding of phenomena from diverse perspectives (Meleis, Isenberg, Koerner, Lacey, and Stern, 1995). Nursing is going public and nurses are much more aware of the power of influencing policies by involving the public. Nursing's history may be the reason why nurse scholars became more aware than other health care scholars of their role as a voice for the voiceless and as advocates for those who are in dire need of their advocacy. Therefore, communicating with the public through such avenues as the media to describe and report nurses' goals and actions is another characteristic of this stage. An example of the gap in this information is nurses' claims of health and well-being as a domain focus and the limited recognition of this mission by members of the other disciplines as well as by the public.

Another significant characteristic of reaching out is manifested in the promotion of collaboration with international colleagues and the increase in published dialogues about phenomena that represent the nursing domain and that represent diverse explanations.

Milestones

Nine milestones were identified in Chapter 3; these are presented below, and a tenth one also is defined.

Prior to 1955—From Florence Nightingale to nursing research
1955–1960—The birth of nursing theory: The Columbia University Teachers College approach
1961–1965—Theory: A national goal in nursing
1966–1970—Theory development: A tangible goal for academics
1971–1975—Theory syntax
1976–1980—A time to reflect
1981–1985—Nursing theories' revival: Emergence of the domain concepts
1986–1990—From metatheory to concept development
1990–1995—Mid-range and situation-specific theories
1995 and beyond—Multidiscipline theories

These milestones represent the development of theoretical nursing from 1955 to 1995 and beyond. At the turn of the century, there is awareness and heightened consciousness of the domain of nursing by nurses in many special clinical and functional fields. The discipline of nursing with its perspective, domain, theories, and research is used as the organizing framework and as substantive content for education, clinical practice, and research. There is less need for advocacy of nursing and a preoccupation with the rationale for nursing theories. Nursing programs discuss and use nursing theories in addition to theories from other disciplines. Graduates of programs where nursing theories are used are aware of the strengths and limitations in utility of nursing theory and the strengths and limitations of theories that were developed to answer questions that are more central and more relevant to other disciplines.

The syntactical debates (theory versus conceptual framework; nursing theory versus borrowed theory; and qualitative versys quantitative methods) are fading and give way to substantive debates (different views of health, environment, client, and communities). Indications of refinement/extension of theories began in the early 1980s and gained momentum at the turn of the 21st century. Relationships between domain concepts were being explored using existing nursing theories and other pertinent theories, such as interpersonal relations and the delivery of nursing care (nursing therapeutics), resulting in theoretical exemplars that could guide nursing research (Kasch, 1984; see examples of theory support in Chaps. 15 through 18; Meleis, 1992b).

Although philosophical discussions and theoretical exchanges are useful, their utility is limited without considering related research as an integral part of these discussions. This view is congruent with the more contemporary view of science (Laudan, 1981). Theorists, researchers, clinicians, and educators explicitly state the theoretical underpinnings of their work and to engage in dialogues with self and others to help in identifying relationships or the lack of them within the nursing domain. Such discussions helped to refine both the domain and the work being done.

Because our scholarly work centers around and emanates from the domain, special interest groups emerged as (what Merton calls) a "community of scholars" who, in turn, helped in the refinement and extension processes (Merton, 1973). These communities of scholars were organized around substantive nursing areas, such as mobility, rest, nursing interventions, quality of care, symptom management, women's health, nursing theories, and nursing diagnosis among others.

While striving for an approach in care and in research that is congruent with holism and nonreductionism, there is acceptance that the limited tools and methodologies have not constrained serious work that may combine reductionism with holism, objectivity with subjectivity, stability with change, and empiricism with historicism. To hold up theoretical and research investigation until all our premises, concepts, propositions, and research are congruent would be to hold up progress. Inconsistencies, paradoxes, and oppositions, if viewed as functions of the time, may still contribute to the goal of total congruence or collaboration. Neither end of the pole (that is, total congruence or total incongruence) is conducive to solving problems in a field. A healthy presence of multiple perspectives, even though sometimes inconsistent, is bound to help us understand the richness of the multiple realities of nursing.

Nursing theories of the past, present, or the future do not answer all the questions that nurses may ask; neither do sociological, psychological, physiologic, or engineering theories. Different theories in each of these disciplines answer different questions, and yet some questions still have not been answered satisfactorily. Other questions that appeared to be answered satisfactorily were being challenged by new data and new competing explanations, for example, Margaret Mead's cultural determinism and Sigmund Freud's seduction theories. These we have learned were not reasons to condescendingly brush away nursing theory or nurses' abilities to develop theories. The next milestone demonstrates a new maturity in the discipline—members of the discipline continue to develop theories; however, they join with other colleagues in developing theories that are of utility to other disciplines. Theories related to symptom management, women's health, and health care for manginalized populations are examples of multidiscipline theories.

The End for Now! On Practical Wisdom

The major goals of this book are to make a contribution to raising the consciousness of the reader about the theoretical development and progress of our discipline, to acknowledge our theoretical history, to place the present in the context of our history, and to develop an awareness of the potential inherent in members of the discipline, men or women. To paraphrase McBride (1986), the future should not be viewed with apologies nor should we be highlighting and focusing on our inadequacies; rather, we should develop and nurture a sense that theoretical nursing has contributed a great deal to the present maturity of the discipline.

Within these goals, the following points were made in this book:

1. Nurses have a fine and useful theoretical heritage that is worthy of analysis. By understanding how and why our heritage evolved as it did, we may be in a better position to consciously and deliberately drive the development of theoretical nursing to meet the mission that we have articulated about our discipline.

2. Nurses have the resources by which they can conceptualize different aspects of their universe for the purpose of facilitating understanding, increasing autonomy in their actions, and enhancing control over their domain for the ultimate objective of providing the kind of quality care they aspire to. The resources and the tools differ, based on education and experience; however, it was proposed here that the clinicians are as valuable as the theoreticians because they articulate their practical wisdom into exemplars that may help to solve other clinical problems.
3. The scientific development of the discipline of nursing has followed a unique path that was charted by members of the discipline to suit its unique features and its nursing care complexities. Sociology of nursing science and philosophy of nursing science are legitimate and significant areas of investigation to discern the progress and development of the discipline. As nurses question the empiricist's view of science and begin to embrace other more dynamic and changing conceptions of science, the behavior of scientists and theoreticians, the processes of selection of research and theories, the historical environment, and the sociocultural context for the development and utility of the discipline's theories become legitimate and central questions.
4. Our theoretical history, our epistemology, and our domain are the bases for our theoretical future. The novice should be acquainted with them, the advanced should explore and question the relationships between the parts and, together with the experienced, they should shape and reshape nursing knowledge. More specifically, I propose four avenues to pursue to begin a pattern of practical wisdom. These are not exhaustive, but should be considered as a beginning for others the reader may identify:
   - A deliberate plan to engage in *theoretical dialogues* should be developed and implemented in educational and clinical institutions. The extent to which the discipline of nursing will continue to evolve with a theoretical base depends on the ability of its members to engage in theoretical discussion and debates at all levels of education and practice. Opportunities for theoretical thinking could be found in the dailiness of students' lives (classroom teaching as well as clinical mentorship), and in clinicians' lives (shift reports as well as supervisory education).
   - Analytical and critical consideration of nursing theories should be a cornerstone of curricula in nursing, from community college to doctoral programs, with different goals at each educational level. For example, a choice of discussion of human beings as nursing clients may be organized around nursing theories that discuss human beings and the different goals of the different perspectives.
   - Consideration of research and clinical exemplars that are related to different domain concepts and questions and beginning attempts at a thorough review may help in creating some coherence and may delineate further avenues of investigation.
   - The advanced clinicians and clinical specialists can be coached to develop and share their wisdom gleaned from their clinical practice in the form of exemplars. Exemplars identify, model, and direct problems of concern to nursing and ways of solving these problems.

What Johnson referred to as "practical wisdom" (1959, p. 294) characterizes nursing at the turn of the century. Practical wisdom is manifested in actions that are theoretically sound and are designed to make a difference in the lives of people and provide some good for them. It includes a deliberate action that is subjected to reflection and analysis. Lauder (1994) differentiated between theoretical knowledge and practical wisdom, with the former ending up with an intellectual conclusion and the latter with action that is morally good for human beings. The age of wisdom encompasses all the properties of the stages that the discipline of nursing has experienced, not in a cumulative way but rather synthetically and developmentally, with experience and practice as its hallmark. There will be more acceptance of the complexity and fluidity of nursing concepts and the significance of the temporal dimension in our research and theory development. Natural turns and detours will be made with ease and comfort, just as Newton made a natural turn to astronomy because, at that time, finding one's way in the sea had been a preoccupation of the time, or just as Kepler turned to astrology and used it during the Thirty Years' War.

Using theories and developing new theories will benefit from temporal experiences. From such use and further development comes wisdom. Although we must not forget Bacon's reasoning for empirical testing or Kant's insistence on *a priori* conceptual schemata independent of experience, a practice discipline such as nursing cannot exist if it forgets Kaplan's advice that the pursuit of wisdom expresses a deep concern with the good that can be achieved in human life. Those benefits resulting from nursing practice have to be conveyed to the public, to whom nursing is ultimately accountable. It is such public awareness and accountability that are the main pillars on which the discipline of nursing will rest.

This book presents our domain as we see it today, and such are the consequences we must nurture during the 21st century. At any particular time, the recognized domain will include many phenomena that are not entirely clear or apparently consequential, or they might create genuine and inquisitive stances. This does not reflect the lack of maturity of a discipline but rather indicates its continuing growth. During the age of wisdom, the bond between scientific endeavors and reflection will become stronger; adaptation and demand will be the key forces of progress instead of structure and inflexibility. We will accept limitations in the discipline of nursing as limitations of the time rather than as the discipline's shortcomings.

Wisdom is the "capacity to take account of all important factors in a problem and to attach to each its due weight" and to know which ends to pursue (Russell, 1957, p. 29). It combines knowledge, feelings, morals, and practice. Wisdom is a sense of proportion. Knowledge can give us nursing therapeutics to enhance self-care, increase mother–infant attachment, increase social support or networks, ease effects of transition, or maintain integrity of the individual. Only wisdom and understanding can ensure their appropriate use for our clients without imposing our own values. Wisdom is a total perspective, seeing an object, event, or idea in all its pertinent relationships. Spinoza defined wisdom as seeing things "*sub specie aeternitatis*," in view of eternity (Copleston, 1963, p. 253); Durant (1957) suggested defining it as seeing things "*sub specie totuis*," in view of the whole. Considering the stages of development of knowledge in nursing and considering nursing as a whole leads to the proposition that nursing is currently encountering a scholarly evolution.

Emerson once said, "To the philosopher, all things are friendly and sacred, all events profitable, all days whole, all men (or women) divine." To nursing, all stages were essential to bring us to the stage of scholarliness, and from all stages will emerge the age of wisdom. "Knowledge is power, but only wisdom is liberty" (Durant, 1957, p. 9). Once there was a there. Now "there" is here. Let us acknowledge and enjoy our accomplishments, but we must also remember that there is no end to what lies ahead because it is the process that is the future.

REFERENCES

Allan, J. and Hall, B. (1988). Challenging the focus on technology: A critique of the medical model in a changing health care system. *Advances in Nursing Science*, 10(3), 22–34.

Allen, D.G. (1987). The social policy statement: A reappraisal. *Advances in Nursing Science*, 10(1), 39–48.

American Nurses Association. (1995). *Nursing's social policy statement* (Publication No. NP-107). Washington, DC: Author.

Anderson, R.A., Dobal, M.T., and Blessing, B. (1992). Theory-based approach to computer skill development in nursing administration. *Computers in Nursing*, 10(4), 152–157.

Batra, C. (1987). Nursing theory for undergraduates. *Nursing Outlook*, 35(4), 189–192.

Bradshaw, A. (1995). What are nurses doing to patients? A review of theories of nursing past and present. *Journal of Clinical Nursing*, 4(2), 81–92.

Brown, S.J. (1996). [Letter to the editor]. *Advances in Nursing Science*, 18(4), vi–vii.

Christmyer, C.S., Catanzariti, P.M., Langford, A.M., and Reiz, J.A. (1988). Bridging the gap: Theory to practice—Part I, clinical applications. *Nursing Management*, 19(9), 42–50.

Copleston, S.J. (1963). *A history of philosophy. Volume 4, Modern philosophy: Descartes to Leibniz.* (Baruch Spinoza, pp. 211–269). Garden City, NY: Image Books.

Dashiff, C. (1988). Theory development in psychiatric mental health nursing: An analysis of Orem's theory. *Archives of Psychiatric Nursing*, 2(6), 366–372.

Davies, B. and Hughes, A.M. (1995). Clarification of advanced nursing practice: Characteristics and competencies. *Clinical Nurse Specialist*, 9(3), 156–160.

DeGroot, H.A., Ferketich, S.L., and Larson, P.J. (1987). Theory development in a non-university service setting. *Journal of Nursing Administration*, 17(4), 38–44.

Dennison, P.D., and Keeling, A.W. (1989). Clinical support for eliminating the nursing diagnosis of knowledge deficit. *Image: Journal of Nursing Scholarship*, 21(3), 142–144.

Dewey, J. (1982). *How we think.* Lexington, MA: Heath (originally published in 1910).

Dickoff, J., James, P., and Wiedenbach, E. (1968). Theory in a practice discipline: Part 1. Practice oriented theory. *Nursing Research*, 17, 415–435.

Durant, W. (1957). What is wisdom? *Wisdom: The Magazine for Knowledge for All America*, 20(8), 25.

Engel, G.L. (1977). The need for a new medical model: A challenge for biomedicine. *Science*, 196, 129–137.

Facione, N.C., Facione, P.A., and Sanchez, C.A. (1994). Critical thinking disposition as a measure of competent clinical judgment. The development of the "California Critical Thinking Disposition Inventory." *Journal of Nursing Education*, 33(8), 345–350.

Gebbie, K.M. and Lavin, M.A. (1975). *Proceedings of the First National Conference on Classification of Nursing Diagnosis.* St. Louis: C.V. Mosby.

Gordon, M. (1979). The concept of nursing diagnosis. *Nursing Clinics of North America*, 14(3), 487–496.

Gordon, M. (1985). Nursing diagnosis. *Annual Review of Nursing Research*, 3, 127–146.

Hall, J.M., Stevens, P.E., and Meleis, A.I. (1994). Marginalization: A guiding concept for valuing diversity in nursing knowledge development. *Advances in Nursing Science*, 16(4), 23–41.

Hays, B.J., Norris, J., Martin, K.S., and Androwich, I. (1994). Informatics issues for nursing's future. *Advances in Nursing Science*, 16(4), 71–81.

Henry, B., Arndt, C., Di Vincenti, M., and Marriner-Tomey, A. (Eds.). (1989). *Dimensions of nursing administration: Theory, research, education, practice.* Boston: Blackwell Scientific Publications.

Iowa Intervention Project. (1993). The NIC taxonomy structure. *Image: Journal of Nursing Scholarship*, 25(3), 187–192.

Iowa Intervention Project. (1995). Validation and coding of the NIC taxonomy structure. *Image: Journal of Nursing Scholarship*, 27(1), 43–49.

Jacobs-Kramer, M. and Huether, S.E. (1988). Curricular considerations for teaching nursing theory. *Journal of Professional Nursing*, 4(5), 373–380.

Jacobson, S. (1987). Studying and using conceptual models of nursing. *Image: Journal of Nursing Scholarship*, 19(2), 78–82.

Jacoby, M.K. (1985). Eliminating the double standard. *American Journal of Nursing*, 85(3), 281, 285.

Jennings, B.M. and Meleis, A.I. (1988). Nursing theory and administration practice: Agenda for the 1990s. *Advances in Nursing Science*, 10(3), 56–69.

Jenny, J.I. (1987). Knowledge deficit: Not a nursing diagnosis. *Image. Journal of Nursing Scholarship*, 19(4), 184–185.

Johnson, D.E. (1959). The nature of a science of nursing. *Nursing Outlook*, 7(5), 291–294.

Karmels, P. (1993). Conundrum game for nursing theorists Neuman, King, and Johnson. *Nurse Educator*, 18(6), 8–9.

Kasch, C. (1984). Interpersonal competence and communication in the delivery of nursing care. *Advances in Nursing Science*, 6(2), 71–88.

Kim, M.J. (1985). Without collaboration, what's left? *American Journal of Nursing*, 85(3), 281–284.

Kim, M.J. (1989). Nursing diagnosis. *Annual Review of Nursing Research*, 7, 117–142.

Kleffel, D. (1996). Environmental paradigms: Moving toward an ecocentric perspective. *Advances in Nursing Science*, 18(4), 1–10.

Kritek, P.B. (1978). The generation and classification of nursing diagnoses: Toward a theory of nursing. *Image: Journal of Nursing Scholarship*, 10(2), 33–40.

Kritek, P.B. (1979). Commentary: The development of nursing diagnosis and theory. *Advances in Nursing Science*, 2(1), 73–79.

Kritek, P.B. (1985). Nursing diagnosis in perspective: Response to a critique. *Image: Journal of Nursing Scholarship*, 17(1), 3–8.

Laudan, L. (1981). A problem solving approach to scientific growth. In I. Hacking (Ed.), *Scientific revolutions*. Oxford, UK: Oxford University Press.

Lauder, W. (1994). Beyond reflection: Practical wisdom and the practical syllogism. *Nurse Education Today*, 14(2), 91–98.

Lenz, E.R., Suppe, F., Gift, A.G., Pugh, L.C., and Milligan, R.A. (1995). Collaborative development of middle-range nursing theories: Toward a theory of unpleasant symptoms. *Advances in Nursing Science*, 17(3), 1–13.

Levine, M.E. (1995). The rhetoric of nursing theory. *Image: Journal of Nursing Scholarship*, 27(1), 11–14.

McBride, A.B. (1986). Theory and research. *Journal of Psychosocial Nursing*, 24(9), 27–32.

McManus, R.L. (1950). Assumptions of functions of nursing. In *Regional planning for nurses and nursing education*. New York: Bureau of Publications, Teachers College, Columbia University.

Meleis, A.I. (1992a). Theoretical thinking progress in the discipline of nursing. In K. Kraus and P. Astedt-Kurki (Eds.), *International perspectives on nursing* (pp. 1–12). Tampere, Finland: University of Tampere Department of Nursing.

Meleis, A.I. (1992b). Directions for nursing theory development in the 21st century. *Nursing Science Quarterly*, 5(3), 112–117.

Meleis, A.I. (1996). Theory development: A blueprint for the 21st century. In P. Hinton Walker and B. Neuman (Eds.), *Blueprint for use of nursing models* (pp. 317–329). New York: National League for Nursing.

Meleis, A.I., Isenberg, M., Koerner, J.E., Lacey, B., and Stern, P. (1995). *Diversity, marginalization, and culturally competent health care issues in knowledge development*. Washington, DC: American Academy of Nursing.

Meleis, A.I. and Jennings, B.M. (1989). Theoretical nursing administration: Today's challenges, tomorrow's bridges. In B. Henry, C. Arndt, M. Di Vincenti, and A. Marriner-Tomey (Eds.), *Dimensions of nursing administration: Theory, research, education, practice*. Boston: Blackwell Scientific Publications.

Meleis, A.I. and Price, M.J. (1988). Strategies and conditions for teaching theoretical nursing: An international perspective. *Journal of Advanced Nursing*, 13, 592–604.

Merton, R.K. (1973). *The sociology of science: Theoretical and empirical investigations*. Chicago: University of Chicago Press.

Nakajima, H. (1995, May 20). Growing inequity is a matter of life and death [editorial]. *Michigan State University IIH, Newsletter*, p. 25.

Rafferty, A.M., Allcock, N., and Lathlean, J. (1996). The theory/practice 'gap': Taking issue with the issue. *Journal of Advanced Nursing*, 23, 685–691.

Reed, P.G. (1995). A treatise on nursing knowledge development for the 21st century: Beyond postmodernism. *Advances in Nursing Science*, 17(3), 70–84.

Russell, B. (1957). The world's need for wisdom. *Wisdom: The Magazine for Knowledge for all America*, 14, 29.

Shamansky, S.L. and Yanni, C.R. (1983). In opposition to nursing diagnosis: A minority opinion. *Image: Journal of Nursing Scholarship*, 15(2), 47–50.

Shaver, J. (1985). A biopsychosocial view of human health. *Nursing Outlook*, 33(4), 186–1101.

Taylor, A.J.W. and Frazer, A.G. (1982). The stress of post-disaster body handling and victim identification work. *Journal of Human Stress*, 8, 4–12.

University of California, San Francisco, School of Nursing Symptom Management Faculty Group. (1994). A model for symptom management. *Image: Journal of Nursing Scholarship*, 26(4), 272–276.

Visintainer, M. (1988). The nature of knowledge and theory in nursing. *Image: Journal of Nursing Scholarship*, 18(2), 32–38.

Wilson, H.S. (1985). *Research in nursing*. Menlo Park, CA: Addison-Wesley.

World Health Organization. (1978). Primary health care. *Report on primary health care*. Alma Ata, USSR; Geneva, Switzerland: Author.

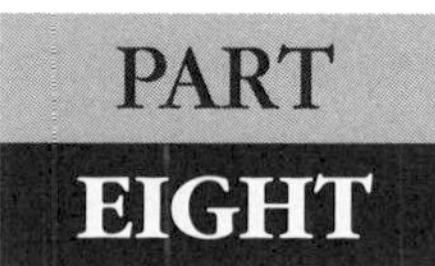

Our Theoretical Literature

Literature in nursing is rich with writings in theory, of theory, and on theory. Some of the writings provided significant milestones in the shaping of the theoretical progress in nursing. Chapters 20 and 21 of this book are organized around these writings. They provide an analytical review of the central literature in metatheory and theory up to the beginning of the 1980s as well as a comprehensive bibliography up to the beginning of the 1990s.

These chapters are offered for students, faculty, clinicians, and researchers. The serious theory student needs analytical familiarity with the significant writing that shaped the progress in the discipline of nursing. The cursory theory student can find these chapters helpful as an overview of the writing related to nursing theory. All concerned with the discipline of nursing will find that the literature relates, in some way, to their specific area of expertise. This literature is a significant component of our heritage without which our practice, teaching, and research are limited.

CHAPTER 20

Analysis of Theoretical Writing in Nursing

To develop, analyze, or critique theories, a theory student, user, or developer needs a background that includes all the significant writings related to theoretical nursing. This chapter provides the reader with a critical assessment of the central writing contained in the nursing literature of the 1980s. With the publication of *Advances in Nursing Science*, as well as other theoretically oriented journals and books, theory literature has developed and proliferated exponentially, and it is therefore no longer possible to include a comprehensive critical assessment of writings in theory. As many as possible of the writings up to the early 1980s that are considered classic in theory are included in this chapter.

The chapter is divided into two sections. **Section I** includes analysis and critique of the metatheory literature. **Section II** includes analysis and critique of the literature on nursing theory, written by the nurse theorists or by others who have used the nursing theory in research, practice, education, and administration. All analytical abstracts are listed alphabetically within the sections.

A reader can use this chapter in many ways: *first*, the reader can use it in conjunction with the contents of various chapters in the book; *second*, when studying a particular theorist's work, the reader can identify citations related to the theorist and can pull out those that have been abstracted for review; *third*, Section I could be read in its entirety as a way to prepare for a general overview of nursing theory; *fourth*, the reader can divide the writings in Section II into those relating to a particular theory or read the abstracts related to each theorist separately; and *fifth*, readers interested in the development of theoretical nursing may wish to have a temporal perspective by reading abstracts according to year of citation.

The intent of the abstracts is to challenge readers to different interpretations and not to critique the writing. *Readers are encouraged to read original writings and to use these analytical abstracts only to provide them with one perspective of the writings.* Finally, the reader should remember that the analyses here include the interpretation of the authors who abstracted them, which may or may not agree with others' interpretations.

SECTION I

Abstracts of Writings in Metatheory, 1960–1984

Ellen Mahoney and Afaf Meleis

Abdellah, F.G. (1969). The nature of nursing science. *Nursing Research*, 18(5), 390–393.

This article seeks to move toward the "identification of a nursing science." History is reviewed, and nursing scientists are exhorted to build on the work of nurse pioneers who were mainly theorists. Nursing science is defined as a body of cumulative scientific knowledge (drawn from the physical, biologic, and behavioral sciences) that is uniquely nursing. Emphasis is on an evolving science. The more that nursing research is directed by scientific theory, the more likely its results will contribute to the development of a nursing science. There are too few nursing scientists (should be 1%), but the numbers are growing. "It is the inescapable role of the nurse–scientist to point the way for change in nursing."

This is a short overview article, but it contains details of nursing history and random observations of interest.

Andreoli, K.G. and Thompson, C.E. (1977). The nature of science in nursing. *Image*, 9(2), 32–37.

The theoretical basis of practice is the science of nursing, and it defines nursing's uniqueness. Science is defined as a system of knowledge based on scientific principles. Its ultimate goal is the discovery of new knowledge, the expansion of existing knowledge, and the reaffirmation of previously held knowledge. Nursing is defined by abstracting the major elements from the conceptions of several nursing theorists. Science in nursing (the body of verified knowledge found within the discipline of nursing) is distinguished from the science of nursing (that body of verifiable knowledge that will be derived from nursing practice, the unique way in which nursing uses borrowed knowledge). Nursing will attain the status of a science once it has clearly identified a verifiable knowledge base that can be contested and corroborated. This knowledge base will come from practice. Specific attention is given to the scientific methodologies of nursing research, conceptual models in nursing, the nursing process, and nursing diagnosis as a means of developing a knowledge base.

The fact that the article offers more than the others in the category is an interesting argument for the integration of basic and applied science and the sections on scientific methodologies in nursing that stress the theory–practice–research link. One might argue that the "unique" elements of nursing presented are really not so unique. The definition of "science" comes from the dictionary; the conceptions of nursing science presented (especially by Johnson and Rogers) should be read in the original.

Batey, M.V. (1972). Values relative to research and to science in nursing as influenced by a sociological perspective. *Nursing Research*, 21(6), 504–508.

Central to the development of a science of nursing is the continuing issue of the function of values in research and in science. This article is a response to the question: How does preparation in one of the disciplines related to nursing bear on the identification and conceptualization of nursing research problems and approaches used to design and carry through an investigation? Batey's response is organized in three topics: (1) an overview of her conceptual and methodological orientation in sociology; (2) illustrations of the research in her work; and (3) contrasting perspectives of science with thought geared toward nursing science. It is to the third topic that the abstract is addressed.

Research is a tool of science; the goal of science is the continuing advancement of an objective body of knowledge. Batey contrasts two perspectives of science: (1) as a social system with values (expressed) as the desired goal toward which science strives (ie, an advancing and objectively verified body of knowledge), *norms* (expected standards of behavior, including disinterest organized skepticism, and communality) and *parteined relations* (the expectation of a competent response to one's creative effort); versus (2) as a means (knowledge for use). An investigator's perspective will influence types of research problems identified as well as the selection of knowledge brought to bear for their conceptualization and research methodologies. In nursing, where knowledge is valued for its use (perspective 2), it is hypothesized that there is a greater emphasis on descriptive studies than on the subsequent stages of the discovery process toward an objectively verified body of knowledge. Until we alter our normative system in nursing relative to science, we can expect little movement toward nursing science.

Whereas a major thrust of the article focuses on the dilemma of conflicting values for nurses educated in other fields, the section "Perspectives of Science" (pp. 507–508) is provocative and well worth reading, particularly after exposure to explications of nursing science and arguments for practice theory. Does the reader agree with Batey's hypothesis that a discipline emphasizing knowledge for use will emphasize descriptive research?

Batey, M.V. (1977). Conceptualization: Knowledge and logic guiding empirical research. *Nursing Research*, 26(5), 324–329

This is an excellent article analyzing functions and processes of research conceptualization. Analyzing a systematic sample of articles published in *Nursing Research*, Batey identified "limiting features" representing problems of: (1) the *conceptual phase* ("fallacies of reasoning, specification of meaning, and use of knowledge in conveying the problem, conceptual framework, and/or purpose"); (2) the *empirical phase* ("technical processes related to the methods and procedures of data production and reduction"); and (3) the *interpretative phase* ("analytical processes related to deriving meanings of findings"). Batey judged that the vast majority of problems are due to limitations of the conceptual phase, particularly the lack of clear definition and inadequate development or utilization of a conceptual framework. Factors contributing to conceptual limitations are identified, as are their consequences.

The remainder of the paper is an explication of the conceptual phase of research to achieve a reduction of the limitations noted. Components of the conceptual phase are: (1) The *problem* determines the context of the study by setting the major parameters of the phenomenon of concern; it includes what, how, why, or under what conditions phenomena occur, and a normative statement; (2) the *conceptual framework* involves background knowledge that delineates the present knowledge state about the problem and that yields the theoretical statement through which the investigator attempts to construct an accurate image of the phenomenon of study; it includes background (review of literature) and rationale (theoretical framework); and (3) the *purpose* is derived from the rationale; the research purpose is the hypothesis to be tested.

The article also includes brief but helpful sections on purposes and methods for literature review, scientific versus common sense meanings of concepts, tips on critical reading, and guidelines for the interpretative phase and its dynamic relation to conceptualization.

There is some overlap and lack of clarity in defining the three components of the conceptual phase, and it would have been appropriate to explicate more on the theoretical background of a study. This article should be read in the context of other articles that address conceptualization and conceptual frameworks. Besides tying these phases together, this article provides useful criteria for the design and evaluation of research.

Becker, C.H. (1983). A conceptualization of concept. *Nursing papers: Perspectives in Nursing*, 15(2), 51–58

The first part of this article is a series of lists. The first list has to do with characteristics of concepts: ambiguity, conventional meaning, dependent on context, neither false nor true, and either significant or nonsignificant. The author inserts an observation: "Concepts arise in the mind of an individual as a result of attempts to make order out of what is observed."

The next list describes modes of concept analysis (from Edel, 1979): Socratic (general and essential), element analysis, genetic (how evolved), functional, systems, pragmatic, logical, operational, phenomenological. A summary list gives the requirements for an appropriate use of concepts in theory development: "(1) concepts have intention; (2) concepts are seen as models of some aspect of reality; (3) the concepts selected are significant; (4) the mode of concept analysis dictates the method of investigation of the concept; (5) the value bias and semantic overtones are inherently present in the concepts selected for study; and (6) concepts are subject to continual analysis and refinement."

Then, micro-concepts are endorsed: "micro-concepts rather than general macro-concepts may have the potential to contribute more to the structuring of nursing knowledge." An example is given: self-esteem (micro) versus personality (macro). The author presents the following reasoning: "Macro-concepts, because of their generalness, have a loose flexibility of meaning. Micro-concepts would not allow this looseness." There are also fewer variables in micro-level concepts: (1) the intention of the author is easily understood; (2) meaning is not so easily distorted; (3) the most appropriate mode of analysis is easily identified; and (4) there is not polarity.

Beckstrand, J. (1978). The notion of a practice theory and the relationship of scientific and ethical knowledge to practice. *Research in Nursing and Health*, 1(3), 131–136

Beckstrand critiques several authors who have supported a "practice theory" (Dickoff and James, Jacox, etc). For such notions to be meaningful, practice knowledge must be shown to be different from scientific knowledge or ethical knowledge, or else "no need for a separate practice theory would exist." Two primary aspects of practice knowledge, the knowledge of how to make changes and the knowledge of what is "good" are examined. First *science*, "the knowledge of lawlike empirical relationships," is studied to determine if it includes the knowledge used to control phenomena in practice. Beckstrand provides an extended summary discussion of the nature of scientific knowledge, relating it to the notion of "control." "The potential for controlling a phenomenon is synonymous with lawlike relationships and the potential for prediction that they provide. . . . Science seeks to establish the knowledge that allows for this kind of control." To make changes one must have some control. Although practice often seeks this control through invalid argument, "functional argument," and empirical generalization, these are "based on the knowledge of scientific laws and lawlike relationships." The controls possible in scientific experimentation are impossible in the practice situation, but despite uncertainty of outcome, practice methodology nonetheless proceeds by valid deduction from scientific laws.

Next is a review of the field of ethics. Ethics is concerned with the knowledge of what is right, good, or obligatory. Both normative ethics and metaethics have relevance to practice. But theories of the moral obligations of practitioners "are identical in form" to other theories of moral obligation; theories of moral value in practice do not represent unique forms of theory. The goals defined in practice are not moral values that may be determined by the methods of ethical philosophy and no others. In short, "it would appear that there is no need for a practice theory distinct from a scientific or ethical theory."

The bulk of the article is Beckstrand's reading in the philosophy of science and ethical theory. Her more abbreviated attempts to apply these readings to Dickoff and colleagues are dependent on crucial unargued and unevidenced assertions. For example, (1) the relation of "practice knowledge," (Beckstrand's term) to "practice theory," which is the focus of the authors she surveys), after all, to have a theory of teaching is not to have the knowledge to teach a course in Russian history; (2) the assertion that practice knowledge can be broken down into two generalizations—"how to make changes" and "what is good"—without oversimplification or distortion; and (3) the assertion that unscientific reasoning and procedures are "based" on scientific reasoning and procedures. Although Beckstrand argues that the knowledge on which practice is based is science-knowledge, she admits outright that the reasoning process in practice is often unscientific, and she ignores experience, tradition, or even nonscientific logic as bases.

Beckstrand emphasizes what might be called "content" with regard to science and practice theory (ie, concern only for the knowledge in science and practice and not the reasoning processes, and concern only for just what information, basically, is used in it and not for the descriptive shape of the activity, its form, nor its outline definition). Beckstrand reverses herself when discussing ethics, saying that although there may be specific ethical obligations or directives especially and uniquely applicable to a practice, the form of the theory is that of an ethical theory. Might one not ask her then, why a theory of practice (although the information used in it may well be the same as ethics and science) cannot remain unique because its shape and its form is that of a practice theory?

Beckstrand, J. (1978). The need for a practice theory as indicated by the knowledge used in the conduct of practice. *Research in Nursing and Health*, 1(4), 175–179

Beckstrand's aim is to extend her previous argument. Her first article said that "much of the knowledge required for practice is the knowledge of science and ethics." Here, she "examines" practice to see if "the theoretical knowledge used in practice is completely defined by science, ethics, and logic." To determine this, she turns to the definition of the purpose of practice: "Practice attempts to *change* an entity or phenomenon in such a way that a greater good is realized." Accomplishing change in practice necessitates the knowledge of both change and action. This knowledge can be reduced to limited categorization, but Beckstrand broadens the base of necessary knowledge here to include "the domain of logic in general."

Following this is the logical analysis of the conduct of practice. First, she discusses conditions. She asserts that "[t]o say that an interaction is meaningful is to say that the interaction has logical implications in relation to existing scientific or ethical knowledge." She argues that although the combination of conditions in each situation can draw on infinite numbers for infinite variance, and that because the "human potential" to perceive or the "personal knowledge" of the practitioner are limited, only a finite number of conditions are attended to or identified, and they are identified in a way "most dependent on the practitioner's scientific and ethical knowledge."

Next under the rubric of "description" of the conduct of practice, Beckstrand discusses values and goals. She restates that the goal of practice is change toward the greater good. Determination of this greater good depends on the values of the practice discipline, values that "reflect normative ethical theories." A practitioner sometimes accepts a hierarchy of values "implicitly and uncritically, but these hierarchies and their implementation represent ethical decisions." She concludes that the knowledge of practice "depends not on some special aspects of practice, but on science and ethics alone."

Immediately in her introduction, Beckstrand, without calling attention to it, puts forward two new factors missing from her first article: "theoretical knowledge" presumably now will bridge her pass from "theory" to "knowledge" (whereas this formulation does not appear at all in her first essay, it is seen three times in this introduction to her second), and "logic" is added (again, without comment) to science and ethics, to subsume practice theory. One might hypothesize that these additions reflect a reaction to criticism (her own or that of others) of the first piece, and therefore that problems are to be addressed. The body of the article never again mentions "theoretical knowledge" but instead substitutes "knowledge" alone, as in the first essay. What is more, because she freely interchanges "theoretical knowledge used in practice" with "knowledge used in practice," one may deduce a confusion in the use of the concept "theoretical." What of the goal to maintain health *against* changes?

In addition, it would have been helpful if Beckstrand had considered, even as an error to be refuted, that a theory of nursing might be as relevant to "nursing ethics" as a theory of ethics. Finally, her conclusion forgets her introduction and its specificities of "theoretical" and "logic." "Thus, the knowledge of practice depends not on some special aspects of practice, but on science and ethics alone." Both articles are thought to be provoking and central readings in metatheory.

Beckstrand, J. (1980). A critique of several conceptions of practice theory in nursing. *Research in Nursing and Health*, 3, 69–79

Although the title and summary suggest a survey of ideas about "practice theory," half of this article (roughly five pages) is devoted to what Beckstrand characterizes as the "set of rules" conception of practice theory, which she attributes to Ada Jacox. Other writers, most notably Dickoff, James, and Wiedenbach, who provide the opening focus of the essay, are given remarkably short shrift The initial section, "The notion of Dickoff et al.," attempts to explain their notion, mixing restatement of their formulations with a series of asserted exemplifications of what they mean: "the articulation of the conceptual frameworks . . . practitioners actually use"; "in changing a flat tire a practice theory is being employed"; an identity between their notions and "technology" (ie, "the totality of a plan of action used to bring about a goal that is presumed desirable").

The big interest for Beckstrand is Jacox (1974). Jacox's is presented as an incorrect interpretation of Dickoff and colleagues—incorrect because Beckstrand appears to interpret Dickoff and James' position in terms of each practitioner having her own practice theory formula. Jacox, according to Beckstrand, suggests a rigid, compulsion-carrying deck of directives, which one shuffles on each occasion to find the right rules of procedure. Nurses are "compelled to conform . . . to a set of rules imposed by an external authority." Under this conception, "prescriptive practice theory becomes a set of universally prescribed rules for practice."

Following this is the longest section of the essay (by far)—an attack on the Jacox position so characterized. Beckstrand produces a discussion of ethics intended to demonstrate that you cannot prescribe a goal without making an unjustifiable value judgment. Then she makes a series of "practical arguments." Prescriptions cannot take into account all the variables in a given situation. Sometimes, two prescriptions will conflict. The practitioner will be forced to make an "arbitrary" decision between them. She takes time to "demonstrate" that you could not have a prescription specific to every situation. She responds to objections by saying that, even under such a theory, scientific and ethical judgment would still be required. Granted this, Beckstrand asserts that the change would be nil. She argues that such a theory will not be valuable in the education of practitioners because she has already shown it is not valuable in practice. Nursing education does not involve prescriptions of this kind because those in education "are not imperatives carrying sanctions for their adoption or violation." Sets of rules for practice are no aid in research because "as prescriptions, they imply no deductively derivable empirically true or false consequences (predictions)."

Other notions of practice theory are briefly examined. Conceptual frameworks of nursing, such as Roy's or Jones' "are not scientific theories but ideologies" because they are "legitimately alterable on the sole basis of personal or public discretion." Beckstrand also differs with those (like Peterson) who wish to try to delineate the bounds of nursing inquiry. In theory development and in research, you do not know *a priori* what is relevant, rather, you let the characterizations and categorizations emerge and evolve from the situation.

In this article, Beckstrand provides a unique interpretation of Dickoff and colleagues and of Jacox. Although the problem with Dickoff and colleagues inevitably represents some difficulties with their exposition, most attempts like this at reduction can be problematic (as they dismiss and refute such approaches in their 1975 article) simply because they fail to include all the elements Dickoff, James, and Wiedenbach insist on (ie, a conceptual framework with built-in goal orientation, prescriptions, and a survey list). The set of rules theory attributed to Jacox also has some flaws. We would assume that Jacox would argue that her proposed system is not intended to be a straightjacket and that provisions for "breaking" rules are made. Beckstrand's arguments against Jacox would seem to apply to any attempts to teach practice, or to any potential contributions from research. She sees the possibility of this objection: "one might argue that if a prescriptive practice theory of the set-of-rules type cannot be justified, then no decision can be made about what to do in practice."

As to her paragraph on metatheory, first, under Carnap's definition, all theories of nursing are metatheories. Second, after all these attempts to discredit practice theory, she says that if you will call it metatheory, it is okay, and Dickoff and colleagues' may be considered a beginning (and worthy) metatheory of nursing practice. Beckstrand notes that because Dickoff and colleagues "did not fully explicate or formalize their theory," they have only offered "undeveloped ideas." Dickoff and colleagues, of course, do not have a theory. (That is to say, they do not have a "practice theory.") These appear to be unfortunate mix-ups. Despite our analytical arguments, we consider Beckstrand's writing stimulating, challenging, and an absolute must for a theory student.

Benoliel, J.Q. (1977). The interaction between theory and research. *Nursing Outlook*, 25(2), 108–113

This essay explores relationships between theory and research as reciprocal elements in an ongoing process through which scientific knowledge relevant to nursing is created, expanded, tested, and refined. Practice can serve as a stimulus to research and can therefore form part of the cyclical process. There is also a brief section on sources of knowledge in nursing.

This is a simple account of the "constantly flowing interchange between the realities of practice, theory development, and scientific investigation." The inductive/deductive cycle is demonstrated, as is an example of building a body of knowledge by the "application of different philosophical approaches to the study of a particular human phenomenon." Better "sources of knowledge" include Rogers, Carper, and Beckstrand.

Berthold, J.S. (1968). Prologue: Symposium on theory development in nursing. *Nursing Research*, 17(3), 196–197

According to the author, no substantive definition of "theory" can be applied with any generality due to the ambiguity and complexity of the concept "theory." Differential use of terms necessitates clear understanding of their use to avoid semantic confusion and to allow for attention to the substance of various positions.

In this introduction to the symposium, Berthold states: "The questions . . . involve a discussion of various positions about and approaches to developing a conceptual structure of knowledge useful and necessary to attain the goals established by nurses." In elaborating on this statement, the author stresses: thought processes that result in theoretical constructs, ordered in a systematic way; knowledge that is verified; theory that is useful in stimulating new observations and insights and in generating propositions concerning relevant events; and goals that are established and controlled by nurses for nursing.

This is a brief overview that succinctly captures the major issues, questions, and debates about nursing theory development addressed in the symposium. (See articles by Schrag, Crowley, Folta, and Brown, as well as Panel Discussion).

Brown, M.I. (1964). Research on the development of nursing theory: The importance of a theoretical framework in nursing research. *Nursing Research*, 13(2), 109–112

Two major questions are addressed: (1) How far have we progressed through research toward the development of an integrated body of nursing theory? and (2) How can we determine if a research project has a theoretical framework that will make possible a contribution to scientific knowledge? Sections of the paper include: the need for nursing theory, concept validation through research, and assessment of the theoretical framework of a research project. A research project that contributes to nursing theory can be identified by certain characteristics, such as: an aim to pursue knowledge for its own sake, the statement of the relationship of the problem to research and nursing literature, the use of established meaningful terms, the association of findings to the work of others, and the logical but creative exposition of implications and further hypotheses for testing.

This early, easy-to-read article is a brief reminder of the theory/research symbiosis. The article emphasizes rationale rather than criteria for selecting theoretical frameworks. Would Brown's conclusions be different if this article were written in the 1980s?

Brown, M.I. (1968). Theory development in nursing: Social theory in geriatric nursing research. *Nursing Research*, 17(3), 213–217

This is an exemplification of Brown's theme—the nature of nursing research and its relation to theory formation. The article is a descriptive account of the use of the concept of socialization in a gerontologic research project.

Although Brown asks how theories of the basic and other applied sciences relate to nursing research, her response stresses problems intrinsic to the theories. Other authors (see especially Klein, Crawford, and Johnson et al) emphasize the implications of "borrowing" theories formulated in other disciplines. The article is part of the 1968 Symposium on Theory Development in Nursing.

Brown, M.L. (1983). Research questions and answers: The use of theory and conceptual frameworks in nursing research and practice. *Oncology Nursing Forum,* 10(2), 111–112

The author presents an initial distinction: "A theory explains the nature of phenomena and a conceptual framework identifies what variables are important." Both are important to "identify, categorize, and expand nursing knowledge in an organized and thoughtful way. A catalog of notions of theory is then offered. The author summarizes: "Theory, then, helps identify the research problem, defines . . . appropriate evidence . . . and determines methods to obtain, organize, and integrate information."

In dealing with conceptual frameworks, on the other hand, the author simply presents a definition: "A conceptual framework is an organized grouping of ideas or concepts that assists in providing overall structure to the research project and the nursing process."

The author follows Derdiarian's delineation of the need for order and systematization in nursing research, education, and practice. Finally, she cites Marino's conceptual framework for cancer nursing.

This article is actually a columnist's response to a question by readers about the terms "theory" and "conceptual framework." More elaborate and somewhat different presentations are available elsewhere in the literature.

Burgess, G. (1978). The personal development of the nursing student as a conceptual framework. *Nursing Forum,* 17(1), 96–92

Burgess proposes "personal development" of the student nurse as a conceptual framework in professional nursing education. Rationales are presented (enhanced potential for professional effectiveness; improved quality of care; criteria for retention of students) as well as means of operationalizing personal development (ability to articulate goals and philosophy and to evaluate accomplishments and needs; change in attitudes; increased sensitivity to others).

A conceptual framework is defined, by analogy, as a unifying central theme that provides the mechanism for articulating and relating all parts of the curriculum. Course objectives are the means of providing attachment to the central theme, and the courses themselves (content plus learning experiences) are "free to respond to currents of movement and creative expression," while maintaining their attachment to the central theme.

The proposed conceptual framework provides a provocative, if controversial, alternative to more common subject or process-oriented curricula. The major value of this article however, is its simple, yet creative and helpful explanation of the characteristics and purposes of the conceptual framework and its emphasis on the need to operationalize concepts.

Bush, H.A. (1979). Models for nursing. *Advances in Nursing Science.* 1(2), 13–21

This article examines types of models, the relationship between models and theories, and the use of models in nursing research, education, and practice.

Models provide a means for ordering, clarifying, and analyzing concepts and their relationships; they provide analogs to reality and stimulate the scientific process by identifying new possibilities. A model primarily expresses structure, whereas a theory provides substance. Models used in nursing must represent the ordered reality of focus on human beings, their environment, their health, and nursing itself (ie., isomorphic). Models are used: (1) in research, to conceptualize the research process itself and to facilitate thinking about concepts and their relationships; (2) in education, to guide curricula planning; and (3) in practice, to guide assessment, intervention, and evaluation.

This article provides a good summary of types of models and their purposes in nursing. More pragmatic information on the development of models may be found in Jacox and McKay.

Carper, B.A. (1978). Fundamental patterns of knowing in nursing. *Advances in Nursing Science*, 1(1), 13–23

A classification of the patterns of knowledge in nursing is presented here. The article addresses the question: "What kinds of knowledge are most valuable to the discipline of nursing?" Answers are meant to provide: (1) perspective and significance to the discipline; (2) awareness of the complexity and diversity of nursing knowledge; and (3) an operational definition of nursing.

Four patterns of knowing are identified:

1. *Empirical* (the science of nursing). The science of nursing is in a healthy but embryonic stage; theoretical models are presenting new perspectives.
2. *Aesthetics* (the art of nursing). Aesthetics is achieved by empathy, "dynamic integration" of parts into the whole, and the recognition of particulars versus universals.
3. *Personal knowledge.* Personal knowledge is concerned with the quality of interpersonal contacts, promoting therapeutic relationships, and individualized care.
4. *Ethics* (the moral component) "what ought to be done." Each individual pattern of knowing is necessary, but not sufficient, for achieving the goals of nursing. It is their interrelationship that defines the whole. These patterns provide structure and boundaries, dictate subject matter for nursing education, and, together, represent a complete approach to the problems and questions of the discipline of nursing.

The reader of this article should consider several points. The "Aesthetics of Nursing" section appears to confuse knowledge with action ("a science teaches us to know, and an art to do") and blurs distinctions between intuition, perception, instinct, and what we more ordinarily call knowledge. Perhaps most important, the identification of aesthetic with *empathy* loses any sense of clear distinction between this and her third category, described as "acceptance." In this case, Carper is rejecting an approach to the client as an "object," and is rejecting establishing "authentic personal relationships."

In addition, the "Ethics of Nursing" obscures a major oversight of this paper (something emphasized by Donaldson and Crowley)—that nursing involves history and philosophy as well as science and art. The delineation of goals, principles, and values and of the hierarchies among these that are specific to nursing are the continuing products of nursing experience and of thought in nursing that is broadly theoretical. The value of this article lies in its provision of a broader perspective of nursing knowledge than has been previously presented in the literature.

Chapman, C.M. (1976). The use of sociological theories and models in nursing. *Journal of Advanced Nursing*, 1, 111–127

Theory development has not kept pace with expanding roles in nursing and does not support nursing actions. Nursing and sociology are similarly defined as interactive processes between individuals, and the author therefore suggests the potential contribution of sociological theories and models to the development of nursing theory.

Social exchange theory is proposed to explain how patients and nurses satisfy their own needs and goals, and organizational theories are considered in the context of their effect on goal achievement, communication, and compliance. Concluding remarks stress that: (1) borrowed theories must be validated in the new situation, and (2) theories in the behavioral sciences can describe and explain more accurately than they can predict due to the variability in human behavior.

The bulk of this article focuses on the effects of organizational structure on nurse roles and behaviors in the United Kingdom. The reader might question comparisons between nursing and sociology and assumptions about nurses and patients. The article emphasizes theories related to the delivery of care and the development of nursing theory that would support clinical practice. Whereas the ideas presented in the conclusions are important, their development is somewhat limited.

Chinn, P.L. and Jacobs, M.K. (1978). A model of theory development in nursing. *Advances in Nursing Science*, 1(1), 1–11

The process of theory development is a means of facilitating the evolution of nursing science and is the most critical task facing the nursing profession. Theory is defined as "an internally consistent body of relational statements about phenomena which is useful for prediction and control." Conceptual frameworks are presented as less developed theoretical statements allowing description and explanation.

The model of theory development contains four separate but interrelated components: (1) examination and analysis of concepts, (2) formulation and testing of relational statements, (3) theory construction, and (4) practical application of theory. These components may be differentiated by the nature of the operations involved: cognitive (1 and 3); empirical (2 and 4); and by their functions: description and explanation (1 and

2); prediction and control (3 and 4). As a whole, the model demonstrates, "how different types of research yield varying types of products, each contributing to the total development of the science." Also included in the model are boundaries that delimit areas of nursing concern, while allowing free exchange of content and processes among sciences, and a central core denoting the influence of history on theory development in nursing. The importance of the theory–practice linkage and the dynamic and contextual nature of the process of theory development are emphasized.

Two major arguments are developed: (1) "The process of theory development has greater value for nursing than the product," and (2) the emphasis in theory development should be prediction and control. These positions should be contrasted with authors who emphasize the preliminary importance of descriptive and explanatory theories, the importance of the "product" for building a science of nursing, and the guiding influence of a clear conception of nursing.

Clark, J. (1982). Development of models and theories on the concept of nursing. *Journal of Advanced Nursing*, 7(2), 129–134

This article aims to show that models and theories in nursing have "practical value for the ordinary clinical nurse." One must relate theoretical work to what nurses actually do, built around concepts that can be operationalized. The failure to do this explains "the relative lack of impact on nursing practice . . . of the work in theory development undertaken in recent years."

Clark presents a "simple model of nursing." The model is a "gross simplification," but deliberately so, as more elaborate models are less universal. Often, models do not easily fit all fields of nursing.

How can such a model help the ordinary practicing nurse? (1) It purports explicitly that there is something called "nursing" that has an identity of its own ("versus those who still see nursing merely as a collection of tasks undertaken on the initiative of . . . doctors"); (2) it stresses the reciprocity of the nurse–patient relationship and the significance of environment; and (3) it stresses cause and effect relationships; "considerably more attention must be paid than in the past to outcomes of nursing care."

The remainder of the article is an application to her own situation. Clark demonstrates by considering her own nursing care in light of the model.

More popularizing than theory or scholarship, the article provides a role model of informal, thoughtful, and conscious practice, and does a good job of presenting serious ideas in attractive and readily understandable ways. It is a well written example of what it argues—relating scholarship in nursing to practice, making it available to "consumers." It is a soft-sell for theory-based practice and is effective.

Cleland, V.S. (1967). The use of existing theories. *Nursing Research*, 16(2), 118–121

Theory serves two major functions: as a tool, it gives direction to empirical investigation; as a goal, it tends to abstract, summarize, and order research findings. The goal function of theory, which is the basis for progression of science, has been less adequately used in nursing. The functional method of research, which begins with a significant problem or question and then searches for relevant theoretical formulations, enables the nurse researcher to take advantage of advances made in other disciplines, while ensuring nursing relevance. It permits the researcher to work inductively from existing empirical data and deductively from other theoretical formulations. An example of this is given to illustrate the inherent limitation of research that has no theoretical framework (and, of course, the superiority of one that does).

This rationale for conceptual frameworks is similar to others on the subject, and may be contrasted with the "grounded" approach (see Quint). Although the authors in this group of articles agree on the values of a framework, consider the integral relationship of this section and the one on theory critique.

Collaizzi, J. (1975). The proper object of nursing science. *International Journal of Nursing Studies,* 12(4), 197–200

The beginning of a science should be a philosophical inquiry into its appropriate domain. In initiating a science of nursing, considerable theoretical ambiguity has resulted from the assumption that nursing science is synthetic. Although we have amassed a body of scientific findings (that can be properly called health technology), what we have failed to do is circumscribe that which is uniquely nursing. Although nursing takes place within both technical and existential dimensions, the proper object of nursing science is the human experience of health and illness. Therefore, the research methods of human science, rather than those of natural science, must be used to investigate the questions that arise within this (existential) dimension.

This article offers an intelligent support of prevalent and influential conceptions of nursing science that emerged in the 1980s.

Collins, R.J. and Fielder, J.H. (1981). Beckstrand's concept of practice theory: A critique. *Research in Nursing and Health,* 4(3), 317–321

The authors find two major flaws in Beckstrand's analysis. First, they attack her claim that "the knowledge nurses need to effect changes is scientific knowledge." Specifically, they follow Toulmin's suggestion that there is a "plurality of different types of medical knowledge," and they quickly collapse it into two "modes." Beckstrand has overlooked or ignored the subjective, the knowledge of the particular, "knowing the client as a particular human being." Several of the authors' statements on this issue are memorable: "The role of the nurse and the biographer are similar; both must turn their attention to knowing individuals in all of the uniqueness and particularity. . . . The nurse's role is perhaps closer to that of the priest, intimate friend, or therapist—seeking not only knowledge of the individual but also the person's well-being. Understanding is not the primary goal, but a way of becoming an effective adviser and advocate for the person's interest."

Second, there are moral issues in nursing that will not be resolved by appeal to ethics but are specific to nursing. The authors point to activities or goals that are not obligatory but that are praiseworthy; these are characterized as, "[M]oral ideal. . . . The questions of which, if any, moral ideals an individual pursues is not answered by an ethical theory. The theory may be used to justify an ideal as a moral ideal, but the choice of which ones to pursue must flow from an individual's concept of what kind of life the person wishes to lead. . . . The profession of nursing has only recently emerged from the role of being the physician's handmaiden and is now in the process of defining itself as a profession in its own right, embodying certain moral ideals. Just what those ideals should be is one of the major elements of a practice theory."

This is an interesting, analytical article. It nicely adjusts and fills out Beckstrand's work, without any excessive negativity. It is a good example of the sense of a shared enterprise: Beckstrand is a colleague whose work is to be built on.

Crawford, G., Dufault, S.K., and Rudy, E. (1979). Evolving issues in theory development. *Nursing Outlook*, 27(5), 346–351

This review of nursing theory literature addresses issues in historical perspective: Is nursing theory borrowed or unique? Is nursing a basic or applied science? Should there be theories *of* nursing or *for* practice? What are the approaches to theory development? The purpose of the article is to redefine these issues in light of Donaldson and Crowley's article.

A strong bias for unique, practice-oriented, "situation-producing" theories is presented. Problems of borrowing are presented (eg, lack of isomorphism). Authors agree with Johnson that the nature of knowledge required for nursing will foster theory development that is unique to nursing.

As defined in the 1968 nursing science conference, basic science supports knowledge for its own sake, whereas applied science demonstrates knowledge with practical aims and applications. Donaldson and Crowley present the need to increase understanding of phenomena (basic), demonstrate applicability of basic knowledge in real situations (applied), and explain how to use knowledge to achieve goals in practice (prescriptive theory). Together, these comprise nursing science.

Regarding the issue of theory *of nursing* (delineation of definition and scope of or about nursing and the nursing process) versus *for practice* (conceptualizations guiding nursing action to achieve desired goals), these authors address the question of unified versus diverse theories, supporting Jacox's "middle-range theories." It is possible that they confuse "unified theory" with the values of a theoretical framework. The complexities of the arguments for and against unified and diverse theories are not addressed.

This approach to theory development lends support to inductive, deductive, historical, and philosophical methods. Theories should be developed to generate new knowledge and to organize knowledge about the discipline of nursing (supporting Donaldson and Crowley). The author states McKay's questions about which methods are most appropriate and what are criteria for acceptance of findings. She also supports Stevens' advice to ask the significant questions and only then to seek appropriate research methodologies.

This article provides a good overview of critical issues in nursing theory development from a historical perspective. Although one is attempting to resolve these issues, the complexities of the arguments and contrasting positions are not always fully addressed, precluding comprehensive, definitive resolution. Nevertheless, this article is a good synthesis of supporting positions and contains an excellent bibliography on theory development in nursing.

Dickoff, J. and James, P. (1968). Researching research's role in theory development. *Nursing Research*, 17(3), 204–205

Research is for the sake of theory and theory is for practice. However, research alone will not produce theory, and theory produced without research has little hope of viability. Research is a tool to be used in conjunction with adequate conceptualization and with a level of precision that, although scientifically sound, does not preclude practical usefulness. The purpose of research (creating or testing theory) should determine the methodology used.

This excellent, humorous, and atypically brief article by Dickoff and James is one of the best articles on the research–theory–practice link available in the literature.

Dickoff, J. and James, P. (1968). A theory of theories: A position paper. *Nursing Research*, 17(3), 197–203

Dickoff and James begin by defining theory as: a conceptual system or framework invented for some purpose. (There are other kinds of theory besides "predictive theory.") Because a profession shapes reality, nursing theory must provide conceptualizations to guide the shaping of reality to nursing's professional purpose. Therefore, nursing theory is at the fourth or highest level—situation-producing theory—because the nursing aim is practice. Nursing has an advantage to offsetting the difficulty of producing so complex a theory, namely, "the privileged and habitual intercourse with empirical reality carried on in a practice discipline," together with the practical wisdom passed on in apprenticeship. (There follows a summary of "Theory in a Practice Discipline"—see abstract of that article for this information.) Natural and social science theories will be offered by contributors, but one should realize that conceptualization at a sophisticated level constitutes the integration of these into nursing theory. The authors' summary indicates that definition and types of theory delineated are the crucial points made. They suggest valuation of their theory or theories to rest on "whether or not the proposed position constitutes a fruitful view of theory."

This is a stimulating introduction to the ideas of Dickoff and James and contains some knowing asides (eg, the authors encourage nurses to persist in theory building despite "the smoother sailing and quicker payoff in status and funds to be found in repetition or imitation of inquiry" in other disciplines). Nevertheless, the article is simply an overview and depends on the more elaborate articulations ("Theory in a Practice Discipline," etc.) for substantive support.

Dickoff, J., James, P., and Wiedenbach, E. (1968a). Theory in a practice discipline: Part I—Practice oriented theory. *Nursing Research*, 17(5), 415–435

This is the first of two articles on the nature and development of theory in a practice discipline. A major thesis is made explicit at the outset: theory is relevant to practice, eory, and both are relevant to research. The movement is delineated from practice t rt/criticism to articulation of a problem, and then to speculative and even-felt disq resolution. This "epitomizes that theory is born in practice and must return tual p" What is theory? Theory is a "conceptual framework to some purpose." to pme discussion of the nature of theory and misconceptions about theory.

Th our levels of theory are: (1) factor-isolating theories; (2) factor-relating theories ive); (3) situation-relating theories (predictive, etc); and (4) situation-producing (prescriptive). Each of these is then described: (1) involves naming, classifying; epicting or "natural-history-stage" theory; (3) extends from predictive theory into oting and inhibiting" theories; (4) is the primary subject of the article, situation-ucing theory. The three essential ingredients of a situation-producing theory are: oal content specified as an aim for activity; (2) prescriptions for activity; and (3) a ey list to serve as a supplement.

Each of these ingredients is discussed, the first two briefly, the survey list at some ngth. As to the first, "No more feeling of reverence to some shadowy high ideal can ubstitute in theory for the conception of goal as goal." As to prescriptions, they are commands giving a directive, aimed at a specified end, and directed toward some specified agent. The survey list accounts for the agent's judgment, experience, and practical insight. It bridges the gap between particular activity and the goal content and prescriptions. Such activity has six salient aspects: agency, patiency, framework, terminus, procedure, and dynamics.

What is nursing theory? It must be a theory at the most sophisticated level, a situation-producing theory. This article suggests what might be expected in a nursing theory. Again, the discussion is structured on the tripartite division—goal, prescription, and survey-list ingredients. The discussion of goal content identifies the goals as "beforehand specifications of situations the theorist deems worthy to produce," as well as "explicit conceptualizations subject to revision." The treatment of the prescription ingredient merely expands with examples of what has been said already. Furthermore, "appropriate specificity of goal content and prescription is an important consideration in any practice theory."

The survey list ingredients are explained and illustrated at some length. Under *agency*, the question is asked, "Who might be agents of activity that realizes the nursing goal?" The conclusion is that there is no theoretical reason that all nursing agents must be nurses or even persons. *Patiency*, similarly, is mainly the extension of that term to cover "[a]ny person or thing that receives the activity of a registered nurse." *Framework* asks: What in the context of activity, practically speaking, is relevant? *Terminus* is activity in terms of outcomes. This and *procedure* are fairly obvious discussions of viewing activity in terms of means and ends. *Dynamics* introduces interesting questions about the motivations of nurses and how these may be influenced. The question is of the "power sources" for successful nursing activity.

The article closes with a brief look at existing nursing theory. Actually, this is mainly a look at nursing literature. Beginning with the observation that there is no existing nursing theory to meet their paradigm, the authors argue nonetheless that extant nursing literature constitutes a contribution to, or preparation for, such a theory. They discuss the difficulties of "would-be" nursing theorists, they observe that there may be more than one good nursing theory, and then they propose to consider types of nursing literature (other than research studies): the "inspirational" literature of nur treatises and text- books, and procedure and policy books. These constitute "a rich m we know how to exploit the veins." The existence of something concrete to be e d critically— written materials and existing practice—is a necessary stepping ston her words, even now, practice is guided in some incipient way by embryonic th

Dickoff and colleagues have much to offer: "As Einstein's the is . . . so is our theory of theories." In fact, it is this very insistence that ducing a *new kind* of theory, substantively different, that provides the ma tivity doubt or dispute. Whereas some parts of this article are dense and full of ro- sections seem diffuse, rambling, simplistic, and often unnecessary. There is raphy. However, their pretensions to metatheory are the main objectionable (except for an occasional condescension to nurses and "would-be" nurse theori is the major substantive article by these authors, and it is a "must read" becaus contagion and impact of their ideas. Critical reading of this article should be fol by reading of the article by Jacox and the series by Beckstrand.

Dickoff, J., James, P., and Wiedenbach, E. (1968b). Theory in a practice discipline: Part II—Practice orien research. *Nursing Research*, 17(6), 545–554

To have a nursing theory, three sources must be tapped: awareness of practice theory, interest in developing it, and "openness to relevant empirical reality." The authors see the first two of these as covered in Part I of this article, which is briefly reviewed. Research and practice are the constituents of the required "openness." The essential aspect of practice as opposed to "mere" research lies in the accomplishment of something in the here-and-now. Research has as its goal "[i]nput to knowledge beyond the immediate particular." Possible research objectives are: to stimulate conception and to validate a conception already formed. "We can say that research has two objectives or that research has theory as its immediate objective but in two different ways." Simply put, though, research tests theory or stimulates theory.

There are two ways to stimulate theory: the researcher "encounters again and again, and with as many variations as possible, empirical reality." This is called planned "staring." A second way is to test theory at the just-preceding level. As for testing, only fourth-level theory testing is considered; it is "fairly well-accepted" that the others can be tested. The purpose of situation-producing theory is threefold: (1) to achieve its goal; (2) that these results be desirable when achieved; and (3) that guiding action by the theory is feasible in terms of cost, etc. Testing means testing all three dimensions: the theory's *coherency* must be tested; its *palatability* must be assessed; and the *feasibility* claim must be evaluated. Research methodology is not absolute and can be expected to vary with the level of theory tested, and with its being strictly "test" *or* stimulation. The conditional nature of methodology is stressed to approach creatively the kind of research needed or to stimulate practice theory for nursing. Summary and conclusions follow. Noteworthy among these observations are:

> "Research is for theory, theory for practice, so that practice fittingly has first place and theory has the mediating role."

"There is a thorough-going, mutual interdependence as among the three activities of practice, theorizing, and research."

"In short, to supply nursing image is to venture a nursing theory."

The authors are mostly to be commended for certain emphases, certain stressed elements, especially concerning the place and importance of theory in nursing. As with their other productions, this article fails to provide any bibliography. This article is not so controversial and seems not so valuable as their other contributions.

Donaldson, S.K. and Crowley, D. (1978). The discipline of nursing. *Nursing Outlook*, 26(2), 113–120

This article poses a series of significant questions. It begins by noting the question of the nature of nursing, but addresses this through a subquestion: What are the recurrent themes in nursing inquiry? These could suggest "boundaries" for systematic study of the discipline of nursing. There follows a long discussion of the nature of classification of disciplines. Nursing is seen as a "professional" discipline. It is noted as a discipline different from nursing science (doctoral training for nursing historians as well as for nursing scientists is endorsed) and different from nursing practice (the discipline should be governing practice instead of vice versa). Finally, the structure of the discipline of nursing is considered, a generalization is offered ("nursing studies the wholeness or health of humans"), and some "major conceptualizations in nursing" are presented.

The article is poorly organized. The opening ideas are not developed and are unrelated to what follows (except for the assertion, not discussed, that they provide "boundaries"). On the second page, the authors state that what is truly important is to define the discipline of nursing. Having discussed the nature and relations of disciplines, one expected the next section to be entitled "The Discipline of Nursing." Instead, the authors launch into a discussion of nursing-as-practice versus the discipline of nursing. The structure (as opposed to the nature or definition?) and nursing's "perspective" are not clearly delineated or related. Definition is never mentioned, and what is given is somewhat vague, broad, and unspecific to nursing, such as "Major conceptualizations in nursing: 1. Distinctions between human and nonhuman beings; 2. Distinctions between living and non-living. . . . 7. Human characteristics . . . such as consciousness, abstraction . . . aging, dying, reproducing."

Nevertheless, this seminal work is challenging, and it has had a wide and significant impact on the theory development literature because of the importance of the topic and its timeliness. It makes the point successfully that nursing is a discipline and gives support to its focus.

Ellis, R. (1968). Characteristics of significant theories. *Nursing Research*, 17(3), 217–222

Significant theories for nursing are those that (1) improve practice by addressing the goal of nursing (represented by Henderson's definition) and (2) include the patient as a component. The purposes of theory development are (1) to distinguish fact from pseudofact, (2) to structure and synthesize facts from other fields, (3) to give direction to practice, and (4) to provide a framework for retrieval and use of generated and stored knowledge.

Seven characteristics of significant theories are enumerated: (1) *Scope* (the number of concepts related). Scope provides framework for ordering observations about a variety of phenomena, and it must include psychological and biologic variables; the broader the scope, the greater the significance. (2) *Complexity* (the notion that theory should treat multiple variables or relationships of a single variable in its full complexity). The strength of this argument is Ellis' admonition that "incomplete conceptualizations lead to hazards of illusory comprehension." (3) *Testability* (focuses chiefly on the importance of recognizing theories as hypothetical constructs, amenable to change). (4) *Usefulness* (the ultimate criterion is that theories help develop and guide clinical practice). (5) *Implicit value* must be recognized and made explicit. (6) *Capability* of generating new information, new ideas, and practices must be there. (7) *Terminology* can be used meaningfully with, or applied to, phenomena observed in nursing.

These "characteristics of significant theories" speak directly or indirectly to evaluative methodologies and criteria for internal and external validity presented elsewhere, providing a succinct presentation of major considerations. Ellis' positions on scope and complexity should be compared with those of Jacox, Hardy, Stevens, Duffey and Muhlenkamp, and Hage. The major area of disagreement between Ellis and other authors is related to the characteristic of testability, which, she states, can be sacrificed in favor of scope, complexity, and clinical usefulness. Ellis she argues that "elegance and complexity of structure are to be preferred to precision in the meaning of concepts in the present state of knowledge." This view should be contrasted with the more prevalent argument for testability as the ultimate determinant of significance.

Fawcett, J. (1980). A framework for analysis and evaluation of conceptual models of nursing. *Nurse Educator*, 5(6), 10–14

The purpose of this article is to provide a clear definition of conceptual models, to delineate the confused distinction between conceptual models and theories, and to develop a framework for analysis and evaluation of conceptual models.

A conceptual model is defined as a set of abstract concepts and the assumptions that integrate them into a meaningful configuration. By identifying relevant phenomena, (person, environment, health, and nursing), a conceptual model provides a perspective for scientists; by describing these phenomena and their interrelationships in general and abstract terms, the model represents the first step in developing the theoretical formulations needed for scientific activities.

A theory is a set of interrelated concepts, definitions, and propositions that present a systematic view of phenomena by specifying relations among variables (Kerlinger). It postulates specific relations among concepts and takes the form of a description, explanation, prediction, or prescription for action. Any theory presupposes a more general abstract conceptual system. The crucial distinction between a conceptual model and a theory is the level of abstraction; a theory is both more precise and more limited in scope than its parent conceptual scheme.

Based on this distinction between conceptual models and theories, different frameworks are required for analysis and evaluation. The remainder of the article is devoted to the presentation of a framework for analysis (philosophical base, context, scope) and evaluation (internal validity, etc) of conceptual models of nursing.

This is an excellent, substantive article that is of value both in its articulation of differences between conceptual models and theories and its eclectic framework.

Gebbie, K. and Lavin, M.A. (1974). Classifying nursing diagnoses. *American Journal of Nursing*, 74(2), 250–253

Report of the First National Conference on the Classification of Nursing Diagnoses. This article describes the process of developing a classification system and a list of tentative nursing diagnoses.

It is an example of what Dickoff and James call a factor-isolating theory. The relationship of nursing diagnoses to theory development, while observed in the article, is made explicit and developed in detail by Kritek (1978).

Gortner, S.R. (1983). The history and philosophy of nursing science and research. *Advances in Nursing Science*, 5(2), 1–8

Only in the past few years have philosophy of science issues attracted serious attention in nursing research, as the research tradition moves into a new phase of development. Questions regarding method, discovery (as opposed to justification or proof), ethics, politics, and so forth are now prompting comment. This article presents an overview of this philosophical component of emerging nursing science and research and does so in part through a historical perspective.

In the early years, practice was the source of knowledge. Efforts to generate a knowledge base for nursing through research have been much more prominent in the past two decades. Early research approaches included development of critical resources, surveys, conferences, studies of procedure, case analyses, and alliance with other disciplines. More recent times have seen the enlargement of critical resources (especially in doctoral education) and public support and new development of colleagueship, communication, and research designs and methods.

On this last subject, Gortner addresses a major point of discussion: "To assume that the choice of research methods used in nursing was influenced by a particular philosophy of science (eg, logical positivism) is to attribute too much deliberation or rationality to what was the result of social, political, and economic events." With doctoral training in other fields than nursing, nursing scientists brought with them methods that had served them well in other fields. They also had to face the pragmatics of funding. "Granting agencies prefer controlled studies in which variables are well-specified and instrumentation is precise." Finally, generalizability has become a critical element because "the capacity to affect practice depends heavily on this factor."

Consensus has emerged about the definition and subject matter of nursing and the research paradigms of its science. However, the philosophical orientation of the science remains chiefly empirical and naturalistic. Attempts to incorporate theoretical propositions are now being made, and the search is on to discover relationships. "Science (empirics), art (esthetics), morality (ethics), and intuition (personal or subjective) all represent sources of knowledge. . . . The profession surely can accommodate multiple paradigms (analytic, humanistic) and modes of inquiry (naturalistic, experimental, historical). In the formation of research questions and the choice of areas of inquiry, it can be expected that inquiry will be of a more fundamental nature in the future than was true in the past. Examples of phenomena that have relevance for nursing include self-care, social support, family functioning, and stress. Two other important areas are clinical therapeutics and investigation of environments.

Gortner concludes that "nursing science will make a major contribution, as science, in the interface of the biological and social sciences concerned with illness and health."

This article is significant because of its comprehensiveness and currency; it points forward to the shape of nursing's future.

Green, J.A. (1979). Science, nursing and nursing science: A conceptual analysis. *Advances in Nursing Science*, 2(1), 57–64

This article examines the term "science" historically, linguistically, and contextually. The scientific method is considered ("science includes both methodology and knowledge"), and the functions of science are indicated. Various definitions are cited (Conant, Nagel, Fischer), and a synthetic definition is offered. The usefulness of this definition of science for nursing is said to be its potential for evaluating the status of nursing science: "It provides a standard to determine whether or not a designated body of knowledge constitutes a science." A distinction is established between science and technology.

A series of definitions of nursing are considered, with attention given to chronological development of the nurse's role (Henderson, Wiedenbach, Yura and Walsh, King, Travelbee). Following Travelbee, an analytical course is set. Nursing is seen as involving content and process. A comparison of nursing and medicine is made. Knowledge drawn from natural, behavioral, social, and medical sciences constitutes the science in nursing. This is then transformed through application in clinical practice. So, a definition of nursing becomes "a service discipline that provides care, concern, and comfort to recipients experiencing a broad range of health–illness phenomena through the synergetic combination of its art and science." This definition precludes separate classification of technical and professional nursing.

The main value of this article is that it collects and presents good basic materials on the questions "What is science?" and "What is nursing?" Green's only argument for "nursing science" is a reference to Gortner and colleagues, who, she says, document its existence. Also, her synthetic definitions seem to be inferior to her citations from other sources.

Hall, B.A. (1981). The change paradigm in nursing: Growth versus persistence. *Advances in Nursing Science*, 3(4), 1–6

Questions of emerging and competing paradigms in nursing theory development are addressed as they relate to shaping the values of the professional. The "change paradigm," which postulates continuous flux, has been pervasive in nursing theory (eg, adaptation, development). It is argued that: (1) a paradigm based on change may not be the most productive departure for the study of humans and health; (2) a focus on change leads to the illusion that things are changing when they are actually staying the same; and (3) nursing's attention may have been drawn to the phenomena of changes at the expense of increasing our understanding of the capacity for stability and persistence.

Hall's attention to the heuristic value of a paradigm is an interesting example of the sociology of science, and her admonitions about the acceptance of unverified assumptions underlying theory are provocative and important. Several interesting questions are raised that are based on Kuhn and have generalizability beyond the specific example: What is the process by which a paradigm is accepted? Why and when does a paradigm's shift occur? What is the relationship between theory and value? Can competing paradigms exist simultaneously, and with what implications?

The presentation of change and stability as competing theoretical notions may be somewhat oversimplified. Although Hall explicitly refrains from dropping models of change, her presentation is strongly biased in the direction of stability (albeit perhaps for the sake of balance). Perhaps change and stability are better viewed as which/when versus either/or phenomena. Kuhn's paradigm, espoused by Hall, would seem to preempt the possibility of dialectical theory development. This article should be read by the student with some background in theory development.

Hardy, M.E. (1978). Perspectives on nursing theory. *Advances in Nursing Science*, 1(1), 37–48

Nursing theory development and evaluation are viewed within the context of stages of scientific development. Applying Kuhn's thesis on the development of scientific knowledge, Hardy argues that nursing is in a "preparadigmatic" stage of theory development, "characterized by divergent schools of thought which, although addressing the same range of phenomena, usually describe and interpret these phenomena in different ways." Nursing needs to struggle through and beyond the preparadigmatic stage of scientific development because confusion, wasted energy, and poorly focused, systematic research result from this lack of a well-defined perspective.

A "metaparadigm," or prevailing paradigm, on the other hand, presents a general orientation that holds the commitment and consensus of the scientists in a particular discipline. It determines the general parameters of the field, it provides focus to scientific endeavor, and it may subsume several "exemplar" paradigms, which are more concrete and specific in directing the activities of scientists. The existence of a prevailing paradigm facilitates the "normal work of science." Research is purposeful, orderly, and raises few unanswerable questions. Whereas the adoption of a metaparadigm cannot be decreed but rather will be based on its scientific credence and its potential for advancing scientific knowledge, nursing scientists can facilitate this process by being well informed in a substantive area and participating actively in theory construction and research.

Subsequent sections of this article address the nature of theory, the relationship between theory and practice, criteria for "borrowing" theory from other disciplines, types (levels) of theory, and criteria for theory evaluation, including logical adequacy, empirical adequacy, usefulness, and significance. Each of these criteria is clearly elaborated.

Whereas Hardy's "perspectives" are not clearly interrelated, they are well worth reading. Before reflecting on the implications of nursing's "preparadigmatic" stage of theory development, consider: (1) the applicability of Kuhn's thesis to nursing and (2) evidence for other conclusions on the status of nursing science. The sections on development and evaluation of theory are excellent. Hardy's criteria should be compared with other taxonomies.

Jacobs, M.K. and Huether, S.E. (1978). Nursing science: The theory-practice linkage. *Advances in Nursing Science,* 1(1), 63–73

Nursing science is defined as both process and product: "the process of nursing science requires that concepts be defined, operationalized, linked into relationships, and verified. From verified conceptual linkages accrue the product, which is theory; and the theory explains and predicts nursing phenomena." The goal of nursing science is to define goals and guide practice; it is prerequisite to professional autonomy and impact.

The complementary and mutually dependent interrelationship of theory and practice are emphasized and demonstrated. Concepts, the building blocks of theory, must be empirically derived and operationalized in a clear and useful manner. They are then linked in theoretical formulations that are subject to empirical verification. Theory without practice is vacuous; practice without theory is intuitive rather than scientific. The contributions of both researchers and practitioners are crucial.

These authors present nursing as an evolving science. The current status of nursing science is illuminated by historical perspective; education and "cohesiveness will facilitate the advancement of nursing science." The article includes brief sections on the nature of science, the structure and function of science, and the process of concept selection and definition. The theory–practice linkage is clearly articulated and appropriately emphasized.

Jacox, A. (1974). Theory construction in nursing: An overview. *Nursing Research*, 23(1), 4–13

Three levels or stages of theory development are discussed: (1) a period of specifying, defining, and classifying the concepts used in describing the phenomena of the field; (2) developing statements or propositions that propose how two or more concepts are related; and (3) specifying how all the propositions are related to each other in a systematic way.

Concepts are abstract representations of reality that indicate the subject matter of a theory. They may vary both in complexity (concepts, "higher-level" concepts, constructs), and in the degree to which they are observable versus symbolic (empirical–theoretical continuum). Precise operational definitions are emphasized.

Propositions are statements of constant relationships between two or more concepts or facts. All scientific propositions are based on empirical generalizations that may be proved false in the future. Types of relational statements include laws, axioms, theorems, hypotheses and principles—differentiated on the basis of degree of tentativeness. Although nursing has made wide use of principles on which to base nursing action, Jacox observes little attempt to relate these principles to one another systematically.

Scientific theory is defined as "a systematically related set of statements, including some law-like generalizations, that is empirically testable." The purpose of theory "to describe, explain, and predict a selected aspect of empirical reality" requires the use of both inductive and deductive reasoning and a close relationship between theory, practice, and research.

Jacox espouses nursing practice theory as that which guides the nurse's actions in attaining nursing goals in patient care. While presupposing and building on theory that explains, describes, and predicts, nursing practice theory must allow the investigator to go beyond these levels to prescribe and control. She describes nursing as a discipline "in which the major concern is *use* of knowledge."

Other topics discussed in this article include: (1) definition and use of models to guide research, (2) arguments for "middle-range theories" in nursing (versus "grand theory" or abstracted empiricism"), and (3) a discussion of the nature and source of knowledge and theory in (of, for) nursing and the proper use of nursing resources in theory development.

This article is a good overview of theory construction, emphasizing the relationships between various elements of theories and emphasizing issues in the development of nursing theory. Jacox's nursing practice theory should be compared with Dickoff and James and the contrasting position of Beckstrand. Comparisons should also be made with Hardy, Donaldson and Crowley, and Green. Reflection on Jacox's description of the "state of the art" of theory construction in nursing is recommended.

Johnson, D.E. (1959). The nature of a science of nursing *Nursing Outlook*, 7(5), 291–294

The basis for the concepts set forth in this article is found in the earlier article by this author on the philosophy of nursing. Here, the focus is on exploring the nature of nursing as a science and as a discipline. Johnson identifies professional disciplines as representing applied sciences. One might be interested in comparing her thoughts on this with a more recent article by Donaldson and Crowley, noting that Johnson and Crowley were colleagues at the University of California, Los Angeles in the mid-1960s and that Crowley was influenced by Johnson (1978).

Johnson believes that the goals of nursing must be established in precise terms to give direction to the search for a body of knowledge. Although nursing shares the ultimate goal held by all health workers, its specific and unique goal is not as clearly understood or as widely accepted as that of medicine. It is through a discussion of nursing's professional goal that Johnson elaborates on her conceptions as a way of illustrating how the development of science can be given direction. Her conception of nursing care is borrowed from general systems theory, and the primary purpose of nursing care is expressed in terms such as tension, equilibrium, and dynamic state.

For nursing to achieve its goals, it is hypothesized that two kinds of knowledge are needed: the knowledge of people, which is shared knowledge common to all health workers; and knowledge of the science of nursing. Furthermore, it is this author's thesis that "the science of nursing is developed through the reformulation of concepts drawn from the basic sciences to yield a body of knowledge fundamental to the development of theories of nursing diagnosis and nursing intervention."

Borrowing theory is a controversial approach to the development of nursing knowledge but is nonetheless a useful one, as demonstrated by a number of other nursing theorists as well as Johnson. Herein Johnson develops a rationale for that approach. We will later see how she does this using systems theory as a prototype to develop her behavioral systems model.

This article makes an important contribution to the early thinking about a science of nursing, in addition to showing us Johnson's early thinking about the behavioral systems model. The writing is clear, and the presentation is logically developed and expressed. This article should be read by those who are interested in Johnson's model, especially by those who wish to see how the model unfolded, and by all who are interested in the development and organization of nursing knowledge. Responses and patterns, part of the lexicon in nursing in the 1980s, were introduced as early as 1959, as is evident in this publication.

Johnson, D.E. (1968). Theory in nursing: Borrowed and unique. *Nursing Research*, 17(3), 206–209

Differentiation of "borrowed" and "unique" theory in nursing may help clarify nursing's appropriate place and focus in theory development. Borrowed theory is defined as that knowledge that is developed in the main by other disciplines and that is drawn on by nurses. Unique theory is defined as that knowledge derived from the observation of phenomena and the asking of questions unlike those that characterize other disciplines.

The question of borrowed and unique is analyzed first in respect to the nature of knowledge required for nursing practice and the availability of the knowledge. This knowledge may be divided into: (1) knowledge of order, that which describes and explains the "normal" state of people and the "normal" scheme of things (this kind of knowledge has been the focus of the basic sciences); (2) knowledge of disorder, that which helps us understand events that pose a threat to the well-being or survival of the individual or society; and (3) knowledge of control, that which allows prescription of a course of action that, when executed, changes the sequence of events in desired ways predicated on the knowledge of disorder and geared toward specified outcomes. Although knowledge of all these types is basic to nursing practice, it is in the area of disorder that efforts at nursing theory development should be concentrated.

A second perspective for analysis of the borrowed/unique issue considers the problem of nursing's objects in scientific investigation. Nursing is ill defined as a field of practice and as a field of inquiry. The lack of definition constitutes a serious obstacle to professional and scientific development. If there is an area for study and theory development unique to nursing, it will evolve only through the study of phenomena and through asking questions in a way that is not characteristic of any other discipline. Behavioral system disorders represent such a focus.

Part of the 1968 Symposium on Theory Development in Nursing. This article is a "must read" because: (1) it is a cogent and effective analysis of one of the major issues in theory development. (2) Johnson's framework of order, disorder, and control is one of the major typologies in the literature; and (3) it serves as an introduction and rationale for Johnson's Behavioral Systems Model.

Johnson, D.E. (1978). Development of theory: A requisite for nursing as a primary health profession. In Chaska, N. (Ed.), *The nursing profession: Views through the mist.* New York: McGraw-Hill

The development of a theoretical body of nursing knowledge is a means of acquiring professional status. Impediments to the development of nursing science are surveyed, and two questions are presented as means of providing direction: For what purpose is a theoretical body of knowledge intended? and What phenomena must be studied and what kinds of questions must be asked to develop the needed knowledge?

In response to these questions, Johnson discusses the evaluation of scientific disciplines and the professions as sciences. Sciences become differentiated on the basis of the distinctive perspective for observation and interpretation of selected phenomena. The focus of any profession's scientific concern is interdependent with its service (social function). Johnson discusses the implication of different conceptual models and alternative routes to theory development and presents three social criteria for evaluating models: congruence (Do nursing decisions and actions that are based on the model fulfill social expectations?); significance (Do nursing decisions and actions based on the model lead to outcomes for patients that make an important difference in their lives or well-being?); and utility (Is the conceptual system on which the model is based sufficiently well developed to provide clear direction for nursing practice, education, and research?).

This is a good theoretical treatise on problems in nursing theory development and the evaluation of solutions to these problems. Direct responses to Johnson's guiding questions, however, must be supplemented from other sources (see sections on philosophy, practice, research, guidelines). Johnson's theory evaluation criteria, based on factors extrinsic to the substance of the model, represent an often neglected yet important dimension.

Kramer, S. (1969). Behavioral science and human biology in medicine. *The New Physician*, 18(11), 965–978

The question is raised whether information in the biologic, behavioral, and medical sciences can be used to develop a comprehensive theory of the human organism. Kramer presents the thesis that "in human development, the social environment, through its influence on genetically determined patterns of behavior together with the normal process of growth, is capable of modifying the development of every individual in characteristic ways." Examples of the interrelated nature of biopsychosocial variables are given, using growth and development as a frame of reference. One major concept—"character structure"—is developed to define psychic, somatic, and social unity of the individual to explain the empirical finding that alterations of behavior in one realm are capable of influencing all other realms (as in stress reactions).

The proposed "medical-ecological model" of the human organism represents an attempt to develop an eclectic "grand theory." The rationale is presented intelligently, and recognition is given to some major obstacles, for example, the fact that individual disciplines use words in different ways and use different units of analysis, ranging from the molecular (physiology) to the molar (behavioral sciences). Implications for conceptualization or viable theory development are left to the reader.

Kritek, P.B. (1978). The generation and classification of nursing diagnosis: Toward a theory of nursing. *Image*, 10(2), 33–40

In building nursing theory, we have skipped the first stage of specifying, defining, and classifying our concepts, and this has led to problems. To the degree that first-level theory (descriptive) is dissonant with or unclear when related to "what is" in nursing, the eventual level-four theory (prescriptive) will be dissonant or unclear. Returning to the level-one theory, building and doing first things first, may be a worthwhile place toward which we could redirect our energies. This is being done through the generation and classification of nursing diagnoses (see Gebbie and Lavin, 1974). This level-one theory is evaluated in terms of Ellis' criteria of a significant theory.

Read this article after Dickoff, James, and Wiedenbach (1968a, 1968b), Ellis (1968), and Gebbie and Lavin (1974). It is most insightful in the application and implications of Dickoff, James, and Wiedenbach's framework. Would you call nursing diagnoses theory?

Leininger, M.M. (1969). Introduction: Nature of science in nursing. *Nursing Research*, 18(5), 388–389

This is a statement of conference goals to explore approaches and methods that will support a scientific discipline and a body of nursing knowledge. There is a core of nurses eager to develop both a scientific and a humanistic discipline of nursing within institutions of higher education. Though "a theory" of nursing is spoken of, it is healthy and desirable that there be multiple theories, models, and conceptual frameworks. An attitude of constructive skepticism and critique of colleagues is urged.

In addition to induction and deduction, an ethnoscientific approach is suggested: a systematic and descriptive documentary study of phenomena through the eyes of people in their situations. Nursing lacks systematic ethnological studies of concrete nurse–patient–other situations.

There is a need to be tolerant of one another's failures and frustrations. Finally, change must be accommodated. Students should be encouraged to explore problems and test ideas that seem "exotic, highly radical, or out-of-this-world." This is a brief overview of concerns facing the conference.

McCarthy, R.T. (1972). A practice theory of nursing care. *Nursing Research*, 21(5), 406–410

Can the format (of Dickoff, James, and Wiedenbach), applied to a real-life situation, produce useful theories of nursing (practice)?

The purpose of this article is to illustrate how a practice theory can be developed on four levels. McCarthy presents data from her survey of postoperative patterns of voiding in patients with spinal anesthesia to demonstrate the four levels of theory as described by Dickoff and colleagues (1968a). Under first-level theory (factor-isolating), she categorizes patients according to type of surgery. Second-level theory (factor-relating) involves analyzing the relationships between need for catheterization, duration of surgery, fluid intake, and so on. So far so good. When we get to the third level we find that "a statement that 'patients who have not voided within 14 hours may have to be catheterized' could be said to constitute predictive theory." The highest level of theory—situation-producing or prescriptive—is a nursing care plan (eg, "note time of last voiding," note when patient expresses desire to void, offer assistance, etc.).

The article also includes an example of a survey list in operation. Is the reader's response to the opening question affirmative or negative? Does your response reflect comment on McCarthy or on Dickoff, James, and Wiedenbach?

McKay, R. (1969). Theories, and models, and systems for nursing. *Nursing Research*, 18(5), 393–400

Theory is the cornerstone of all scientific work because the understanding, which is the goal of science, is expressed in terms of theoretical formulations. The article gives much space to defining various senses of the term "theory." Nursing, at present, should use the word in a modest sense. "Models" are defined and analyzed. Models vary in two ways: level of abstraction and metaphor used. Two metaphors have been dominant—the machine and the organism. The organism is currently the dominant model in many fields, and, for both philosophic and practical reasons, it is dominant in nursing.

The concept of "systems" is the ultimate central focus of the article. Various definitions of systems are offered. Open and closed systems are discussed. Properties of open systems are articulated, and the suggestion is made that nursing could be represented by such a systems approach. Theorems or propositions based on general systems theory developed by James Miller are endorsed as particularly appropriate for nursing. Finally, a systems approach to the study of nursing education is proposed for the study of students and of curricula.

This is a valuable treatment of the subjects considered. Its value is due in great part to the many clear and careful definitions and to its detailed application of systems theory to nursing. There is a crucial question about models and metaphor: Is the model merely a restatement in other terms or does it accomplish extension or clarification? The late Dr. McKay was a central figure in metatheory. This represents a fine example of her writing.

McKay, R.C. (1977). What is the relationship between the development and utilization of a taxonomy and nursing theory? *Nursing Research*, 26(3), 222–224

This essay is a brief description of the purposes and principles of classification schemes. The definition and arrangement of concepts in a taxonomy, presuming it reflects the natural system, is a descriptive model of reality and can be considered a theoretical design (factor-isolating or naming). The value of taxonomies for clinicians and educators are briefly listed.

It is another example of first-level theory; how it relates to the second level is not discussed. This article is really McKay's response to a reader's question.

Menke, E.M. (1978). Theory development: A challenge for nursing. In N.L. Chaska (Ed.), *The nursing profession: Views through the mist*. New York: McGraw-Hill

Menke considers three issues related to theory development in nursing: the importance of theory development, the present status of theory development, and strategies to facilitate theory development in nursing.

Theory development is important for any discipline because it prescribes the conceptual framework for describing, explaining, and predicting phenomena. It serves as a means to isolate and classify facts, and it points to gaps in the available knowledge. Definitions and components of theories are discussed, as well as levels (Dickoff and James) or stages (Jacox) of theory development. The importance of lower-level theory development as a sound basis is emphasized, and consideration of theories about nursing rather than of nursing is proposed. Lack of theory development may have been caused by the lack of systematic direction and collaboration among theory developers. An eclectic approach to theory development is advocated.

This is an excellent, well-written, and substantive review of major issues in theory development.

Moore, M.A. (1968). Nursing: A scientific discipline? *Nursing Forum*, 7(4), 340–348

Moore argues that in our eagerness to break away from the apprenticeship tradition, nurses are trying to develop a scientific discipline without setting the foundation that is characteristic of every well-structured discipline. The fallacies and shortcomings of such practices as searching for a theory of nursing; borrowing concepts, tools, methods, and even questions from other disciplines; and allowing values to interfere with science are discussed, along with their ramifications. The only sensible basis for the development of a content area to be labeled "nursing" involves empirical generalizations regarding the effects on the patient of the activities we carry out as nurses.

This short, easy-to-read article should be read early in a nursing theorist's career because it provides an excellent overview of major issues and pitfalls in the development of nursing theory and nursing science. Moore's emphasis on clear, precise definition of terms is refreshing. Although you can, now or later, argue about "the only sensible basis . . . ," Moore is obviously interested in the theory-practice-research linkage.

Murphy, S.A. and Hoeffer, B. (1983). Role of the specialties in nursing science. *Advances in Nursing Science*, 5(4), 31–39

There is some conceptual movement away from specialization in nursing. Three trends have impact in this regard: (1) defining nursing as a discipline separate from medicine, (2) educating entry-level generalists, and (3) developing conceptual frameworks.

As to the first, perspectives of the two professions—medicine and nursing—are now clearly different. Medicine has become more specialized in an attempt to keep abreast of technological changes and increased knowledge, whereas nursing has become more generalized and holistic in its approach to health care.

Second, medical-surgical nursing was disease-based, psychiatric nursing was patient-based, and community health nursing was locus-based. Many schools determined that using specialty departments as organizing components of the curriculum was no longer efficient; many now offer a series of concepts basic to nursing, along with the nursing process, and they loosely refer to these as an integrated curriculum. One of the outcomes is that the specialties are no longer clearly distinguishable. Also, movement from the hospital setting to the university, as well as changing patterns of illness, have reinforced this direction.

Third, the new conceptual system in nursing provides direction for practice and education. However, none have delineated the role of the specialties. The role of nursing specialties is supported, nonetheless. The authors bring to their aid the social policy statement on nursing by the ANA: "The effectiveness of the profession is increased when specialists are available to focus their efforts on a particular aspect of clinical nursing, to test application of newly available theory to conditions germane to that clinical aspect, and to translate those theory applications into nursing approaches considered more useful than prevailing ones."

It appears that nursing specialties can best contribute to nursing science by generating and testing middle-range or limited-size theories. This type of theory is more directly relevant for addressing practice concerns. As practice-relevant theory was developed and refined in each specialty from its particular vantage point, the specialty would contribute to nursing science through both cumulative and didactic processes.

The article concludes with a brief discussion of the theory development process (inductive, deductive, adapted) and a sustained example drawn from mental health nursing, where a concept from nursing, "mutual withdrawal," is identified and traced through its history.

This article is especially important for its focus on a perhaps as yet unassimilated consequence of recent developments in nursing: the de-emphasis of the specialties.

Newman M.A. (1972). Nursing's theoretical evolution. *Nursing Outlook,* 20(7), 449–453

Following a brief discussion of the evolution of nursing science, Newman elabor on three main approaches to the discovery of nursing knowledge that emerged du the 1960s: (1) the borrowing of theory from other disciplines with an intent to inte it into a science of nursing; (2) an analysis of nursing practice situations in sea the theoretical underpinnings; and (3) the creation of a conceptual system from theories could be derived. While limitations and difficulties in the first two appr are discussed, Rogers is credited with initiating the third phase. The clear-cut del of the individual as the focus of nursing gave direction to the development that is basic to nursing.

Newman cites Hempel to evidence the value of the Rogerian approac comparing Rogers with other nurse theorists, concludes that a conceptual nursing is evolving and does provide meaningful direction for research. Whether the theory evolves inductively from ideas conceived in clinical practice or deductively from broad generalizations within the theoretical framework does not seem particularly important. What is important is that the nursing investigator should determine the relationship of her study question to the overall conceptual system in nursing and should therefore expand and elaborate the system by the testing of theories that have derived from it. Nursing is coming of age.

Newman's article should be contrasted with that of Hardy, who sees nursing in a "preparadigmatic" stage (from Kuhn). She cites the problem of the past as a dearth of nursing knowledge while "the problem of the future will be an acceleration of that knowledge." Has this prediction been realized in the 20 years since this article was written? How does your answer attest to the veracity of Newman's characterization?

Notter, L.E. (1975). The case for nursing research. *Nursing Outlook,* 23(12), 70–763

Slow progress in nursing research is attributed to views of nursing and women, too little cumulative effort, and the relatively new idea of nursing as an intellectual profession. The following are areas for concentrated effort: the need for more research based on theories consonant with nursing's domain of responsibility; the need for replication; the need for postdoctoral research and for individual researchers who select a problem area and continue to study it over time; and the need for more service agencies to develop clinical research programs that encourage staff participation in research.

ayne, G. (1973). Comparative sociology: Some problems of theory and method. *British Journal of Sociology,* 1), 13–29

Comparative sociology is a method of inquiry that allows "explicit testing of sociological theories with data from various sources" and that examines "the nature of society as revealed by . . . the operation and interrelation of key processes in different societies, r areas of societies (historical, geographical, social)" (p. 13). The interrelationship of eory and method in the generation of social theory is examined, with emphasis on hodological issues in comparative analysis.

ocieties that are similar in regard to a specific variable (*e.g.,* form, function, or e) are studied to generate laws that explain that one type of society only. Prob- erent in this approach are categorization (defining categories and determining ble level of similarity) and generalization (producing theories that have more application). The purpose of comparing dissimilar societies is to yield uni- Defining and determining the appropriate scope of variables, as well as cific, meaningful hypotheses, are major difficulties. In both approaches, p in selecting study variables and studying them outside of their cul- ertheless, the comparative method provides not only understanding a means of verifying theory and developing a science of sociology. ent, substantive article on a particular methodology for develop- ence. Issues and problems of comparative study are addressed, and insight is given on the relationship of theory and methodology. What is missing in clarity of expression in this article is more than counterbalanced by the salience of ideas and the potential for applicability to nursing science development.

Payne, L. (1983). Health: A basic concept in nursing theory. *Journal of Advanced Nursing,* 8(5), 393–395

The article traces the historical evolution of the concept of health. For centuries, disease has been the central focus for the examination of the phenomenon of health. Only one major formulation (Sigerist's in 1941) preceded the critical turning point statements in the constitution of the World Health Organization (1958): "Health is a state of complete physical, mental, and social well-being and not merely the absence of disease and infirmity."

Various paradigms have subsequently been developed: the ecological model, based on the relationship of people to the total environment (Blum, 1974; Rogers, 1960), and the equilibrium model, based on the body's self-regulatory powers to maintain constancy of the internal milieu (Dubos, 1965). Psychosocial models came later: sociocultural, philosophical, or relating health to notions or normality. A new emphasis on quality of life and high-level wellness emerged (Dunn, 1959) due to people's dissatisfaction with life despite their affluence; the idea of holism, originating in Gestalt theory, grew to a multidimensional approach, emphasizing self-responsibility, the whole person, and the process of care-giving; and the "salutogenic" model of health (Antonovsky, 1979) originated, in which "the origin of health lies in a 'sense of coherence,' that is, the way in which one sees life as meaningful, manageable, and comprehensible."

Assumptions based on traditional paradigms have bound nursing curricula and practice to the negative view of health in terms of absence of disease. "The concept of health constitutes a basic building block for nursing theory. . . . If the goal of nursing is the promotion of health, making this concept operational is essential for nursing practice." Finally, a definition of health is offered (a nursing concept of health): "Health is the effective functioning of self-care resources that ensures the operation and adequacy of self-care actions."

The article combines some history, some popularization, some commonplace information, and perhaps some helpful reminders.

Peterson, C.J. (1977). Questions frequently asked about the development of a conceptual framework. *Journal of Nursing Education,* 16(4), 22–32

The relationship between theory and conceptual frameworks in nursing is examined. A conceptual framework is defined as "a loosely organized set or complex of ideas . . . that provides the overall structure of a curriculum (p. 25)." A theory is defined as a group of systematically interrelated propositions that provides organization to a body of content and, by allowing explanation and prediction, provides a guide for practice. A conceptual framework is an earlier evolutionary step that may be developed into theory, generating testable hypotheses.

Essential elements of a conceptual framework include: the nature of the service provided (nursing/nursing process), goal or outcome (health), rationale for services (nonhealth or illness), characteristics of the care-giver (nursing practitioner), characteristics of the recipient (patient/client), and context for service (care setting or environment). Explanations of the relationships of these concepts provide the framework.

The relationship of the conceptual framework to borrowed theories, program philosophy and objectives, and curricular threads, as well as its role in the development of a nursing curriculum, are also addressed.

This is an excellent article that demystifies the conceptual framework in a thorough, organized, and articulate manner. While emphasizing the use of conceptual frameworks in nursing curricula, the article provides much useful material on theory components (including simple but excellent definitions) and theory development. Excellent figures summarize major points. Peterson's selection of concepts may be compared with those of Dickoff and James, and her presentation of the conceptual framework should be contrasted with that of Torres and Yura.

Phillips, J.R. (1977). Nursing systems and nursing models. *Image,* 9(1), 4–7

Because the primary goal of nursing theory is the generation of knowledge specific to nursing, the process of theory building must be couched in a nursing frame of reference. Otherwise, the obtained knowledge will not be nursing knowledge that can be used to build or expand nursing science or that can be used for nursing education, practice, or research. Models that nursing has borrowed (medical, psychological, ecological, social) are criticized on the grounds that not one of them views the person as a totality in interaction with the environment. Models of Rogers and Johnson are proposed as frameworks for nursing theory construction.

There are many agreements between the arguments of this article and one by Newman (1972). Although some good points are made about the shortcomings (*e.g.,* of the medical model), many of the arguments could be further developed. Are there any legitimate prototypes outside of nursing?

Putnam, P. (1965). A conceptual approach to nursing theory. *Nursing Science,* 3, 430–442

A theoretical framework is valuable as a stimulus in the development of nursing science. In the absence of adequate theory, nursing is limited by the concrete here and now; nursing then becomes restricted to immediate impressions and is unable to explain the past, evaluate the present, or predict the future. Despite the clear necessity of a generalized theory, development has been slow and piecemeal; contributing factors include complexity of the subject matter, the proximity (and therefore influence) of the scientist to the empirical data, and the necessity of delimiting a knowledge base that will encompass changing objects in changing environmental fields.

A key to the conceptual maze is the identification of the unique domain of nursing. The knowledge base of the nursing process, nursing science, is at least a four-dimensional synthesis of knowledge relating to biological function, psychological function, social function, and variations in organization of these factors. The operational identification of the intermixture of components in the synthesis, defined and tested through nursing research, would be a genuine contribution to science. Nurses make it possible for patients to accomplish their own energy exchanges with the external environment. The abstraction of the idea of how nursing makes these exchanges possible is an essential step in theory construction. The constant interplay between theory, practice, and research is stressed.

Although other articles provide more cogent arguments for the value of nursing theory, more enlightened definitions of nursing, or more pragmatic suggestions for theory development, Putnam is particularly eloquent on the problems of lack of adequate theory, the characteristics of conceptual difficulties in nursing theory, and the need to identify the unique domain of nursing.

Quint, J.C. (1967). The case for theories generated from empirical data. *Nursing Research,* 16(2), 109–114

This work discusses a research approach in which a given problem area is studied for the purpose of developing a conceptual framework. Sections are devoted to the research problem and its overall design, the collection and analysis of data, and the reporting and interpretation of the findings.

This article is the precursor of an approach that has gained increased interest and credibility in the ensuing years.

Rogers, M.E. (1963). Some comments on the theoretical basis of nursing practice. *Nursing Science,* 1, 11–13, 60–61

This substantive article contains many of the elements that are later to be incorporated into Rogers' *Introduction to the theoretical basis of nursing* (1970). It is recommended that this be read prior to reading the book, but it is not a requisite to understanding the theory.

There is a mix of philosophy, definitions, concepts, and goals—all about life, human beings, nursing, and nursing science. Elements of the prototype theory—systems theory—are also present. These are presented not as a theoretical basis of the nursing process but rather "to stimulate logical and creative thinking concerning its identification and development." Despite Rogers' intent, however, a rudimentary structure of the future theory appears to be taking shape here.

First, the philosophical statements and beliefs are presented, along with assumptions about human beings. Nursing is defined as a process and the goal of nursing is also stated. The concept-building process is discussed, with one concept—the life process—presented. Principles rest on the definitions of the concepts, and principles are integral to nursing science. As an example of a basic principle in nursing science, the adaptive mechanism in human beings is identified. Rogers states, "The human organism has an amazing, innate capacity to adapt: physically, biologically, socially." (An assumption!) What is the purpose of a principle is not discussed in detail.

Finally, Rogers says that the theoretical basis of nursing practice must include a philosophy and a concept of death as well as life. However, she does not undertake that task. Furthermore, though the term "health" was used, it was not defined. Nor does

Rogers discuss the role of nursing as it relates to or interfaces with other health care givers. These, then, are a few limitations of this article.

The purpose of this article is to stimulate thinking concerning the identification and development of nursing science—the theoretical basis of nursing practice. Nursing science is a body of scientific knowledge characterized by descriptive, explanatory, and predictive principles about the life process of human beings. These principles rest on the review of the person as a unified "biophysicalpsychosocial" phenomenon in constant interaction with all parts of the environment. The body of knowledge develops through synthesis and resynthesis of selected information from the humanities and the biological, physical, and social sciences in order to form new concepts and understanding about the person and environment. It assumes its own "unique scientific mix" through selection and patterning of this information. The focus of nursing science is central to the formation and understanding of its theories. This focus is elaborated in the remainder of the article.

This is one of the original and most influential articles by one of nursing's true sages. This article, along with that of Johnson (1959), ushered in the era of nursing theory and nursing science. Rogers' characterization of nursing science has been a source of challenge and inspiration, and sometimes of conflict, to all subsequent nurse philosophers and theorists.

For its historical importance and strength of argument, this article should definitely be read. An introduction to Rogers' theory is an added bonus.

Rubin, R. (1968). A theory of clinical nursing. *Nursing Research,* 17(13), 210–212

This article is part of the 1968 Symposium on Theory Development in Nursing. It is a brief and simple example of development of a model and its use in research.

Silva, M.C. (1977). Philosophy, science, theory: Interrelationships and implications for nursing research. *Image,* 9(3), 59–63

This is an overview of the relationships among philosophy, science, and theory, with implications for the conduct of nursing research. Science developed into specializations; philosophy "unifies scientific findings so that man as a holistic being might emerge." Science aims to describe, understand, predict, control, or explain phenomena. Theory refers to a set of related statements that have been derived from scientific data and from which plausible hypotheses can be deduced, tested, and verified.

Implications for nursing research: (1) all nursing theory and research is derived from or leads to philosophy, (2) philosophical introspection and intuition are legitimate methods of scientific inquiry, and (3) nursing knowledge arrived at by the scientific method too often sacrifices meaningfulness for rigor.

The author argues that no real distinctions are made between different kinds of knowledge until the Industrial Revolution; Darwin and Freud set off a proliferation of knowledge. This appears to ignore much great work, including the obvious contributions of Francis Bacon. Silva's comparisons of the realms of philosophy, science, and theory are good beginnings in nursing. Her pleas for the recognition of nonscientific ways of knowing deserve attention.

Silva, M.C. and Rothbart, D. (1984). An analysis of changing trends in philosophies of science on nursing theory development and testing. *Advances in Nursing Science,* 6(2), 1–13

Philosophy of science and nursing theory are in states of transition. Has nursing theory kept pace with new trends in the philosophy of science?

Two competing schools in the philosophy of science are traced and examined: logical empiricism (1940s–1960s) and historicism (1960s–present). The schools are compared in terms of their views of science: (1) its components, (2) its characterization, and (3) its outcomes.

Components: For logical empiricism—deductive system, theories linked to and tested through empirically observable properties; for historicism—research tradition that includes many theories, ontological commitments, and methodological commitments.

Characterization: For logical empiricism—product, scientific knowledge, theory validation; for historicism—the human activity of working scientists, theory discovery.

Outcome: For logical empiricism—verification leading to a body of truth; for historicism—problem-solving effectiveness.

There follows a review of the literature in nursing theory. Three time periods are examined: 1964–1969, 1970–1975, and 1976–present.

1964–69: Logical empiricist position everywhere (*e.g.,* Dickoff and James, Abdellah. The exception—Leininger offered an ethnoscience research methodology.

1970–75: Culmination of logical empiricism in Jacox and Hardy; conceptual frameworks; "The irony is that . . . the logical empiricist viewpoints espoused were being strongly repudiated by a growing number of philosophers of science. . . . [N]ursing's theoretical link to philosophy of science was . . . about a decade behind the times."

1976–present: Continued commitment to logical empiricism; a beginning trend toward historicism (*e.g.,* in Newman, Hardy); revisions of conceptual frameworks and introduction of new ones, moving more explicitly toward logical empiricism; questioning of strictly quantitative methods.

Implications: (1) There should not be a single conceptual framework for nursing; (2) there will never emerge a static set of eternal truths; (3) historicism strongly encourages a careful study of actual practices, belief systems, and external factors; (4) the assessment of progress will be more practical (*i.e.,* problem solving).

Important recommendations: (1) Cooperation among nursing theorists, researchers, clinicians, and scholars; (2) exploration of innovative qualitative methods.

Because this article presents itself as expository rather than argumentative, the major questions are: Should one, after all, be trendy and in line with the latest fashion in the philosophy of science? In what ways do the ultimate recommendations differ from what Dickoff and James would suggest?

Stainton, M.C. (1982). The birth of nursing science. *The Canadian Nurse,* 78(10), 24–28.

"The birth of nursing science" celebrates the coming-to-terms of the new science by reviewing its history and describing the conditions necessary for its development. The history is detailed despite its brevity and is told in a lively style, with the added perspective of the author's Canadian nationality and focus.

The list of developmental requirements includes: a perception of nursing as a developing science in the minds and hearts of all nurses; a sense of the significance of each nurse's contribution; a cadre of nursing scientists; the conceptualization of nursing as a science; nursing research teams; monies; the introduction of nursing science to science in general; research and facilities in major centers of nursing; collaboration and international networks; replication of studies; nursing education at all levels of career development; an individual goal of professionalism; and an expectation that one day a nurse will be the recipient of the Nobel Prize for excellence in contributing to science.

The significance of this article should be considered in terms of its effects on the intended readership.

Tinkle, M.B. and Beaton, J.L. (1983). Toward a new view of science: Implications for nursing research. *Advances in Nursing Science,* 5(2), 27–36

This article begins by pointing to two oppositions: the "hard" versus the "soft" science debate and the opposition between traditional historians of science and the "historicist" revisionists, such as Kuhn and Laudan. These oppositions are associated and identified in Sampson's formulation as Paradigm I versus Paradigm II. "Context-free generalizations" comprise the object of Paradigm I; research guided by the view of Paradigm II is "often conducted in naturalistic settings, using observational methods."

The authors further contend that the dominance of Paradigm I science is a result of "nourishment it has received from a male-dominant, Protestant-ethic-oriented, middle-class, liberal, and capitalistic society." The implications for nursing are multiple. If scientific truth is acontextual, then little attention is likely to be paid to the values and biases underlying research endeavors, so methodological biases or determinations of proper research subjects may go unexamined.

Further, nursing is, at its most basic level, a relational profession. However, acontextual study is not likely to focus on interpersonal or person—situation interactions. Such studies are apt to lack "ecological validity" and to be removed from the "real world."

The overarching conceptualization of nursing that can be abstracted from nursing theory is centered around the view of a human being as a holistic being. Nursing involves each person's unique bio-psycho-social context. The impact of the environment is a recurrent theme. Sociocultural context is stressed. However, the experimental method is also held in the highest regard.

"What is proposed is a blending of both methodologies to produce a science that retains a critical concern for objectivity while ensuring that the research it produces has validity in the real world and the influence of contextual variables is acknowledge."

This article suffers from the very problems it indicts. It is too abstract and general (*i.e.,* it rarely provides *examples* of the kinds of studies it talks about), and when, as in two references to women's studies in psychology, it moves toward some specificity, the work is simply alluded to. It is also too far from real life; the proposal for blending the two methodologies in a future state moves toward the mystical: "This new synthesis will not consist of the use of Paradigm II methods in the context of discovery and the use of Paradigm I in matters of verification. Rather, a convergence will involve the higher organization of the opposites in both paradigms."

Nevertheless, the point of the article—that we must have an explicit awareness of the assumptions and biases underlying our methods (particularly, in this case, sexist ones)—commands our assent.

Tucker, R.W. (1979). The value decisions we know as science. *Advances in Nursing Science,* 1(2), 1–12

Tucker argues that the processes of science necessarily involve the making of value judgments (versus the ubiquitous image of science as "value-free"). After classifying value judgments along the dimensions: rationale (personal versus objective), subscribership (individual versus "market") and explicitness (formal versus contextual), he discusses the "value decision-making contexts in research." Tucker's position is that each step of the research process—from selection of a problem, theoretical framework, and methodology to analyzing and reporting data—involves value judgments. The principal activity of science is to make well-supported value judgments.

Tucker encourages an explicit awareness of "the value decisions we know as science." There are some valuable insights in this article—if you can avoid getting hung up on the PVJs, CVJs, and VDMCRs.

Wald, F.S. and Leonard, R.C. (1964). Toward development of a nursing practice theory. *Nursing Research,* 13(4), 309–313

Nursing practice theory—based on the empirical approach of building knowledge directly from systematic study of nursing—is proposed as an alternative to "making borrowed concepts fit." In developing its own theories, nursing would become an independent discipline in its own right. In freeing themselves from the burden of looking only for applications of the basic sciences in their practice, nurses would at the same time take on the responsibility of developing their own science. This calls for the development of nursing practice theory.

Major sections of this article deal with: (1) the fallacy of nursing as an applied science ("accepted" principles may be invalid or inappropriate to nursing, nursing problems are being rephrased as social science cues rather than cues of practice); (2) characteristics of research methods for practice versus descriptive science (the difference lies in the selection of variables and the kind of hypotheses that are entertained); (3)

characteristics of practice versus descriptive theory (practice must contain causal hypotheses); and (4) barriers to the development of research of practice theory in nursing (related to research attitudes, need to generalize, and skill in research methods).

This is the first article written on practice theory in nursing and should definitely be read. Those interested in nursing theory should certainly contrast "the fallacy of nursing as an applied science" with the more prevalent view of how nursing science is developed. In addition, consider the process of development of practice theory presented by Wald and Leonard (p. 311) that is clearly a precursor to the influential work of Dickoff, James, and Wiedenbach.

Weatherston, L. (1979). Theory of nursing: Creating effective care. *Journal of Advanced Nursing,* 4(7), 365–375

Effective nursing care requires a *theory of nursing*—a phrase that connotes the interdependence of the two concepts. Conceptual analysis of "nursing," using Wilson's "model case" method is presented as a way to determine the "essence of nursing," and provides a basis for deciding what nursing theory is. The purpose of theory is to explain, predict, or control phenomena. In order to be a theory of nursing "the theory must be created and used with reference to the unique functions and intentions of nursing and the nature of nursing activity." The relationship of "microtheory" and "paradigmatic theory" are described. A model is developed to demonstrate the relationship of theory, practice, and education.

This article addresses several key issues, including the "essence" of nursing; the relationships among theory, practice, and education; and the rationale for and process of theory building in nursing. However, more sophisticated treatments of each of these subjects are available elsewhere, and should be read first. Many of the article's shortcomings are related to the nonevaluative use of several frameworks and definitions: Wilson's Model Case method, Peter's criteria for education, and conceptions of nursing that do not stress its scientific aspects.

SECTION II

Abstracts of Writings in Nursing Theory, 1960–1984

Afaf Meleis and Sandra Scheetz

The citations abstracted in this section pertain to selected central writings related to only six of the nurse theorists presented in this text (Johnson, Levine, Orem, Rogers, Roy, and Travelbee). Only selected writings related to each of the theorists and others' writings (based on theories) were described and analyzed below. The abstracts presented in this section are organized alphabetically according to theorist and author. This section is best used in conjunction with Chapter 3 and with the corresponding chapters in the text that focus on the analysis of the particular theory (Chapters 12, 15, 16, 17, and 18).

Dorothy Johnson

Auger, J.R. and Dee, V. (1983). A patient classification system based on the behavioral system model of nursing: Part 1. *Journal of Nursing Administration,* 13, 38–43

This first article of a two-part series focused on the development of a patient classification system based on a nursing model and was presented from the combined perspectives of administration and clinical practice. Part 2 (Dee and Auger), to follow, focused on the implementation of the classification system in the clinical setting. The nursing model used was Johnson's behavioral system model and the clinical setting was psychiatric.

The specific intent of such a classification system was for use "as a clinical measure of patient progress in addition to the administrative determination of staffing levels" (p. 38). The importance of a framework common to both was stressed. The rationale for such a classification system versus the use of an existing classification system was discussed.

The rationale for using the Johnson behavioral systems model as the theoretical framework for the classification system in this psychiatric setting was threefold: (1) it could be used with the existing programs based on social learning theory; (2) it could be applied to all clinical settings because of the emphasis on bio-psychosociocultural factors; and (3) it identified universal patterns of behavior applicable to all individuals. The model addresses the eight subsystems outlined by Johnson that include ingestive, eliminative, sexual, dependency, affiliative, achievement, aggressive-protective, and restorative. These subsystems of behavior are "assumed to be universal and of primary significance to all persons" (p. 39).

Integrated with the nursing process, the model provided a focus for the assessment phase and is intended to link specific patient behaviors with the corresponding nursing interventions. Furthermore, the model allows for use in clinical settings other than psychiatry.

The development of the classification tool began by certain people addressing the nursing care requirements for patients admitted to either the adult or child psychiatric units of the agency where it was developed. Therefore, the tool had to be both comprehensive and flexible enough to describe behaviors reflective of a wide variety of diagnoses and age groups. To meet this challenge, a group of expert clinicians and nursing administrators was organized to develop the tool.

The criteria for item inclusion reflected several dimensions. First, each of the eight subsystems of the Johnson behavioral system model were operationalized in terms of both adaptive and maladaptive behaviors. The behavioral statements had to meet four criteria: "measurable, relevant to the clinical setting, observable, and specific to the subsystem" (p. 39). A panel of experts then evaluated the statements to make certain that they met the four criteria. The behaviors were also ranked in one of three categories according to their level of adaptiveness, with one being the most adaptive and three being the least adaptive, or maladaptive. Nursing interventions were also ranked according to requirements for intensity and frequency of nursing contact. A fourth level was included to reflect the intensity of one-to-one nursing care required for extremely maladaptive behavior.

After the initial set of critical behaviors were formulated, they were tested by letting a sample of 28 registered nurses, in pairs, serve as observers on seven inpatient units. "Each pair of observers was asked to rate each subsystem of behavior for all patients present on the unit during the shift. In addition, the observers rated the overall level of behavior for each patient" (pp. 39–40). Several exhibits were included to illustrate some components of the process thus far: first, the eight subsystems, definitions of behaviors, and critical behavior characteristics; second, characteristic patient behaviors and the requisite nursing intervention; and third, samples of level three (maladaptive) patient behaviors and nursing interventions for the eliminative and affiliative subsystems.

The implementation of the system was described briefly, with mention of the steps taken. The description did not provide adequate information if someone had been trying to duplicate the process. However, more depth was included in Part 2.

Preliminary testing of the tool revealed that there were several problem areas associated with patient assessment. There were disagreements among staff about ratings of patient behaviors, although it was recognized that these reflected difficulties inherent in defining and measuring behaviors. Observer bias was also an uncontrolled variable associated with measurement of patient behaviors. The two subsystems with the highest level of agreement were eliminative and sexual, probably because these required the least inference on the part of the observers. The subsystems of affiliative, dependency, and achievement—requiring a higher level of observer inference—were found to have lower levels of observer agreement in this preliminary testing.

The importance of minimizing the influence of observer interpretation was recognized, but only one suggestion about how to accomplish this was made, other than through the use of a model to structure the observed behaviors. The suggestion was for staff to "consistently identify and discuss their observations of patient behavior to develop a common frame of reference and achieve a higher degree of agreement (p. 43)." Instrument testing, (specifically, measures of content validity), reliability, and improving interrater reliability would also be important contributions to theory validation. In the long run, these would do more to contribute to the overall theory development and concept measurement. This is the next important step to be taken with the work done this far on the classification tool.

A number of administrative benefits of the classification tool were listed. They all reflected factors influencing decisions that considered cost-effectiveness and quality of care issues.

Broncatello, K.F. (1980). Auger in action: Application of the model. *Advances in Nursing Science,* 2(2), 13–23

It has long been proposed that continued development of conceptual models is an important part of the development of nursing as a science; it is also a given that a part of the continued development of models is application of the models in a variety of practices. However, what has become increasingly apparent in the 1980s is that application of the model to practice is insufficient for refinement of theory. This article is a good example; although it demonstrates application to practice, it does not offer extension or refinement, neither of which are possible in single-case application.

There are several other limitations. After giving a fairly extensive review (summary) of Auger's application of the Johnson behavioral system model to the chronically ill hemodialysis patient, the author attempts to apply the model using new concepts that are not central to either Johnson's or the extension offered by Auger. The section about applying the model begins with a discussion of self-concept and body image. A reader could rightfully question the fit of these concepts with the behavioral systems model.

Stressors are identified that could be extrapolated from the model, including: diet, which affects the eliminative subsystem, and dependence on a machine, which sounds as if it were related to the aggressive-protective subsystem, though logically, it is more directly a problem of the dependence subsystem. Careful analysis of relationships with Auger were better provided in the next section on the model in practice. Here, the author proposes to examine the consequences of hemodialysis on the eight subsystems outlined by Auger. The reader may continue to remain at a loss as to where body image and self-concept fit in the analysis.

This article provides labeling of nursing problems experienced by the chronically ill hemodialysis patient. The author also discusses interventions within the Johnson-Auger subsystems.

Dee, V. and Auger, J.R. (1983). A patient classification system based on the behavioral system model of nursing: Part 2. *Journal of Nursing Administration,* 13(May), 18–23

The patient categorization tool (see Auger and Dee, Part 1), a major component of the classification system outlined in Part 1, provided a basis for the clinical application in terms of the nursing process in a child psychiatry inpatient setting. It was designed to be both comprehensive and flexible enough to allow for use with clients with a variety of diagnoses as well as a wide age range. (How this was implemented was the subject of Part 1.) What was required by way of inpatient unit revisions has been the focus of this second part.

The plan for development of materials and teaching strategies required revision of nursing assessment forms, teaching materials, staff seminars, and orientation of new employees. First of all, inpatient unit nursing assessment forms had to be revised to reflect the model. What had previously been two six-page assessment forms were replaced by four-page forms designed to assess patient factors or behaviors based on the Johnson model. Whereas the earlier forms had been specific to the patient populations, the new assessment form was specific to the Johnson model and was therefore useful in all clinical settings. In view of the fact that nurses vary in levels of education, clinical experience, and abilities, an interview guide was constructed to assist the nurses in eliciting information from the patient and family. The questions included reflected content from the eight subsystems of the Johnson Behavior System Model (JBSM) as they related to the specific psychiatric setting and patient population.

The clinical nurse specialists (CNS) and the nursing coordinators (NC) of each unit developed a package of the teaching materials to illustrate the clinical application of the model. "The materials consisted of samples of completed nursing assessment forms, nursing care plans, and a list of recommended readings pertinent to the behavioral systems model and each subsystem" (Dee and Auger, 1983, p. 19).

Two exhibits contribute to the overall presentation of the teaching materials developed and stand alone, not needing additional narrative to describe them to the reader. Exhibit 1 illustrates two pages of the nursing assessment form (with sample data) developed for one of the specific inpatient units; Exhibit 2 shows portions of a sample nursing care plan based on the assessment.

Staff seminars conducted totaled four hours and were required for all nursing staff on each unit. These were followed up by actual application on the units. All newly admitted patients were assessed, and care plans were developed based on the model using the new materials. Integration and follow-up of the nursing process was provided by the CNS through weekly nursing care plan meetings or individual clinical supervision.

The orientation of new employees consisted of didactic presentations of purpose and theory, audiovisual materials of examples of different levels of patient behaviors and the corresponding nursing intervention, and unit orientation. Subsequently, the orientee was required to complete a nursing assessment and care plan with supervision from an experienced R.N.

While theoretical advantages of using the model were anticipated, the practical advantages were realized only with continued use. There were many practical advantages. Some of the clinical advantages included: more systematic patient behavioral assessment resulting in a comprehensive baseline of behavior at time of hospitalization, more specific and expedited nursing care plans, a focus on patient strengths versus pathology, and improved monitoring of patient behavior over the course of hospitalization. These factors consequently provided more objective means for evaluating the quality of nursing care.

Administrative advantages included improved ability to determine required levels of staffing based on more accurate assessment of patient behaviors, and also a more appropriate assignment of new admissions to a unit based on the level of patient need and level of staffing available; thus achieving a better match of patient needs with staff resources. The corollary would then be that as the overall identified need rose and fell, staffing levels could be raised or lowered accordingly; affecting (conversely influencing) scheduling, budgeting, and nursing hours. Overall efficiency in the integration and balance of scheduling, budgeting, and nursing hours would be improved, resulting in more cost-effective management.

Although the work was written primarily for administrators and clinicians, this scholarly approach to applying theory to practice demonstrates the utility of the JBSM for practice in various inpatient psychiatric units and gives direction to research. It also provides a working model of the "how to" in implementing theory in a practice setting and provides a blueprint for those who might choose to implement this or another theoretical model. (See more recent publications by Dee under Johnson references in Chapter 21.)

Derdiarian, A.K. (1983). An instrument for theory and research development using the behavioral systems model for nursing: The cancer patient, Part I. *Nursing Research,* 32(4), 196–201

Clearly stated by the author in the introduction are both the main purposes of the research carried out and the scope and content of each of a two-part series. The purpose was to develop a valid and reliable research tool to describe the behavioral changes of cancer patients as perceived by them. The research was conceptualized from the behavioral system perspective, and therefore much of the content of Part I is a synopsis of the Johnson behavioral systems model for nursing. For a reader who is unfamiliar with the model, this is an excellent review. The author's concise writing style makes the theoretical overview quite understandable, and the author remains true to Johnson's original work. Each of the seven subsystems (achievement, affiliation, aggressive-protective, dependence, eliminative, ingestive, and sexual) and the eighth subsystem that was added later (restorative) are reviewed, terms are defined, and relationships between concepts are spelled out. The goal of nursing is also stated.

In the rest of the article, the author reviews the support from the literature for the existence of each subsystem, both from work by Johnson and Auger as well as from others writing on the same topic. The author then identifies the major dimensions extrapolated for each of the subsystems. The impact of cancer on each subsystem is then described using previously reported research. The Johnson model provides a conceptual reservoir within which research findings find a coherent existence.

This is a fine example of how theory can be used to guide research findings. The author then presents a table containing each subsystem, the determinants of behavior, and behavioral manifestations. It is upon these that the variables of interest for measurement were based. These then comprised the items of the instrument developed by the author. The development of the items and the frequencies in the table are not clear to the reader and are incongruent with the theoretical discussion. The table fits in with Part II of the article, published in the next issue, where it is discussed and described.

Derdiarian, A.K. and Forsythe, A.B (1983). An instrument for theory and research development using the behavioral systems model for nursing: The cancer patient, Part II. *Nursing Research,* 32, 260–267

The focus and scope of Part II of this two-article series is on the process of establishing validity and reliability for an instrument that will test perceived behavioral changes of cancer patients, based on Johnson's Behavioral Systems Model. One hundred twenty-one change items, based on each subsystem, were delineated from previous research and were given to a homogeneous sample of 163 cancer patients. The criteria for inclusion and exclusion of subjects are listed. The authors' rationale for the "limitation of selection criteria was to maximize the homogeneity of the sample in terms of salient intervening variables such as visible, extensive body disfigurement, level of awareness, comprehension, absence of additional stress caused by a new treatment or procedure, and variables of adult life cycle (p. 261)." What is not clear is why there are such broad parameters for inclusion of subjects. The extreme age variation (20–70), various cancer diagnoses, and range of treatments do not logically suggest a homogeneous sample to achieve the desired results.

Patients were asked to identify changes they perceived happening due to or since they became ill and to add or subtract changes. They were also asked to indicate quantitatively and quantitatively the extent of the changes and, finally, their perceptions of the consequences of the changes. Figure 1 in Part I presents frequency distribution of responses. The authors did not discuss what decisions they made based on these frequency distributions.

Several approaches were used to estimate content validity and reliability of the instrument. What appears to be the first step was to use an expert panel of six members, divided into two groups. "The first group evaluated the comprehensiveness of the theoretical framework and its consistency with known theories, and the consistency of the operational definitions with the theoretical framework. The second group evaluated the consistency of the operational definitions with the categories and the times. The panel judged independently" (p. 262). A supplemental assessment of empirical validity was done using the theta coefficient estimation, which was derived from a factor analysis.

Described later in the "method" section are two other methods of evaluation of comprehensiveness. Here, a panel of three clinical nurse specialists in oncology independently judged the "other" changes added by the patients (p. 262). Because of these various methods used to evaluate comprehensiveness, some confusion is generated about the sequential timing of these evaluations as well as about when the pilot testing and the reliability testing were completed.

The Derdiarian behavioral system model (DBSM) instrument was pilot tested after construction and estimation of content validity, using three male and three female subjects. Test-retest reliability was assessed by administering the instrument to, apparently, all 163 subjects. The instrument did not have identifying information on it, and "a randomized permutation schedule always places a subsystem questionnaire designed for retesting for reliability in the third place in the sequence of the subsystem questionnaires" (p. 262). Time to complete the instrument as reported by subjects was approximately 1.75 hours. After a 15-minute respite, the patient was asked to complete the retest subsystem questionnaire.

Also evaluated in the overall process was the performance of each of the eight trained research assistants. Interviewer reliability was an ongoing concern as manifested by regular review of the tapes and rating of the interviewer behavior by two independent raters who were not involved in the data-gathering process.

Grubbs, J. (1980). An interpretation of the Johnson behavioral system model for nursing practice. In J.P. Riehl and C. Roy (Eds.), *Conceptual models for nursing practice*. New York: Appleton-Century-Crofts

The purpose of this article is an attempt to operationalize the model so that it could be used as a systematic guide to nursing practice. The author indicates that this is her own interpretation of the Johnson behavioral system model.

The most obvious difference between Grubbs' interpretation and the original model is the addition of the restorative subsystem, with its goal being "to relieve fatigue and/or achieve a state of equilibrium by reestablishing or replenishing the energy distribution among the other subsystems" (p. 228). The additional subsystem was articulated by faculty members at the University of California, Los Angeles after long discussions and debates. Johnson continued to remind the faculty that restoration is a requirement for each subsystem, and its addition may therefore be teleological and tautological. Also described are the functional requirements, which are better defined in Auger (1976).

An important contribution this article makes to the reader is the use of this model in the prospective development of tools (*e.g.*, sample flow sheet and work sheet, which illustrate use of the model to guide the nursing process). There is even an appendix describing items, by systems, that should be included in the assessment. Furthermore, the language and terminology used in the examples are consistent both with systems theory in general and with the behavioral system model more specifically.

Overall, this article is a contribution to the understanding of the behavioral system theory and, if read with Johnson's own account of her theory in the same book, will help to clarify the theory components. The process demonstrated here shows thought and solid construction based on the model.

Holaday, B. (1980). Implementing the Johnson model for nursing practice. In J.P. Riehl and C. Roy (Eds.), *Conceptual models for nursing practice* (2nd ed.). New York: Appleton-Century-Crofts

The focus of this article, which follows the Grubbs article, is the operationalization of the model and application of the nursing process to care of the individual patient, using Johnson's model. The author designed a new assessment tool and synthesized Piaget's definition of cognition with Johnson's view of a human being as a system of behavior.

This author devotes the entire article to cognition—not even one of the behavioral subsystems—and to the eliminative system, which was defined by Johnson to include the excretion of physiological wastes and which was expanded by Grubbs (and the faculty of UCLA) to include the expulsion of one's feelings, beliefs, and emotions.

Had the author developed a rationale for incorporating Piaget's theory and refined the integration of it within either a subsystem or a cultural or psychological variable, the argument would have been more defensible.

Overall, the article is limited because of the narrow focus on the redefined eliminative subsystem, even though the author does follow through with each phase of the nursing process in accord with the purpose of the article. The article offers some clarification of the use of the behavioral systems model in practice. Refinement and extension were not provided.

Johnson, D.E. (1959). A philosophy of nursing. *Nursing Outlook,* 7(4), 198–200

At the time this article was written, the author had identified factors impinging on nursing that resulted in a confusion of goals and the division of nursing into two camps. The camps were divided into those who believed the professional nurse of the future would have largely supervisory and managerial responsibilities and, on the other side, those who believed that nursing could and would take its place as a professional discipline in relation to direct service to people who are "in need of nursing care."

Johnson belonged to the latter camp: the science of nursing and the art of nursing. The first of these—the discussion of the science of nursing, centered around the patient, the recipient of care—is phenomenal in that it is as relevant today as it was in the late 1950s. In fact, the discussion might almost be considered prophetic because three decades later, the client was identified as one of the nursing phenomenon. Nursing process, nursing diagnosis, and nursing science are no longer as esoteric as they seemed in 1959 when Johnson's article was published. Nursing art, to Johnson, represented ministration of the basic unmet needs of the patient. Also identified are those activities that are delegated and controlled by the physician.

A sociological analysis of the nursing role is used as a vehicle for understanding the division of labor between nurses and physicians. We will also see, much later in time, just how much of an impact this sociological analysis has had on Johnson's own theory.

Johnson, D.E. (1961). The significance of nursing care. *Nursing Outlook,* 61(11), 63–66

This is a very significant, indeed, classic work in nursing knowledge. Here, Johnson introduces the notion of stability rather than change as the goal of nursing. Meeting the needs of the patient helps bring about that stability.

Because of pressures from the medical and hospital management on nursing to take on non-nursing tasks, Johnson believes that the view of nursing as a direct and individualized service has become less goal-oriented and more blurred. Three major components or types of nursing services were identified: (1) nursing care, (2) delegated medical care, and (3) health care. Of the three, only one—nursing care—has "no well-delineated theoretical framework or conceptual basis to give it meaning or direction (p. 64)."

The purpose of this article, then, is to delineate such a framework within the context of nursing's distinctive contribution to patient welfare and the specific purpose of nursing care.

Using concepts of physiological homeostasis borrowed from Cannon and stability in patterns of social interaction from Parsons, Johnson synthesized them and related them to individuals who are ill. Instability causes tension; if tension is intense, an individual experiences discomfort and displeasure.

Speculating from these, Johnson attempted to evolve a basis for nursing care, using concepts of equilibrium, stress, and tension. Each of these is defined in general terms and then as it applies to an individual patient (or group) or how the nurse might identify or assess stress, tension, or equilibrium. The conceptualization of equilibrium, stress, and tension presents a way of viewing the nature of disturbances that a patient might have as well as the purpose of nursing care, or what might be considered nursing's specific responsibility in nursing care.

Two nursing interventions within this framework are also suggested. First, reduction of the stressful stimuli through the management of the physical and psychological environment, and second, support of the patient's "natural defenses and adaptive processes" through "protective and sustaining measures." The focus of nursing is on immediate situations, universal needs, and patterns that belong to the patient and are gratifying to him. The seeds for Johnson's theory were planted in this writing.

Johnson, D.E. (1980). The behavioral system model for nursing. In J.P. Riehl and C. Roy (Eds.), *Conceptual models for nursing practice* (2nd ed.). New York: Appleton-Century-Crofts

Dorothy Johnson, for the first time in writing, clearly presents the whole of her theory. Much of her unpublished work had been alluded to by her protegees and, though available in manuscript form, it suffered from limited distribution. This was the first time the original behavioral systems theory for nursing was published in its entirety.

According to its author, the behavioral systems model has its origins in a philosophical perspective and has been supported by an expanding empirical and theoretical base (*i.e.,* systems theory). (It would be helpful to read three of the author's early publications, two in 1959 and one in 1961, in conjunction with this one.) It is Johnson's perspective that both nurses and physicians theoretically have viewed a human being as a system. However, nurses view the patient as a behavioral system, whereas physicians view him as a biological system. It is the nursing view of the human being as a behavioral system that underlies this model. A review of this article shows that the underlying assumptions of the model are explicit. The concepts are embedded in the context and are not specifically defined. The system is identified as having seven subsystems, which are briefly defined. The four structural elements of each subsystem are listed and discussed.

The basic elements of the model that are briefly touched upon and that are implicit rather than explicit include values, goal of action, patiency, and source of difficulty. The latter is discussed only minimally; noticeably missing is a discussion of intervention.

In summarizing, the author indicated that the behavioral systems model "seems defensible and promising by three criteria." The criteria were named in the 1974 article and are social congruence, social significance, and social utility. She also said that the model has "proved its utility in providing clear direction for practice, education, and research." Although the present work does not provide any evidence to support this, some available documentation exists and is discussed in the section on Johnson in this book.

Despite these limitations of the model—that is, underdevelopment of some of the elements and lack of supportive evidence for the model's utility—this theoretical model for nursing is one of the major contributions to nursing theory development in the past two decades. Furthermore, Johnson's thinking has impacted on a great number of graduate students in nursing who have since gone on to develop other theoretical models. Johnson's stimulus for progress should not be underestimated; it has resulted in the advancement of nursing as a science.

Lovejoy, N.C. (1983). The leukemic child's perceptions of family behaviors. *Oncology Nursing Forum,* 10(4), 20–25

Contributing to theory development and testing through the development of instruments to measure concepts is of utmost importance to the advancement of nursing science.

The author states that the Johnson model was selected as the theoretical framework "because of its basic premise that human behavior in health and illness is the independent domain of nursing" (Lovejoy, 1983, p. 20). In table form as part of the background materials, the author presented a comparison of the Johnson behavioral system model (JBSM) goals by subsystem and by theorist, showing differences between theorists. The theorists compared are Johnson, Grubbs, Auger, and Lovejoy; all of whom have elaborated upon and used the model. This provides a helpful summary and review of the subsystems for the reader familiar with the model. It is assumed, however, that the reader has some knowledge of the model. The author notes the disparity among the theorists regarding the scope of the goal-directed behaviors of the subsystems, but concludes that "the goals used in this research appeared to parsimoniously and discretely define special domains of behavior (Lovejoy, 1983, p. 21)." The reader is left wondering where the support for such a conclusion is. Little additional elaboration of or support for "discretely defined domains of behavior" was given.

The Family Relations (FR) test, the instrument upon which the family assessment instrument was modeled, was then described. The FR test situation was designed as a play situation in which the child was to decide what feelings fit what members of the family. The family assessment instrument (Lovejoy) consists of 47 items apparently designed to reflect the eight subsystems of the JBSM. The number of questions ranges from four to eight for each subsystem. No explanation is provided for having a variable number of items per subsystem. The items are shown in Table 2 and stand alone without additional explanation. Items for the assessment tool were generated and formulated based on a review of major growth and development theorists and a review of chronic illness research. Statements reflecting functional and dysfunctional family member behaviors were formulated from this review. The statements describing these behaviors were then placed on individual cards for later test administration. Noticeably missing was reference to how items were formulated to reflect the eight subsystems of the JBSM. This is an important omission given that the author purported that the instrument was "based on the Johnson Model for nursing (1983, p. 20)."

There are several major limitations with this instrument. First, there is little or no evidence of content validity and face validity within the context of either growth and development theory or the Johnson model. No evidence is presented indicating that the items were subjected to a review by experts either in growth and development or the Johnson model. This was also true of the review of the scoring guide, as discussed previously. Although it is a time-consuming and arduous task, some attempt to develop content validity is crucial, even for initial instrument development, and was overlooked in the development of this instrument.

Second, the scoring guide and the method of scoring described suggest that the rating of 0 to 2 is a scale, with equal distances between each measure. In application, these appear to be discrete categories and therefore not conducive to the summation-scoring method used.

It may be more appropriate to standardize the instrument by developing norms for each age group.

Rawls, A.C. (1980). Evaluation of the Johnson behavioral model in clinical practice: Report of a test and evaluation of the Johnson theory. *Image,* 12, 13–16

In the introduction, the author clearly identifies the importance of model testing for the future of nursing in general and, specifically, her rationale for choosing to evaluate the application of the Johnson theory. The purpose and scope of the report are also identified. The title might suggest that the "test" was research when, actually, it was an exercise in whether or not the theory was clinically useful.

As background for the study, a brief history and an overview of other authors' contributions to the model is presented. Johnson's model is briefly reviewed to provide readers with an outline of how the model was used as a framework by the author. The subsystems and their components and the structure and function of the theory are all defined. For purposes of discussion only, the structure, function, and functional requirements of the subsystems are discussed in detail. After clarification of a few other components of the model, the use of the Johnson model (JM) as a guide for the nursing process is illustrated.

Each stage of the nursing process—assessment through evaluation—is described within the context of the JM subsystems using the Grubbs assessment tool and nursing process worksheet. These process and description are similar to those described by Janelli (1980) with Roy's model. Prior to the beginning of the "study," variables that may have influenced the outcome were explored. Four were identified: "limited knowledge of Johnson's theory," "lack of experience in utilizing Grubbs' assessment tool and nursing process worksheet," and patient's response to the researcher, to the assessment tool, and to the plan of care developed. Time available for the study and the size of the study group were also identified. The author chose to limit the sample size to one "due to the variables cited previously (Rawls, 1980 p. 13)."

The study focused on a case presentation of one subject, beginning with patient background, followed by first- and second-level assessment. The patient selected for the study was a white male who had been hospitalized for evaluation of an accidental injury, resulting in painful amputation of the left hand and distal phalanges approximately six months earlier. The first level assessment appeared to be more in keeping with the medical model in that information about past and present history of the problem, psychological assessment, family, and social, environmental, and development history were reviewed.

From the perspective of the JM, no examples of assessments of subsystems were presented. An exception was a statement indicating that because no problems were noted in the review to that point, a complete review of the behavior subsystems was conducted using Grubbs' assessment tool. Two problem areas in the achievement subsystem were identified. Because there were problem areas in only this one subsystem, the discussion was limited to that one. Second-level assessment proceeded from there. One concept—the concept of body image—was explored in depth.

The assessment phase was followed by a plan for care, again focusing on intervention for the two problems in the achievement subsystem only. The plan focused on how the patient's loss of his left hand and its function prevented him from meeting the conceptual goal of the achievement subsystem (*i.e.,* to achieve or master). Variables that might have influenced the patient's care were explored and identified. "The developmental, psychological, sociological, and level-of-wellness variables were all viewed as influencing variables that could be manipulated to benefit the patient" (Rawls, 1980, p. 16).

The next step was the identification of nursing problems. This step may be confusing in that problems were identified earlier in the assessment phases of the nursing process. Furthermore, the author did not clarify why this additional step of problem identification was necessary. Further reading led me to conclude that these additional problems were refinements of previously identified problems in the achievement subsystem. The nursing interventions for these problems were detailed, with numerous examples used for illustration. Both long-term and short-term goals of nursing intervention were formulated. The plan of care was evaluated and found to be appropriate, as measured by changes consistent with the short-term goals. The plan of care, with minor revisions, was also found to be appropriate to the patient's postoperative course.

The author's "evaluation of the Johnson Model" was more of an evaluation of the usefulness of the model for clinical practice than a critical review of the model itself. The author recommended that the model be tested further in a variety of settings with clients who have a variety of complex problems in each of the subsystems. To have stated this limitation is to the author's credit. Disadvantages of the model as perceived by the author included complex and unique terminology and the requirement of knowledge of systems theory in order to use the model more effectively. The author concluded that the advantages of the model for practice, in essence, outweighed the disadvantages; she believed that the Johnson model "offers the nurse a tool which will allow her to accurately predict the results of nursing interventions prior to care," and "formulate standards for care" (1980, p. 16).

The nursing educator who is interested in teaching the JM or in demonstrating the application of theory to practice (as well as the nursing theorist concerned about the utility of the model for practice) would find this article of some interest. The beginnings of the elaboration of the concept of body image as it relates to the achievement subsystem are present in this author's assessment phase.

Small, B. (1980). Nursing visually impaired children with Johnson's model as a conceptual framework. In J.P. Riehl and C. Roy (Eds.), *Conceptual models for nursing practice* (2nd ed.). (pp. 264–273). New York: Appleton-Century-Crofts

Although nursing research that tests hypotheses of nursing theories is critical for the advancement of a particular theory, this study does not test hypotheses evolving from Johnson's theory, but it demonstrates that the theory could be utilized in working with visually impaired children.

The report of a research study is the first of two parts of this chapter. The second includes implications for nursing. The major assumptions underlying the theoretical framework of the study were derived from Piaget and cognitive developmental psychology. Two null hypotheses were tested and rejected. The first stated that "there would be no significant difference between the perceived body image of visually impaired and normally sighted preschool children." The second stated that there would be no significant difference between the spatial awareness of visually impaired preschoolers and those who were normally sighted.

The author explains results of the study using Johnson's theory. Vision plays an important role in the development of object permanence and the relation of objects in space. These two concepts are necessary for the development of a child's body image and for his awareness of his body in space. Therefore, if a child is visually handicapped, the implications are that nurses can intervene to meet his needs and to facilitate the development of his self-concept.

Once this line of reasoning was developed, and once a brief description of Johnson's model was presented, the author tended to focus more on interventions with the parents than with the child, therefore supporting Johnson's recommendations for intervention: manipulation of the environment to reduce tension.

Myra Levine

Esposito, C.H. and Leonard, M.K. (1980). Myra Estrin Levine. In the Nursing Theories Conference Group, *Nursing theories: A base for professional practice* (pp. 150–163). Englewood Cliffs, NJ: Prentice-Hall

The content of this article is organized to include a summary of the components of Levine's theory, its application to the nursing process, and the relationship of the theory to five major concepts (humanity, society, health, learning, and nursing). In addition, a brief case study is included to demonstrate application to practice (*i.e.*, the utility of the theory for clinical practice).

One of the major contributions of this chapter is the identification of the explicit assumptions underlying Levine's theory. This is helpful because the assumptions are implicit in Levine's writing.

There is one important omission in this discussion of Levine's theory: the major theoretical underpinnings, namely systems theory, is not identified. Given that systems theory is not acknowledged, it becomes clearer why Levine's theory is identified as having a close kinship to Maslow's hierarchy of needs. One might agree that parallels could be drawn between the conservation principles and Maslow's levels of needs, but Maslow's theory must not be construed as the prototype for Levine's principles. Nowhere in Levine's writing is there any reference to Maslow's needs hierarchy.

Two potential problems in this chapter are the lack of identification of what is Levine's and what are Esposito's and Leonard's additions and that the parallels between Maslow's hierarchy of needs and conservation principles (tenuous at best) may be accidental and therefore do not justify this as a prototype paradigm. More support could be given to system or adaptations as guiding paradigms.

Hirschfeld, M.J. (1976). The cognitively impaired older adult. *American Journal of Nursing,* 76(12), 1981–1984

In a very straightforward discussion of the possible cognitive impairments of older adults, and in the only published work on utilization of Levine's theory in practice, Hirschfeld demonstrates how Levine's four principles of conservation can be applied to give direction to nursing interventions when impairments are present. The goal of the interventions is specified as trying to keep remaining cognitive capacities intact and in use.

Each conservation principle, and examples demonstrating problems in the area it covered, were discussed separately. For example, a variety of problems are described wherein the balance of activity and rest were disturbed. Focusing on conservation of energy in this case gave the nurse direction for intervention.

Levine, M.E. (1966). Adaptation and assessment: A rationale of nursing intervention. *American Journal of Nursing,* 66(11), 2450–2453

Levine introduced "trophicognosis" as an alternative concept to replace "nursing diagnosis" (Levine, M.E. [1966]. Trophicognosis: An alternative to nursing diagnosis. In *Exploring progress in medical surgical nursing practice* [pp. 55–70]. New York: American Nurses Association. A series of papers presented at the 1965 Regional Clinical Conferences, November 3–5, 1965, Washington, D.C.). The latter conjures up medicine and disease orientation, whereas the former focuses attention on judgments related to nursing care utilizing the scientific method. In that earlier writing, it becomes apparent that Levine is interested in delineating nursing goals and differentiating them from medical goals.

In this second of four articles that precede the publishing of her book, *Introduction to Clinical Nursing,* Levine further demonstrates her conceptualization of nursing as utilizing the scientific method and as a coherent theory in guiding its actions. She argues that nursing practice and education have long been influenced by the prevailing beliefs about health and disease. As a result of a carry-over or a carry-through of earlier theories, nursing care has become "an unsynthesized "total," a sum of many disparate parts" (p. 2451). Thus there is an urgent need, as Levine sees it, for a restatement of the theoretical basis for nursing practice. This is what she attempted to do in this article.

Drawing from a variety of sources—philosophy, physiology, and sociology—a few basic ideas about human beings become implicit assumptions of the theory. Central ideas are (1) a human being's life is multidimensional, (2) a human being is in constant interaction with the environment, (3) a human being's internal environment is integrated and is dynamically balanced, (4) a human being responds to forces in the environment in a unique but integrated manner, (5) health and disease are patterns of adaptive change, and (6) the nurse is part of every patient's environment. One sees here the influence of systems theory: wholeness of human being, dynamic equilibrium, human being-environment interactions, and adaptation.

The author revived Nightingale's ideas of multicausality of illness, disease as a "reparative process," and nursing's goal as establishing a health environment that would enhance healing and reparative processes. Levine refocused nursing's attention on the wholeness of human beings, the uniqueness of each human being, and on the fact that a broad knowledge base is required by the nurse in order to give nursing care.

Levine's discussion of adaptation raises some questions. Adaptation is introduced but not really defined per se. For example, "all the processes of living are processes of adaptation," "diseases represent patterned responses or adaptations," "health and disease are patterns of adaptive change" (p. 2452). But what is adaptation? Levine indicates that a criterion of successful adaptation is the attainment of social well-being, which is neither defined nor related to the preceding physiological discussion.

The major ideas expressed about nursing are that the nurse is an agent who intervenes between a patient and his environment to facilitate adaptation and that the interventions are based on coherent and systematic knowledge and a scientific process in collecting data about the patient.

Levine, M.E. (1967). The four conservation principles of nursing. *Nursing Forum*, 6(1), 45–59

This article is the third that this author wrote in an attempt to lay down a framework for nursing intervention. It is helpful to read this after reading the first two on trophicognosis and on adaptation and assessment in order to fully understand the process that Levine used in theory development: redefining central concepts, reconceptualization of nursing goals, and then nursing actions. She identified central concepts, stated assumptions, and proposed four central propositions.

The concept of adaptation as developed by Levine in her earlier article remains undefined. In the introduction alone, adaptation may be conceived or interpreted in three different ways. First, one can infer that it "can be manifested in patterns" and "has a course." One could also infer that adaptation is an outcome because it can be measured by "renewed social well-being." Third, in another context, one can infer that adaptation can be a capability or a characteristic of a person.

Aside from adaptation, the major focus of this article and Levine's major contribution to theory is the introduction of four conservation principles that are central to the mission of nursing. Levine identifies nursing principles as "fundamental assumptions which provide a unifying structure for understanding a wide variety of nursing activities" (p. 45). Here, each principle (labeled assumptions, but they may be the theory's propositions) is listed separately along with a statement about nursing intervention and is then followed by a discussion that supports the principle and the rationale for it. Clinical examples are included as supportive evidence. The four principles are all conservation principles. Conservation is defined as "keeping together," but the author emphasizes that this "should not imply minimal activity," especially on the part of the nurse.

The four principles are: "(1) The Principle of the Conservation of Patient Energy, (2) The Principle of the Conservation of Structural Integrity, (3) The Principle of Conservation of Personal Integrity, (4) The Principle of Conservation of Social Integrity." For each of these, nursing intervention is based on the conservation of the particular patient's need in focus. The four principles evolved from an assumption of the unity and integrity of the individual; they are well-developed and supported with clinical examples; and they are, in part, consistent with some assumptions from the systems theory.

Three critical questions are raised: (1) How did the author come to the point of identifying four and only four principles? (2) In principle 2, given the complex interrelationships of human structure and function (which Levine does discuss), why is the principle not stated in terms of both structural and functional integrity, or why weren't two separate principles for these developed? What is the rationale for focusing on structural integrity versus both structure and function? (3) Why aren't personal integrity and social integrity specifically defined?

Considering the dearth of theoretical frameworks for nursing available in the late 1960s, this framework made a substantial contribution to the science of nursing. Levine proved herself to be an insightful, forward-looking theorist.

Levine, M.E. (1969). The pursuit of wholeness. *American Journal of Nursing,* 69(1), 93–98

Consistent with the first three articles and with systems theory, Levine views a human being as a system in constant interaction with the environment: "patients are complete persons, not groups of parts."

This article provides a view of the human being from a nursing perspective, as a system in a constant dynamic interchange with the environment and as part of a larger ecosystem. Information is exchanged between the human system and the larger ecosystem—by way of the perceptual subsystem. Disturbances in the perceptual subsystem, as well as the levels of organismic response used to protect the organism as it responds to the environment, give direction to nursing.

When the environment changes, the human being must change. Levine makes a fairly succinct theoretical statement here about what adaptation is. This process of change "whereby the individual retains his integrity—his wholeness—within the realities of his environment" is labeled adaptation (p. 95). The goal of the individual is to defend his wholeness.

There are at least four levels of organismic response, each physiologically predetermined. (This is an implicit assumption on Levine's part.) The responses are used to protect the organism so that it can make a viable adaptation to the environment. The four levels include: response to fear, inflammatory response, response to stress, and sensory response. These four levels are fairly well-documented.

Alone, this article does not contribute substantially to our understanding of Levine's theory; it must not be read in isolation. In the context of earlier articles and ones that come later, the perspective of this one becomes clearer.

Levine, M.E. (1971). Holistic nursing. *Nursing Clinics of North America,* 6(2), 253–264

No new material is presented here. This is more of a synthesis of previously published material, which contributes to a better general understanding of the theory. The author brings together all the ideas, the separate parts, of the earlier four articles into a whole. The parts of Levine's theory—the assumptions, central concepts, definitions of person (who is the nursing client), goals of nursing, and nursing intervention—are put together, and the interrelationships between parts are then described.

Levine views holistic nursing as the challenge before nurses. This approach to nursing takes place at the interface between the organism (human being) and the environment. In other words, nursing is an interaction, and the nurse, in a sense, mediates between the organism and his environment, whether the environment in question is the organism's internal environment or external environment.

For the person desiring an overview of the theory, or some help in piecing together the earlier parts of the theory, this article could be most helpful and should then be read before the first four articles.

Levine, M.E. (1971). Time has come to speak of . . . health care. *AORN Journal,* 13, 37–43

In a speech to the annual congress of the Association of Operating Room Nurses (AORN), focusing on the concerns of that group for viability, Levine indirectly presents arguments in support of her theoretical framework for nursing. Ostensibly, the focus of the speech is the threat of increased technological change and innovation to the roles of nurses. especially with the concomitant requirement for technicians to manage the machinery. The health care field has responded to the technological advances by increasing the number of technicians. Although operating room nurses were the first to be threatened by the influx. their area is not the only one inundated by technicians. For example, there are now ICUs, CCUs, trauma, dialysis, burn, coma, respiratory, and hyperbaric units.

Nevertheless, Levine argues that in all these settings there are both technical and professional roles to be filled. She further argues that situations continue to arise in which there are new threats of new technicians; however, her real concern is for the quality of care to patients. What will happen if the new physician assistants, for example, go into underserved areas and provide a second-class kind of medical care? If this is a trend, then nursing must make itself heard to prevent these inadequacies from occurring. Those in society who are now already underserved, already suffering, would be most affected by these inadequacies of health care.

Confusion in the roles of workers, both professional and technical, has been a result of all the changes in health care. However, there still remains one need that nurses can recognize and sustain: self-respect and humanity of the patient. The nurse traditionally has been and must remain the patient's advocate. Unless the effort is made to reach out and establish human contact, the patient will just become another part of the elaborate machinery of the technology. The technical role in this situation is supportive and essential, but it is the professional nurse who must be the patient's advocate, the humanizing agent, the one who brings "compassion, protection, and commitment to the bedside."

Given the changes in health care, the education of nurses must change too. In order to be the professional nurse, as described previously, Levine believes that tl achievement of the education of a patient's advocate requires knowledge and skills (a global kind. Furthermore, there needs to be a conceptualization of nursing. She pr sents her formulations as valid forms of nursing intervention. She also suggests that t concepts inherent in the generalizations can be readily applied to all kinds of nurs intervention. It is here that we see Levine's support for her theoretical framework nursing as one way to counter the threat of technological advances to nursin patients, and to health care.

Dorothea Orem

Allison, S.E. (1973). A framework for nursing action in a nurse-conducted diabetic management clinic. *Journal of Nursing Administration,* 3(4), 53–60

This article is based on and follows the 1974 Backscheider article, although this one was published first. The author provides a comprehensive picture of the health care system, using the self-care model as a basis for the nurse-conducted diabetic management clinic. The author synthesizes some of Orem's and Backscheider's concepts: universal self-care, health deviation self-care (Orem), and mental, physical, motivational, emotional, and orientational capacities to follow a therapeutic regimen (Backscheider). The article provides a highly useful example of the use of Orem's ideas in a nurse-run diabetic clinic. Three models—self-care, health status, and environment—are offered as a framework for assessment and intervention. The author provides a very useful discussion of areas of responsibility and differentiates between traditional nursing roles (administrative) and practitioner roles (clinically oriented) as shared and as delineated for nursing, medicine, and other health services. Although this is an ideal setting for theory testing, the focus of the article is on application.

Anna, D.J., Christensen, D.G., Hohn, S.A., Ord, L., and Wells, S.R. (1978). Implementing Orem's conceptual framework. *Journal of Nursing Administration,* 8(11), 8–11

The authors present a descriptive account of the implementation of Orem's model by a group of graduate students in a nursing home setting for adult patients (geriatric setting). In doing so, the authors provide a short summary of the theory, the use of the nursing process according to Orem, the strategies the students used in implementing the theory in the setting, and the obstacles preventing implementation by students, patients, and nursing staff. Difficulties experienced by the students in shifting to Orem's conceptualization (terminology, concept definitions, mechanization) are those that could be universal and could apply to all initial attempts at implementing any nursing theory. The conceptualization of a patient's role as that of a significant decision maker and eventually a performer of self-care activities presented another obstacle. Patients felt more comfortable as recipients of care. As expected, the nursing staff was resistant to change initiated by a group of temporary students. Evaluation of the implementation process was done by review of students' personal diaries. Themes were an increase in patient participation, motivation, and cooperation.

. (1974). Self-care requirements, self-care capabilities, and nursing systems in the diabetic t clinic. *American Journal of Public Health,* 64(12), 1138–1146

or provides a conceptualization of the diabetic-related component of thera- -care, encompassing a set of patient responsibilities (related to the patient's own condition and therapy and to the effects of his condition and therapy) and a set of action capabilities (physical, mental, motivational, emotional, and orientational). Nursing care is needed when a patient has limited capability to meet the therapeutic self-care (self-care deficit). Nursing is a mediating system and is divided into four types. Nursing care (nursing system) is focused on the patient as a one-time guidance or teaching, on long-term assistance that is oriented toward maintenance and support, on more permanent compensatory care oriented toward some changes in the patient, or on compensatory care using changes in the environment.

When a given health care deviation occurs, the capabilities essential to meet that portion of the therapeutic self-care are determined first and foremost. Criteria can then be established. The nurse can assess the patient's capabilities against the established criteria to determine whether or not the patient can meet the self-care demands. This is a more positive approach, a more scientific one to establishing nursing interventions than by estimating the patient's abilities or limitations.

This is an important article to read in relation to the theory of self-care. It demonstrates the interaction between practice and theory development and shows potential for researchable questions.

Bromley, B. (1980). Applying Orem's self-care theory in enterostomal therapy. *American Journal of Nursing,* 80(2), 245–249

The author, an enterostomal therapist, begins with a discussion of her own personal philosophy of nursing practice, with the most useful tool being the nurse. Her choice of Orem's theory was made because of the apparent congruency between hers and Orem's philosophies. The usefulness of this article lies in the author's synthesis of her perceptions of Orem's theory and the use of an exemplar to demonstrate the theory–practice fit, particularly around nursing interventions. The author writes clearly and does a particularly nice job of showing how the nursing systems of self-care are implemented in an inpatient (hospital) setting. Using an example, she shows how she has moved from a wholly compensatory system, through the partly compensatory system, to the supportive–educative system with a client.

For those interested in the appropriateness of Orem's model for inpatient practice in a surgical setting, this is a good example because the author followed the theory closely throughout.

Buckwalter, K.C. and Kerfoot, K.M. (1982). Teaching patients self-care: A critical aspect of psychiatric discharge planning. *Journal of Psychiatric Nursing and Mental Health Services,* 20(5), 15–20

While ostensibly presenting clinical applications under the umbrella of Orem's self-care framework, this article is about discharge planning and teaching; it appears that the notion of self-care has been added after the fact. The abstract clues us in to the fact that self-care is not an integral part of the conceptualization of the discharge planning.

The content includes the following topics: understanding the diagnosis, stressors, signs and symptoms, resocializing issues, community support, and medication compliance. Each topic is briefly described and illustrated with clinical examples. A sample standardized protocol for depressives and their families is included.

The only references to Orem are the use of her definition of self-care and two references to kinds of nursing assistance, namely teaching and self-care guidance. Self-care concepts are not applied to the content. To be consistent with the theoretical framework, the content must also follow. For example, the summary of the five areas to be covered with patient and family in the discharge planning interview (p. 16) lend themselves to the six health deviation self-care requisites as elaborated by Orem (1980, pp. 48–51).

This article covers an important topic of present concern for all mental health practitioners—not just nurses—regarding maintaining the mentally ill in the community. Overall, the article is written in a straightforward and understandable style and presents important clinical content. What is of concern is that the authors state that they are using Orem's perspective. Although they do include topics under the rubric of self-care, Orem's framework in fact does not guide the conceptualization of the teaching and guidance plan.

Caley, J.M., Dirkensen, M., Engally, M., and Hennrich, M.L. (1980). The Orem self-care nursing model. In J.P. Riehl and C. Roy (Eds.), *Conceptual models for nursing practice* (2nd ed.). (pp. 302–314). New York: Appleton-Century-Crofts

The intent of the chapter is to offer an example of the use of Orem's theory in a psychiatric setting, using a suicidal patient as the case study. The discussion of the model, brief and limited, is organized around the goal of action, patiency, actor's role, source of difficulty, intervention focus/mode, and consequences, both intended and otherwise.

It would be helpful for a theory novice who is focused on a theory-psychiatric practice link to read this chapter in conjunction with Orem's work, with the understanding that it is a limited expose and does not do complete justice to Orem's theories. The authors freely used concepts from Backscheider (1971; 1974) and the Nursing Development Conference Group (1973) in addition to Orem (1971).

Chang, B.L. (1980). Evaluation of health care professionals in facilitating self-care: Review of the literature and a conceptual model. *Advances in Nursing Science,* 3(1), 43–58

The purpose of this article is stated in terms of needs. "A need exists for the evaluation of health professionals in facilitating self-care. Such an evaluation must take into account lay persons' judgments regarding the health care received. A conceptual framework is needed for the evaluation of the role of health professionals in facilitating self-care" (p. 44). The "why" of this, the importance, is not spelled out.

The author states that the derivation of her framework for the evaluation of health professionals is in part from Orem's work and in part from other literature related to the evaluation of quality of care. The dimensions of the framework are listed as "(1) patient or layperson characteristics, (2) health care professional characteristics, and (3) patient outcomes" (p. 44). A diagram illustrates the relationship of these dimensions and serves to introduce the components of these dimensions. The diagram contains all the dimensions and their components and the direction of the linkages. The third and last dimension, influenced by the preceding two, is the focus of the review of literature. Why only the third dimension—evaluation of outcomes of self-care—is reviewed in detail is not stated.

Although the author has presented a broad definition of self-care, a strong statement about the overall importance of the topic and why this particular definition of self-care was chosen over others commonly used in the literature has thus far not been presented.

There are numerous opportunities to use Orem's framework to guide the conceptualization of the model proposed, and they are not taken advantage of. In the review of the literature on evaluation of outcomes of self-care, specifically the three components, the author appears to have neglected to use important articles relevant to the framework presented. Examples of this include writings by Allison (1973), who addresses nurses and other health team members and their role in assisting patients to perform self-care regarding diabetic management, and by Backscheider (1974), who also addresses the role of nurses in assisting with the self-care practices of diabetics and the self-care competencies required by ambulatory diabetics.

Although the author may have accomplished her overall goals of presenting a conceptual model and reviewing some literature related to evaluation of health care professionals, conceptual linkages between the different dimensions, are missing.

Coleman, L.J. (1980). Orem's self-care concept of nursing In J.P. Riehl and C. Roy (Eds.), *Conceptual models for nursing practice* (2nd ed.). (pp. 315–328). New York: Appleton-Century-Crofts

The primary purpose of this article is to describe the implementation of Orem's theory in one nursing service department of a large metropolitan hospital. Therefore, Orem's model is first summarized by the author, with particular emphasis on those concepts and ideas that would be most useful for the nursing service department of a hospital (*e.g.*, nursing assistance, nursing process). The language of the chapter, to be sure, is the language of nursing administration, such as classification of patients, techniques essential for nursing practice, utilization of nursing personnel, and operational documents. The author then described what was involved in revising operational documents of a nursing service, including departmental philosophy and goals, departmental policies, divisional philosophy and objectives, position descriptions, nursing tools, and nursing care evaluation instruments in the process of operationalizing Orem's model. Also briefly described was the preparation of the nursing personnel for understanding and using Orem's concepts.

This chapter offers a "how to" contribution to the nursing administrator who wishes to implement the theory in practice.

Dickson, G.L. and Lee-Villasenor, H. (1982). Nursing theory and practice: A self-care approach. *Advances in Nursing Science,* 5, 29–40

The stated purpose of this article is "to bridge the gaps between theory and practice through the research of the application of an evolving theory" (p. 29). The authors also present a “new nursing model in which to “think nursing’ ”’ (p. 30). The findings described were from a field study carried out by the authors in their own independent practice settings using their own clients.

The framework of self-care developed by Orem and modified by Kinlein was chosen as the theoretical model for practice and research because the beliefs underlying the model were in keeping with the authors’ philosophy. The authors adequately describe and document these background materials sufficiently for those familiar with the model. For those unfamiliar with the model, the review is not adequate.

A nonexperimental, descriptive design was used. The source of data was the written recording of nurse–patient interactions from 35 time periods of four clients. Although the authors describe the four female subjects, they do not tell us why eight other prospective subjects were not included.

The research process proceeded as follows: during the clients’ appointments and during the process of providing nursing care, the nursing researchers recorded their clients’ words. At the time that a “need” was expressed, the nurse then identified self-care assets, the self-care demands, and the self-care measures with the client. The next step was a period of introspection for reflection on the nursing phenomena observed. Operational definitions were established, and four research questions were generated.

The data analysis yielded four categories of care: (1) the client’s expression of need, (2) self-care asset, (3) self-care demand, and (4) self-care measures. These were analyzed using content analysis from the grounded field theory methodology. Further analysis, in keeping with the inductive method of research being used (Glaser and Strauss), focused on the integration of categories and their properties. Specifically, data were analyzed to determine properties of expressions of need and self-care assets. The latter were found to be similar to the indicators of self-care agency as identified by Kearney and Fleischer (1979).

In summary, the authors reflect on the limitations of the research, namely sample size and bias, implications for practice and research, and directions for future research. The authors demonstrate clarity in describing both the procedures and the process of their experiences in relating theory to practice and research. The complex helical relationship of the three is clearly illustrated and the scholarliness of their approach and writing adds to the overall readability. The model was their guide for practice and research and, with the model in mind, it helped to maintain their focus on their goals. For these reasons, this study would be of interest to theorists, researchers, and clinicians alike who espouse the self-care framework. More important, the article provides an exemplar for theory development using the practice-theory strategy.

Karl, C.A. (1982). The effect of an exercise program on self-care activities for the institutionalized elderly. *Journal of Gerontological Nursing,* 8, 282–285

Although the title of this short report of a research study includes the concept of self-care, and although Orem is mentioned in the section, “Program Background,” the self-care framework does not seem to guide the conceptualization of the study. The review of the research literature focuses on general topics of feelings of well-being and physiological benefits of exercise rather than on self-care. Furthermore, liberties are taken with Orem's framework when the author states that "the theoretical defense for a study of the positive effects an exercise program can have on the institutionalized elderly and their ability to care for themselves has been formulated by Orem in her theory of self-care" (p. 283). Also misstated were the "assumptions"; in fact, these are really the hypotheses tested by the study.

Miller, J.F. (1980). The dynamic focus of nursing: A challenge to nursing administration. *Journal of Nursing Administration,* 10(1), 13–18

Although the title of this article suggests that the focus will be on nursing administration, and despite the introductory statement that "nursing administrators are challenged to establish a climate that facilitates the use of appropriate frameworks to guide nursing" (p. 13), this article is really about the application of a nursing framework—Orem's—to acute care. However, there is very little evidence of the self-care theory, which the author purports to use. What the author did, in fact, was to pull out the idea of changes in the health/illness continuum, suggesting that nurses focus on changes in the patient's health status as a model to guide intervention. The author presents three conceptual phases for acute care patients (acute illness, convalescence, and restored health), problems and nursing care strategies related to each, and a patient case study to demonstrate application. Only phases 2 and 3 are linked to patient development of self-care skills.

Although it takes into account where the person is on the health/illness continuum (which phase), the proposed "model for dynamic nursing practice" essentially ignores Orem's nursing systems, which give direction for nursing intervention based on the person's health self-care needs or self-care deficits regardless of where he is on the health/illness continuum. Therefore, this article offers a very limited application of Orem's theory.

Miller, J.F. (1982). Categories of self-care needs of ambulatory patients with diabetes. *Journal of Advanced Nursing,* 7, 25–31

The stated purpose of this paper is to report a study of the identification of need categories of ambulatory diabetic patients within the context of the self-care nursing framework. The title of the article reflects this purpose. The method used to discover the categories of self-care needs was that of participant observation. The need for the research was identified, but why the self-care framework is "especially appropriate" (p. 25) was not explained.

The sample of 65 men and women, ranging in age from 22 to 83, came from different socioeconomic classes and were from various cultural backgrounds. No rationale for sample selection was presented. The clinic where the subjects were treated used the self-care concept for nursing practice. Data collection initially involved an assessment of the patient's self-care agency using an instrument designed by the researcher and published elsewhere.

Additional self-care evaluation was completed during later patient contacts, with all patients in the study having a minimum of three contacts. "The evaluation consisted of four parts: an interview, physical assessment, interpretation of findings, and mutually determined goals." (p. 26) During this process, nursing care was provided during the contact. "Data gathered were recorded on a care plan and collection continued until no new categories were discovered and each category had been saturated with examples" (p. 27). Ten categories of needs were identified: "acquire skills for self-care management, receive feedback regarding self-care management, become aware of own resources, have feelings of self-esteem enhanced, grieve over losses, work towards acceptance of chronic disease, have new or continuing health concerns evaluated, obtain services from various support agencies, alleviate physical and mental discomforts, identify positive role of the health care agency and feel like a full participant in determining care goals, and maintain family solidarity and support or assist ill member" (p. 27).

These findings reveal an interesting contrast to the findings of Dickson and Lee-Villasenor (1982), who similarly used the method of participant observation. The latter also made observations in a clinical setting with a quite different sample and gleaned their need categories from statements of needs as expressed by their subjects.

In the discussion and conclusions, there is a certain eagerness to apply the findings to the practice setting as the next step. Here, that application is premature. More appropriate to the present stage of theory development of Orem is the phase of reanalysis and refinement of the self-care need categories for this subpopulation.

This study makes an important contribution to nursing science by using the theoretical formulations of Orem to guide the organization of the observations made of 65 ambulatory diabetic clients into the need categories. These data and categories contribute important information for continued theory development, for the inductive approach, and, more specifically, for the development of the concept of self-care needs.

Murphy, P.P. (1981). A hospice model and self-care theory. *Oncology Nursing Forum,* 8(2), 19–21

This brief article describes how Orem's self-care framework was used as a guide for nursing practice in a hospice setting. The focus of the article is on the role of nursing in this setting, using the three basic systems of nursing care described by Orem: (1) supportive–educative, (2) partially compensatory, and (3) wholly compensatory. Examples of level of interaction between the nurse and the patient for each system and a diagram illustrate how the hospice team operates using the self-care framework.

Although this article is not based on research but rather on clinical application, and although it does not provide any new insights or interpretations of Orem's work, it does demonstrate that the self-care framework is a useful guide for practitioners in a setting with terminally-ill patients.

Petrlik, J.C. (1976). Diabetic peripheral neuropathy. *American Journal of Nursing,* 76, 1794–1797

While this article does not mention Orem's theory as a basis for the discussion of self-care, it is based on the earlier article by Backscheider on self-care requirements and self-care abilities and should be read in conjunction with it. In this case, the author focused on assessment of the self-care abilities of patients who have peripheral neuropathy and the concomitant long-term problems. The theory-practice analysis is useful in helping the reader delineate some research propositions.

Porter, D., and Shamian, J. (1983). Self care in theory and practice. *Canadian Nurse,* 79(8), 21–23

Self-care as theory originated in the early 1950s. Orem was perceived as visionary, and the theory was labeled as revolutionary by the authors. Self-care was defined, and the assumptions of the theory and the goal of nursing were identified; the scope of practice—the role of nurse in relation to the client—was also discussed. How nurses might achieve the goal of nursing according to Orem was also explored in this article.

The basic needs of clients, which nurses assist in meeting, are classified by Orem as universal, developmental, and health deviational. While these are consistent with Orem's theory, only brief listings suggest what makes up each of these categories of needs. Citing Orem, the authors suggested that nursing interventions corresponding to the first two categories of needs could be considered primary prevention. Secondary and tertiary prevention would be those interventions related to health deviation self-care needs.

Within the context of Orem's theory, nursing care planning is facilitated by the development of nursing systems. Nursing system was defined, and the hierarchical components of the nursing system were outlined. These included wholly compensatory, partly compensatory, and supportive–educative; all of which were defined indirectly within the context of examples. Patients were to be categorized into one of these three systems through the nursing process when the nurse planned care.

The nursing process within the context of self-care theory included the identification of a number of factors influencing a person's ability to perform self-care. Some were listed. This concluded the brief description of the assessment phase. Likewise, the intervention phase was only briefly described.

Intervention is required when self-care abilities are inadequate to meet self-care demands. Nursing measures that help the client to achieve the goal of self-care as defined by Orem include: (1) acting or doing for; (2) guiding; (3) teaching; (4) supporting; and (5) providing a developmental environment. None of these was discussed by the authors. The meanings of major terms and concepts were illustrated within the context of a clinical situation and were offset for emphasis. This clinical example was titled "Self-care theory in practice at the JGH" (Jewish General Hospital).

Overall, the authors' description was in keeping with the theory, and the few omissions of concepts were not significant in terms of the model. The article provides a clear distillation or synopsis of the theory presented in an easy reading style, and although it is merely informative, it might be of interest to the newcomer to Orem's model. It might also be of interest to clinicians wishing a quick overview of the model and its potential utility in the practice setting.

Smith, M.C. (1979). Proposed metaparadigm for nursing research and theory development: An analysis of Orem's self-care theory. *Image,* 11(3), 75–79

The purpose of this article is to "propose a classification scheme to structure the analysis of existing research and the design of future research in nursing." The author uses Orem's theory to illustrate the proposed scheme. The ultimate purpose using the proposed scheme is to "formulate a cohesive, organized body of knowledge for theory building and development in nursing" (p. 75) as well as to organize existing research and design future research studies from a nursing framework.

Having developed a scheme and labeled a metaparadigm, the author illustrated how the premises and propositions of this particular nursing theorist are or can be classified. The author acknowledges and makes explicit her personally biased assumptions regarding the *sine qua non* of professional nursing practice.

This article is relevant to discussions of central phenomena in nursing and to the relationship between nursing research, theory development, and nursing practice.

Sullivan, T.J. (1980). Self-care model for nursing. In *New directions for nursing in the '80s*. Kansas City, MO: American Nurses' Association

The introduction to this article is very broad, discussing the issues for nursing and society for the 1980s. This leads the reader to the present focus of self-care, the appropriateness of it for clients and for the nursing profession, specifically because of the values it embraces and their similarity to those embedded in our American sociocultural value system. Nowhere in the introduction is the reader made aware that the author has taken what she perceived to be a broad, abstract, and otherwise static grand-level theory and operationalized the concept of self-care to make it more usable. She undertook to organize a body of knowledge for nursing the aged, which resulted in a self-care model for nursing the aged.

More than one-half of the article focuses on a review of Orem's self-care model. This review includes a fairly comprehensive picture of the model and description of its components. The nature, philosophy (including four underlying assumptions), and conceptual framework of the self-care model are all presented. The conceptual framework includes definitions of the three major conceptual constructs: therapeutic self-care demand, self-care agency, and nursing agency. The relationships between these parts of the framework are also explicated. Nursing agency is defined, and the hierarchical systems and their hierarchical subsystems—technological, interpersonal, and social—of nursing care are further described and linkages noted.

In the author's discussion of the philosophy of self-care—more specifically within the discussion of the nurse-patient relationship—the author has taken what she described as a "lawlike generalization" and restated it as a proposition. Another statement of a corollary could also have been restated as a propositional statement. These statements were almost incidental to the purpose of this paper, yet they are what are critically needed to move this theory to the point of being tested by research. Elaboration of the concepts, development of propositional statements, and subsequent hypothesis generation are basic requirements for validation of the self-care model. This author's brief discussion provides an important step in this direction.

The development of the self-care model for the aged was accomplished following "analysis and review of nursing literature on the aged and self-care." The outcome was a self-care model for nursing the aged. The four levels of the self-care system that emerged were listed and discussed. Conclusions that were reached following identification of these four self-care systems were also listed. The author also addressed the reality that clients might be functioning partly on one level and partly on another and that the four levels of the self-care system are therefore fluid; they represent a continuum. The model also allows for movement over time, indicating that clients may move vertically from one level of self-care to another as well, in several identifiable directions.

The technological and interpersonal subsystems of the nursing systems overlap in the process of accomplishing the goals of self-care. These were discussed, and approaches for applying methods of assistance to the aged emerged as a result of the study. These approaches were listed from the highest level to the lowest level of client capability for self-care. Also listed from the highest level of client capability to the lowest were four interpersonal subsystems. The social subsystem dimension of the nursing subsystem was also briefly discussed. Horizontal linkages with the model were also discussed. The author noted that, while it was not within the scope of the paper to present the concrete referents identified in the model, they had been identified.

Implications for use of the self-care theory in general, and the self-care model for nursing the aged more specifically, were succinctly summarized. Implications for model development for nursing groups other than the aged, for nursing practice with an emphasis on health versus illness, for hypothesis generation leading to research, for nursing leadership roles in health care, and for issues in nursing such as accountability, legal and ethical, were all presented.

This article would be of interest to practitioners, educators, and researchers who desire to use the self-care model for any of those areas—and is recommended reading. For the student of the self-care model, it would be helpful reading as a succinct summary of the model, with examples of statements of propositions. It would also be of interest to those working with the elderly and those who are interested in the self-care model. Furthermore, for students of epistemology, it illustrates the process of model development through the operationalization of a grand-level theory. The article is clearly written and logically developed; overall, it is a scholarly work that suggests that the model can be used as a curriculum model for gerontological nursing.

Martha Rogers

Egbert, E. (1980, January). Concept of wellness. *JPN and Mental Health Services,* 18(1), 9–12

Based on the opening sentence in this article, it appears that Rogers' use of the term *health* (not wellness) in a statement about what nursing is was the stimulus for developing the concept of wellness. At no other time is there any reference to Rogers' work, nor is the concept of wellness, as it is developed, related back to her theory.

The concept of wellness as developed here was, in essence, distilled from a variety of definitions as a result of a review of the literature. Based on the review, the author determined that wellness could not be clearly defined. Instead, she delineated a list of characteristics of wellness from the conceptions described by several authors and institutions that attempted to define health, such as Freud, Maslow, Jourard, Perls, Jahoda,

Wu, and the World Health Organization. The author suggested that although health and wellness could not be clearly defined, the list, a synthesis of many definitions, could provide guidelines for nursing intervention and prevention.

This article does not contribute to our understanding of Rogers' theory but provides us with a summary of some of the definitions of health.

Falco, S.M. and Lobo, M.L. (1980). Martha E. Rogers. In the Nursing Theories Conference Group, *Nursing theories: The base for professional nursing practice.* Englewood Cliffs, NJ: Prentice-Hall

Consistent with the other chapters in this edited volume, there is a brief history about the theoretician whose theory is presented. This summary of Rogers' *Theoretical basis of nursing* by Falco and Lobo is generally written clearly and concisely.

The authors present Rogers' definition of nursing and the five major assumptions about human beings that underlie the nursing science explicated by Rogers. What are not listed by these authors are the more general, broader assumptions underlying the four principles of homeodynamics, which are explicitly stated by Rogers. The second set of assumptions, similar to those about human beings, are grounded in systems theory. The four principles of homeodynamics are identified and elaborated on by the authors.

In the remainder of the article, the authors compare Rogers' theory with other theories, present clinical examples, and demonstrate the principles of homeodynamics, and then show how the principles might be used in the nursing process. This illustration shows the potential application of the model to clinical practice. Examples include series of questions to be used in the assessment phase to reflect each of the principles of homeodynamics. There are also examples of nursing diagnoses, planning, and implementation within the framework. Tables illustrate the relationship of the principles of homeodynamics to the nursing process. This use of Rogers' principles in the nursing process is only one of two known uses that are published (see also Whelton, 1979) and is an important contribution to the theory.

The authors also discuss limitations of Rogers' principles (*i.e.,* that they are too abstract and that terms have not been sufficiently operationalized).

For the reader unfamiliar with Rogers' *Theoretical basis of nursing,* this article presents a brief overview and summary. The examples of application to practice using the nursing process show the utility of the theory for practice, and this makes it more useful for the practitioner. In this way, the article contributes to our understanding and use of this theory and therefore to the science of nursing.

Katz, V. (1971) Auditory stimulation and developmental behavior of the premature infant. *Nursing Research,* 20(3), 196–201

It has never been explicitly stated by the author; however, because she was a student in Martha Rogers' program and because this research was based on other research carried out at the same institution, it is assumed that Katz's study was developed based on assumptions of Rogers' theory. If this is correct, not presenting the theoretical framework would be a limitation.

If one were to try to guess which assumptions of Rogers underlie this study, the following might be included: (1) a human being and his environment are continuously exchanging matter and energy with one another, (2) the life process evolves irreversibly and unidirectionally along the space/time continuum, (3) pattern and organization identify a human being and reflect his innovative wholeness (Rogers, 1970).

"The focus of this study was to determine whether a variation in the environment of the low-birth-weight premature infant by the introduction of the maternal voice can influence behavior." (p. 196) The design of the study was quasi-experimental with a control group; it had a sample size of 62. The major statistical analysis was an analysis of variance, comparing those premature infants who received a regimen of auditory stimulation with those who did not. The behavioral outcomes measured were motor, tactile-adaptive, auditory, visual, muscle-tension, and irritability responses. All the tools used had reliability and validity data available.

The same two raters (not the investigator) who were used to test all infants were blind as to which groups the infants were in. Interscorer agreement between the raters and the investigator was obtained after the raters were trained. These and other measures are important safeguards that were used in this study to reduce the potential for bias in the data. In general, based on the write-up, it appears that the study was well-designed.

The study supported previous findings that had indicated that variations in behavioral development are evident after changes are made in sensory input in low-birth-weight premature infants. More important, and consistent with Rogers' belief that the purpose of nursing as an empirical science is to describe and explain the phenomena central to its concern (*i.e.*, person) and to predict about them, this study provides empirical data from which nursing intervention can then be planned. In Rogers' terms, "the identification of relationship between events provides for an ordering of knowledges and for the development of nursing's hypothetical generalizations and unifying principles (1980, pp. 84–85)."

For these reasons, this study supports Roger's theory and contributes both to empirical validation of it as well as to the science of nursing in general by the rigor of the research. An important omission in the write-up, however, was that the researcher did not indicate other potentially testable hypotheses generated by this research.

Porter, L.S. (1972). The impact of physical-physiological activity on infants' growth and development. *Nursing Research,* 21(3), 210–219

This rigorous experimental study was explicitly based on two assumptions of Martha Rogers' theory: (1) the human organism is an open system in constant interaction with the environment, and (2) growth and developmental processes are unitary and integrative. The study was developed with the conceptualization that the human organism is an energy field in continuous motion. The researcher postulated a direct relationship between environmentally imposed motion and a speeding up of infant growth and development.

The research was built on earlier studies that also used Rogers' theory as a conceptual framework as well as the researcher's own earlier study of infants. Because the researcher believed that the results of her earlier study were not generalizable enough, this study was undertaken as a follow-up study to corroborate the earlier findings. (An earlier study by the author, Luz Sobong, tested Johnson's proposition of stimulation and growth.)

The study is methodically and systematically described, clearly enough so as to be reproducible. Background, hypotheses, methodology, data collection, and results are all described in detail. Tables showing the data are included as well as a summary of the analyses performed on the six measures of growth and development used in the study. The six measures of growth and development were gains in weight, length, motor, adaptive, language, and personal-social behavior. The design of the study was experimental, with random assignment of subjects who were then matched with a control group. One limitation in the data collection was that the investigator collected the data and was not blind to whether the subjects were in the experimental group or the control group (or so it appears from the write-up).

A question is raised here regarding the data analysis. For example, the subjects were pretested on the six measures. Results presented showed that the heaviest control subject initially weighed 325 ounces, while the corresponding experimental subject weighed 369 ounces. There is a difference between these two of 44 ounces. In the discussion, the author indicated that there was "no important initial difference" (p. 216) between the groups. The question is, Is this a significant difference between the two groups? A t-test would have provided this information and, although it may have been done by the investigator, the results were not reported here.

This research study has contributed to the science of nursing not only by contributing to knowledge about infants with implications for nursing intervention but also by providing support for the assumptions upon which it was based, namely those of Martha Rogers. This was a rigorous study and a scholarly report.

Rogers, M.E. (1970). *An introduction to the theoretical basis of nursing.* Philadelphia: F.A. Davis

It is in this book that Martha Rogers first presents her ideas about the theoretical basis of nursing in a formal way. Some of the origins of her ideas, her earlier thinking, is seen in her 1963 article, which it is helpful to read either prior to or in conjunction with this book. (Rogers uses "man" to refer to the nursing client in this early writing.)

Essentially, the book is divided into three main sections. In the first section, "Book of modern nursing," she presents background material related to man's beginnings, the evolution of man's thinking, and theories of this century about how man and life originated. "The phenomenon of man: Nursing's concern" is the second section. Here Rogers states what it is she sees as the central concern of nursing: man in his entirety. Man as a whole, man as a system, is the prototypic theory used to present the underlying assumptions Rogers makes about man. The assumptions are explicitly numbered and labeled as such. Five assumptions upon which nursing science builds are identified.

In the third section, "Nursing's conceptual system," Rogers clearly points out the aims of nursing, nursing's conceptual model, the principle of nursing science, the principles of homeodynamics, evidence to support the concepts, ideas about formulating testable hypotheses, ways in which to translate the conception into practice and, finally, some ideas about the future. The essence of the theory is expressed in the first part of this section. The assumptions about man, the focus of nursing, were identified in the earlier section, but it is here that the concepts and principles are defined—the internal structure, aspects of the goals and consequences, and some dimensions of the theory are outlined.

An important chapter in this section relates to the potential of this theory for research. In fact, a whole body of research attempting to verify the principles of the real world (being carried out by doctoral students under Rogers' direction) is presented. The limitation in this chapter discussing the findings is that about 95% of it includes unpublished doctoral dissertations and is not generally available. Nevertheless, the important thing is that numerous studies, including cluster studies, have been and continue to be undertaken in attempts to accumulate evidence in support of the principles postulated by Rogers. This fact alone makes Rogers' formulations stand out from all of the other nursing theories and models, even to this day. Furthermore, implications of many of the studies give direction for practice as well as provide direction for additional research.

The major limitations of Rogers' formulations are well known. These are that the principles of homeodynamics—reciprocity, synchrony, helicy, and resonance—are all quite abstract and have not been adequately operationalized. Some would say that because the principles are not easily understood, they are difficult to translate into practice. Also, because of the lack of operational definitions, the research carried out to verify the principles provides questionable results. The major counter argument, if one were to think along the lines of Rogers' theory and writing, is that research must focus on the range of human phenomena and that this will give substance to nursing's abstract system. There is, to a degree, an element of inductive reasoning, and an inductive approach is suggested; that is, the principles provide the framework, the direction for research, but the research results really provide the substance of the theory.

A chapter in the third section, in addition to discussing research, addresses the potential of the theory for practice. With the exception of citing four research studies suggesting direction for nursing practice, the discussion is more or less an abstract discussion of nursing interventions that purportedly are based on the different principles of homeodynamics. It does not indicate whether or not the theory is actually used in any practice settings.

In closing, we would recommend to anyone interested in Rogers' theory to read, at the minimum, the third section of the book; then for additional understanding of the assumptions about human beings, the second section, and for background in general, the first. The book is clearly and logically developed and very readable. In general, reading the whole book, elegant in its simplicity, sophisticated in its presentation, and erudite as its author, is highly recommended. Rogers stands out among the nursing theorists, and her work in theorizing, research, and education presents a major contribution to nursing as a science.

Rogers, M.E. (1975). Euphemisms in nursing's future. *Image,* 7(2), 3–9

The focus of this paper is an argument against the many forms of nursing services parading under the guise of nice-sounding titles, when in fact they are cover-ups for physicians' assistants. This controversy was at its height in the early to mid-1970s, and Rogers was strongly opposed to the development of new roles or any new title, such as the family health practitioner, pediatric associate, and primary care nurse. She believed these were cover-ups for the physician's assistant, were "perpetrated to deny a future to nurses and nursing" (p. 3), and were coined to enhance the economic gains of the physicians.

This article bears little if any relevance to Rogers' theoretical basis of nursing per se. What comes through are her beliefs about roles and levels of education needed to prepare nurses and what the scope of nursing is. Her theme that a baccalaureate preparation for nursing is important is repeated here.

For those unfamiliar with the more personal side of the professional Martha Rogers, this article provides a touch of that side. It gives one a feel for the spontaneous way in which she makes her arguments and for the strength of her convictions. Her wit, sense of humor, and a touch of cynicism are well demonstrated in this article. For this alone, this article is worth reading.

Rogers, M.E. (1980). Nursing: A science of unitary man. In J.P. Riehl and C. Roy (Eds.), *Conceptual models for nursing practice* (2nd ed.). New York: Appleton-Century-Crofts

In this chapter, Rogers brings us up to date on her thinking about nursing and a conceptual system in nursing. She in fact presents a few changes in the underlying assumptions and in the principles of homeodynamics, compared with her earlier book (1970). No explanation is set forth as to why the changes were made. In essence, no specific assumptions about man are identified. Rather, Rogers states that four building blocks are essential in the conceptual system presented in this paper. They are: (1) energy fields, (2) universe of open systems, (3) pattern and organization, and (4) four-dimensionality. Each is briefly discussed.

The principles of homeodynamics have been reduced from four to three, and one of the three is different from the original. The original four were the principles of reciprocity, synchrony, helicy, and resonance. The new three are the principles of helicy, resonance, and complementarity. The first two remain essentially the same in definition. The principles of complementarity have elements of the original principle of reciprocity with the added idea of interaction between man and environment.

There are some elements of the theory that appear to have been updated; for example, the title. Here the underlying assumptions are broadened to include more than those five assumptions about the human being. Here, they are also described as building blocks rather than assumptions. As already discussed, the principles of homeodynamics have changed somewhat.

Also updated are the theories deriving from the proposed conceptual system. Only a few of these are discussed. These include theory of accelerating evolution, explanations of par ormal events, and rhythmical correlates of change. The implications that advances echnology have for change are also taken into account by Rogers.

The of these updates are in the discussion of implications for practice. Changes in nur practice must result from changes in man, such as the evolutionary emer- ew behavior patterns (eg, hypertension and hyperactivity), new knowledge, ges in values. This is an interesting point that Rogers makes and, indeed, one mmonly mentioned by most theorists.

is recommended that this chapter be read in conjunction with Rogers' 1970 book.

Whelt 979). An operationalization of Martha Rogers' theory throughout the nursing process. *Inter- nati al of Nursing Studies*, 16, –20

This is the second of only two known articles referring to situations in which Rogers' theory is used throughout the nursing process. This whole article essentially focuses on that, whereas Falco and Lobo (1980) only present the nursing process in a section of their chapter.

The introduction clearly states the purpose of the paper and describes the content to be covered and then, clearly and precisely, the authors carry out their plan. This makes the paper very readable.

The version of Rogers' theory used here is the earlier (1970) version rather than the 1980 updates. In the presentation of the theory, the structural components are clearly spelled out; that is, basic assumptions about man, the five nursing concepts (stated more explicitly than Rogers really did), and the nursing principles of homeodynamics derived from the concepts. The five nursing concepts identified by this author are wholeness, openness, pattern and organization, unidirectionality, and sentience and thought.

The clinical population of interest identified to be the focus of the operationaliza- tion of Rogers' theory are those patients with decreased cardiac output and impaire neurological function. For example, the assessment of these patients would include da related to the five general concepts already mentioned. Tables are included that sh what is assessed under each of these categories. For example, under wholeness, ph ical integrity and psychological integrity are listed. Then in a later table for a pa with impaired neurological functioning, the subitems are listed.

The general format is carried out in detail through each phase of the nursing pr here identified as assessment, nursing diagnosis, plan of care (including goal), and mentation and evaluation. Detailed tables present an actual nursing care plan s diagnosis, plan, and goal. No examples are given for implementation and evalu

At least one example in this area would have complemented the other p summarizing, Whelton indicates that assessment tools will vary with the patie tion. However, it is not entirely reasonable to have an assessment tool for each different patient population. Therefore, the tool described here could be d more general terms and could thus be more generalizable to other patient

This article has contributed significantly to the applicability of Rog practice by making the somewhat abstract notions of the theory more c operationalizing the theory within the nursing process.

Sister Callista Roy

Brower, H.T. and Baker, B.J. (1976). Using the adaptation model in a practitioner cu[illegible]m. *Nursing Outlook*, 24(11), 686–689

The practitioner curriculum described here is a geriatric nurse practitione[illegible] uses the adaptation model of Roy. The authors forthrightly state that Roy's [illegible] the following criteria: it outlines the features of the discipline and provides d[illegible]l that practice, research, and education; it considers the values and goals of nursing, [illegible]ets and practitioner interventions; and, in essence, it is a theory at the prescriptive or si[illegible] producing level. Because these criteria were met, the model was incorporated int[illegible] curriculum.

Another important aspect of the model identified was that it was helpful in diffe[illegible]entiating between those aspects of care unique to nursing versus medical practice within the context of Roy's four modes of adaptation. Furthermore, in describing the application of the model, it appeared that examples used are the authors' interpretation of Roy's model. Although the potential of the model for practice is supported (eg, another area of practice is covered), the application offers neither refinement nor extension. On the other hand, some insights in the form of interventions for nursing are suggested. For example, to promote client adaptation, nursing interventions might include facilitation of adaptive tasks of aging through counseling, effective communication techniques, health education, active manipulation, providing support, and identifying resources. However, here the points of entry for the nursing intervention are not clearly spelled out. It is stated: "If inadequate adaptation is occurring, the practitioner can attempt to modify or manipulate focal stimuli, thereby making a positive response pos[illegible]ble" (p. 687). This example simply is not specific enough; it suggests where to inter[illegible] but not when.

[illegible]he third focus in this article is curriculum application. In this section, there is an [illegible]tion of the content taught that provides information about what these authors [illegible] from other fields and other theoretical models for a knowledge base as it [illegible]is model. For example, crisis intervention theory, health anthropology, atti[illegible]iew, stage theory, and role theory are all included. This information may [illegible]o those who want to plan a similar practitioner program.

[illegible]blems with nursing home application for elderly persons: An application of [illegible] *Journal of Advanced Nursing*, 6(5), 363– 368

[illegible]the outset that the elderly are often dependent on significant [illegible]plementary to home care for them to remain at home. The [illegible]n, was to "assess the life circumstances surrounding nurs[illegible]rly people" (p. 364), and the Roy adaptation model was [illegible]ganize data collected about adaptation problems of [illegible]ant others.

Three research questions were identified:

1. "In what way can a conceptual framework in nursing provide for the understanding of adaptation problems of elderly persons and significant others which contribute to nursing home applications?
2. If two groups of elderly persons are receiving at least one home care service, what similarities and differences exist in adaptation problems that allow one group to remain at home while the other group must apply for admission to a nursing home?
3. To what extent do the adaptation problems on the part of the elderly person of those persons closest to him contribute to the nursing home application for the elderly person?" (p. 364)

The discussion of the conceptual framework that followed those research questions briefly presented the underlying beliefs of the Roy adaptation model and identified the four adaptive modes and what was considered an "adaptive response." The nurse's role within the model was identified as promoting adaptation that involved two factors in the nursing process: assessment and intervention. Other than this brief overview, the author assumed that the reader was familiar with the model. Only one study was cited that documented characteristics or problems of elderly applicants to long-term care facilities, and no research, related to adaptation or to use of the adaptation model, was cited.

In the purpose statement, the general purpose to assess factors associated with nursing home application was repeated. A general statement that five hypotheses were formulated and tested was made, and a statement was made that they related to "overall adaptation problems, powerlessness, role reversal guilt, and knowledge and utilization of services, but the hypotheses were not explicitly stated. Furthermore, no theoretical connections between the hypotheses and the Roy model were explicated. It is not clear that all the hypotheses flowed from the research question. This led me to conclude that the conceptualization of this research within the Roy model was extremely limited; that is, it was conceptually inadequate.

The study group and the control group were described, but criteria for each subject group were not specific.

The method used in this study was described as an *ex post facto* design, appropriate to this population because admission to a nursing home is not a variable that can be controlled. Statistical analyses were completed using Chi-square. Both the elderly subjects and their significant others were interviewed in their homes.

The limitations of this research outweigh the contributions it might have made to the testing of the Roy adaptation model. What is more, in the conclusion, neither the limitations of the research nor the implications for future research are discussed.

Galligan, A.C. (1979). Using Roy's concept of adaptation to care for young children. *American Journal of Maternal Child Nursing*, 4(1), 24–28

Given the psychosocial as well as the physical needs of children while they are hospitalized, this author has chosen Roy's concept of adaptation "as a means of guiding nurses in a more conscious effort to assist the child during hospitalization." Rationale for the choice of this model was not provided.

The author has divided the hospital stay into four different stages: prehospitalization, preoperative, postoperative, and discharge. The rationale for these divisions was that because "man" (child?) is in constant interaction with a changing environment, the nursing assessment and appropriate interventions must be revised periodically during the patient's stay. Each stage is briefly discussed regarding the potential for assessment and intervention. Then, to illustrate how the Roy adaptation model might be used to assess and intervene with a young child, a hypothetical case was presented.

For three of the four stages of hospitalization, omitting discharge, each mode is discussed with examples of assessment—including focal, contextual, and residual stimuli—and intervention. In the second and third stages, the dimensions of diagnosis and evaluation were added. The discharge stage was discussed only very briefly, indicating that the child should be evaluated again in each of the four adaptive modes, and a discharge plan should be formulated.

For those interested in the applicability of the model for practice, especially with patients other than adults, this is an important contribution, demonstrating that the model is useful in the nursing care of children. On the whole, however, it does not increase our understanding of the Roy model itself.

Janelli, L.M. (1980). Utilizing Roy's adaptation model from a gerontological perspective. *Journal of Gerontological Nursing*, 6(3), 140–150

The title of this article clearly indicates the focus, but more specifically, the author discusses two purposes. The first is general background about how the author came to use the theory and an overview of the model. Selye's stress theory was identified as the paradigmatic origin of the theory. The second purpose of the article is to present use of the model with specific clinical examples in gerontologic nursing.

As far as contributions to the theory, the author presents her conception, in diagrammatic form, of a human being as a biopsychosocial being interacting with the environment. Although the Roy adaptation model is basically a systems model, Roy does not use the word "tension" as it is used in this description. Other than the diagram, this article does not substantially add to our understanding of the model. It does, or at least did in this case, provide enough direction for practice with an elderly clientele.

This article is useful for those interested in gerontologic nursing. Tables of needs and the schematic presentation of the human being–environment interactions are also useful.

Jones, P.S. (1978). An adaptation model for nursing practice. *American Journal of Nursing*, 78(11), 1900–1906

The adaptation model described here is not related to the Roy adaptation model and, in fact, uses a different prototype theory as a basis for its development. The author suggested that having this second framework based on the idea of adaptation (in this case modeled after Selye) might be confusing, but she thought her model might have more to offer than other theories. She suggested that there were difficulties with other existing theories; however, the difficulties were not identified.

In addition to using Selye's theory as a prototype, Maslow's hierarchy of needs was also used "to provide structure and guidance for assessing all needs." Based on the hierarchy, the author developed an elaborate assessment tool.

In terms of the structural components of the model, assumptions and concepts were explicit. Eight underlying assumptions were listed. The major concepts used included wholeness, needs, adaptability, illness, and wellness. The author did not specifically develop propositional statements that described the relationship of the concepts.

On the whole, this article does not contribute to our understanding of Roy's adaptation model, although it may have contributed another perspective to the concept of the health/illness continuum (in this case, illness/wellness continuum), which is not terribly clear in Roy's model. Jones illustrates her model using a triangle to demonstrate the interaction of the three variables in an average person. This conceptualization helps to determine wellness when the person is physically ill but "well" in other areas, a problem in Roy's model.

Mastal, M.F. and Hammond, H. (1980). Analysis and expansion of the Roy adaptation model: A contribution to holistic nursing. *Advances in Nursing Science*, 2(4), 71–81

Although believing that the Roy adaptation model has much to offer nursing by way of providing a framework to organize its body of nursing knowledge, these authors are highly critical of the model in its present form. Specifically, the criticisms focus on a lack of explicit theoretical components of assumptions and concepts, simple propositions, and relational propositions (criticisms noted in earlier critiques also).

The purpose, then, of this article is to make up for some of the above deficits. Assumptions underlying the mode, heretofore implicit, are explicitly stated. (Roy's 1980 edition of *Conceptual Models* was not yet published when this article was written because in that edition, the assumptions are outlined by Roy. Readers are encouraged to compare the two sets of assumptions.)

The five major concepts within the framework are identified, summarized, and discussed. These include: (1) person, (2) environment, (3) adaptation, (4) health/illness, and (5) nursing.

The authors focus on the lack of theoretical and operational definitions as well as on the narrow scope of health/illness. In attempting to elucidate this concept and to answer some questions, a continuum is defined, a new idea of transition is introduced, and nursing assessment along the continuum is clarified. This addition is justified on the basis that it expands the model's scope. However, based on this brief discussion, this is a critical addition to the concept of health/illness.

Two other major additions to the theory are a diagram depicting the relationships between the major concepts of the model and a set of propositional statements. The latter is a particularly important contribution because it is what the model was lacking at the time this article was published.

Overall, the article is clearly written and adds to our understanding of the theory. The contribution of propositional statements adds to the researchability of the theory, and ultimately to nursing as a science.

Mastal, M.F., Hammond, H., and Roberts, M.P. (1982). Theory into hospital practice: A pilot implementation. *Journal of Nursing Administration,* 12(6), 9–15

This article describes both the process involved when the Roy adaptation model was implemented in one unit of a small community hospital, and how the process contributed to the validation of nursing theory. The description of the process is detailed enough to give guidance to clinicians or administrators who might choose to implement a theoretical model. Each step of the process is outlined and described.

Adequate review and understanding of any theoretical model to be used in a clinical setting is requisite. In this case, the review revealed that not all components (philosophical basis, assumptions, concepts, and propositions) had been specifically identified and defined. This led the authors to pursue this end directly with the theorist, Sister Callista Roy. From this, specific components were clarified, and what were perceived by the authors to be the model's components were depicted visually. This effort was later used to make the model understandable and usable for the hospital's nursing staff. (This process of clarification of the components of the model and the communications with Sister Roy would also make another significant contribution to the validation of the theory.) Once components of the model had been clarified, the administrative processes were initiated.

Planning and organizing were the major steps required administratively to start the pilot. Approval was sought, starting with the top levels of hospital and nursing administration. Congruence with the hospital philosophy, standards of patient care, and cost effectiveness were all explored. One unit was selected for the pilot with justification for that choice outlined.

Organization was based on Di Vincenti's theoretical framework for change and required three major steps: (1) establishing the change structure, (2) developing appropriate procedures, and (3) determining requirements and allocating resources. Each of these steps was described and was discussed in some detail. In the change structure, shared power was the category of "how" to change. Group problem solving and group decision making, as part of shared power, was emphasized. Open communication and a method for addressing problems in an ongoing way was also important to the success of the project.

The development of procedures included review of existing forms and required revision of nursing assessment, although not of the nursing care plan. Procedures affecting unit function required guidelines for the following: "(1) using the assessment and planning tools, (2) nursing reports and rounds, (3) patient care conferences, (4) nursing documentation, (5) orientation of new personnel, (6) standards of performance and job descriptions for nurses involved in the project, and (7) audit criteria" (p. 13). Costs for these services and required materials were assumed by the hospital. The planning and organizational phase was reported to have taken five months.

Staff education required the next major block of time. One-hour sessions weekly for a period of 15 weeks were structured for all the staff—RNs and LVNs—on the pilot unit. Cooperation of the head nurse and other departmental heads to cover staffing on the unit during this time period was critical to the success of the classes.

The authors believed that the overall components of success of the pilot implementation were authority, leadership, and communication. Clear lines of authority and administrative sanction for the implementation of the adaptation model were critical. Furthermore, open communication was fostered and facilitated through weekly group meetings, through frequent one-to-one talks between project directors and staff nurses, and through the use of an on-unit community log book for staff to express feelings.

Outcomes were measured indirectly both by improved patient care and by nurses' satisfaction with enhanced professional practice. Since then, patient satisfaction is being documented by conducting further research. There were more concrete measures of enhanced nursing practice. Namely, the development of a new tool to assess the biopsychosocial status of patients (illustrated by Exhibit 1), more complete nursing care plans phrased in terms consistent with the model, and greater collegial sharing and rapport were reported.

This report was written clearly in a conversational style, without sacrificing scholarliness and thoroughness. It would be of interest to theorists, researchers, and clinicians alike who are interested in the Roy model because it clearly illustrates the helical nature of theory, research, and practice. What is more, it makes an important contribution to the science of nursing by demonstrating application to practice and by stimulating research.

Roy, C. (1970). Adaptation: A conceptual framework for nursing. *Nursing Outlook*, 18(3), 42–45

The purpose of this article is to describe the framework of a conceptual model for nursing that was in the early stages of development by a nursing faculty group. Implications of the model for nursing science, practice, and education are suggested.

Implicit in the section, "Theoretical Model," are the functional components of assumptions and concepts. Examples of the underlying assumptions are: (1) man is a biopsychosocial being, (2) man is constantly interacting with a changing environment, and (3) man has both innate and acquired coping mechanisms. The major concepts of the model are adaptation and coping, health and illness, and man and the environment. However, Roy, in this first publication on her theory, does not yet explicitly identify either the assumptions or the concepts.

In the discussion of the concepts, the major concept of adaptation is described in terms of its origin in the physiologic theory of Harry Helson. The definition is technical and somewhat tautological and does not answer the questions raised by the author, which are: "How does this adaptation take place?" and "What is behind the process?" These are difficult questions, and it was too early to answer them. Furthermore, when the author tries to answer the question about how the concept of adaptation applies to nursing, the answer is in terms of the function of nursing, which is "to support and promote patient adaptation."

Although the term "elements," as applied to conceptual models, was not used at the time this article was published, except in a course taught by Dorothy Johnson at the University of California, Los Angeles, where Roy was studying for her master's degree, this analysis reveals that the following elements are present: *goal of action*—to support and promote patient adaptation; *actor's role*—to assess and intervene and to promote adaptation. Less clear are the elements of *patiency*, which is when the nurse becomes involved with the patient on the health/illness continuum, and the *source of difficulty* (although it is similar to patiency). The recipient of nursing care is the human being. The *intervention focus* or *mode* is to promote adaptation by changing the person's response potential. Specific examples are given. Understanding man in health and illness is the essential focus of adaptation nursing.

That this developing theoretical model presents rudimentary outlines of a nursing science is an overstatement on the part of the author. However, considering that this is one of the earlier theoretical models developed in nursing, it is an important contribution to the growth of nursing as a science. This is a useful article to read for those interested in analyzing the development of theoretical thinking in nursing.

Roy, C. (1971). Adaptation: A basis for nursing practice. *Nursing Outlook*, 19(4), 254–257

This article picks up where the earlier one (1970) left off; it is helpful to read both together. It offers a description of man as an adaptive system with four modes of coping. Assumptions underlying the model are offered; the four modes of adaptation and their components as well as examples are listed. The four modes—later called effector modes—are physiologic needs, self-concept, role mastery (later, role function), and interdependence. All four modes were identified based on samples of behavior collected by nursing students of the author as well as on a synthesis of work done by other nurses. The other nursing sources included Abdellah and McCain. Ultimately, it appears that the categories are a synthesis of several sources, which may raise some questions about the validity of the categories. What data and what research supported these four choices? Are there other modes, such as the cognitive mode, which might be included?

A more rigorous approach that may have helped in the development of nursing knowledge would have been for the author to develop a research orientation and a scientific approach rather than a curricular one. Hindsight aside, the leap was immediately made to clinical application. Within the context of clinical application, new concepts then came up that had had insufficient elaboration. Examples of these included health/illness continuum, "positive" responses versus "negative" needs, and a diagram/figure describing the nursing process and first-level assessment.

The nursing goal, clearly stated, is "to bring about an adapted state in the patient, which frees him to respond to other stimuli which may be present." This remains a nursing goal of the theory in 1984 and continues to raise questions about what the nature of the adapted state is and the intended consequences (being [in 1984] the quality of life and the integrity of the individual).

To demonstrate the applicability of the model of adaptation to nursing, two case studies were presented. In each, the nurse used the model as a basis for assessment and intervention. Because it is clearly stated that the nurse establishes a nursing care plan and later evaluates it, and because the nursing process as it was known at the time encompasses four stages—assessment, planning, intervention, and evaluation—one wonders why Roy chose instead to use a nursing process including only two of the four—assessment and intervention. That question aside, the steps grew to six in 1984.

Although there is a discussion about planning, the "how to" of choosing nursing approaches is left to the process of nursing judgment outlined by McDonald and Harms. Additionally, the unintended consequences of the nursing intervention are not discussed.

Overall, this article continues to contribute to our understanding of processes, strategies, and phases of theory development in nursing.

Roy, C. (1976). The Roy adaptation model: Comment. *Nursing Outlook*, 24(11), 690–691

Sister Callista Roy, who developed the Roy adaptation theory, herein presents her reactions to two articles by Brower and Baker (1976) and by Wolfer (1976). She thinks that the authors did a fine job in implementing ideas from her writings, considering that they used only her published material as a basis.

After more general reactions to Brower and Baker's article regarding the importance of a nursing model as a basis for role identification, Roy goes on to clarify her views, to identify what could be considered limitations, and to acknowledge difficulties with the model. Among these are the fact that the model "has not yet been submitted to the rigors of clinical research that will be necessary to establish its validity," and that the model is a deductive one and has not been developed by formal theory construction methods.

This interaction and feedback is an important process for the growth of nursing knowledge, and the thinking of scholars was evident later on in the development of Roy's theory.

Roy, C. (1979). Relating nursing theory to education: A new era. *Nurse Educator*, 4(2), 16–21

This article examines the relationship between nursing theory and nursing education, from the meaning of theory to mechanisms of theory utilization, within a department of nursing.

Roy, C. (1980). The Roy adaptation model. In J.P. Riehl and C. Roy (Eds.), *Conceptual models for nursing practice* (2nd ed.). New York: Appleton-Century-Crofts

Notably still missing in this updated version of the Roy model are data from research, a decade after the first publication appeared in *Nursing Outlook*.

Presented here is the more formal theory construction work that was promised in the earlier "Comment" (1976). Clearly presented and labeled as such are the basic assumptions underlying the model and the elements of the model, namely, values, goal of action, patiency, source of difficulty, and intervention. What is still missing is an elaboration of the major concepts and the propositions, or those statements that show the relationship between the concepts. This important omission is not acknowledged by the author. More seriously at issue here is that the model is now 10 years old, is widely used as a curricular framework and in nursing practice settings, and yet research is still not being carried out.

There is a new diagram depicting the "source of difficulty," which is not clarified in the text. The source of difficulty is first "described as the originating point of deviations from the desired state or condition." However, the discussion continues in the vein of how the modes and coping mechanisms are called into play (ie, like a feedback system) rather than truly defining the source of difficulty. The discussion closes with this summary explanation: " 'The source of difficulty,' then, is coping activity that is inadequate to maintain integrity in the face of a need deficit or excess." This does not match the diagram that shows that there can exist either adaptive or maladaptive behaviors. The question unanswered by either the diagram or the text description is: When does a source of difficulty really exist? and, particularly and more important, When does the nurse intervene, at the originating point of deviation or at a later time, when the coping mechanisms called up are inadequate? The diagram is somewhat confusing in light of the discussion in the text.

In summarizing, the author points to areas in which "continuing development" is needed, such as validation of assumptions, explication of values, and clarification of elements.

Schmitz, M. (1980). The Roy adaptation model: Application in a community setting. In J.P. Riehl and C. Roy (Eds.), *Conceptual models of nursing practice* (2nd ed.) (pp. 193–206). New York: Appleton-Century-Crofts

The Roy adaptation model was applied here in the home setting, which is different from the inpatient setting where it has heretofore exclusively been applied. This necessitated an expansion of the concept of client from individual with an identified need to include the "family of care." If this broadened definition of the client is accepted, and it seems appropriate to do so, this will be an important contribution to the model.

In the introduction, the author is careful to identify differences between the home and hospital, especially in terms of nursing goals and nursing interventions. Also identified in the home setting were variables influencing care. The introductory remarks laid the groundwork for a detailed case study, with a family requiring home nursing care, which was the major focus of the study.

The care presentation included six detailed tables describing the client behaviors with focal, contextual, and residual stimuli for each mode and an accompanying nursing care plan for each.

The author summarized how the Roy adaptation model was used to assess and intervene with a family. Application of the model was the focus of this article. A more theoretical discussion would also have been appropriate because an expansion of the concept of client resulted from the thinking and work of this author, which is an important theoretical contribution.

Starr, S.L. (1980). Adaptation applied to the dying client. In J.P. Riehl and C. Roy (Eds.), *Conceptual models for nursing practice* (2nd ed.). New York: Appleton-Century-Crofts.

In this brief descriptive article, the author has elaborated on "elements of adaptive death" within four modes (Roy's): (1) physiologic mode, (2) self-concept mode, (3) role mode, and (4) interdependence mode. Within each mode, adaptive behaviors of the dying client are identified, stimuli affecting the behaviors are listed, and the nursing goal and interventions appropriate to each mode are presented.

Although this article is included in a set of three articles about the Roy adaptation model, there is no direct reference to Roy's work by the author. If one assumes that this is an application of the Roy model to practice, it is clear that it is timely, that the model can be applied to this group of patients, and that it is appropriate to nursing practice in this area. However, the article does not extend the Roy adaptation model.

Wagner, P. (1976). The Roy adaptation model: Testing the adaptation model in practice. *Nursing Outlook*, 24(11), 682–685

The potential for practice in both episodic and distributive settings using the Roy adaptation model has been realized, according to this author. Graduate students who tested the feasibility of the model for practice concluded that "the model provided a good framework for ordering a variety of observations" and using the model for nursing enhanced assessment and intervention as well as the overall nursing process.

Before field testing the model, the graduate students reviewed materials published about the model. They found discrepancies between sources and also, although not stated directly, they found limitations in the original assessment tools. They also identified limitations with a tool they subsequently developed even though their tool met the criterion that it was both theoretical and practical. These authors also expressed concern with overlap between the four modes as developed by Roy.

The author gives an indication that the model provides enough direction to affect practice in a variety of settings. Who is acted upon is not as clearly described as where or in what setting the person is acted upon. We are not any clearer as to the focus of the theory, nor are any definitions clarified such as health/illness, modes, positive and negative behavior, and adaptation.

Wagner added two dimensions—nursing diagnosis and evaluation—to Roy's nursing process of assessment and intervention. These later (1984) became an integral part of Roy's nursing process.

Overall, this article supports the notion that the conceptual model currently applies to practice and that it does have relevance for the way nursing is practiced today.

Joyce Travelbee

Travelbee, J. (1963). What do we mean by rapport? *American Journal of Nursing*, 63(2), 70–72

This article provides an excellent example of an attempt to conceptualize a phenomenon. It could be used as an early exemplar in concept development. However, the lack of clinical referents limits its wide utility and curtails its research potential. The term "rapport" is commonly used in nursing but had previously been neither conceptualized, operationally defined, nor researched. Frequently, rapport is defined by what it is not rather than by what it is. The explicit assumption underlying this development is that a controlled type of emotional involvement with the patient is allowed to establish and maintain rapport. Implicit in this is the value judgment that rapport is good or positive and to be valued.

Rapport is described in a number of ways here. It is a process in the way people perceive and relate to each other. It is an entity with empathy, compassion, and sympathy as components. It is also an outcome, being the ability to communicate creatively and intelligently to others. To establish rapport, certain ingredients are essential. A patient has to feel a sense of trust in the nurse. The nurse's needs should have been met in the past to be able to give of herself, but a bit of previous "suffering" would help nurses in understanding others. Stages of rapport development begin with empathy, then sympathy (equated in 1964 with caring), and then rapport.

Travelbee's major concepts that later evolved into her theory were introduced in this article.

CHAPTER 21

Metatheory and Theory Bibliography

The purpose of this chapter is to provide the reader with a comprehensive bibliography related to nursing theory and theorizing in nursing. The chapter is divided into 53 sections. Sections 1 through 12 include literature related to metatheory and theorizing in nursing. Sections 13 through 37 include nursing theories organized alphabetically by theorist. Sections 38 through 48 include major paradigms that have influenced nursing or have been used in nursing. Sections 49 through 53 include videotapes and audiotapes on theory. More specifically, the sections are:

THEORY AND THEORIZING IN NURSING

NURSING THEORY AND THEORISTS

There are several points to remember when using the bibliography.

1. Citations preceded by *asterisks* refer to works that have been abstracted in Chapter 18, Section I. Citations preceded by *daggers* refer to works that have been abstracted in Chapter 18, Section II.
2. Most of the abstracts in Chapter 18 are expansions of citations in Chapter 19, Sections 3, 6, 7, 8, 10, and 11. The emphasis was on providing a comprehensive view of literature cited in Sections 3 and 11.

3. There are many ways to use the bibliography, such as systematically reading within a section, reading within chronological themes, selecting readings according to years or decades of publication, and reading sections in conjunction with appropriate book chapters.

Theory and Theorizing in Nursing

1. Philosophy and Methods

Barber, B. and Hirsch, W. (Eds.). (1962). *The sociology of science.* New York: Free Press of Glencoe.

Benner, P. (2000). Links between philosophy, theory, practice, and research. *Canadian Journal of Nursing Research*, 32(2), 7–13.

Bennis, W.G., Benne, K.D., and Chin, R. (1976). *The planning of change* (3rd ed.). New York: Holt, Rinehart & Winston.

Blake, R.M., Ducasse, C.J., and Madden, E.H. (1960). *Theories of scientific method: The Renaissance through the nineteenth century.* Seattle, WA: University of Washington Press.

Blalock, H.M. (1969). *Theory construction.* Englewood Cliffs, NJ: Prentice-Hall.

Blumer, H. (1954). What is wrong with social theory? *American Sociological Review*, 19(1), 3–10.

Boykin, A., Parker, M.E., and Schoenhofer, S.O. (1994). Aesthetic knowing grounded in an explicit conception of nursing. *Nursing Science Quarterly*, 7, 158–161.

Brodbeck, M. (1956). The philosophy of science and educational research. *Review of Educational Research*, 26(5), 427–441.

Brodbeck, M. (1959). Models, meanings, and theories. In L. Gross (Ed.), *Symposium on sociological theory* (pp. 373–403). Evanston, IL: Row, Peterson & Co.

Brody, J.K. (1988). Virtue ethics, caring, and nursing. *Scholarly Inquiry for Nursing Practice,* 2(2), 87–96.

Bruner, R.S. (1966). The social construction of social theory In R.S. Rudner (Ed.), *Philosophy of social science.* Englewood Cliffs, NJ: Prentice-Hall.

*Burgess, G. (1978). The personal development of the nursing student as a conceptual framework. *Nursing Forum*, 17(1) 96–102.

Campbell, N. (1953). The structure of theories. In H. Feigl and M. Brodbeck (Eds.), *Readings in the philosophy of science* (pp. 288–308). New York: Appleton-Century-Crofts.

Carnap, R. (1966). *An introduction to the philosophy of science.* New York: Basic Books.

Chafetz, J.S. (1978). *A primer on the construction and testing of theories in sociology.* Itasca, IL: F.E. Peacock Publisher.

*Chapman, C.M. (1976). The use of sociological theories and models in nursing. *Journal of Advanced Nursing*, 1, 111–127.

Clarke, D.J. and Holt, J. (2001). Philosophy: A key to open the door to critical thinking. *Nurse Education Today*, 21(1), 71–78.

Cohen, M.R. and Nagel, E. (1962). *An introduction to logic and the scientific method* (Rev. ed.). New York: Harcourt Brace Jovanovich.

Copi, I.M. (1972). *Introduction to logic* (4th ed.). New York: Macmillan. (Note especially: Chapter 3, "Informal Fallacies," and Chapter 6, "Categorical Syllogisms.")

Copleston, F. (1963). *A history of philosophy: Vol. 8. Modern philosophy: Bentham to Russel, Part II, Idealism in America. The Pragmatic movement, the revolt against idealism.* Garden City, NJ: Image Books.

Costner, H. (1969). Theory, deduction, and rules of correspondence. *American Journal of Sociology,* 75, 245–263.

Costner, H. and Leik, R.K. (1964). Deductions from axiomatic theory. *American Sociological Review,* 29, 819–835.

Darbyshire, P., Diekelmann, J., and Diekelmann. N. (1999). Reading Heidegger and interpretive phenomenology: A response to the work of Michael Crotty. *Nursing Inquiry,* 6(1), 17–25.

Davis, K. and Glass, N. (1999). Contemporary theories and contemporary nursing—Advancing nursing care for those who are marginalized. *Contemporary Nurse,* 8(2), 32–38.

Denisoff, R.S., Callahan, O., and Levine, M.H. (1974). *Theories and paradigms in contemporary sociology.* Itasca, IL: F.E. Peacock Publisher.

deRaeve, L. and Wainwright, P. (2001). Conference report. Philosophy of nursing: Theory and evidence, Swansea, 18–20 September 2000. *Nursing Philosophy,* 21(1), 95–97.

Dewey, J. (1958). *Experience and nature* (Rev. ed.). New York: Dover Publications.

Dewey, J. (1964). *Reconstruction in philosophy* (Rev. ed.). Boston: Beacon Press.

Dewey, J. (1980). *The quest for certainty* (Rev. ed.). New York: Perigee Books.

DiBartolo, M.C. (1998). Philosophy of science in doctoral nursing education revisited. *Journal of Professional Nursing,* 14(6), 350–360.

Dubin, R. (1978). *Theory building.* New York: Free Press.

Durbin, P.R. (1968). *Philosophy of science: An introduction.* New York: McGraw-Hill.

Edwards, S. (1997). Philosophy in nursing. *Nursing Times,* 93(51), 48–49.

*Ellis, R. (1968). Characteristics of significant theories. *Nursing Research,* 17(3), 217–222.

Fry, S.T. (1999). The philosophy of nursing. *Scholarly Inquiry in Nursing Practice,* 13(1), 5–15.

Gadow, S. (1988). Covenant without cure: Letting go and holding on in chronic illness. In J. Watson and M. Ray (Eds.), *The ethics of care and the ethics of cure. Synthesis in chronicity* (pp. 5–14). New York: National League for Nursing.

Gastaldo, D. and Holmes, D. (1999). Foucault and nursing: A history of the present. *Nursing Inquiry,* 6(4), 231–240.

Gibbs, J. (1972). *Sociological theory construction.* Hinsdale, IL: Dryden Press.

Gibson, Q. (1960). *The logic of social inquiry.* New York: Humanities Press.

Goode, W.J. and Hatt, P.K. (1952). *Methods in social research.* New York: McGraw-Hill. (Note especially: Chapter 5, pp. 41–55, "Basic Elements of the Scientific Method: Concepts.")

Gouldner, A.W. (1961). Theoretical requirements of the applied social sciences. In H.J. Bennis, K.D. Benne, and R. Chin (Eds.), *The planning of change* (2nd ed.). New York: Holt, Rinehart & Winston.

Grinker, R.R. (Ed.). (1967). *Toward a unified theory of human behavior: An introduction to general systems theory* (2nd ed.). New York: Basic Books.

Habermas, J. (1984). *The theory of communicative action: Vol. 1. Reason and the rationalization of society.* London: Heinmann.

Hage, J. (1972). *Techniques and problem of theory construction in sociology.* New York: John Wiley & Sons.

Hall, J. M. (1990). Towards a psychology of caring. *British Journal of Clinical Psychology,* 29, 129–143.

Hardy, M.E. (1974). Theories: Components, development, evaluation. *Nursing Research,* 23(2), 100–107.

Harris, S. (1977). What's so funny about science? (Rev. ed.). Los Altos, CA: William Kaufmann.

Hempel, C.G. (1952). *Fundamentals of concept formation in empirical science.* Chicago: University of Chicago Press.

Hempel, C.G. (1965). *Aspects of scientific exploration and other essays in the philosophy of science.* New York: Free Press.

Heslop, L. (1997). The (im)possibilities of poststructuralist and critical social nursing inquiry. *Nursing Inquiry,* 4(1), 48–56.

Holmes, C.A. and Warelow, P.J. (2000). Some implications of postmodernism for nursing theory, research, and practice. *Canadian Journal of Nursing Research,* 32(2), 89–101.

Husserl, E. (1962). *Ideas: General introduction to pure phenomenology* (Rev. ed.). (Trans. W.R. Boyce Gibson). New York: Collier Books.

Inkeles, A. (1964). *What is sociology?* Englewood Cliffs, NJ: Prentice-Hall. (Note especially: "Models of Society in Sociological Analysis," pp. 28–67.)

Johnson, J.L. (1991). Nursing science: Basic, applied, or practical? Implications for the art of nursing. *Advances in Nursing Science,* 14(1), 7–16.

Johnson, J.L. (1994). A dialectical examination of nursing art. *Advances in Nursing Science,* 17(1), 1–14.

Kaplan, A. (1964). *The conduct of inquiry: Methodology for behavioral science.* San Francisco: Chandler.

*Kramer, S. (1969). Behavioral science and human biology in medicine. *The New Physician,* 18(11), 965–978.

Kuhn, T.S. (1970). The structure of scientific revolutions. In Neurath O. (Ed.), *International encyclopedia of unified science* (2nd ed., Vol. 2). Chicago: University of Chicago Press.

Kuhn, T.S. (1977). *The essential tension: Selected studies in scientific tradition and change.* Chicago: University of Chicago Press.

Lachman, R. (1963). The model in theory construction. In Melvin H. Marx (Ed.), *Theories in contemporary psychology.* New York: Macmillan.

Laudan, L. (1977). *Progress and its problems: Toward a theory of scientific growth.* Berkeley, CA: University of California Press.

Lemaire, G., Macleod, R., Mulkay, M., and Weingart, P. (Eds.). (1976). *Perspectives on the emergence of scientific disciplines.* Chicago: Aldine.

Lister, P. (1997). The art of nursing in a "postmodern" context. *Journal of Advanced Nursing,* 25(1), 38–44.

Losee, J. (1980). *A historical introduction to the philosophy of science* (2nd ed.). Oxford, England: Oxford University Press.

MacKinnon, C.A. (1982). Feminism, Marxism, method, and the state: An agenda for theory. *Signs: Journal of Women in Culture and Society,* 7, 515–544.

Maris, R. (1970). The logical adequacy of Homan's social theory. *American Sociological Review,* 35, 1069–1081.

Marx, M.H. (1963). *Theories in contemporary psychology.* New York: Macmillan. (Note especially "The General Nature of Theory Construction," pp. 4–46.)

McCall, R.J. (1963). *Basic logic: The fundamental principles of formal deductive reasoning* (2nd ed.). New York: Barnes & Noble.

*McKay, R. (1969). Theories, models and systems for nursing. *Nursing Research,* 18(5), 393–399.

Merton, R.K. (1973). *The sociology of science: Theoretical and empirical investigations* (edited with an introduction by N.W. Storer). Chicago: University of Chicago Press.

Merton, R.K. (1977). *The sociology of science: An episodic memoir.* Carbondale, IL: Southern Illinois University Press.

Miller, E.F. (1980). Epistemology and political inquiry: Comment on Kress' "Against epistemology." *Journal of Politics,* 42, 1160–1167.

Monti, E.J. and Tingen, M.S. (1999). Multiple paradigms of nursing science. *Advances in Nursing Science,* 21(4), 64–80.

Morgan, G. (1982). Cybernetics and organizational theory: Epistemology or technique? *Human Relations,* 35, 521–538.

Mulholland, J. (1997). Assimilating sociology: Critical reflections on the "sociology in nursing" debate. *Journal of Advanced Nursing,* 25(4), 844–852.

Murphy, J.F. (Ed.). (1971). *Theoretical issues in professional nursing.* New York: Appleton-Century-Crofts. (Note especially Chapters 1, 2, and 3.)

Nolan, P.W., Brown, B. and Crawford, P. (1998). Fruits without labour: The implications of Friedrich Nietzsche's ideas for the caring professions. *Journal of Advanced Nursing,* 28(2), 251–259.

Northrup, F.S.C. (1965). *The logic of the sciences and the humanities* (Rev. ed.). New York: The World Publishing Co.

Paley, J. (1998). Misinterpretive phenomenology: Heidegger, ontology and nursing research. *Journal of Advanced Nursing,* 27(4), 817–824.

Parsons, C. (1995). The impact of postmodernism on research methodology: Implications for nursing. *Nursing Inquiry,* 2(1), 22–28.

Paul, R.W. and Heaslip, P. (1995). Critical thinking involving nursing practice. *Journal of Advanced Nursing,* 22, 40–47.

*Payne, G. (1973). Comparative sociology: Some problems of theory and method. *British Journal of Sociology,* 24(1), 13–29.

*Peterson, C.J. (1977). Questions frequently asked about the development of a conceptual framework. *Journal of Nursing Education,* 16(4), 22–32.

Pierson, W. (1999). Considering the nature of intersubjectivity within professional nursing. *Journal of Advanced Nursing,* 30(2), 294–302.

Polanyi, M. (1962). *Personal knowledge.* New York: Harper & Row.

Popper, K.R. (1959). *The logic of scientific discovery.* New York: Basic Books.

Popper, K.R. (1971). *The open society and its enemies: The spell of Plato* (Rev. ed.). Princeton, NJ: Princeton University Press.

Popper, K. (1976). *Unended quest: An intellectual autobiography.* La Salle, IL: Open Court.

Reed, P.G. (1995). A treatise on nursing knowledge development for the 21st century: Beyond postmodernism. *Advances in Nursing Science,* 17(3), 70–84.

Reynolds, P.D. (1971). *A primer in theory construction.* New York: Bobbs-Merrill.

Rolfe, G. (1999). The pleasure of the bottomless: Postmodernism, chaos and paradigm shifts . . . Reconstructing nursing: Evidence, artistry and the curriculum. *Nurse Education Today,* 19(8), 668–672.

Roy, C.L. (1995). Developing nursing knowledge: Practice issues raised from four philosophical perspectives. *Nursing Science Quarterly,* 8(2), 79–85.

Rudner, R.S. (1966). *Philosophy of social science.* Englewood Cliffs, NJ: Prentice-Hall. (Note especially: "The Construction of Social Theory.")

Russell, B. (1965). *On the philosophy of science.* New York Bobbs-Merrill.

Rutty, J.E. (1998). The nature of philosophy of science, theory and knowledge relating to nursing and professionalism. *Journal of Advanced Nursing,* 28(2), 243–250.

Sahakian, W.S. (1968). *History of philosophy from the earliest times to the present.* New York: Barnes & Noble.

Sarter, B. (1988). Philosophical sources of nursing theory. *Nursing Science Quarterly,* 1(2), 52–59.

Schoenhofer, S.O. (2002). Theoretical concerns. Philosophical underpinnings of an emergent methodology for nursing as caring inquiry. *Nursing Science Quarterly,* 15(4), 275–280.

Schultz, P.R. and Meleis, A.I. (1988). Nursing epistemology: Traditions, insights, questions. *Image: Journal of Nursing Scholarship,* 20(4), 217–221.

Sheridan, A. (1980). *Michel Foucault: The will to truth.* New York: Tavistock.

Shils, E. (Ed.) (1968). *Criteria for scientific development, public policy, and national goals.* Cambridge, MA: MIT Press.

Sidorsky, D. (Ed.) (1977). *John Dewey: The essential writings.* New York: Harper Torch-books.

Simon, H.A. and Newell, A. (1963). The uses and limitations of models. In M.H. Marx (Ed.), *Theories in contemporary psychology* (pp. 89–104). New York: Macmillan.

*Silva, M.C. (1977). Philosophy, science, theory: Interrelationships and implications for nursing research. *Image: Journal of Nursing Scholarship,* 9(3), 59–63.

Silva, M.C. and Rothbart, D. (1984). An analysis of changing trends in philosophies of science on nursing theory development and testing. *Advances in Nursing Science,* 6(2), 1–13.

Silva, M.C., Sorrell, J.M., and Sorrell, C.D. (1995). From Carper's patterns of knowing to ways of being: An ontological philosophical shift in nursing. *Advances in Nursing Science,* 18(1), 1–13.

Sorrell, J.M. (1994). Remembrance of things past through writing: Esthetic patterns of knowing in nursing. *Advances in Nursing Science,* 17(1), 60–70.

Stacy, J. and Thorne, B. (1985). The feminist revolution in sociology. *Social Problems,* 32(4), 301–315.

Stein, K.F., Corte, C., Colling, K.B., and Whall, A. (1998). A theoretical analysis of Carper's ways of knowing using a model of social cognition. *Scholarly Inquiry in Nursing Practice,* 12(1), 43–60.

Stevenson, J.S. and Woods, N.F. (1986). Nursing science and contemporary science: Emerging paradigms. In G.E. Sorensen (Ed.), *Setting the agenda for the year 2000: Knowledge development in nursing* (Publication No. G-a170, 3M, 5/86). Kansas City, MO: American Nurses Association.

Stinchcombe, A.L. (1968). *Constructing social theories.* New York: Harcourt Brace Jovanovich.

Suppe, F. and Jacox, A.K. (1989). Philosophy of science and the development of nursing theory. *Annual Review of Nursing Research*, 3, 241–267.

Torres, G. and Yura, H. (1974). *Today's conceptual framework: Its relationship to the curriculum development process* (Publication No. 15–1529). New York: National League for Nursing.

Toulmin, S. (1977). *Human understanding: The collective use and evolution of concepts.* Princeton, NJ: Princeton University Press.

Toulmin, S. (1981). The tyranny of principles. *Hastings Center Report*, 11, 31–39.

Traynor, M. (1997). Postmodern research: No grounding or privilege, just free-floating trouble making. *Nursing Inquiry*, 4(2), 99–107.

Van Laer, P.H. (1956). *Philosophy of science: Part One—Science in general.* Pittsburgh, PA: Duquesne University Press.

Van Laer, P.H. (1962). *Philosophy of science: Part Two—A study of the division and nature of various groups of sciences.* Pittsburgh, PA: Duquesne University Press.

Wainwright, S.P. (1997). A new paradigm for nursing: The potential of realism. *Journal of Advanced Nursing*, 26(6), 1262–1271.

Wallace, W. (1971). Theories: Logical deduction, hypothesis, interpretation, instrumentation, scaling, and sampling. In *The logic of science in sociology* (pp. 63–74). New York: Aldine Atherton.

Warms, CA. and Schroeder, C.A. (1999). Bridging the gulf between science and action: The "new fuzzies" of neopragmatism. *Advances in Nursing Science*, 22(2), 1–10.

Watson, J. (1995). Postmodernism and knowledge development in nursing. *Nursing Science Quarterly*, 8, 60–64.

Weaver, W. (1970). *Science of change: A lifetime in American science.* New York: Charles Scribner's Sons.

White, J. (1995). Patterns of knowing: Review, critique, and update. *Advances in Nursing Science*, 17(4), 73–86.

Wolfer, J. (1993). Aspects of "reality" and ways of knowing in nursing: In search of an integrating paradigm. *Image: Journal of Nursing Scholarship*, 25, 141–146.

Wolman, B.B. and Nagel, E. (Eds.). (1965). *Scientific psychology: Principles and approaches.* New York: Basic Books.

2. Nursing Theory: General

Algase, D.L. and Whall, A.F. (1993). Rosemary Ellis' views on the substantive structure of nursing. *Image: Journal of Nursing Scholarship*, 25, 69–72.

Barnum, B.J.S. (1994). *Nursing theory: Analysis, application and evaluation* (4th ed.). Philadelphia: J.B. Lippincott.

Beckerman, A. (1994). A personal journal of caring through esthetic knowing. *Advances in Nursing Science*, 17(1), 71–79.

Beeber, L.S. and Schmitt, M.H. (1986). Cohesiveness in groups: A concept in search of a definition. *Advances in Nursing Science*, 8, 1–11.

Benner, P. (1984). *From novice to expert: Excellence and power in clinical nursing practice.* Menlo Park, CA: Addison-Wesley.

Benner, P. (Ed.). (1994). *Interpretive phenomenology: Embodiment, caring, and ethics in health and illness.* Thousand Oaks, CA: Sage.

Benner, P. and Wrubel, J. (1989). *The primacy of caring.* Menlo Park, CA: Addison-Wesley.

Bjork, I.T. (1995). Neglected conflicts in the discipline of nursing: Perceptions of the importance and value of practical skill. *Journal of Advanced Nursing*, 22, 6–12.

Booth, K., Kenrick, M., and Woods, S. (1997). Nursing knowledge, theory and method revisited. *Journal of Advanced Nursing*, 26(4), 804–811.

Bottorff, J.L. (1991). Nursing: A practical science of caring. *Nursing Science*, 14(1), 26–39.

Cash. K. (1997). Social epistemology, gender and nursing theory. *International Journal of Nursing Studies*, 34(2), 137–143.

Chinn, P.L. (1983). *Advances in nursing theory development.* Rockville, MD: Aspen Systems.

Chinn, P.L. (Ed.). (1986). *Nursing research methodology issues and implementation.* Rockville, MD: Aspen Systems.

Chinn, P.L. (1994). *Developing substance: Mid-range theory in nursing* [Preface]. Gaithersburg, MD: Aspen Systems

Chinn, P.L. and Jacobs, M. (1987). *Theory and nursing: A systematic approach* (2nd ed.). St. Louis, MO: C.V. Mosby.

Chinn, P.L. and Kramer, M.K. (1991). *Theory and nursing: A systematic approach* (3rd ed.) St. Louis, MO: C.V. Mosby.

Clift, J. and Barrett, E. (1998). Testing nursing theory cross-culturally. *International Nursing Review*, 45(4), 123–126.

Cull-Wilby, B.L. and Pepin, J.I. (1987). Towards a coexistence of paradigms in nursing knowledge development. *Journal of Advanced Nursing*, 12(4), 515–521.

Dean, J.M. and Mountford, B. (1998). Innovation in the assessment of nursing theory and its evaluation: A team approach. *Journal of Advanced Nursing*, 28(2), 409–418.

Dudley-Brown, S.L. (1997). The evaluation of nursing theory: A method for our madness. *International Journal of Nursing Studies*, 34(1), 76–83.

Edwards, S.D. (1998). The art of nursing. *Nursing Ethics*, 5(5), 393–400.

Engebretson, J. (1997). A multiparadigm approach to nursing. *Advanced Nursing Science*, 20(1), 21–33.

Fawcett, J. (1993). *Analysis and evaluation of nursing theories.* Philadelphia: F.A. Davis.

Fawcett, J. (1995). *Analysis and evaluation of conceptual models of nursing* (3rd ed.). Philadelphia: F.A. Davis.

Fawcett. J. (1995). Notes on book review of analysis and evaluation of nursing theories. *Nursing Science Quarterly*, 8, 58–59.

Fawcett, J., Watson, J., Neuman, B., Walker, P.H., and Fitzpatrick, J.J. (2001). On nursing theories and evidence. *Image: Journal of Nursing Scholarship,* 33(2), 115–119.

Fitzpatrick, J. and Whall, A. (1989). *Conceptual models of nursing: Analysis and application* (2nd ed.). East Norwalk, CT: Appleton & Lange.

Fitzpatrick, J., Whall, A., Johnston, R., and Floyd, J. (1982). *Nursing models and their psychiatric mental health applications.* Bowie, MD: Robert J. Brady Co.

Funk, S.G., Tornquist, E.M., Champage, M.T., Copp, L.A., and Wiese, R.A. (Eds.). (1990). *Key aspects of recovery: Improving nutrition, rest, and mobility.* New York: Springer.

Gastaldo, D. and Holmes, D. (1999). Foucault and nursing: A history of the present. *Nursing Inquiry,* 6(4), 231–240.

Gebbie, K. (Ed.). (1976, March 4–7). *Summary of the second national conference: Classification of nursing diagnosis.* 1310 South Boulevard, St. Louis, MO 63104.

Gioiella, E.C. (1996). The importance of theory guided research and practice in the changing health care science. *Nursing Science Quarterly,* 9(2), 47.

Hagerty, B.M., Lynch-Sauer, J., Patusky, K.L., and Bouwsema, M. (1993). An emerging theory of human relatedness. *Image: Journal of Nursing Scholarship,* 25(4), 291–296.

Harden, J. (2000). Language, discourse and the chronotope: Applying literary theory to the narratives in health care. *Journal of Advanced Nursing,* 31(3), 506–512.

Hilton, P.A. (1997). Theoretical perspectives of nursing: A review of the literature. *Journal of Advanced Nursing,* 26(6), 1211–1220.

Holmes, C.A. and Warelow, P.J. (1997). Culture, needs and nursing: A critical theory approach. *Journal of Advanced Nursing,* 25(3), 463–470.

Holmes, C.A. and Warelow, P.J. (2000). Some implications of postmodernism for nursing theory, research, and practice. *Canadian Journal of Nursing Research,* 32(2), 89–101.

Im, E.O. and Meleis, A.I. (1999). A situation-specific theory of Korean immigrant women's menopausal transition. *Image: Journal of Nursing Scholarship,* 31(4), 333–338.

Im, E.O. and Meleis, A.I. (1999). Situation-specific theories: Philosophical roots, properties, and approach. *Advances in Nursing Science,* 22(2), 11–24.

Johnson, J. (1994). A dialectical examination of nursing art. *Advances in Nursing Science,* 17(1), 1–14.

Kahn, S. and Fawcett, J. (1995). Continuing the dialogue: A response to Draper's critique of Fawcett's 'Conceptual models and nursing practice: The reciprocal relationship.' *Journal of Advanced Nursing,* 22, 188–192.

Ketefian, S. and Redman, R.W. (1997). Nursing science in the global community. *Image: Journal of Nursing Scholarship,* 29(1), 11–15.

Kim, H.S. (1983). *The nature of theoretical thinking in nursing.* Norwalk, CT: Appleton-Century-Crofts.

Kim, H.S. (1994). Practice theories in nursing and a science of nursing practice. *Scholarly Inquiry for Nursing Practice,* 8, 145–166.

Kolcaba, K.Y. and Kolcaba, R. (1991). An analysis of the concept of comfort. *Journal of Advanced Nursing,* 16, 1301–1310.

Laurent, C.L. (2000). A nursing theory for nursing leadership. *Journal of Nursing Management,* 8(2), 83–87.

Lauver, D. (1992). A theory of care-seeking behavior. *Image: Journal of Nursing Scholarship,* 24, 281–287.

Lenz, E.R., Suppe, F., Gift, A.G., Pugh L.C., and Milligan, R.A. (1995). Collaborative development of middle-range nursing theories: Toward a theory of unpleasant symptoms. *Advances in Nursing Science*, 17(3), 1–13.

Liaschenko, J. and Fisher, A. (1999). Theorizing the knowledge that nurses use in the conduct of their work. *Scholarly Inquiry for Nursing Practice*, 13(1), 29–41.

Liehr, P. and Smith, M.J. (1999). Middle range theory: Spinning research and practice to create knowledge for the new millennium. *Advances in Nursing Science*, 21(4), 81–91.

Lundh, U., Soder, M., and Waerness, K. (1988). Nursing theories: A critical view. *Image: Journal of Nursing Scholarship*, 20, 36–40.

Maeve, M. K. (1994). The carrier bag theory of nursing practice. *Advances in Nursing Science*, 16, 9–22.

Manias, E. and Street, A. (2000). Possibilities for critical social theory and Foucault's work: A toolbox approach. *Nursing Inquiry*, 7(1), 50–60.

Marck, P. (1990). Therapeutic reciprocity: A caring phenomenon. *Advances in Nursing Science*, 13(1), 49–59.

Marriner-Tomey, A. (1989). *Nursing theorists and their work* (2nd ed.). St. Louis, MO: C.V. Mosby.

McCance, T.V. (1999). Caring: Theoretical perspectives of relevance to nursing. *Journal of Advanced Nursing*, 30(6), 1388–1395.

Meleis, A.I. (1992). Directions for nursing theory development in the 21st century. *Nursing Science Quarterly*, 5(3), 112–117.

Meleis, A.I. (1996). Theory development: A blueprint for the 21st century. In P. Hinton Walker and B. Neuman (Eds.), *Blueprint for use of nursing models*. New York: National League for Nursing.

Mischel, M.H. (1990). Reconceptualizing of the uncertainty in illness theory. *Image: Journal of Nursing Scholarship*, 22, 256–262.

Monti, E.J. and Tingen, M.S. (1999). Multiple paradigms of nursing science. *Advances in Nursing Science*, 21(4), 64–80.

Morse, J.M., Anderson, G., Bottorff, J.L., Yonger, O., O'Brien, B., Solberg, S.M., and Hunter Mcllveen, K. (1992). Exploring empathy: A conceptual fit for nursing practice? *Image: Journal of Nursing Scholarship*, 24, 273–280.

Morse, J.M., Bottorff, J., Neander, W., and Solberg, S. (1991). Comparative analysis of conceptualizations and theories of caring. *Image: Journal of Nursing Scholarship*, 23, 119–126.

Morse, J.M., Miles, M.W., Clark, D.A., and Doberneck, B.M. (1994). "Sensing" patient needs: Exploring concepts of nursing insight and receptivity used in nursing assessment. *Scholarly Inquiry for Nursing Practice*, 8, 233–254.

Morse, J.M., Solberg, S.M., Neander, W.L., Bottorff, J.L., Johnson, J.L. (1990). Concepts of caring and caring as a concept. *Advances in Nursing Science*, 13(1), 1–14.

Newman, M. (1979). *Theory development in nursing*. Philadelphia: F.A. Davis.

Nicoll, L.H. (Ed.). (1992). *Perspectives on nursing theory* (2nd ed.). Philadelphia: J.B. Lippincott.

Nolan, M., Lundh, U. and Tishelman, C. (1998). Nursing's knowledge base: Does it have to be unique? *British Journal of Nursing*, 7(5), 270–276.

Norris, C. (Ed.). (1969). *Proceedings: Second Nursing Theory Conference.* University of Kansas Medical Center, Department of Nursing Education, October 9–10, 1969.

Nursing Development Conference Group. (1977). *Concept formalization in nursing: Process and product.* Boston: Little, Brown.

Nursing's metaparadigm concepts: Disimpacting the debates. (1998). *Journal of Advanced Nursing,* 27(6), 1257–1268.

Oberst, M. T. (1995). To what end theory? *Research in Nursing & Health,* 18, 83–84.

Parse, R.R. (1987). *Nursing science: Major paradigms, theories, and critiques.* Philadelphia: W.B. Saunders.

Parse, R.R. (1995). Nursing theories and frameworks: The essence of advanced practice nursing. *Nursing Science Quarterly,* 8, 1.

Reed, P.G. (1997). Nursing: The ontology of the discipline. *Nursing Science Quarterly,* 10(2), 76–79.

Riehl-Sisca, J.P. (1989). *Conceptual models for nursing practice* (3rd ed.). East Norwalk, CT: Appleton & Lange.

Rutty, J.E. (1998). The nature of philosophy of science, theory and knowledge relating to nursing and professionalism. *Journal of Advanced Nursing,* 28(2), 243–250.

Sarvimki A. and Stenbock-Hult, B. (1992). *Caring: An introduction to health care from a humanistic perspective.* Helsinki, Finland: Foundation for Nursing Education.

Severinsson, E.I. (1998). Bridging the gap between theory and practice: A supervision programme for nursing students. *Journal of Advanced Nursing,* 27(6), 1269–1277.

Silva, M.C. (1987). Conceptual models of nursing. *Annual Review of Nursing Research,* 5, 229–246.

Simpson. J. (1998). The perplexities of conceptual frameworks. *Canadian Nurse,* 94(10), 51.

Taylor, J.S. (1997). Nursing ideology: Identification and legitimation. *Journal of Advanced Nursing,* 25(3), 442–446.

Thompson, C. (1999). A conceptual treadmill: The need for "middle ground" in clinical decision making theory in nursing. *Journal of Advanced Nursing,* 30(5), 1222–1229.

Thorne, S.E., Kirkham, S.R., and Henderson, A. (1999). Ideological implications of paradigm discourse. *Nursing Inquiry,* 6(2), 123–131.

Tierney, A.J. (1998). Nursing models: Extant or extinct? *Journal of Advanced Nursing,* 28(1), 77–85.

Timpson, J. (1996). Nursing theory: Everything the artist spits is art? *Journal of Advanced Nursing,* 23, 1030–1036.

Torres, G. (1986). *Theoretical foundations of nursing.* Norwalk, CT: Appleton-Century-Crofts.

University of California, San Francisco, School of Nursing Symptom Management Faculty Group. (1994). A model for symptom management. *Image: Journal of Nursing Scholarship,* 26, 272–276.

Vicenzi, A.E. (1994). Chaos theory and some nursing considerations. *Nursing Science Quarterly,* 7(1), 36–42.

Wainwright, P. (2000). Towards an aesthetics of nursing. *Journal of Advanced Nursing,* 32(3), 750–756.

Walker, L.O. and Avant, K.C. (1995). *Strategies for theory construction in nursing* (3rd ed.). East Norwalk, CT: Appleton & Lange.

Winstead-Fry, P. (1986). *Case studies in nursing theory*. New York: National League for Nursing.

Younger, J.B. (1991). A theory of mastery. *Advances in Nursing Science*, 14(1), 76–89.

Zbilut, J.P. and Staffileno, B. (1994). Chaos theory and nursing revisited. *Nursing Science Quarterly*, 7(4), 150–152.

3. Metatheory and Theory Development in Nursing

Algase, D.L. and Whall, A.F. (1993). Rosemary Ellis' views on the substantive structure of nursing. *Image: Journal of Nursing Scholarship*, 25, 69–72.

Allan, H. (1998). Issues in infertility nursing: Broadening the debate. *Nursing Standard*, 12(27), 39–41.

Allchin-Petardi, L. (1998). Weathering the storm: Persevering through a difficult time. *Nursing Science Quarterly*, 11(4), 172–177.

Allen, D.G. (1987). The social policy statement: A reappraisal. *Advances in Nursing Science*, 10(1), 39–48.

American Nurses Association. (1995). *Nursing's social policy statement* (Publication No. NP-107). Washington, DC: Author.

Andershed, B. and Ternestedt, B.M. (2001). Development of a theoretical framework describing relatives' involvement in palliative care. *Journal of Advanced Nursing*, 34(4), 554–562.

Anderson, R.A., Dobal, M.T., and Blessing, B. (1992). Theory-based approach to computer skill development in nursing administration. *Computers in Nursing*, 10(4), 152–157.

Avant, K.C. (1993). The Wilson method of concept analysis. In B.L. Rodgers and Knafl, K.A. (Eds.), *Concept development in nursing* (pp. 51–60). Philadelphia: W.B. Saunders.

Baker, C. (1999). From chaos to order: A nursing-based psycho-education program for parents of children with attention-deficit hyperactivity disorder. *Canadian Journal of Nursing Research*, 31(2), 71–75.

Banks-Wallace, J. (2000). Womanist ways of knowing: Theoretical considerations for research with African American women. *Advances in Nursing Science*, 22(3), 33–45.

Barker, P. (1998). The future of the theory of interpersonal relations? A personal reflection on Peplau's legacy. *Journal of Psychiatric and Mental Health Nursing*, 5(3), 213–220.

Barker. P.J., Reynolds, W., and Stevenson, C. (1997) The human science basis of psychiatric nursing: Theory and practice. *Journal of Advanced Nursing*, 5(4), 660–667.

Barnett, K. (1972). A theoretical construct of the concepts of touch as they relate to nursing. *Nursing Research*, 21(2), 102–110.

Barrett, E.A. and Caroselli, C. (1998) Methodological ponderings related to the power as knowing participation in change tool. *Nursing Science Quarterly*, 11(1), 17–22.

*Batey, M.V. (1977). Conceptualization: Knowledge and logic guiding empirical research. *Nursing Research*, 26(5), 324–329.

Baumann, S.L. (1997). Contrasting two approaches in a community-based nursing practice with older adults: The medical model and Parse's nursing theory. *Nursing Science Quarterly*, 10(3), 124–130.

*Becker, C.H. (1983). A conceptualization of concept. *Nursing Papers: Perspectives in Nursing*, 15(2), 51–58.

*Beckstrand, J. (1978). The notion of a practice theory and the relationship of scientific and ethical knowledge to practice. *Research in Nursing and Health*, 1(3), 131–136.

*Beckstrand, J. (1978). The need for a practice theory as indicated by the knowledge used in conduct of practice. *Research in Nursing and Health*, 1(4), 175–179.

*Beckstrand, J. (1980). A critique of several conceptions of practice theory in nursing. *Research in Nursing and Health*, 3(2), 69–80.

Bell, A., Horsfall, J., and Goodin, W. (1998) The Mental Health Nursing Clinical Confidence Scale: A tool for measuring undergraduate learning on mental health clinical placements. *Australian and New Zealand Journal of Mental Health Nursing*, 7(4), 184–190.

Bergenson, B.S. (1971). Adaptation as a unifying theory. In J.F. Murphy (Ed.), *Theoretical issues in professional nursing.* New York: Appleton-Century-Crofts.

*Berthold, J.S. (1968). Prologue: Symposium on theory development in nursing. *Nursing Research*, 17(3), 196–197.

Bibace, R. and Walsh, M.E. (1982). Conflict of roles: On the difficulties of being both scientist and practitioner in one life. *Professional Psychology*, 13, 389–395.

Blegen, M.A. and Tripp-Reimer, T. (1997). Implications of nursing taxonomies for middle-range theory development. *Advances in Nursing Science*, 19(3), 37–49.

Blix, A. (1999). Integrating occupational health protection and health promotion: Theory and program application. *Official Journal of the American Association of Occupational Health Nurses*, 47(4), 168–171.

Bohny, B.J. (1980). Theory development for a nursing science. *Nursing Forum*, 19(1), 50–67.

Botha, M.E. (1989). Theory development in perspective: The role of conceptual frameworks and models in theory development. *Journal of Advanced Nursing*, 14(1), 49–55.

Bournes, D.A. and DasGupta, T.L. (1997). Professional practice leader: A transformational role that addresses human diversity. *Nursing Administration Quarterly*, 21(4), 61–68.

Boutain. D.M. (1999). Critical nursing scholarship: Exploring critical social theory with African American studies. *Advances in Nursing Science*, 21(4), 37–47.

Bowers, R. and Moore, K.N. (1997). Bakhtin, nursing narratives, and dialogical consciousness. *Advances in Nursing Science*, 19(3), 70–77.

Boychuk Duchscher, J.E. (1999). Catching the wave: Understanding the concept of critical thinking. *Journal of Advanced Nursing*, 29(3), 577–583.

*Brown, M.I. (1964). Research on the development of nursing theory: The importance of a theoretical framework in nursing research. *Nursing Research*, 13(2), 109–112.

*Brown, M.I. (1968). Theory development in nursing: Social theory in geriatric nursing research. *Nursing Research*, 17(3), 213–217.

*Brown, M.L. (1983). Research questions and answers: The use of theory and conceptual frameworks in nursing research and practice. *Oncology Nursing Forum*, 10(2), 111–112.

Bunkers, S.S. (1998). Considering tomorrow: Parse's theory-guided research. *Nursing Science Quarterly*, 11(2), 56–63.

Burks, K.J. (2001). Intentional action. *Journal of Advanced Nursing*, 34(5), 668–675.

*Bush, H.A. (1979). Models for nursing. *Advances in Nursing Science*, 1(2), 13–21.

*Carper, B.A. (1978). Fundamental patterns of knowing in nursing. *Advances in Nursing Science*, 1(1), 13–23.

Carr, J.M. (1998). Vigilance as a caring expression and Leininger's theory of cultural care diversity and universality. *Nursing Science Quarterly*, 11(2), 74–78.

Carson, M.G. and Mitchell, G.J. (1998). The experience of living with persistent pain. *Journal of Advanced Nursing*, 28(6), 1242–1248.

Carter, P.A. (1998). Self-care agency: The concept and how it is measured. *Journal of Nursing Measurement*, 6(2), 195–207.

*Chapman, C.M. (1976). The use of sociological theories and models in nursing. *Journal of Advanced Nursing*, 1, 111–127.

*Chinn, P.L. and Jacobs, M.K. (1978). A model for theory development in nursing. *Advances in Nursing Science*, 1(1), 1–11.

*Clark, J. (1982). Development of models and theories on the concept of nursing. *Journal of Advanced Nursing*, 7(2), 129–134.

Cleary, F. (1971). A theoretical model: Its potential for adaptation to nursing. *Image: Journal of Nursing Scholarship*, 4(1), 14–20.

*Cleland, V.S. (1967). The use of existing theories. *Nursing Research*, 16(2), 118–121.

Clift, J. and Barrett, E. (1998). Testing nursing theory cross-culturally. *International Nursing Review*, 45(4), 123–126.

Cohen, S.S. and Milone-Nuzzo, P. (2001). Advancing health policy in nursing education through service learning. *Advances in Nursing Science*, 23(3), 28–40.

*Colaizzi, J. (1975). The proper object of nursing science. *International Journal of Nursing Studies*, 12(4), 197–200.

*Collins, R.J. and Fielder, J.H. (1981). Beckstrand's concept of practice theory: A critique. *Research in Nursing and Health*, 4(3), 317–321.

Conway, M.E. (1985). Toward greater specificity in defining nursing's metaparadigm. *Advances in Nursing Science*, 7(4), 73–81.

Cooley, M.E. (1999). Analysis and evaluation of the Trajectory Theory of Chronic Illness Management. *Scholarly Inquiry in Nursing Practice*, 13(2), 75–95.

Copnell, B. (1998). Synthesis in nursing knowledge: An analysis of two approaches. *Journal of Advanced Nursing*, 27(4), 870–874.

Cormack, D.F.S. and Reynolds, W. (1992). Criteria for evaluating the clinical and practical utility of models used by nurses. *Journal of Advanced Nursing*, 17, 1472–1478.

Cowley, S. and Billings, J.R. (1999). Resources revisited: Salutogenesis from a lay perspective. *Journal of Advanced Nursing*, 29(4), 994–1004.

Cowling, W.R., III. (2000). Healing as appreciating wholeness. *Advances in Nursing Science*, 22(3), 16–32.

*Crawford, G., Dufault, S.K., and Rudy, E. (1979). Evolving issues in theory development. *Nursing Outlook*, 27(5), 346–351.

Croom, S., Procter, S., and Couteur, A.L. (2000). Developing a concept analysis of control for use in child and adolescent mental health nursing. *Journal of Advanced Nursing*, 31(6), 1324–1332.

Crossan, F. and Robb, A. (1998). Role of the nurse: Introducing theories and concepts. *British Journal of Nursing*, 7(10), 608–612.

Crow, R. (1982). Frontiers of nursing in the 21st century: Development of models and theories on the concept of nursing. *Journal of Advanced Nursing*, 7, 111–116.

Cull-Wilby, B.L. and Pepin, J.I. (1987). Towards a coexistence of paradigms in nursing process. *Journal of Advanced Nursing*, 12, 515–521.

Deatrick, J.A., Knafl, K.A., and Murphy-Moore, C. (1999). Clarifying the concept of normalization. *Image: Journal of Nursing Scholarship*, 31(3), 209–214.

DeMong, N.C. and Assie-Lussier, L.L. (1999). Continuing education: An aspect of staff development relating to the nurse manager's role. *Journal of Nurses Staff Development*, 15(1), 19–22.

Derdiarian, A.K. (1979). Education: A way to theory construction in nursing. *Journal of Nursing Education*, 18(2), 36–47.

DeSantis, L. and Ugarriza, D.N. (2000). The concept of theme as used in qualitative nursing research. *Western Journal of Nursing Research*, 22(3), 351–372.

DiBartolo, M.C. (1998). Philosophy of science in doctoral nursing education revisited. *Journal of Professional Nursing*, 14(6), 350–360.

*Dickoff, J. and James, P. (1968). A theory of theories: A position paper. *Nursing Research*, 17(3), 197–203.

Dickoff, J. and James, P. (1971). Clarity to what end? *Nursing Research*, 20(6), 499–502.

*Dickoff, J., James, P., and Wiedenbach, E. (1968). Theory in practice discipline: Part I. Practice oriented theory. *Nursing Research*, 17(5), 415–435.

*Dickoff, J., James, P., and Wiedenbach, E. (1968). Theory in practice discipline: Part II. Practice oriented theory. *Nursing Research*, 17(6), 545–554.

Dierckx de Casterle, B., Roelens, A., and Gastmans, C. (1998). An adjusted version of Kohlberg's moral theory: Discussion of its validity for research in nursing ethics. *Journal of Advanced Nursing*, 27(4), 829–835.

Dluhy, N.M. (1995). Mapping knowledge in chronic illness. *Journal of Advanced Nursing*, 21, 1051–1058.

Dolan, K. (1997). Children in accident and emergency. *Accident and Emergency Nursing*, 5(2), 88–91.

*Donaldson, S.K. and Crowley, D. (1978). The discipline of nursing. *Nursing Outlook*, 26(2), 113–120.

Donnelly, G.F. (1986). Nursing theory: Evolution of a sacred cow. *Holistic Nursing Practice*, 1(1), 1–7.

Dubin, R. (1978). *Theory building*. New York: Free Press.

*Ellis, R. (1968). Characteristics of significant theories. *Nursing Research*, 17(3), 217–222. (See Section 2.)

Ellis, R. (1971). Commentary on Walker's "Toward a clearer understanding of the concept of nursing theory." *Nursing Research*, 20(6), 493–494.

Ellis, R. (1982). Conceptual issues in nursing. *Nursing Outlook*, 30(7), 406–410.

Emden, C. (1998). Conducting a narrative analysis. *Collegian*, 5(3), 34–39.

Engebretson, J. (1997). A multiparadigm approach to nursing. *Advances in Nursing Science*, 20(1), 21–33.

Fawcett, J. and Boubonniere, M. (2001). Utilization of nursing knowledge and the future of the discipline. In N.L. Chaska (Ed.), *The nursing profession—Tomorrow and beyond* (pp. 311–320). Thousand Oaks, CA: Sage.

Fealy, G.M. (1997). The theory-practice relationship in nursing: An exploration of contemporary discourse. *Journal of Advanced Nursing*, 25(5), 1061–1069.

Fernandez, E. (1997). Just 'doing the observations': Reflective practice in nursing. *British Journal of Nursing*, 6(16), 939–943.

Fisher, M.A. and Mitchell, G.J. (1998). Patients' views of quality of life: Transforming the knowledge base of nursing. Comment in: *Clinical Nurse Specialist*, (1998) 12(3), 98. *Clinical Nurse Specialist*, 12(3), 99–105.

Flaskerud, J.H. and Halloran, E.J. (1980). Areas of agreement in nursing theory development. *Advances in Nursing Science*, 3(1), 1–7.

Flaskerud, J.H. and Halloran, E.J. (1981). Areas of agreement in nursing theory development. *Advances in Nursing Science*, 3(3), 31–42.

Freshwater, D. (1998). From acorn to oak tree: A neoplatonic perspective of reflection and caring. *Australian Journal of Holistic Nursing*, 5(2), 14–19.

Fry, S.T. (1999). The philosophy of nursing. *Scholarly Inquiry in Nursing Practice*, 13(1), 5–15.

Gaberson, K.B. (1997) What's the answer? What's the question? *Journal of the Association of periOperative Registered Nurses*, 66(1), 148–151.

Gassner, L.A., Wotton, K., Clare, J., Hofmeyer, A., and Buckman, J. (1999). Evaluation of a model of collaboration: Academic and clinician partnership in the development and implementation of undergraduate teaching. *Collegian*, 6(3), 14–21.

Gastaldo, D. and Holmes. D. (1999). Foucault and nursing: A history of the present. *Nursing Inquiry*, 6(4), 231–240.

Geanellos, R. (1997). Nursing knowledge development: Where to from here? *Collegian*, 4(1), 13–21.

*Gebbie, K. and Lavin, M.A. (1974). Classifying nursing diagnoses. *American Journal of Nursing*, 74(2), 250–253.

Goode, W.J. and Hatt, P.K. (1952). Science: Theory and fact. In W.J. Goode and P.K. Hatt (Eds.), *Methods in social research* (pp. 7–17). New York: McGraw-Hill.

Gordon, N.S. (1998). Influencing mental health nursing practice through the teaching of research and theory: A personal critical review. *Journal of Psychiatric and Mental Health Nursing*, 5(2), 119–128.

Gormley, K.J. (1997). Practice write-ups: An assessment instrument that contributes to bridging the differences between theory and practice for student nurses through the development of core skills. *Nurse Education Today*, 17(1), 53–57.

*Gortner, S.R. (1983). The history and philosophy of nursing science and research. *Advances in Nursing Science*, 5(2), 1–8.

Gottlieb, L.N. and Gottlieb B. (1998). Evolutionary principles can guide nursing's future development. *Journal of Advanced Nursing*, 28(5), 1099–1105.

Gramling, L.F., Lambert, V.A., and Pursley-Crotteau, S. (1998), Coping in young women: Theoretical retroduction. *Journal of Advanced Nursing*, 28(5), 1082–1091.

Greenwood, J. (1998). Establishing an international network on nurses' clinical reasoning. *Journal of Advanced Nursing*, 27(4), 843–847.

Greenwood, J. (2000). Critical thinking and nursing scripts: The case for the development of both. *Journal of Advanced Nursing*, 31(2), 428–436.

Gulzar, L. (1999). Access to health care. *Image: Journal of Nursing Scholarship*, 31(1), 13–19.

Haas, B.K. (1999). Clarification and integration of similar quality of life concepts. *Image: Journal of Nursing Scholarship*, 31(3), 215–220.

Haase, J.E., Britt, T., Coward, D.D., Leidy, N.K., and Penn, P.E. (1992). Simultaneous concept analysis of spiritual perspective, hope, acceptance and self-transcendence. *Image: Journal of Nursing Scholarship*, 24, 141–147.

Hadley, B.J. (1969). Evolution of a conception of nursing. *Nursing Research*, 18(5), 400–405.

*Hall, B.A. (1981). The change paradigm in nursing: Growth versus persistence. *Advances in Nursing Science*, 3(4), 1–6.

Hall, J.M., Stevens, P.E., and Meleis, A.I. (1994). Marginalization: A guiding concept for valuing diversity in nursing knowledge development. *Advances in Nursing Science*, 16(4), 23–41.

Hardy, L.K. (1986). Janforum: Identifying the place of theoretical frameworks in an evolving discipline, the nursing profession. *Journal of Advanced Nursing*, 11(1), 103–107.

Hardy, M.E. (1974). The nature of theories. In M.E. Hardy (Ed.), *Theoretical foundations for nursing* (pp. 10–22). New York: MSS Information Corp.

*Hardy, M.E. (1978). Perspectives on nursing theory. *Advances in Nursing Science*, 1(1), 37–48.

Harris, I.M. (1971). Theory building in nursing: A review of the literature. *Image: Journal of Nursing Scholarship*, 4(1), 6–10.

Hart, M.A and Foster, S.N. (1998). Self-care agency in two groups of pregnant women. *Nursing Science Quarterly*, 11(4), 167–171.

Hawley, P., Young, S., and Pasco, A.C. (2000). Reductionism in the pursuit of nursing science: (In)congruent with nursing's core values? *Canadian Journal of Nursing Research*, 32(2), 75–88.

Henderson, D. (1997). Intersecting race and gender in feminist theories of women's psychological development. *Issues in Mental Health Nursing*, 18(5), 377–393.

Herbert, C.L. (1997). "To be or not to be"—An ethical debate on the not-for-resuscitation (NFR) status of a stroke patient. *Journal of Clinical Nursing*, 6(2), 99–105.

Herth, K. (1998). Hope as seen through the eyes of homeless children. *Journal of Advanced Nursing*, 28(5), 1053–1062.

Hinshaw, A.S. (1987). Response to "Structuring the nursing knowledge system: A typology of four domains." *Scholarly Inquiry for Nursing Practice*, 1(2), 11–114.

Hisama, K.K. (1999). Towards an international theory of nursing. *Nursing and Health Sciences*, 1(2), 77–81.

Holmes, C.A. and Warelow, P.J. (1997). Culture, needs and nursing: A critical theory approach. *Journal of Advanced Nursing*, 25(3), 463–470.

Holmes, C.A. and Warelow, P.J. (2000). Some implications of postmodernism for nursing theory, research, and practice. *Canadian Journal of Nursing Research*, 32(2), 89–101.

Hopkinson, J.B. (1999). A study of the perceptions of hospice day care patients: My phenomenological methodology. *International Journal of Nursing Studies*, 36(3), 203–207.

Horsburgh, M.E. (1999). Self-care of well adult Canadians and adult Canadians with end stage renal disease. *International Journal of Nursing Studies*, 36(6), 443–453.

Hurley, B.A. (1979). Why a theoretical framework in nursing research? *Western Journal of Nursing Research*, 1(1), 28–41.

Jaarsma, T., Halfens, R., Senten, M., Abu Saad, H.H., and Dracup, K. (1998). Developing a supportive-educative program for patients with advanced heart failure within Orem's general theory of nursing. *Nursing Science Quarterly*, 11(2), 79–85.

Jacobs-Kramer, M.K. and Chinn, P.L. (1988). Perspectives on knowing: A model of nursing knowledge. *Scholarly Inquiry for Nursing Practice*, 2(2), 129–139.

Jacobson, M. (1971). Qualitative data: As a potential source of theory in nursing. *Image: Journal of Nursing Scholarship*, 4(1), 10–14.

*Jacox, A. (1974). Theory construction in nursing: An overview. *Nursing Research*, 23(1), 4–13.

Janes, N.M. and Wells, D.L (1997). Elderly patients' experiences with nurses guided by Parse's theory of human becoming. *Clinical Nursing Research*, 6(3), 205–222.

Jennings, B.M. (1987). Nursing theory development: Successes and challenges. *Journal of Advanced Nursing*, 12(1), 63–69.

*Johnson, D.E. (1959). The nature of a science of nursing. *Nursing Outlook*, 7(5), 291–294.

*Johnson, D.E. (1968) Theory in nursing: Borrowed and unique. *Nursing Research*, 17(3), 206–209.

Johnson, D.E. (1974). Development of theory: A requisite for nursing as a primary health profession. *Nursing Research*, 23(5), 372–377.

*Johnson, D.E. (1978). Development of theory: A requisite for nursing as a primary health profession. In N. Chaska (Ed.), *The nursing profession: Views through the mist.* New York: McGraw-Hill.

Johnson, D.E., et al. (1978). *Theory development: What, why, how?* (Publication No. 15–1708). New York: National League for Nursing.

Jonas-Simpson, C. (1997). Living the art of the human becoming theory. *Nursing Science Quarterly*. 10(4), 175–179.

Kaplan, A. (1964). *The conduct of inquiry: Methodology for behavioral science.* San Francisco: Chandler.

Kelley, L.S. (1999). Evaluating change in quality of life from the perspective of the person: Advanced practice nursing and Parse's goal of nursing. *Holistic Nursing Practice*, 13(4), 61–70.

Ketefian, S. (1987). A case study of theory development: Moral behavior in nursing. *Advances in Nursing Science*, 9(2), 10–19.

Ketefian, S. and Redman, R.W. (1997). Nursing science in the global community. *Image Journal of Nursing Scholarship*, 29(1), 11–15.

Kidd, P. and Morrison, E.F. (1988). The progression of knowledge in nursing: A sear for meaning. *Image: Journal of Nursing Scholarship*, 20(4), 222–224.

Kim, H.S. (1987). Structuring the nursing knowledge system: A typology of four domains. *Scholarly Inquiry for Nursing Practice*, 1(2), 111–114.

Kim, H.S. (1999). Critical reflective inquiry for knowledge development in nursing practice. *Journal of Advanced Nursing*, 29(5), 1205–1212.

Kim, H.S. (2001). Directions for theory development in nursing. In N.L. Chaska (Ed.), *The nursing profession—Tomorrow and beyond* (pp. 272–285). Thousand Oaks, CA: Sage.

Kim, M.S., Shin, K.R., and Shin, S.R. (1998). Korean adolescents' experiences of smoking cessation: A prelude to research with the human becoming perspective. *Nursing Science Quarterly*, 11(3), 105–109.

King, I.M. (1964). Nursing theory: Problems and prospect. *Nursing Science*, 10, 394–403.

King, I.M. (1971). *Toward a theory for nursing.* New York: John Wiley & Sons.

King, I.M. (1978). The "why" of theory development. In J. G. Paterson (Ed.), *Theory development: What, why, how?* (Publication No. 15–1708, pp. 11–16) New York: National League for Nursing.

Kirkevold, M. (1997). Integrative nursing research—An important strategy to further the development of nursing science and nursing practice. *Journal of Advanced Nursing*, 25(5), 977–984.

Klein, J.F. (1978). Theory development in nursing. In N.L. Chaska (Ed.), *The nursing profession: Views through the mist.* New York: McGraw-Hill.

Knight, M.M. (2000). Cognitive ability and functional status. *Journal of Advanced Nursing*, 31(6), 1459–1468.

Kramer, M.K. (1993). Concept clarification and critical thinking: Integrated processes. *Journal of Nursing Education*, 32(9), 406–414.

Krawczyk, R.M. (1997). Teaching ethics: Effect on moral development. *Nursing Ethics*, 4(1), 57–65.

Kristjanson, L.J., Tamblyn, R., and Kuypers, J.A. (1987). A model to guide development and application of multiple nursing theories. *Journal of Advanced Nursing*, 12, 523–529.

*Kritek, P.B. (1978). The generation and classification of nursing diagnoses: Toward a theory of nursing. *Image: Journal of Nursing Scholarship*, 10(3), 33–40.

Kulbok, P.A., Gates, M.F., Vicenzi, A.E., and Schultz, P.R. (1999). Focus on community: Directions for nursing knowledge development. *Journal of Advanced Nursing*, 29(5), 1188–1196.

Kulig, J.C. (2000). Community resiliency: The potential for community health nursing theory development. *Public Health Nursing*, 17(5), 374–385.

Kuss, T., Proulx-Girouard, L., Lovitt. S., and Katz, C.B., (1997). A public health nursing model. *Kennelly P. Public Health Nursing*, 14(2), 81–91.

Lancaster, W. and Lancaster, J. (1980). Models and model building in nursing. *Advances in Nursing Science*, 3(1), 1–7.

auder, W. (2001). The utility of self-care theory as a theoretical basis for self-neglect. *Journal of Advanced Nursing*, 34(4), 545–551. Comment in *Journal of Advanced Nursing* (2001), 34(4), 552–553.

(1998). An analysis and evaluation of Casey's conceptual framework. *International* *rnal of Nursing Studies*, 35(4), 204–209.

Leenerts, M.H. and Magilvy, J.K. (2000). Investing in self-care: A midrange theory of self-care grounded in the lived experience of low-income HIV-positive white women. *Advances in Nursing Science*, 22(3), 58–75.

Legault, F. and Ferguson-Pare, M. (1999). Advancing nursing practice: An evaluation study of Parse's theory of human becoming. *Canadian Journal of Nursing Leadership*, 12(1), 30–35.

*Leininger, M.M. (1969). Introduction: Nature of science in nursing. *Nursing Research*, 18(5), 388–389.

Lerdal, A. (1998). A concept analysis of energy: Its meaning in the lives of three individuals with chronic illness. *Scandinavian Journal of Caring Sciences*, 12(1), 3–10.

Levesque, L., Ricard, N., Ducharme, F., Duquette, A., and Bonin, J.P. (1998). Empirical verification of a theoretical model derived from the Roy adaptation model: Findings from five studies. *Nursing Science Quarterly*, 11(1), 31–39.

Levine, M.E. (1988). Antecedent from adjunctive discipline: Creative of nursing theory. *Nursing Science Quarterly*, 1(1), 16–21.

Liehr, P. and Smith, M.J. (1999). Middle range theory: Spinning research and practice to create knowledge for the new millennium. *Advances in Nursing Science*, 21(4), 81–91.

MacGregor, J. and Dewar, K. (1997). Opening up the options: Making the inflexible into a flexible framework. *Nurse Education Today*, 17(5), 502–507.

Madden, B.P. (1990). The hybrid model for concept development: Its value for the study of therapeutic alliance. *Advances in Nursing Science*, 12(3), 75–87.

Markovic, M. (1997). From theory to perioperative practice with Parse. *Canadian Operating Room Nursing Journal*, 15(1) 13–19.

Martin, P.J. (2000). Hearing voices and listening to those that hear them. *Journal of Psychiatric and Mental Health Nursing*, 7(2),135–141.

Matas, K.E. (1997). Human patterning and chronic pain. *Nursing Science Quarterly*, 10(2), 88–96.

Mathwig, G. (1971). Nursing science: The theoretical core of nursing knowledge. *Image: Journal of Nursing Scholarship*, 4(1), 20–23.

McCance, T.V., McKenna, H.P., and Boore, J.R. (1999). Caring: Theoretical perspectives of relevance to nursing. *Journal of Advanced Nursing*, 30(6), 1388–1395.

*McCarthy, R.T. (1972). A practice theory of nursing care. *Nursing Research*, 21(5), 406–410.

McHolm, F.A. and Geib, K.M. (1998). Application of the Neuman Systems Model to teaching health assessment and nursing process. *Nursing Diagnosis*, 9(1), 23–33.

*McKay, R. (1969). Theories, models, and systems for nursing. *Nursing Research*, 18(5), 393–400.

*McKay, R.C. (1977). What is the relationship between the development and utilization of a taxonomy and nursing theory? *Nursing Research*, 26(3), 222–224.

McKenna, B. and Roberts R. (1999). Bridging the theory-practice gap. *Nursing New Zealand*, 5(2), 14–16.

McKenna, H. (1999). The role of reflection in the development of practice theory: A case study. *Journal of Psychiatric and Mental Health Nursing*, 6(2), 147–151.

McMurry, P.H. (1982). Toward a unique knowledge base in nursing. *Image: Journal of Nursing Scholarship*, 14(1), 12–15.

Meleis, A.I. (1985). International nursing for knowledge development. *Nursing Outlook,* 33(3), 144–147.

Meleis, A.I. (1987). ReVisions in knowledge development: A passion for substance. *Scholarly Inquiry for Nursing Practice,* 1(1), 5–19.

Meleis, A.I. (1987). Theoretical nursing: Today's challenges, tomorrow's bridges. Nursing papers: Perspectives in nursing. *Canadian Journal of Nursing Research,* 19(1), 45–56.

Meleis, A.I. (1992). Theoretical thinking progress in the discipline of nursing. In K. Kraus and P. Astedt-Kurki (Eds.), *International Perspectives on Nursing* (pp. 1–12). Tampere, Finland: University of Tampere Department of Nursing.

Meleis, A.I. (1998). ReVisions in knowledge development: A passion for substance. *Scholarly Inquiry in Nursing Practice,* 12(1), 65–77.

Meleis, A.I., Sawyer, L.M., Im, E.O., Hilfinger Messias, D.K., and Schumacher, K. (2000). Experiencing transitions: An emerging middle-range theory. *Advances in Nursing Science,* 23(1), 12–28.

*Menke, E.M. (1978). Theory development: A challenge for nursing. In N.L. Chaska (Ed.), *The nursing profession: Views through the mist.* New York: McGraw-Hill.

Miller, M.E. and Dzurec, L.C. (1993). The power of the name. *Advances in Nursing Science,* 15(3), 15–22.

Miller, S.K. (1999). Nurse practitioners in the county correctional facility setting: Unique challenges and suggestions for effective health promotion. *Clinical Excellence in Nurse Practice,* 3(5), 268–272.

Moccia, P. (1986). *New approaches to theory development.* New York: National League for Nursing.

Mohr, W.K. (1999). Beyond cause and effect: Some thoughts on research and practice in child psychiatric nursing. *Journal of Child and Adolescent Psychiatric Nursing,* 12(3), 118–127.

Mohr, W.K. and Naylor, M.D. (1998). Creating a curriculum for the 21st century. *Nursing Outlook,* 46(5), 206–212.

Monti, E.J. and Tingen, M.S. (1999). Multiple paradigms of nursing science. *Advances in Nursing Science,* 21(4), 64–80.

*Moore, M. (1968). Nursing: A scientific discipline. *Forum,* 7(4), 340–348.

Morse, J. M. (1995). Exploring the theoretical basis of nursing using advanced techniques of concept analysis. *Advances in Nursing Science,* 17, 31–46.

Murphy, J.D. (1978). Toward a philosophy of nursing. In N.L. Chaska (Ed.), *The nursing profession: Views through the mist.* New York: McGraw-Hill.

Murphy, J.F. (Ed.). (1971). *Theoretical issues in professional nursing.* New York: Appleton-Century-Crofts. (Note especially Chapters 1, 2, and 3.)

*Murphy, S.A. and Hoeffer, B. (1983). Role of the specialties in nursing science. *Advances in Nursing Science,* 5(4), 31–39.

Neal, L.J. (1999). Facilitating the growth of nursing staff case management in PPS. *Caring,* 18(10), 46–48.

Neill, S.J. (1998). Developing children's nursing through action research. *Journal of Child Health Care,* 2(1), 11–15.

Nelson, S. (1997). Reading nursing history. *Nursing Inquiry,* 4(4), 229–236.

Newman, M. (1977). *Theory development in nursing.* Philadelphia: F.A. Davis.

*Newman, M.A. (1972). Nursing's theoretical evolution. *Nursing Outlook,* 20(7), 449–453.

Nicoll, L. (1992). *Perspectives on nursing theory* (2nd ed.). Philadelphia: J.B. Lippincott.

Noble-Adams, R. (1999). Ethics and nursing research. 1: Development, theories and principles. *British Journal of Nursing*, 8(13), 888–892.

Nolan, M., Lundh, U., and Tishelman, C. (1998). Nursing's knowledge base: Does it have to be unique? *British Journal of Nursing*, 7(5), 270–276.

Norris, C.M. (Ed.). (1969, 1970). *Proceedings, first, second, and third nursing theory conference*. Kansas City. MO: University of Kansas Medical Center, Department of Nursing Education.

Norris, C.M. (1982). *Concept classification in nursing*. Rockville, MD: Aspen Systems.

Northrup, D.T. and Cody, W.K. (1998). Evaluation of the human becoming theory in practice in an acute care psychiatric setting. *Nursing Science Quarterly*, 11(1), 23–30.

*Notter, L.E. (1975). The case for nursing research. *Nursing Outlook*, 23(12), 760–763.

Nursing Development Conference Group. (1979). *Concept formalization in nursing: Process and product*. Boston: Little, Brown.

O'Brien, B. and Pearson, A. (1993). Unwritten knowledge in nursing: Consider the spoken as well as the written word. *Scholarly Inquiry for Nursing Practice*, 7, 111–127.

O'Connell, B., Rapley, P., and Tibbett, P. (1999). Does the nursing diagnosis form the basis for patient care? *Collegian*, 6(3), 29–34.

Ohashi, J.P. (1985). The contributions of Dickoff and James to theory development in nursing. *Image: Journal of Nursing Scholarship*, 17(1), 17–20.

Olson, J. and Hanchett, E. (1997). Nurse-expressed empathy, patient outcomes, and development of a middle-range theory. *Image: Journal of Nursing Scholarship*, 29(1), 71–76.

Panel Discussion. (1968). Theory development in nursing. *Nursing Research*, 17(3), 223–227.

Parse, R.R. (1997). Transforming research and practice with the human becoming theory. *Nursing Science Quarterly*, 10(4), 171–174.

Parse, R.R. (1999). Nursing science: The transformation of practice. *Journal of Advanced Nursing*, 30(6), 1383–1387.

Paul, R.W. and Heaslip, P. (1995). Critical thinking and intuitive nursing practice. *Journal of Advanced Nursing*, 22, 40–47.

*Payne, L. (1983). Health: A basic concept in nursing theory. *Journal of Advanced Nursing*, 8(5), 393–395.

Peden, A.R. (1998). The evolution of an intervention—The use of Peplau's process of practice-based theory development. *Journal of Psychiatric and Mental Health Nursing*, 5(3), 173–178.

Perry, J. (1985). Has the discipline of nursing developed to the stage where nurses do "think nursing?" *Journal of Advanced Nursing*, 10(1), 31–37.

*Peterson, C.J. (1977). Questions frequently asked about the development of a conceptual framework. *Journal of Nursing Education*, 16(4), 22–23.

*Phillips, J.R. (1977). Nursing systems and nursing models. *Image: Journal of Nursing Scholarship*, 9(1), 4–7.

Piccinato, J.M. and Rosenbaum, J.N. (1997). Caregiver hardiness explored within Watson's theory of human caring in nursing. *Journal of Gerontological Nursing*, 23(10), 32–39.

Polk, L.V. (1997). Toward a middle-range theory of resilience. *Advances in Nursing Science*, 19(3), 1–13.

Priest, H. and Roberts, P. (1998). Assessing students' clinical performance. *Nursing Standard*, 12(48), 37–41.

*Putnam, P. (1965). A conceptual approach to nursing theory. *Nursing Science*, 3, 430–442.

*Quint, J.C. (1967). The case for theories generated from empirical data. *Nursing Research*, 16(2), 109–114.

Ramos, M. (1987). Adopting an evolutionary lens: An optimistic approach in discovering strength in nursing. *Advances in Nursing Science*, 10(1), 19–26.

Rankin, S.H. (2000). Life-span development: Refreshing a theoretical and practice perspective. *Scholarly Inquiry in Nursing Practice*, 14(4), 379–388.

Rankin, S.H. and Weekes, D.P. (2000). Life-span development: A review of theory and practice for families with chronically ill members. *Scholarly Inquiry in Nursing Practice*, 14(4), 355–373.

Rask, M. and Hallberg, I.R. (2000). Forensic psychiatric nursing care—Nurses apprehension of their responsibility and work content: A Swedish survey. *Journal of Psychiatric and Mental Health Nursing*, 7(2), 163–177.

Ream, E. and Richardson. A. (1999). From theory to practice: Designing interventions to reduce fatigue in patients with cancer. *Oncology Nursing Forum*, 26(8), 1295–1303. Comment in *Oncology Nursing Forum* (2000), 27(3), 425–426.

Reed, P.G. (1989). Nursing theorizing as an ethical endeavor. *Advances in Nursing Science*, 11(3), 1–9.

Reed, P.G. (1998). A holistic view of nursing concepts and theories in practice. *Journal of Holistic Nursing*, 16(4), 415–419.

Relf, M.V. (1997). Illuminating meaning and transforming issues of spirituality in HIV disease and AIDS: An application of Parse's theory of human becoming. *Holistic Nursing Practice*, 12(1), 1–8.

Richardson, L. (1994). Writing: A method of inquiry. In N.K. Denzin and Y.S. Lincoln (Eds.), *Handbook of qualitative research*. Thousand Oaks, CA: Sage.

Rinehart, J.M. (1978). The "how" of theory development in nursing. In J.G. Paterson (Ed.), *Theory development: What, why, how?* (Publication No. 15–1708, pp. 67–74). New York: National League for Nursing.

Roberts, D. (1997). Liaison mental health nursing: Origins, definition and prospects. *Journal of Advanced Nursing*, 25(1), 101–108.

Rodgers, B.L. (1989). Concepts, analysis, and the development of nursing knowledge: The evolutionary cycle. *Journal of Advanced Nursing*, 14, 330–335.

Rodgers, B.L. (1991). Using concept analysis to enhance clinical practice and research. *Applied Research*, 10, 28–34.

Rodgers, B.L. and Knafl, K.A. (1993). *Concept development in nursing: Foundations, techniques, and applications.* Philadelphia: W.B. Saunders.

*Rogers, M.E. (1963). Some comments on the theoretical basis of nursing practice. *Nursing Science*, 1, 11–13, 60.

Rothrock, J.C. and Smith, D.A. (2000). Selecting the perioperative patient focused model. *Journal of the Association of periOperative Registered Nurses*, 71(5), 1030–1034.

*Rubin, R. (1968). A theory of clinical nursing. *Nursing Research*, 17(3), 210–212.

Running, A. (1997). Snapshots of experience: Vignettes from a nursing home. *Journal of Advanced Nursing*, 25(1), 117–122.

Sanford, R.C. (2000). Caring through relation and dialogue: A nursing perspective for patient education. *Advances in Nursing Science*, 22(3), 1–15.

Sasmor, J.L. (1968). Toward developing theory in nursing. *Nursing Forum*, 7(2), 191–200.

Scanlan, J.M. and Chernomas, W.M. (1997). Developing the reflective teacher. *Journal of Advanced Nursing*, 25(6), 1138–1143.

Schafer, P.J. (1987). Philosophic analysis of a theory of clinical nursing. *Maternal-Child Nursing Journal*, 16(4), 289–368.

Schlotfeldt, R.M. (1988). Structuring nursing knowledge: A priority for creating nursing's future. *Nursing Science Quarterly*, 1(1), 35–38.

Schlotzhauer, M. and Farnham, R. (1997). Newman's theory and insulin dependent diabetes mellitus in adolescence. *Journal of Scholarly Nursing*, 13(3), 20–23.

Schultz, P. (1987). Toward holistic inquiry in nursing: A proposal for synthesis of patterns and methods. *Scholarly Inquiry for Nursing Practice*, 1(2), 135–146.

Schultz, P.R. (1987). When client means more than one: Extending the foundational concept of person. *Advances in Nursing Science*, 10(1), 71–80.

Schultz, P. and Meleis, A.I. (1988). Nursing epistemology: Traditions, insights, questions. *Image: Journal of Nursing Scholarship*, 20(4), 217–221.

Schwartz-Barcott, D. and Kim, H.S. (1993). An expansion and elaboration of the hybrid model of concept development. In B.L. Rodgers and K.A. Knafl (Eds.), *Concept development in nursing* (pp. 107–133). Philadelphia: W.B. Saunders.

Severinsson, E.I. (1999). Ethics in clinical nursing supervision—An introduction to the theory and practice of different supervision models. *Collegian*, 6(3), 23–28.

Severinsson, E.I. (1998). Bridging the gap between theory and practice: A supervision programme for nursing students. *Journal of Advanced Nursing*, 27(6), 1269–1277.

Shih, F.J. (1998). Triangulation in nursing research: Issues of conceptual clarity and purpose. *Journal of Advanced Nursing*, 28(3), 631–641. Comment in *Journal of Advanced Nursing* (1999), 30(3), 775.

*Silva, M.C. and Rothbart, D. (1984). An analysis of changing trends in philosophies of science on nursing theory development and testing. *Advances in Nursing Science*, 6(2), 1–13.

Simko, L.C. (1999). Adults with congenital heart disease: Utilizing quality of life and Husted's nursing theory as a conceptual framework. *Critical Care Nursing Quarterly*, 22(3), 1–11.

Simon, H. (1971). Logical, empirical approach to developing a body of knowledge. In J. Murphy (Ed.), *Theoretical issues in professional nursing*. New York: Appleton-Century-Crofts.

Smith, M.J. and Liehr, P. (1999). Attentively embracing story: A middle-range theory with practice and research implications. *Scholarly Inquiry in Nursing Practice*, 13(3), 187–204.

Smoyak, S.A. (1969). Toward understanding nursing situation: A transaction paradigm. *Nursing Research*, 18(5), 405–411.

Sorenson, G. (Ed.). (1986). *Setting the agenda for the year (2000): Knowledge development in nursing*. Kansas City, MO: American Academy of Nursing.

Sorrell, J.M. (1994). Remembrance of things past through writing: Esthetic patterns of knowing in nursing. *Advances in Nursing Science*, 17(1), 60–70.

Spouse, J. (2001). Bridging theory and practice in the supervisory relationship: A sociocultural perspective. *Journal of Advanced Nursing,* 33(4), 512–522.

*Stainton, M.C. (1982). The birth of nursing science. *Canadian Nurse,* 78(10), 24–28.

Stark, S., Cooke, P., and Stronach, I. (2000). Minding the gap: Some theory-practice disjunctions in nursing education research. *Nurse Education Today,* 20(2), 155–163.

Stein, K.F., Corte, C., Colling, K.B., and Whall, A. (1998). A theoretical analysis of Carper's ways of knowing using a model of social cognition. *Scholarly Inquiry in Nursing Practice,* 12(1), 43–60.

Stember, M.L. (1986). Model building as a strategy for theory development. In P.L. Chinn (Ed.), *Nursing research methodology* (pp. 103–117). Rockville, MD: Aspen Systems.

Stevenson, J.S. and Woods, N.F. (1986). Nursing science and contemporary science: Emerging paradigms. In G. Sorenson (Ed.), *Setting the agenda for the year (2000): Knowledge development in nursing.* Kansas City, MO: American Academy of Nursing.

Suppe, F. and Jacox, A. (1985). Philosophy of science and the development of nursing theory. *Annual Review Nursing Research,* 3, 241–267.

Thorne, S.E., Kirkham, S.R., and Henderson. A. (1999). Ideological implications of paradigm discourse. *Nursing Inquiry,* 6(2), 123–131.

*Tinkle, M.B. and Beaton, J.L. (1983). Toward a new view of science: Implications for nursing research. *Advances in Nursing Science,* 5(2), 27–36.

Tracy, J.P. (1997). Growing up with chronic illness: The experience of growing up with cystic fibrosis. *Holistic Nursing Practice,* 12(1), 27–35.

Tritsch, J.M. (1998). Application of King's theory of goal attainment and the Carondelet St. Mary's case management model. *Nursing Science Quarterly,* 11(2), 69–73.

*Tucker, R.W. (1979). The value decisions we know as science. *Advances in Nursing Science,* 1(2), 1–12.

Turner, S.L. and Bentley, G.W. (1998). A meaningful health assessment course for baccalaureate nursing students. *Nursing Connections,* 11(2), 5–12.

Verran, J.A. (1997). The value of theory-driven (rather than problem-driven) research. *Seminars for Nurse Managers,* 5(4), 169–172.

Villarruel, A.M. and Denyes, M.J. (1997). Testing Orem's theory with Mexican Americans. *Image: Journal of Nursing Scholarship,* 29(3), 283–288.

Visintainer, M.A. (1986). The nature of knowledge and theory in nursing. *Image: Journal of Nursing Scholarship,* 18(2), 32–38.

Wainwright, P. (2000). Towards an aesthetics of nursing. *Journal of Advanced Nursing,* 32(3), 750–756.

*Wald, F.S. and Leonard, R.C. (1964). Toward development of nursing practice theory. *Nursing Research,* 13(4), 309–313.

Walker, L.O. (1971). Toward a clearer understanding of the concept of nursing theory. *Nursing Research,* 20(5), 428–435.

Walker, L.O. (1972). Rejoinder to commentary: Toward a clearer understanding of the concept of nursing theory. *Nursing Research,* 21(1), 59–62.

Walker, L.O. and Avant, K.C. (1995). *Strategies for theory construction in nursing* (3rd ed.). East Norwalk, CT: Appleton & Lange.

*Weatherston, L. (1979). Theory of nursing: Creating effective care. *Journal of Advanced Nursing,* 4(7), 365–375.

Wellard, S. (1997). Constructions of family nursing: A critical exploration. *Contemporary Nurse*, 6(2), 78–84.

Wenzel, L.S., Briggs, K.L., and Puryear, B.L. (1998). Portfolio: Authentic assessment in the age of the curriculum revolution. *Journal of Nursing Education*, 37(5), 208–212.

West, P. and Isenberg, M. (1997). Instrument development: The Mental Health-Related Self-Care Agency Scale. *Archives of Psychiatric Nursing*, 11(3), 126–132.

Westbrook, L.O. and Schultz, P.R. (2000). From theory to practice: Community health nursing in a public health neighborhood team. *Advances in Nursing Science*, 23(2), 50–61.

Whitener, L.M., Cox, K.R., and Maglich, S.A. (1998). Use of theory to guide nurses in the design of health messages for children. *Advances in Nursing Science*, 20(3), 21–35.

Whittemore, R. and Roy, C. (2002). Adapting to diabetes mellitus: A theory synthesis. *Nursing Science Quarterly*, 15(4), 311–317.

Wilde, M.H. (1999). Why embodiment now? *Advances in Nursing Science*, 22(2), 25–38. Comment in *Advances in Nursing Science* (2000), 23(1), vi–vii.

Williams, A.M. (1998). The delivery of quality nursing care: A grounded theory study of the nurse's perspective. *Journal of Advanced Nursing*, 27(4), 808–816.

Wilshaw, G. (1999). Perspectives on surviving childhood sexual abuse. *Journal of Advanced Nursing*, 30(2), 303–309.

Wilson, John (1963). *Thinking with concepts*. Cambridge, England: Cambridge University Press.

Wuest, J. (1994). A feminist approach to concept analysis. *Western Journal of Nursing Research*, 16(5), 577–586.

Wynne, N., Brand, S., and Smith, R. (1997). Incomplete holism in pre-registration nurse education: The position of the biological sciences. *Journal of Advanced Nursing*, 26(3), 470–474.

Yamashita, M. and Tall, F.D. (1998). A commentary on Newman's theory of health as expanding consciousness. *Advances in Nursing Science*, 21(1), 65–75. Comment in *Advances in Nursing Science*, (1999), 21(3), vii–viii; *Advances in Nursing Science*, (1999), 21(3), viii–ix; *Advances in Nursing Science*, (1999), 22(1), vi–vii.

Yegdich, T. (1998). How not to do clinical supervision in nursing. *Journal of Advanced Nursing*, 28(1), 193–202.

Younger, J. B. (1990). Literary works as a mode of knowing. *Image: Journal of Nursing Scholarship*, 22, 39–43.

4. Forces and Constraints in Theory Development: Women as Scientists

Abramson, J. (1975). *The invisible woman: Discrimination in the academic profession*. San Francisco: Jossey-Bass.

Andreoli, K. (1977). The status of nursing in academia. *Image: Journal of Nursing Scholarship*, 9(3), 52–58.

Arditti, R, Brennan, P., and Cavrak, S. (1980). *Science and liberation*. Boston: South End Press.

Armeger, B. (1974). Scholarship in nursing. *Nursing Outlook*, 22(3), 162–163.

Astin, H.S. (1967). Factors associated with the participation of women doctorates in the labor force. *Personnel and Guidance Journal*, 46(3), 240–246.

Bachtold, L.M. and Werner, E.E. (1972). Personality characteristics of women scientists. *Psychological Reports*, 31, 391–396.

Benoliel, J. (1975). Scholarship—A women's perspective. *Image: Journal of Nursing Scholarship*, 7(2), 22–27.

Bissel, M. (1978). Equality for women scientists. *Grants Magazine*, 4, 331–334.

Blankenship, V. (1973). The scientist as a "political man." *British Journal of Sociology*, 24(3), 269–287.

Briscoe, A.M. and Pfafflin, S.M. (Eds.). (1979). Expanding the role of women in the sciences. *Annals of New York Academy of Science*, 323.

*Brown, C. (1975). Women workers in the health service industry. *International Journal of Health Services*, 5(2), 173–184.

Bullough, B. (1975). Barriers to the nurse practitioner movement: Problems of women in a woman's field. *International Journal of Health Services*, 5(2), 225–233.

Bullough, B. (1978). The struggle for women's rights in Denver: A personal account. *Nursing Outlook*, 26(9), 566–567.

Chafetz, J.S. (1978). *Masculine/feminine or human? An overview of the sociology of sex roles.* Itasca, IL: F.E. Peacock Publisher.

Cleland, V. (1974). To end sex discrimination. *Nursing Clinics of North America*, 9(3), 563–571.

Cole, J.R. (1979). *Fair science: Women in the scientific community.* New York: Free Press.

Cole, J.R. (1981). Women in science. *American Scientist*, 69(4), 385–391.

Conant, L.H. (1968). On becoming a nurse researcher. *Nursing Research*, 17(1), 68–71.

Curran, L. (1980). Science education: Did she drop out or was she pushed? In L. Birke et al. (Eds.), *Alice through the microscope.* London, England: Virgo.

Epstein, C.F. (1973). Positive effects of the multiple negative: Explaining the success of black professional women. *American Journal of Sociology*, 78(4), 912–935.

Fausto-Sterling, A. (1981). Women in science. *Women Science International Forum*, 4, 41–50.

Feulner, P.A. (1979). *Women in the professions: A social psychological study.* Palo Alto, CA: R & E Research Association.

Fitzpatrick, M.L. (1977). Nursing: Review essay. *Signs: Journal of Women in Culture and Society*, 2(4), 818–833.

Grier, M.R. and Schnitzler, C.P. (1979). Nurses' propensity to risk. *Nursing Research*, 28(3), 186–191.

Grissum, M. and Spengler, C. (1976). *Woman power and health care.* Boston: Little, Brown.

Humphreys, S.M. (1982). *Women and minorities in science: Strategies for increasing participation.* Boulder, CO: Westview Press.

Jaquette, J.S. (1976). Political science: Review essay. *Signs: Journal of Women in Culture and Society*, 2(1), 147–176.

Keller, M.C. (1979). The effect of sexual stereotyping on the development of nursing theory. *American Journal of Nursing*, 79(9), 1584–1586.

Loomis, M.E. (1974). Collegiate nursing education: An ambivalent profession. *Journal of Nursing Education*, 39–48.

MacDonald, M.R. (1977). How do men and women students rate in empathy? *American Journal of Nursing*, 77(6), 998.

Martin, B.R. and Irvine, J. (1982). Women in science: The astronomical brain drain. *Women's Studies International Forum*, 5, 41–68.

May, K.M., Meleis, A.I., and Winstead-Fry, P. (1982). Mentorship for scholarliness: Opportunities and dilemmas. *Nursing Outlook*, 30, 22–28.

McCain, G. and Segal, E.M. (1977). *The game of science.* Monterey, CA: Brooks/Cole. (Note especially pp. 74–78.)

Meleis, A.I. and Dagenais, F. (1981). Sex role identity and perception of professional self in graduates of three programs. *Nursing Research*, 30(3), 162–167.

Meleis, A.I. and May, K. (1981). Nursing theory and scholarliness in the doctoral program. *Advances in Nursing Science*, 4(2), 31–41.

Meleis, A.I. and May, K. (1982). Mentorship for scholarliness. *Proceedings for Doctoral Forum* (held in Seattle, Washington, 1981). Seattle, WA: University of Washington.

Meleis, A.I., Wilson, H.S., and Chater, S. (1980). Toward the socialization of a scholar: A model. *Research in Nursing and Health*, 3, 115–124.

Merchant, C. (1980). *The death of nature: Women, ecology and the scientific revolution.* San Francisco: Harper & Row.

Moore, D., Decker, S., and Down, M.W (1978). Baccalaureate nursing students' identification with the women's movement. *Nursing Research*, 27(5), 291–295.

Neusner, J. (1977, May 31) The scholars' apprentice. *The Chronicle of Higher Education Point of View*, p. 40.

Roe, A. (1951). A psychological study of eminent biologists. *Psychological Monographs*, 65, 1–67.

Roe, A. (1963). *The making of a scientist.* New York: Dodd Mead.

Roe, A. (1966). Women in science. *Personnel and Guidance Journal*, 54, 784–787.

Rossi, A. (1972). Women in science: Why so few? In C. Safilios-Rothchild (Ed.), *Toward a sociology of women* (pp. 141–153). New York: Xerox Corp.

Rossiter, M.W. (1982). *Women scientists in America: Struggles and strategies in 1940.* Baltimore: Johns Hopkins Press.

Seiden, A. (1976). Overview: Research on the psychology of women. I and II. Gender differences and sexual and reproductive life. *American Journal of Psychiatry*, 133(10), 1111–1118.

Speizer, J.J. (1981). Role models, mentors and sponsors: The elusive concepts. *Signs: Journal of Women in Culture and Society*, 6, 692–712.

Stroller, E.P. (1978). Perceptions of the nursing role: A case study of an entering class. *Journal of Nursing Education*, 17(6), 2–14.

Stromborg, M.F. (1976). Relationship of sex-role identity to occupational image of female nursing students. *Nursing Research*, 25(5), 363–369.

Vaughter, R. (1976, Autumn). Psychology: Review essay. *Signs: Journal of Women in Culture and Society*, 2(1), 120–146.

Wallsgrove, R. (1980). The masculine face of science. In L. Birke et al. (Eds.), *Alice through the microscope.* London, England: Virgo.

Watson, J.D. (1968). *The double helix.* New York: New American Library.

White, M.S. (1972). Psychological and social barriers to women in science. In C. Safilios-Rothchild (Ed.), *Toward a sociology of women.* New York: Xerox Corp.

5. Forces and Constraints in Theory Development: Nursing Profession

Ashley, J.A. (1980). Power in structured misogyny: Implications for the politics of care. *Advances in Nursing Science,* 2(3), 3–22.

Ashley, J. (1976). *Hospital paternalism and the role of the nurse.* New York: Teachers' College Press.

Aydelotte, M.K. (1968). Issues of professional nursing: The need for clinical excellence. *Nursing Forum,* 7(1), 72–86.

Babich, K.S. (1968). The perception of professionalism: Equality. *Nursing Forum,* 7(1), 14–20.

Barber, B. (1963, Fall). Some problems in the sociology of professions. *Daedalus,* 92(4), 669–688.

Bixler, G. and Bixler, R.W. (1959). The professional status of nursing. *American Journal of Nursing,* 59(8), 1142–1147.

Brown, E.L. (1948). *Nursing for the future.* New York: Russel Sage Foundation. (Especially note pp. 669–688.)

*Brown, M.I. (1964). Research in the development of nursing theory. *Nursing Research,* 13(2), 109–112.

Caplow, T. (1954). *The sociology of work.* Minneapolis, MN: University of Minnesota Press. (Especially note p. 139.)

Cogan, M.L. (1955, January). The problem of defining a profession. *Annals of the American Academy of Political and Social Sciences,* 297, 105–111.

Colodarci, A. (1963). What about the word "profession"? *American Journal of Nursing,* 63(10), 116–118.

Conant, L.H. (1968). On becoming a nurse researcher. *Nursing Research,* 17(1), 68–72.

Cox, C. (1979). Who cares? Nursing and sociology: The development of symbiotic relationship. *Journal of Advanced Nursing,* 4, 237–252.

Devereux, G. and Weiner, F. (1950, October). The occupational status of nurses. *American Sociological Review,* 15, 628–634.

Dilworth, A. (1963, May). Goals in nursing. *Nursing Outlook,* 11, 336–340.

Ellison, M., Diers, D., and Leonard, R. (1965). The use of the behavioral sciences in nursing: Further comment. *Nursing Research,* 14, 71–72.

Feldman, H.R. (1980). Nursing research in the 1980s: Issues and implications. *Advances in Nursing Science,* 3(1), 85–92.

Feldman, H.R. (1981). A science of nursing—To be or not to be? *Image: Journal of Nursing Scholarship,* 13, 63–66.

Fox, D. (1964, Winter). A proposed model for identifying research areas in nursing. *Nursing Research,* 13, 29–36.

Goode, W.J. (1959). Community within a community: The professions. *American Sociological Review,* 194–200. (Bobbs-Merrill Reprint S-99.)

Goode, W.J. (1960, December). Encroachment, charlatanism, and the emerging profession: Psychology, sociology, and medicine. *American Sociological Review*, 25, 902–914.

Gouldner, A. (1961). Theoretical requirements of the applied social sciences. In W.G. Bennis, K.D. Benne, and R. Chin (Eds.), *The planning of change*. New York: Holt, Rinehart & Winston.

Hughes, E.C. (1958). *Men and their work*. Glencoe, IL: Free Press. (Especially note p. 133.)

Hughes, E.C. (1963, Fall). Professions. *Daedalus*, 655–668.

Hurley, B.A. (1979). Why a theoretical framework in nursing research. *Western Journal of Nursing Research*, 1(1), 28–41.

Johnson, M. and Martin, H. (1958). A sociological analysis of the nurse role. *American Journal of Nursing*, 58(3), 373–377.

Lipton, N. (1968). Nursing education as a challenge to the professionalization of nursing. *Nursing Forum*, 7(2), 201–214.

Martin, H.W. (1958, October). The behavioral sciences and nursing education. *Social Forces*, 37, 61–67.

Masipa, A.L. (1996). Nursing theory development. *Curationis: South African Journal of Nursing*, 19(1), 61–64.

McGlothlin, W.J. (1960). *Patterns of professional education*. New York: G.P. Putnam's Sons. (Especially note pp. 1–25.)

McGlothlin, W.J. (1961, April). The place of nursing among the professions. *Nursing Outlook*, 9, 216.

Mead, M. (1956). Nursing—Primitive and civilized. *American Journal of Nursing*, 56(8), 948–950.

Meleis, A.I. and May, K. (1981). Nursing theory and scholarliness in the doctoral program. *Advances in Nursing Science*, 4(1), 31–41.

Nolan, M., Lundh, U., and Tishelman, C. (1998). Nursing's knowledge base: Does it have to be unique? *British Journal of Nursing*, 7(5), 270–276.

Montag, M. (1959). *Community college education for nursing*. New York: McGraw-Hill.

Parsons, T. (1939). The professions and social structure. *Social Forces* (S-219). The College Book Co. (Especially note pp. 457–467.)

Parsons, T. (1965). *Essays in sociological theory*. New York: Free Press.

Pierson, W. (1999). Considering the nature of intersubjectivity within professional nursing. *Journal of Advanced Nursing*, 30(2), 294–302.

Reissman, L. and Rorher, J.H. (Eds.). (1957). *Change and dilemma in the nursing profession*. New York: G.P. Putnam's Sons.

Rogers, M. (1975). Euphemisms in nursing's future. *Image: Journal of Nursing Scholarship*, 7(2), 3–9.

Rutty, J.E. (1998). The nature of philosophy of science, theory and knowledge relating to nursing and professionalism. *Journal of Advanced Nursing*, 28(2), 243–250.

Sills, G.M. (1998). Peplau and professionalism: The emergence of the paradigm of professionalization. *Journal of Psychiatric and Mental Health Nursing*, 5(3), 167–171.

Tyler, R. (1952, April). Distinctive attributes of education for the professions. *Social Work Journal*, 33, 55–62.

Van Maanen, J.M.T., Mussallen, H.K., McGilloway, F.A., Cormack, D., Clarke, M., Bergman, R. and King, P. (1979). Janforum: The nursing profession: Ritualized, routinized or research-based? *Journal of Advanced Nursing*, 1, 87–89.

Wolensky, R.P. (1981). The graduate student's double bind: A professional socialization problem in sociology. *Sociological Spectrum*, 1, 393–414.

6. Theory and Science

*Abdellah, F.G. (1969). The nature of nursing science. *Nursing Research*, 18(5), 390–393.

*Andreoli, K.G. and Thompson, C.E. (1977). The nature of science in nursing. *Image: Journal of Nursing Scholarship*, 9(2), 32–37.

Barber, B. and Hirsch, W. (Eds.). (1962). *The sociology of science.* New York: Free Press of Glencoe.

Bernstein, J. (1978). *Experiencing science.* New York: Basic Books. (Especially note p. 87.)

Bilitski, J.S. (1981). Nursing science and the laws of health: The test of substance as a step in the process of theory development. *Advances in Nursing Science*, 4(1), 15–29.

Blume, S. (Ed.) (1977). *Perspectives in the sociology of science.* New York: John Wiley & Sons.

Bohny, B. (1980). Theory development for a nursing science. *Nursing Forum*, 19(1), 50–67.

Cody, W. K. (1994). The language of nursing science: If not now, when? *Nursing Science Quarterly*, 7, 98–99.

*Colaizzi, J. (1975). The proper object of nursing science. *International Journal of Nursing Studies*, 12(4), 197–200.

Crowley, D.M. (1968). Perspective of pure science. *Nursing Research*, 17(6), 497–501.

Danto, A. and Morgenbesser, S. (Eds.). (1966). Laws and theories. In *Philosophy of Science.* New York: World Publishing (Especially note pp. 177–287.)

Fawcett, J., Watson, J., Neuman, B., Walker, P.H., and Fitzpatrick, J.J. (2001). On nursing theories and evidence. *Journal of Nursing Scholarship*, 33(2), 115–119.

Gortner, S.R. (1980). Nursing science in transition. *Nursing Research*, 29(3), 180–183.

*Green, J.A. (1979). Science, nursing and nursing science: A conceptual analysis. *Advances in Nursing Science*, 2(1), 57–64.

Huch, M. H. (1995). Nursing science as a basis for advanced practice. *Nursing Science Quarterly*, 8, 6–7.

*Johnson, D.E. (1959). The nature of a science of nursing. *Nursing Outlook*, 7(5), 291–294.

*Leininger, M.M. (1969). Introduction: Nature of science in nursing. *Nursing Research*, 18(5), 388–389.

Longino, H.E. (1981). Scientific objectivity and feminist theorizing. *Liberal Education*, 67, 187–195.

Mathwig, G. (1971). Nursing science: The theoretical core of nursing knowledge. *Image: Journal of Nursing Scholarship*, 4(1), 20–23.

O'Brien, B.O. and Pearson, A. (1993). Unwritten knowledge in nursing: Consider the spoken as well as the written word. *Scholarly Inquiry for Nursing Practice*, 7(2), 111–127.

Phillips, J.R. (2001). Beyond a decade of research: Moving to the while hole of unitary science. *Nursing Science Quarterly*, 10(1), 6–7.

Ravetz, J.R. (1971). *Scientific knowledge and its social problems.* New York: Oxford University Press. (Especially note pp. 152, 162.)

*Rogers, M.E. (1963). Some comments on the theoretical basis of nursing practice. *Nursing Science*, 1, 11–13, 60.

Sarvimki A. (1994). Science and tradition in the nursing discipline. *Scandinavian Journal of Caring Sciences*, 8, 137–142.

Schrag, C. (1968). Science and the helping professions. *Nursing Research*, 17(6), 486–496.

Schumacher, K.L. and Gortner, S.R. (1992). (Mis)conceptions and reconceptions about traditional science. *Advances in Nursing Science*, 14(4), 1–11.

Schwab, J.J. (1966). The teaching of science as inquiry. In P.F. Brandwern (Ed.), *Elements in a strategy for teaching science in the elementary school.* Cambridge, MA: Harvard University Press. (Especially note pp. 12, 15, 17.)

Shermis, S.S. (1962, November). On becoming an intellectual discipline. *Phi Delta Kappa*, 84–86.

*Tucker, R.W. (1979). The value decisions we know as science. *Advances in Nursing Science*, 1(2), 1–12.

What is nursing science? An international dialogue. (1997). *Nursing Science Quarterly*, 10(1), 10–3.

Younger, J.B. (1990). Literary works as a mode of knowing. *Image: Journal of Nursing Scholarship*, 22(1), 39–43.

7. Theory and Research

Ader, R. (1980). Psychosomatic and psychoimmunologic research. *Psychosomatic Medicine*, 42(3), 307–321.

Allan, J.D. (1988). Knowing what to weigh: Women's self-care activities related to weight. *Advances in Nursing Science*, 11(1), 47–60.

*Batey, M. (1972). Values relative to research and to science in nursing as influenced by a sociological perspective. *Nursing Research*, 21(6), 504–508.

*Benoliel, J.Q. (1977). The interaction between theory and research. *Nursing Outlook*, 25(2), 108–113.

*Brown, M.I. (1964). Research on the development of nursing theory. *Nursing Research*, 13(2), 109–112.

Cheek, J. and Porter, S. (1997). Reviewing Foucault: possibilities and problems for nursing and health care. *Nursing Inquiry*, 4(2), 108–119.

Chinn, P. (1985). Debunking myths in nursing theory and research. *Image: Journal of Nursing Scholarship*, 17(2), 45–49.

Clarke, P.N. (1998). Nursing theory as a guide for inquiry in family and community health nursing. *Nursing Science Quarterly*, 11(2), 47–48.

Compton, P. (1989). Drug abuse. A self-care deficit. *Journal of Psychosocial Nursing and Mental Health Services*, 27(3), 22–26.

Cressler, D.L. and Tomlinson, P.S. (1988). Nursing research and the discipline of etiological science. *Western Journal of Nursing Research*, 10(6), 743–756.

Curtin, L.L. (1984). Who or why or which or what? . . . is nursing. *Nursing Management*, 15(11), 7–8.

*Dickoff, J. and James, P. (1968). Researching research's role in theory development. *Nursing Research*, 17(3), 204–205.

Dierckx de Casterle, B., Roelens, A., and Gastmans, C. (1998). An adjusted version of Kohlberg's moral theory: Discussion of its validity for research in nursing ethics. *Journal of Advanced Nursing,* 27(4), 829–835.

Fawcett, J. (1988). Conceptual models and theory development. *Journal of Obstetric, Gynecologic, and Neonatal Nursing,* 17(6), 400–403.

Fawcett, J. and Downs, F.S. (1986). *The relationship of theory and research.* Norwalk, CT: Appleton-Century-Crofts.

Fawcett, J. (1978). The relationship between theory and research: A double helix. *Advances in Nursing Science,* 1(1), 49–62.

Feldman, H.R. (1980). Nursing research in the 1980s: Issues and implications. *Advances in Nursing Science,* 3(1), 85–92.

Fitzpatrick, J.J. (1988). How can we enhance nursing knowledge and practice? *Nursing and Health Care,* 9(9), 517–521.

Ford-Gilboe, M., Campbell, J., and Berman, H. (1995). Stories and numbers: Coexistence without compromise. *Advances in Nursing Science,* 18(1), 14–26.

Gunter, L.J. (1962). Notes on a theoretical framework for nursing research. *Nursing Research,* 11(4), 219–222.

Haller, K.B. (1988). Beyond idle speculation. *MCN, The American Journal of Maternal Child Nursing,* 13(5), 386.

Hardy, L.K. (1982). Nursing models and research: A restrictive view? *Journal of Advanced Nursing,* 7, 447–451.

Henderson, D.J. (1995). Consciousness-raising in participatory research: Method and methodology for emancipatory nursing inquiry. *Advances in Nursing Science,* 17(3), 58–69.

Hupcey, J.E. (1998). Clarifying the social support theory-research linkage. *Journal of Advanced Nursing,* 27(6), 1231–1241.

Hurley, B.A. (1979). Why a theoretical framework in nursing research? *Western Journal of Nursing Research,* 1(1), 28–41.

Hyrkas, K., Koivula, M., and Paunonen, M. (1999). Clinical supervision in nursing in the 1990s—Current state of concepts, theory and research. *Journal of Nursing Management,* 7(3), 177–187.

Ingram, M.R. (1988). Origins of nursing knowledge. *Image: Journal of Nursing Scholarship,* 20(4), 233.

Jezewski, M.A. (1995). Evolution of a grounded theory: Conflict resolution through culture brokering. *Advances in Nursing Science,* 17(3), 14–30.

Johnson, M. (1983). Some aspects of the relation between theory and research in nursing. *Journal of Advanced Nursing,* 8, 21–28.

Kidd, P. and Morrison, E.F. (1988). Comment. The progression of knowledge in nursing: A search for meaning. *Image: Journal of Nursing Scholarship,* 20(4), 222–224.

Kirkevold, M. (1997). Integrative nursing research—An important strategy to further the development of nursing science and nursing practice. *Journal of Advanced Nursing,* 25(5), 977–984.

Lindeman, C.A. (1985). Theory and research as basic to nursing practice [pamphlet]. (Publication. No. NP-68C, pp. 1–19). Kansas City, MO: American Nurses Association.

Lowenberg, J. S. (1994). The nurse-patient relationship reconsidered: An expanded research agenda. *Scholarly Inquiry for Nursing Practice*, 8, 167–190.

Ludemann, R. (1979). Editorial comment: The paradoxical nature of nursing research. *Image: Journal of Nursing Scholarship*, 11(1), 2–8.

MacPherson, K.I. (1983). Feminist methods: A new paradigm for nursing research. *Advances in Nursing Science*, 5, 17–26.

McBride, A.B. (1986). Theory and research. *Journal of Psychological Nursing*, 24(9), 27–32.

McElmurry, B.J. (1995). Theory in nursing research . . . Editorial on theory in nursing research. *Research in Nursing and Health*, 18(4), 377.

McFarlane, J.K. (1976). Role of research in the development of nursing. *Journal of Advanced Nursing*, 1, 443–451.

McQuiston, C.M. and Campbell, J.C. (1997). Theoretical substruction: A guide for theory testing research. *Nursing Science Quarterly*, 10(3), 117–123.

Mischel, M.H. (1990). Reconceptualizing of the uncertainty in illness theory. *Image: Journal of Nursing Scholarship*, 22, 256–262.

Mitchell, G. J. (1994). Discipline-specific inquiry: The hermeneutics of theory-guided nursing research. *Nursing Outlook*, 42, 224–228.

Moch, S.D. (1990). Personal knowing: Evolving research and practice. *Scholarly Inquiry for Nursing Practice*, 4(2), 155–170.

Moody, L.E., Wilson, M.E., Smith, K., Schwartz, R., Tittle, M., and Van Cott, M.L. (1988). Analysis of a decade of nursing practice research: 1977–1986. *Nursing Research*, 37(6), 374–379.

Munhall, P.L. (1989). Philosophical pondering on qualitative research methods in nursing. *Nursing Science Quarterly*, 2(1), 20–28.

Murdaugh, C.L. (1989). Nursing research. The use of grounded theory methodology to study the process of life-style changes. *Journal of Cardiovascular Nursing*, 3(2), 56–58.

Nagle, L.M. and Mitchell, G. J. (1991). Theoretic diversity: Evolving paradigmatic issues in research and practice. *Advances in Nursing Science*, 14(1), 17–25.

Newshan, G. (1999). Nursing theory and nursing research: What's in it for me? *ASPMN-Pathways*, 8(4), 7, 10.

*Notter, L.E. (1975). The case for nursing research. *Nursing Outlook*, 23(12), 760–763.

Oiler, C. (1982). The phenomenological approach in nursing research. *Nursing Research*, 31(3), 178–181.

Orcutt, J. (1972). Toward a sociological theory of drug effects: A comparison of marijuana and alcohol. *Sociology and Social Research*, 56(2), 243–253.

Parse, R.R. (1989). Qualitative research: Publishing and funding [Editorial]. *Nursing Science Quarterly*, 2(1), 1–2.

*Payne, G. (1973). Comparative sociology: Some problems of theory and method. *British Journal of Sociology*, 24(1), 13–29.

Phillips, J.R. (1989). Qualitative research: A process of discovery. *Nursing Science Quarterly*, 2(1), 5–6.

Phillips, J.R. (1989). Science of unitary human beings: Changing research perspectives. *Nursing Science Quarterly*, 2(2), 57–60.

Phillips, J.R. (1995). Nursing theory-based research for advanced nursing practice. *Nursing Science Quarterly*, 8, 4–5.

*Quint, J.C. (1967). The case for theories generated from empirical data. *Nursing Research*, 16(2), 109–114.

Roberts, K.L. (1999). Through a looking glass: Nursing theory and clinical nursing research. *Clinical Nursing Research*, 8(4), 299–301.

Rubin, R. and Erickson, F. (1978). Research in clinical nursing. *Journal of Advanced Nursing*, 3(2), 131–144.

Salsberry, P.J., Smith, M.C., and Boyd, C.O. (1989). Phenomenological research in nursing: Commentary and responses. *Nursing Science Quarterly*, 2(1), 9–19.

Santopinto, M.D. (1989). The relentless drive to be ever thinner: A study using the phenomenological method. *Nursing Science Quarterly*, 2(1), 29–36.

Schlotfeldt, R.M. (1975). The conceptual framework of nursing research: The need for a conceptual framework. In P.J. Verhonick (Ed.), *Nursing research*. Boston: Little, Brown.

Seng, J.S. (1998). Praxis as a conceptual framework for participatory research in nursing. *Advances in Nursing Science*, 20(4), 37–48.

*Silva, M.C. (1977). Philosophy, science, theory: Interrelationships and implications for nursing research. *Image: Journal of Nursing Scholarship*, 9(3), 59–63.

Treece, E.W. and Treece, J.W. (1977). Theory and method. In *Elements of research in nursing* (2nd ed.). St. Louis, MO: C.V. Mosby.

Verran, J.A. (1997). The value of theory-driven (rather than problem-driven) research. *Seminars for Nurse Managers*, 5(4), 169–172.

Whitney, J.D. (1999). Spotlight on research. Thoughts on theory. *Journal of Wound, Ostomy, and Continence Nursing*, 26(5), 228–229.

Williamson, G.J. (2000). The test of a nursing theory: A personal view. *Nursing Science Quarterly*, 13(2), 124–128.

Willman, A. (2000). Nursing theory in education, practice, and research in Sweden. *Nursing Science Quarterly*, 13(3), 263–265.

Zelauskas, B.A., Howes, D.G., Christmyer, C.S., and Dennis, K.E. (1988). Bridging the gap: Theory to practice-Part II, Research applications. *Nursing Management*, 19(9), 50–52.

8. Theory and Practice

Adam, E. (1983). Frontiers of nursing in the 21st century: Development of models and theories on the concept of nursing. *Journal of Advanced Nursing*, 8, 41–45.

Aggleton, P. and Chalmers, H. (1987). Models of nursing, nursing practice and nursing education. *Journal of Advanced Nursing*, 12(5), 573–581.

Alligood, M.R. (1997). Models and theories: Critical thinking structures. In M .R. Alligood et al. (Eds.), *Nursing theory: Utilization and application* (pp. 31–45). St. Louis, MO: Mosby Year Book.

Alligood, M.R. (1997). Models and theories in nursing practice. In M.R. Alligood et al. (Eds.), *Nursing theory: Utilization and application* (pp. 15–30). St. Louis, MO: Mosby Year Book.

Anderson, K.H. (2000). The Family Health System approach to family systems nursing. *Journal of Family Nursing*, 6(2), 103–119.

Arndt, C. and Huckabay, L.M.D. (1975). Administrative theory within a systems' frame of reference. In *Nursing administration: Theory for practice with a systems approach* (pp. 18–44). St. Louis, MO: C.V. Mosby.

Aveyard, H. (2000). Is there a concept of autonomy that can usefully inform nursing practice? *Journal of Advanced Nursing*, 32(2), 352–358.

Baer, E.D. (1987). "A cooperative venture" in pursuit of professional status: A research journal for nursing. *Nursing Research*, 36(1), 18–25.

Baines, L. (1998). Researchers must reach across the practice-theory divide. *Nursing Times*, 94(38), 21.

Barker, P.J., Reynolds, W., and Stevenson, C. (1997). The human science basis of psychiatric nursing: Theory and practice. *Journal of Advanced Nursing*, 25, 660–667.

Barnard, K.E. (1980). Knowledge for practice: Directions for the future. *Nursing Research*, 29(4), 208–212.

Barton, J.A. and Brown, N.J. (1995). Home visitation to migrant farm worker families: An application of Zerwekh's family caregiving model for public health nursing. *Holistic Nursing Practice*, 9(4), 34–40.

Baumann, S.L. and Carroll, K. (2001). Human becoming practice with children. *Nursing Science Quarterly*, 14(2), 120–125.

*Beckstrand, J. (1978). The notion of a practice theory and the relationship of scientific and ethical knowledge to practice. *Research in Nursing and Health*, 1(3), 131–136.

*Beckstrand, J. (1978). The need for a practice theory as indicated by the knowledge used in the conduct of practice. *Research in Nursing and Health*, 1(4), 175–180.

*Beckstrand, J. (1980). A critique of several conceptions of practice theory in nursing. *Research in Nursing and Health*, 3, 69–79.

Bellin, C., Gagnon, M., Mich, M., Plemmons, S., and Watanabe-Hayami, C. (1997). Ecologic health nursing for community health: Applied chaos theory. *Complexity and Chaos in Nursing*, 3, 13–22.

Bergen, A. (1995). Clinical notes. Theory and practice: Maintaining and facilitating the links after qualifying—The lecturer's view. *Journal of Clinical Nursing*, 4(1), 4.

Berragan, L. (1998). Nursing practice draws upon several different ways of knowing. *Journal of Clinical Nursing*, 7(3), 209–217.

Billings, J.R. (1995). Bonding theory-tying mothers in knots? A critical review of the application of a theory to nursing. *Journal of Clinical Nursing*, 4, 207–211.

Bottorff, J.L. (1991). Nursing: A practical science of caring. *Advances in Nursing Science*, 14(1), 26–39.

Boykin, A. and Schoenhofer, S. (1990). Caring in nursing: Analysis of extant theory. *Nursing Science Quarterly*, 3, 149–155.

Boykin, A. and Schoenhofer, S. O. (1991). Story as link between nursing practice, ontology, epistemology. *Image: Journal of Nursing Scholarship*, 23, 245–248.

Boykin, A. and Schoenhofer, S. (1994). Nursing as caring: A model for transforming practice. *Nursing Science Quarterly*, 7, 183–185.

Bradshaw, A. (1995). What are nurses doing to patients? A review of theories or nursing past and present. *Journal of Clinical Nursing*, 4, 81–92.

Brasell-Brian, R. and Wong, R.Y. (2002). Fears and worries associated with hypoglycaemia and diabetes complications: Perceptions and experience of Hong Kong Chinese clients. *Journal of Advanced Nursing,* 39(2), 155–163.

Brophy, M.S.S. (2001). Nurse advocacy in the neonatal unit: Putting theory into practice. *Journal of Neonatal Nursing,* 7(1), 10–12.

Buchanam, B.F. (1987). Conceptual models: An assessment framework. *Journal of Nursing Administration,* 17(10), 22–26.

Buchmann, W.F. (1997). Adherence: A matter of self-efficacy and power. *Journal of Advanced Nursing,* 26(1), 132–137.

Burns, C., Archbold, P., Stewart, B., and Shelton, K. (1993). New diagnosis: Caregiver role strain. *Nursing Diagnosis,* 4(2), 70–76.

Byers, J.F. and Smyth, K.A. (1997). Application of a transactional model of stress and coping with critically ill patients. *Dimensions of Critical Care Nursing,* 16(6), 292–300.

Carr, E.C.J. (1996). Reflecting on clinical practice: Hectoring talk or reality? *Journal of Clinical Nursing,* 5(5), 289–295.

Cassidy, C.A. (1999). Using the transtheoeretical model to facilitate behavior change in patients with chronic illness. *Journal of the American Academy of Nurse Practitioners,* 11(7), 281–287.

Chapman, J.S., Mitchell, G.J., and Forchuk C. (1994). A glimpse of nursing theory-based practice in Canada. *Nursing Science Quarterly,* 7, 104–112.

Clarke, M. (1986). Action and reflection: Practice and theory in nursing. *Journal of Advanced Nursing,* 11, 3–11.

Clarke, P.N. and Cody, W.K. (1994). Nursing theory-based practice in the home and community: The crux of professional nursing education. *Advances in Nursing Science,* 17, 41–53.

Clifford, C. (1995). Caring: Fitting the concept to nursing practice. *Journal of Clinical Nursing,* 4, 37–41.

Cody, W.K. (1994). Nursing theory-guided practice: What it is and what it is not. *Nursing Science Quarterly,* 7, 144–145.

Cody, W.K. (2001). Bearing witness-not bearing witness as a synergistic individual-community becoming. *Nursing Science Quarterly,* 14(2), 94–100.

Cohen, J.A. (1991). Two portraits of caring: A comparison of the artists, Leininger and Watson. *Journal of Advanced Nursing,* 16(8), 899–909.

Christmyer, C.S., Catanzariti, P.M., Langford, A.M., and Reitz, J.A. (1988). Bridging the gap: Theory to practice—Part I, Clinical applications. *Nursing Management,* 19(8), 42–43, 46–48, 50.

Craig, S.L. (1980). Theory development and its relevance for nursing. *Journal of Advanced Nursing,* 5, 349–355.

Creamer, E. (2000). Examining the care of patients with peripheral venous cannulas. *British Journal of Nursing,* 9(20), 2128, 2130, 2132.

Curtin, L.L. (1988). Thought-full nursing practice [Editorial]. *Nursing Management,* 19(10), 7–8.

Daly, J. and Jackson, D. (1999). On the use of nursing theory in nurse education, nursing practice, and nursing research in Australia. *Nursing Science Quarterly,* 12(4), 342–345.

Davhana-Maselesele, M. Tjallinks, J.E and Norval, M.S. (2001). Theory-practice integration in selected clinical situations. *Curationis: South African Journal of Nursing*, 24(4), 4–9.

Davies, C., Welham, V., Glover, A., Jones, L., and Murphy F. (1999). Teaching in practice. *Nursing Standard*, 13(35), 33–38.

Davis, A.J. (1978). The phenomenological approach. In N.L. Chaska (Ed.), *The nursing profession: Views through the mist*. New York: McGraw-Hill.

Davies, B. and Hughes, A.M. (1995). Clarification of advanced nursing practice: Characteristics and competencies. *Clinical Nurse Specialist*, 9(3), 156–160.

DeGroot, H.A., Ferketich, S.L., and Larson, P.J. (1987). Theory development in a non-university service setting. *Journal of Nursing Administration*, 17(4), 38–44.

Derstine, J.B. (1989). The development of theory-based practice by graduate students in rehabilitation nursing. *Rehabilitation Nursing*, 14(2), 88–89.

DeSocio, J. and Sebastian, L. (1988). Towards a theoretical model for clinical nursing practice at Menningers. *Kansas Nurse*, 63(12), 4–5.

Dhasaradhan, I. (2001). Application of nursing theory into practice. *Nursing Journal of India*, 92(10), 224, 236.

Dickinson, J.K. (1999). A critical social theory approach to nursing care of adolescents with diabetes. *Issues in Comprehensive Pediatric Nursing*, 22(4), 143–152.

*Dickoff, J., James, P., and Wiedenbach, E. (1968). Theory in a practice discipline: Part I. Practice oriented theory. *Nursing Research*, 17(5), 415–435.

*Dickoff, J., James, P, and Wiedenbach, E. (1968). Theory in a practice discipline: Part II. Practice oriented research. *Nursing Research*, 17(6), 545–554.

Dodd, M.J. and Miaskowski, C. (2000). The PRO-SELF program: A self-care intervention program for patients receiving cancer treatment. *Seminars in Oncology Nursing*, 16(4), 300–314.

Duffy, K. and Scott, P.A. (1998). Viewing an old issue through a new lens: A critical theory insight into the education-practice gap. *Nurse Education Today*, 18(3), 183–189.

Edwards, S.D., Benner, P., and Wrubel, J. (2001). Benner and Wrubel on caring in nursing. *Journal of Advanced Nursing* 33(2), 167–174.

Emblen, J. and Pesut, B. (2001). Strengthening transcendent meaning: A model for the spiritual nursing care of patients experiencing suffering. *Journal of Holistic Nursing*, 19(1), 42–56.

Fawcett, J. (1980). A declaration of nursing independence: The relation of theory and research to nursing practice. *Journal of Nursing Administration*, 10(6), 36–39.

Fawcett, J., Watson, J., Neuman, B., Walker, P.H., and Fitzpatrick, J.J. (2001). On nursing theories and evidence. *Journal of Nursing Scholarship*, 33(2), 115–119.

Fealey, G. (1997). The theory-practice relationship in nursing: An exploration of contemporary discourse. *Journal of Advanced Nursing*, 25, 1061–1069.

Fealey, G. (1999). The theory-practice relationship in nursing: The practitioners' perspective. *Journal of Advanced Nursing*, 30(1), 74–82.

Feldman, M.E. (1993). Uncovering clinical knowledge and caring practices. *Journal of Post Anesthesia Nursing*, 8(3), 159–162.

Field, P.A. (1987). The impact of nursing theory on the clinical decision making process. *Journal of Advanced Nursing*, 12(5), 563–571.

Field, L., and Winslow, E.H. (1985). Moving to a nursing model. *American Journal of Nursing,* 85(10), 1100–1101.

Fielding, R.G. and Llewelyn, S.P. (1987). Communication in nursing may damage your health and enthusiasm: Some warnings. *Journal of Advanced Nursing Science,* 12(3), 281–290.

Fitzpatrick, J.J. (1988). How can we enhance nursing knowledge and practice? *Nursing and Health Care,* 9(9), 517–521.

Flaskerud, J.H. (2000). Building excellence and scholarship with vulnerable populations: Overview . . . 33rd Annual Communicating Nursing Research Conference/14th Annual WIN Assembly, "Building on a Legacy of Excellence in Nursing Research," held April 13–15, 2000 at the Adam's Mark Hotel, Denver, Colorado. *Communicating Nursing Research,* 33, 102.

Forbes, D.A., King, K.M., Kushner, K.E., Letourneau, N.L., Myrick, A.F., and Profetto-McGrath, J. (1999). Warrantable evidence in nursing science. *Journal of Advanced Nursing,* 29(2), 373–379.

Friedmann, M.L. (1989). Closing the gap between grand theory and mental health practice with families. Part I: The framework of systemic organization for nursing of families and family members. *Archives of Psychiatric Nursing,* 3(1), 10–19.

Friedmann, M.L. (1989) The concept of family nursing. *Journal of Advanced Nursing,* 14(3), 211–216.

Frissell, S. (1988). So many models, so much confusion. *Nursing Administration Quarterly,* 12(2), 13–17.

Gaudine, A.P. (2001). Demonstrating theory in practice: Examples of the McGill Model of Nursing. *Journal of Continuing Education in Nursing,* 32(2), 77–85.

Geden, E.A, Isaramalai, S., and Taylor, S.G. (2001). Self-care deficit nursing theory and the nurse practitioner's practice in primary care settings. *Nursing Science Quarterly,* 14(1), 29–33.

Gendron, D. (1994). The tapestry of care. *Advances in Nursing Science,* 17(1), 25–30.

Goode, H. (1998). The theory-practice gap and student nurses. *Journal of Child Health Care,* 2(2), 86–90.

Gordon, M., Murphy, C. P., Candee, D., and Hiltunen, E. (1994). Clinical judgment: An integrated model. *Advances in Nursing Science,* 16(4), 55–70.

Gottlieb, L. and Lowat, K. (1987). The McGill model of nursing: A practice-derived model. *Advances in Nursing Science,* 9(4), 51–61.

Gottlieb, L.N. and Feeley, N. (1996). The McGill Model of Nursing and children with a chronic condition: "Who benefits, and why?" *Canadian Journal of Nursing Research,* 28(3), 29–48.

Green-Hernandez, C. (1997). Application of caring theory in primary care: A challenge for advanced practice. *Nursing Administration Quarterly,* 21(4), 77–82.

Greenwood, E. (1961). The practice of science and the science of practice. In W.G. Bennis, K.D. Benne, and R. Chin (Eds.), *The planning of change.* New York: Holt, Rinehart & Winston.

Gruending, D.L. (1986). Nursing theory: A vehicle of professionalization. *Journal of Advanced Nursing Science,* 10(6), 553–558.

Hampton, D.C. (1994). Expertise: The true essence of nursing art. *Advances in Nursing Science,* 17(1), 15–24.

Hanchett, E.S. and Clark, P.N. (1988). Nursing theory and public health science: Is synthesis possible? *Public Health Nursing*, 5(1), 2–6.

Harbison J. (2001). Clinical decision making in nursing: Theoretical perspectives and their relevance to practice. *Journal of Advanced Nursing*, 35(1), 126–133.

Harrell, J.S. (1986). Needed nurse engineers to link theory and practice. *Nursing Outlook*, 34(4), 196–198.

Harrison, J., Saunders, M.E., and Sims, A. (1977). Integrating theory and practice in modular schemes for basic nurse education. *Journal of Advanced Nursing*, 2, 503–519.

Hathaway, D. and Strong, M. (1988). Theory, practice, and research in transplant nursing. *American Nephrology Nurses Association Journal*, 15(1), 9–12.

Henderson, B. (1978). Nursing diagnosis: Theory and practice. *Advances in Nursing Science*, 1(1), 75–82.

Hinshaw, A.S. (1987). Response to "Structuring the nursing knowledge system: A typology of four domains." *Scholarly Inquiry for Nursing Practice*, 1(2), 111–114.

Holmes, C.A. and Warelow, P.J. (2000). Some implications of postmodernism for nursing theory, research, and practice. *Canadian Journal of Nursing Research*, 32(2), 89–101.

Hopkins, S. and McSherry, R. (2000).Is there a great divide between nursing theory and practice? *Nursing Times*, 96(17), 16.

Horsfall, J. (1997). Women's depression: Nursing theory and practice. *Contemporary Nurse*, 6(3–4), 129–135.

Hsieh, H. (2001). Letter to the editor . . . "The role of nursing theory in standards of practice: A Canadian perspective." *Nursing Science Quarterly*, 14(4), 367–368.

Huggins, E.A. and Scalzi, C.C. (1988). Limitations and alternatives: Ethical practice theory in nursing. *Advances in Nursing Science*, 10(4), 43–47.

Jacobs, B.B. (2001). Respect for human dignity: A central phenomenon to philosophically unite nursing theory and practice through consilience of knowledge. *Advances in Nursing Science*, 24(1), 17–35.

*Jacobs, M.K. and Huether, S.E. (1978) Nursing science: The theory-practice linkage. *Advances in Nursing Science*, 1(1), 63–73.

Jameton, A. and Fowler, M.D. (1989). Ethical inquiry and concept of research. *Advanced Nursing Science*, 11(3), 11–24.

Jennings, B.M. and Meleis, A.I. (1988). Nursing theory and administrative practice: Agenda for the 1990s. *Advances in Nursing Science*, 10(3), 56–69.

Jenny, J. and Logan, J. (1992). Knowing the patient: One aspect of clinical knowledge. *Image: Journal of Nursing Scholarship*, 24, 254–258.

Johnson, D. (1987). Evaluating conceptual models for use in critical care nursing practice. *Dimensions of Critical Care Nursing*, 6(4), 195–197.

Johnson, J.L. (1994). A dialectical examination of nursing art. *Advances in Nursing Science*, 17(1), 1–14.

Johnson, S.E. (1989). A picture is worth a thousand words: Helping students visualize a conceptual model. *Nurse Educator*, 14(3), 21–24.

Jones, S. (1989). Practice and theory. Is unity possible? *Nursing Standard*, 3(18), 22–23.

Kasch, C. (1984). Interpersonal competence and communication in the delivery of nursing care. *Advances in Nursing Science*, 6(2), 71–88.

Kathol, D.D., Geiger, M.L., and Hartig, J.L. (1998). Clinical correlation map. A tool for linking theory and practice. *Nurse Educator*, 23(4), 31–34.

Ketefian, S. (1987). A case study of theory development: Moral behavior in nursing. *Advances in Nursing Science*, 9(2), 10–19.

Khatib, H.M. and Ford, S. (1999). The theory-practice gap receives much attention in the press and in discussions—What does it mean? *Journal of Child Health Care*, 3(2), 36–38.

Kim, H.S. (1987). Response to "Structuring the nursing knowledge system: A typology of four domains." *Scholarly Inquiry for Nursing Practice*, 1(2), 111–114.

Kim, H.S. (1993). Putting theory into practice: Problems and prospects. *Journal of Advanced Nursing*, 18, 1632–1639.

Kim, H.S. (1994). Action science as an approach to develop knowledge for nursing practice. *Nursing Science Quarterly*, 7, 134–140.

Kim, HS. (1999). Critical reflective inquiry for knowledge development in nursing practice. *Journal of Advanced Nursing*, 29(5), 1205–1212.

Kite, K. and Pearson, L. (1995). A rationale for mouth care: The integration of theory with practice. *Intensive and Critical Care Nursing*, 11(2), 71–76.

Kristjanson, L.J., Tamblyn, R., and Kuypers, J.A. (1987). A model to guide development and application of multiple nursing theories. *Journal of Advanced Nursing*, 12(4), 523–529.

Landers, M. (2001). The theory/practice gap in nursing: The views of the students. *All Ireland Journal Nursing Midwifery*, 1(4), 142–147.

Laurent, C.L. (2000). A nursing theory for nursing leadership. *Journal of Nursing Management*, 8(2), 83–87.

Lewis, T. (1988). Leaping the chasm between nursing theory and practice. *Journal of Advanced Nursing*, 13(3), 345–351.

Litchfield, M. (1999). Practice wisdom. *Advances in Nursing Science*, 22(2), 62–73.

Lo, R. and Brown, R. (1999). The importance of theory in student nurses' psychiatric practicum. *International Journal of Psychiatric Nursing Research*, 5(1), 542–552.

Long, G.E. (1985). Professional advancement: Theory development through practice and research. *ANA Journal*, 12(1), 35–38.

Mathwig, G. (1971). Nursing science: The theoretical core of nursing knowledge. *Image: Journal of Nursing Scholarship, 4(1), 20–23.*

McBride, A.B. and McBride, W.L. (1981). Theoretical underpinnings for women's health. *Women and Health*, 6, 37–55.

*McCarthy, R.T. (1972). A practice theory of nursing care. *Nursing Research*, 21(5), 406–410.

McFarlane, J.K. (1977). Developing a theory of nursing: The relationship of theory to practice, education, and research. *Journal of Advanced Nursing*, 2(3), 261–270.

McIver, M. (1987). Putting theory into practice. *Canadian Nurse*, 83(10), 36–38.

McKenna, B. and Roberts, R. (1999). Bridging the theory-practice gap. *Nursing New Zealand*, 5(2), 14–16.

Meleis, A.I., Isenberg, M., Koerner, J.E., Lacey, B., and Stern, P. (1995). *Diversity, marginalization, and culturally competent health care issues in knowledge development.* Washington, DC: American Academy of Nursing.

Miller, S.R. (1978). Have we dichotomized theory and practice in nursing? *Nursing Leadership*, 1(1), 34–36.

Mitchell, G.J., Closson, T., Coulis, N., Flint, F., and Gray, B. (2000). Patient-focused care and human becoming thought: Connecting the right stuff. *Nursing Science Quarterly*, 13(3), 216–224.

Moch, S. D. (1990). Personal knowing: Evolving research and practice. *Scholarly Inquiry for Nursing Practice*, 4, 155–165.

Moody, L.E., Wilson, M.E., Smith, K., Schwartz, R., Tittle, M., and Van Cott, M.L. (1988). Analysis of a decade of nursing practice research: 1977–1986. *Nursing Research*, 37(6), 374–379.

Moore, M.A. (1968). Nursing: A scientific discipline? *Nursing Forum*, 7(4), 340–348.

Morse, J. M., Bottorff, J., Neander, W., and Solberg, S. (1991). Comparative analysis of conceptualizations and theories of caring. *Image: Journal of Nursing Scholarship*, 23, 119–126.

Morse, J.M., Solberg, S.M., Neander, W.L., Bottorff, J.L., and Johnson, J.L. (1990). Concepts of caring and caring as concept. *Advances in Nursing Science*, 13(1), 1–14.

Mulhall, A. (1997). Nursing research: Our world not theirs? *Journal of Advanced Nursing*, 25(5), 969–976.

Munhall, P.L. (1989). Philosophical pondering on qualitative research methods in nursing. *Nursing Science Quarterly,* 2(1), 20–28.

Munhall, P. L. (1993). Unknowing: Toward another pattern of knowing in nursing. *Nursing Outlook*, 41, 125–128.

Munnukka, T., Pukuri, T., Linnainmaa, P., and Kilkku, N. (2002). Integration of theory and practice in learning mental health nursing. *Journal of Psychiatric and Mental Health Nursing*, 9(1), 5–14.

Neal, J.E. (2001). Patient outcomes: A matter of perspective. *Nursing Outlook*, 49(2), 93–99.

Newman, M. A. (1994). Theory for nursing practice. *Nursing Science Quarterly*, 7(4), 153–157.

O'Brien, B. and Pearson, A. (1993). Unwritten knowledge in nursing: Consider the spoken as well as the written word. *Scholarly Inquiry for Nursing Practice*, 7, 111–127.

Olson, T. C. (1993). Laying claim to caring: Nursing and the language of training, 1915–1937. *Nursing Outlook*, 41, 68–72.

Patistea, E. (1999). Nurses' perceptions of caring as documented in theory and research. *Journal of Clinical Nursing*, 8(5), 487–495.

Pearson, A. (2002). Nursing in theory and in practice. *International Journal of Nursing Practice*, 8(3), 117.

Phillips, R., Donald, A. Mousseau-Gershman, Y. and Powell, T. (1998). Applying theory to practice—The use of "ripple effect" plans in continuing education. *Nurse Education Today*, 18(1), 12–19.

Raudonis, B.M. and Acton, G.J. (1997). Theory-based nursing practice. *Journal of Advanced Nursing,* 26(1), 138–145.

Raymond, D.P. (1995). Esthetic and personal knowledge through humanistic nursing. *N&HC Perspectives on Community*, 16(6), 332–336.

Rawnsley, M. (1990). Of human bonding: The context of nursing as caring. *Advances in Nursing Science*, 13(1), 41–48.

Rew, L., Stuppy, D., and Becker, H. (1988). Construct validity in instrument development: A vital link between nursing practice, research, and theory. *Advances in Nursing Science*, 10(4), 10–22.

Robb, Y.A. (1997). Have nursing models a place in intensive care units? *Intensive and Critical Care Nursing*, 13(2), 93–98.

Rodgers, J.A. (1976). Today's preparation for tomorrow's practice. The Lehman College nursing program. *Journal of Advanced Nursing*, 1(4), 311–322.

Rodgers, S.J. (2000). The role of nursing theory in standards of practice: A Canadian perspective. *Nursing Science Quarterly*, 13(3), 260–262.

Rolfe, G. (1997). Beyond expertise: Theory, practice and the reflexive practitioner. *Journal of Clinical Nursing*, 6(2), 93–97.

Rolfe, G. (1998). The theory-practice gap in nursing: From research-based practice to practitioner-based research. *Journal of Advanced Nursing*, 28(3), 672–679.

Romeo, J.H. (2000). Comprehensive versus holistic care: Case studies of chronic disease. *Journal of Holistic Nursing*, 18(4), 352–361.

Roper, N. (1966). A model for nursing and nursology. *Journal of Advanced Nursing*, 1(2), 219–227.

Rosswurm, M.A. and Larrabee, J.H. (1999). A model for change to evidence-based practice. *Image: Journal of Nursing Scholarship*, 31(4), 317–322.

Roy, C. and Obby, S.M. (1978). The practitioner movement: Toward a science of nursing. *American Journal of Nursing*, 78(10), 1698–1702.

Saewyc, E.M. (2000). Nursing theories of caring: A paradigm for adolescent nursing practice. *Journal of Holistic Nursing*, 18(2), 114–128.

Santopinto, M.D. (1989). The relentless drive to be ever thinner: A study using the phenomenological method. *Nursing Science Quarterly*, 2(1), 29–36.

Sarter, B. (1987). Evolutionary idealism: A philosophical foundation for holistic nursing theory. *Advances in Nursing Science*, 9(2), 1–9.

Schafer, P.J. (1987). Philosophic analysis of a theory of clinical nursing. *Maternal-Child Nursing Journal*, 16(4), 289–363.

Schultz, P.R. (1987). When client means more than one: Extending the foundational concept of person. *Advances in Nursing Science*, 10(1), 71–86.

Schutzenhofer, K. K. (1991). Scholarly pursuit in the clinical setting: An obligation of professional nursing. *Journal of Professional Nursing*, 7, 10–15.

Schwartz-Barcott, D., Patterson, B.J., Lusardi, P., and Farmer, B.C. (2002). From practice to theory: Tightening the link via three fieldwork strategies. *Journal of Advanced Nursing*, 39(3), 281–289.

Severinsson, E.I. (1998). Bridging the gap between theory and practice: A supervision programme for nursing students. *Journal of Advanced Nursing*, 27(6), 1269–1277.

Shouli, C. (2001). Letter to the editor . . . "Nursing theory-guided practice: What it is and what is it not" by William K. Cody (1994). *Nursing Science Quarterly*, 14(2), 175.

Simpson, P., Chan, M.C., Cheung, L.Y., Hui, T.S., Li, K.Y., Tang, H.T., Tong, N.H., Wong, S.K., and Wong P.M. (2002). Primary health care theory to practice: Experience of first-year nursing students in Hong Kong. *Journal of Nursing Education*, 41(7), 302–309.

Smith, M.C. (1995). The core of advanced practice nursing. *Nursing Science Quarterly*, 8, 2–3.

Spouse, J. (2001). Bridging theory and practice in the supervisory relationship: A sociocultural perspective. *Journal of Advanced Nursing*, 33(4), 512–522.

Stark, S., Cooke, P., and Stronach, I. (2000). Minding the gap: Some theory-practice disjunctions in nursing education research. *Nurse Education Today*, 20(2), 155–163.

Street, A.F. (1992). *Inside nursing: A critical ethnography of clinical nursing practice.* Albany, NY: State University of New York Press.

Taylor-Piliae, R.E. (1998). Establishing evidence-based practice: Issues and implications in critical care nursing. *Intensive and Critical Care Nursing*, 14(1), 30–37.

Timpson, J. (1996). Nursing theory: Everything the artist spits is art? *Journal of Advanced Nursing*, 23(5), 1030–1036.

Titler, M.G., Buckwalter, K.C., and Maas, M.L. (1993). Critical issues for the development of clinical nursing knowledge. *Advances in Clinical Nursing Research*, 28(2), 475–477.

Topham, D.L. and DeSilva, P. (1988). Evaluating congruency between steps in the research process. A critique guide for use in clinical nursing practice. *Clinical Nurse Specialist*, 2(2), 97–102.

Upton, D.J. (1999). How can we achieve evidence-based practice if we have a theory-practice gap in nursing today? *Journal of Advanced Nursing*, 29(3), 549–555.

Visintainer, M.A. (1986). The nature of nursing and theory in nursing. *Image: Journal of Nursing Scholarship*, 18(2), 32–38.

Wald, F.S. and Leonard, R.C. (1971). Toward development of nursing practice theory. *Nursing Research*, 20(5), 428–435.

Welch, J.L., Jeffries, P.R., Lyon, B.L., Boland, D.L., and Backer, J.H. (2001). Experiential learning: Integrating theory and research into practice. *Nurse Educator*, 26(5), 240–243.

Welford, C. (2002). Transformational leadership in nursing: Matching theory to practice. *Nursing Management*, 9(4), 7–11.

Westbrook, L.O. and Schultz, P.R. (2000). From theory to practice: Community health nursing in a public health neighborhood team. *Advances in Nursing Science*, 23(2), 50–61.

Wilcox, V. (1995). Theory and practice: Maintaining and facilitating the links after qualifying-the practitioner's view. *Journal of Clinical Nursing*, 4, 3–4.

Yian, L.G. (2002). Theory-practice quandary. *Singapore Nursing Journal*, 29(1), 21–26.

Young, J. (1995). Bridging the theory-practice gap: Strategies to reduce the gap between research and practice in neonatal intensive care. *Journal of Neonatal Nursing*, 1(2), 16–20.

Zelauskas, B.A., Howes, D.G., Christmyer, C.S., and Dennis, K.E. (1988). Bridging the gap: Theory to practice—Part II, Research applications. *Nursing Management*, 19(8), 42–43, 46–48, 50.

9. Theory and Nursing Taxonomies: Diagnosis and Intervention

Auvil-Novak, S.E. (1997). A middle-range theory of chronotherapeutic intervention for postsurgical pain. *Nursing Research*, 46(2), 66–71.

Barker, P.J., Keady, J., Croom, S., Stevenson, C., Adams, T., and Reynolds, W. (1998). The concept of serious mental illness: Modern myths and grim realities. *Journal of Psychiatric and Mental Health Nursing*, 5(4), 247–254.

Barker, P.J., Reynolds, W., and Stevenson, C. (1997). The human science basis of psychiatric nursing: Theory and practice. *Journal of Advanced Nursing*, 25(4), 660–667.

Barry, P. (1996). Integrating the Barry holistic system an the NANDA nursing diagnosis models. In P.D. Barry (Ed.), *Psychological nursing: Care of the physically ill patients and their families* (3rd ed.). Philadelphia: Lippincott.

Batra, C. (1996). Nursing theory and nursing process in the community. In J.M. Cookfair (Ed.), *Nursing care in the community* (pp. 85–124). St. Louis, MO: Mosby Year Book.

Blegen, M.A. and Tripp-Reimer, T. (1997). Implications of nursing taxonomies for middle-range theory development. *Advances in Nursing Science*, 19(3), 37–49.

Bliss-Holtz, J. (1996). Using Orem's theory to generate nursing diagnoses for electronic documentation. *Nursing Science Quarterly*, 9(3), 121–125.

Brown, R. (2000). Describing a model of nursing as a focus for psychiatric nursing care. *International Journal of Psychiatric Nursing Research*, 6(1), 670–682.

Buckingham, C.D. and Adams, A. (2000). Classifying clinical decision making: Interpreting nursing intuition, heuristics and medical diagnosis. *Journal of Advanced Nursing*, 32(4), 990–998.

Burns, C., Archbold, P., Stewart, B., and Shelton, K. (1993). New diagnosis: Caregiver role strain. *Nursing Diagnosis*, 4(2), 70–76.

Burrell, M. and Hurm, R. (1999). Care of the patient with interstitial cystitis: Current theories and management. *Journal of PeriAnesthesia Nursing*, 14(1), 17–22.

Canuso, R. (1997). Rethinking behavior disorders: Whose attention has a deficit? *Journal of Psychosocial Nursing and Mental Health Services*, 35(4), 24–29.

Carlson-Catalano, J. (1997). Nursing diagnoses and interventions for post-acute phase battered women. In M.J. Rantz et al. (Eds.), *Classification of nursing diagnoses: Proceedings of the twelfth conference, North American Nursing Diagnosis Association*, p. 209.

Carpenito, L.J. (1997). Defining nursing expertise in a multidiscipline health care arena. In M.J. Rantz et al. (Eds.), *Classification of nursing diagnoses: Proceedings of the twelfth conference, North American Nursing Diagnosis Association*, pp. 48–56.

Cavendish, R., Luise, B.K., Horne, K., Bauer, M., Medefindt, J., Gallo, M.A., Calvino, C., and Kutza, T. (2000). Opportunities for enhanced spirituality relevant to well adults. *Nursing Diagnosis*, 11(4), 151–163.

Chambers, M. (1998). Interpersonal mental health nursing: Research issues and challenges. *Journal of Psychiatric and Mental Health Nursing*, 5(3), 203–211.

Chater, K. (1999). Risk and representation: Older people and noncompliance. *Nursing Inquiry*, 6(2), 132–138.

Clark, D.J. (1997). The International Classification for Nursing Practice: A progress report. *Studies in Health Technologies and Informatics*, 46, 62–68.

Conley, V.M. (1998). Beyond knowledge deficit to a proposal for information-seeking behaviors. *Nursing Diagnosis*, 9(4), 129–135.

Cutler, L. (2000). Reflection on diagnosing as a nurse in ITU, including commentary by Johns, C. (2000). *Nursing in Critical Care*, 5(1), 22–30.

Daly, J.M. (1997). How nursing interventions classification fits in the patient information system Patient Core Data Set. *Computers in Nursing*, 15(2 Suppl), S77-S81.

Daly, J.M., Maas, M.L., and Johnson, M. (1997). Nursing outcomes classification. An essential element in data sets for nursing and health care effectiveness. *Computers in Nursing*, 15(2 Suppl), S82-S86.

Davis, P. (1999). Using models and theories in orthopaedic nursing. *Journal of Orthopaedic Nursing*, 3, Suppl. 1, 3–8.

Davis, R. (2000). Holographic community: Reconceptualizing the meaning of community in an era of health care reform. *Nursing Outlook*, 48(6), 294–301.

Dijkstra, A., Buist, G., and Dassen, T. (1998). Operationalization of the concept of "nursing care dependency" for use in long-term care facilities. *Australian and New Zealand Journal of Mental Health Nursing*, 7(4), 142–151.

Dougherty, C.M., Jankin, J.K., Lunney, M.R., and Whitley, G.G. (1993). Conceptual and research based validation of nursing diagnoses: 1950 to 1993. *Nursing Diagnosis*, 4(4), 156–165.

Durand, M. and Prince, R. (1966). Nursing diagnostics: Process and decision. *Nursing Forum*, 5(4), 50–64.

Eisenhauer, L.A. (1994). A typology of nursing therapeutics. *Image: Journal of Nursing Scholarship*, 26, 261–264.

Elliot, T. (1995). Impaired adjustment related to inappropriate utilization of resources: A down under diagnosis . . . "Implementation strategies and use of nursing diagnosis in tertiary institutions and major teaching hospitals throughout Australia." In M.J. Rantz et al. (Eds.), *Classification of nursing diagnoses: Proceedings of the eleventh conference, North American Nursing Diagnosis Association*, pp. 189–198.

Fagerstrom, L. and Engberg, I.B. (1998). Measuring the unmeasurable: A caring science perspective on patient classification. *Journal of Nursing Management*, 6(3), 165–172.

Fagerstrom, L, Rainio, A.K., Rauhala, A., and Nojonen, K. (2000). Validation of a new method for patient classification, the Oulu Patient Classification. *Journal of Advanced Nursing*, 31(2), 481–490.

Fishel, A.H. (1998). Nursing management of anxiety and panic. *Nursing Clinics of North America*, 33(1), 135–151.

Fitzpatrick, J.J. and Zanotti, R. (1995). Where are we now? Nursing diagnosis internationally. *Nursing Diagnosis*, 6(1), 42–47.

Fredericks, D.W. and Williams, W.L. (1998). New definition of mental retardation for the American Association of Mental Retardation. *Image: Journal of Nursing Scholarship*, 30(1), 53–56.

Frisch, N. (1995). Nursing diagnosis and nursing theory—What does it really mean to combine the two? *Nursing Diagnosis*, 6(2), 51.

Frisch, N.C. (2001). Nursing as a context for alternative/complementary modalities. *Online Journal of Issues in Nursing*, 6(2), 2.

Frisch, N.C. and Kelley, J.H. (2002). Nursing diagnosis and nursing theory: Exploration of factors inhibiting and supporting simultaneous use. *Nursing Diagnosis*, 13(2), 53–61.

Gaberson, K.B. (1997). What's the answer? What's the question? *Journal of the Association of periOperative Registered Nurses*, 66(1), 148–151.

Gagan, M.J., Badger, T.A., and de Leon Baker, M. (1999). Nurse practitioner interventions for domestic violence. *Clinical Excellence in Nurse Practice*, 3(5), 273–278.

Gigliotti, E. (1998). You make the diagnosis. Case study: Integration of the Neuman Systems Model with the theory of nursing symptom in postpartum nursing, including commentary by Lunney, M. *Nursing Diagnosis*, 9(1), 14, 34–38.

Gill, J., Hopwood-Jones, L., Tyndall, J., Gregoroff, S., LeBlanc, P., Lovett, C., Rasco, L., and Ross, A. (1995). Incorporating nursing diagnosis and King's theory in the O.R. documentation. *Canadian Operating Room Nursing Journal*, 13(1), 10–14.

Gordon, M. (1979). The concept of nursing diagnosis. *Nursing Clinics of North America*, 14(3), 487–496.

Gordon, M. (1998, September 30). Nursing nomenclature and classification system development. *Online Journal of Issues in Nursing*. Available at: http://www.nursingworld.org/ojin/tpc7/tpc7-1.htm

Gordon, M. (1998). President's reflection. *Nursing Diagnosis*, 9, Suppl. 2, 5–6.

Gordon, M.D. (1985). Nursing diagnosis. *Annual Review of Nursing Research*, 3, 127–146.

Gordon, M., Murphy, C.P., Candee, D., and Hiltunen, E. (1994). Clinical judgment: An integrated model. *Advances in Nursing Science*, 16(4), 55–70.

Gordon, M. and Sweeny, M.A. (1979). Methodological problems and issues in identifying and standardizing nursing diagnosis. *Advances in Nursing Science*, 2(1), 1–15.

Gordon, M., Sweeny, M.A., and McKeehan, K. (1980). Nursing diagnosis: Looking at its use in the clinical area. *American Journal of Nursing*, 80, 672–674.

Grant, J., Kinney, M., and Guzzetta, C. (1990). A methodology for validating nursing diagnoses. *Advances in Nursing Science*, 12(3), 65–74.

Griffiths, P. (1998). An investigation into the description of patients' problems by nurses using two different needs-based nursing models. *Journal of Advanced Nursing*, 28(5), 969–977.

Grobe, S.J. (1990). Nursing intervention lexicon and taxonomy study: Language classification methods. *Advances in Nursing Science*, 13 (2), 22–33.

Grobe, S.J., Hughes, L.C., Robinson, L., Adler, D.C., Nuamah, I., and McCorkle, R. (1997). Nursing intervention intensity and focus: Indicators of process for outcomes studies. *Studies in Health Technologies and Informatics*, 46, 8–14.

Guzzetta, C.E. and Dossey, B.M. (1983). Nursing diagnosis: Framework, process, and problems. *Heart and Lung*, 12(3), 281–291.

Harbison, J. (2001). Clinical decision making in nursing: Theoretical perspectives and their relevance to practice. *Journal of Advanced Nursing*, 35(1), 126–133.

Hassell, J.S. (1996). Improvement management of depression through nursing model application and critical thinking. *Journal of the American Academy of Nurse Practitioners*, 8(4), 161–166.

Henderson, B. (1978). Nursing diagnosis: Theory and practice. *Advances in Nursing Science*, 1(1), 75–83.

Henry, S.B. and Mead, C.N. (1997). Evaluating standardized coding and classification systems for clinical practice: A critical review of the nursing literature in the United States. *Studies in Health Technologies and Informatics*, 446, 15–20.

Higuchi, K.A., Dulberg, C., and Duff, V. (1999). Factors associated with nursing diagnosis utilization in Canada. *Nursing Diagnosis*, 10(4), 134–147.

Hogston, R. (1997). Nursing diagnosis and classification systems: A positive paper. *Journal of Advanced Nursing*, 26(3), 496–500.

Hoskins, L.M. (1999). Sailing the course to advance professional practice with nursing diagnosis: The tenth and eleventh conferences. In M.J. Rantz et al. (Eds.), *Classification of nursing diagnoses: Proceedings of the thirteenth conference, North American Nursing Diagnosis Association. Celebrating the 25th* anniversary of NANDA, pp. 53–58.

Idvall, E., Rooke, L., and Hamrin, E. (1997). Quality indicators in clinical nursing: A review of the literature. *Journal of Advanced Nursing,* 25(1), 6–17.

Iowa Intervention Project. (1993). The NIC taxonomy structure. *Image: Journal of Nursing Scholarship,* 25(3), 187–192.

Iowa Intervention Project. (1995). Validation and coding of the NIC taxonomy structure. *Image: Journal of Nursing Scholarship,* 27(1), 43–49.

Irvin, S.M. and Harrison, S.A. (1996). Case study: High acuity to long term. *SCI Nursing,* 13(4), 88–95.

Jennings-Dozier, K. (1999). Predicting intentions to obtain a Pap smear among African American and Latina women: Testing the theory of planned behavior. *Nursing Research,* 48(4), 198–205.

Jenny, J. (1995). Advancing the science of nursing. In M.J. Rantz et al. (Eds.), *Classification of nursing diagnoses: Proceedings of the eleventh conference, North American Nursing Diagnosis Association,* pp. 73–81.

Johnstone, M.J. (1999). Reflective topical autobiography: An under utilised interpretive research method in nursing. *Collegian,* 6(1), 24–29.

Hardiker, N. and Kirby, J. (1997). A compositional approach to nursing terminology. *Studies in Health Technologies and Informatics,* 46, 3–7

Kajbjer, K. (1997). European standardization in healthcare informatics and the need for increased involvement of healthcare professionals. *Studies in Health Technologies and Informatics,* 46, 269–274.

Kathol, D.D., Geiger, M.L., and Hartig, J.L. (1998). Clinical correlation map: A tool for linking theory and practice. *Nurse Educator,* 23(4), 31–34.

Kerr, M.E., Hoskins, L.M., Fitzpatrick, J.J., Warren, J.J., Avant, K.C., Carpenito, L.J., Hurley, M.E., Jakob, D., Lunney, M., Mills, W.C., and Rottkamp, B.C. (1992). Development of definitions for taxonomy II. *Nursing Diagnosis,* 3(2), 65–71.

Kim, M. (1998). Physiologic nursing diagnosis: Its role and place in nursing taxonomy . . . from Classification of Nursing Diagnoses: Proceedings of the Fifth National Conference (placed on the page in an organized way, 60–62). Copyright 1984 by C.V. Mosby. Reprinted with permission. *Nursing Diagnosis,* 9, Suppl. 2, 32–38.

Kim, M.J. (1989). Nursing diagnosis. *Annual Review of Nursing Research,* 7, 117–142.

Kleinbeck, S.V. (2000). Dimensions of perioperative nursing for a national specialty nomenclature. *Journal of Advanced Nursing,* 31(3), 529–535.

Klemm, P.R. and Guarnieri, C. (1996). Cervical cancer: A developmental perspective. *Journal of Obstetric, Gynecologic and Neonatal Nursing,* 25(7), 629–634.

Kolcaba, K.Y. (1991). A taxonomic structure for the concept comfort. *Image: Journal of Nursing Scholarship,* 23, 237–244.

Kritek, P.B. (1978). The generation and classification of nursing diagnosis: Toward a theory of nursing. *Image: Journal of Nursing Scholarship,* 10(2), 33–40.

Kritek, P.B. (1985). Nursing diagnosis in perspective: Response to a critique. *Image: Journal of Nursing Scholarship*, 17(1), 3–8.

Kritek, P.B. (1985). Nursing diagnosis: Theoretical foundations. *Occupational Health Nursing*, 33(8), 393–396.

Lacko, L., Bryan, Y., Dellasega, C., and Salerno, F. (1999). Changing clinical practice through research: The case of delirium. *Clinical Nursing Research*, 8(3), 235–250.

Logue, G.A. (1997). An application of Orem's theory to the nursing management of pertussis. *Journal of School Nursing*, 13(4), 20–25.

Mackenzie, S.J. and Laschinger, H.K.S. (1995). Correlates of nursing diagnosis quality in public health nursing. *Journal of Advanced Nursing*, 21(4), 800–808.

Madsen, I. and Jytte Burgaard, S.A. (1997). The Danish Health Classification system—Nursing Interventions Classification—A part of a common Danish Health Care Classification. *Studies in Health Technologies and Informatics*, 46, 32–36.

Mason, G.M.C. and Attree, M. (1997). The relationship between research and the nursing process in clinical practice. *Journal of Advanced Nursing*, 26(5), 1045–1049.

McHolm, F.A. and Geib, K.M. (1998). Application of the Neuman Systems Model to teaching health assessment and nursing process. *Nursing Diagnosis*, 9(1), 23–33.

Mitchell, G.J. (1991). Nursing diagnosis: An ethical analysis. *Image: Journal of Nursing Scholarship*, 23, 99–103.

Modrcin-McCarthy, M.A., McCue, S., and Walker, J. (1997). Preterm infants and STRESS: A tool for the neonatal nurse. *Journal of Perinatal and Neonatal Nursing*, 10(4), 62–71.

Moen, A., Henry, S.B., and Warren, J.J. (1999). Representing nursing judgments in the electronic health record. *Journal of Advanced Nursing*, 30(4), 990–997.

Moorhead, S., Head, B., Johnson, M., and Maas, M. (1998). The nursing outcomes taxonomy: Development and coding. *Journal of Nursing Care Quality*, 12(6), 56–63.

Moreira, A.S.P. (1997). Nursing diagnoses and social representation: A methodological approach. In M.J. Rantz et al. (Eds.), *Classification of nursing diagnoses: Proceedings of the twelfth conference, North American Nursing Diagnosis Association*, p. 377.

Nolan, M., Lundh, U., and Tishelman, C. (1998). Nursing's knowledge base: Does it have to be unique? *British Journal of Nursing*, 7(5), 270–276.

Nuamah, I.F., Cooley, M.E., Fawcett, J., and McCorkle, R. (1999). Testing a theory for health-related quality of life in cancer patients: A structural equation approach. *Research in Nursing and Health*, 22(3), 231–242.

O'Connell, B. (1998). The clinical application of the nursing process in selected acute care settings: A professional mirage. *Australian Journal of Advanced Nursing*, 15(4), 22–32.

O'Connell, B., Rapley, P., and Tibbett, P. (1999). Does the nursing diagnosis form the basis for patient care? *Collegian*, 6(3), 29–34.

Paredes, A.S., Furegato, A.R., and Coler, M.S. (1999). Nursing diagnosis and social representation: A methodology of diagnostic formulation. In M.J. Rantz et al. (Eds.), *Classification of nursing diagnoses: Proceedings of the thirteenth conference, North American Nursing Diagnosis Association. Celebrating the 25th anniversary of NANDA*, p. 591.

Peck, S.D. (1998). The efficacy of therapeutic touch for improving functional ability in elders with degenerative arthritis. *Nursing Science Quarterly*, 11(3), 123–132.

Pollack, L.E. and Cramer, R.D. (1999). Patient satisfaction with two models of group therapy for people hospitalized with bipolar disorder. *Applied Nursing Research*, 12(3), 143–152.

Porter, E.J. (1985). Validating a diagnostic label. *Nursing Clinics in North America*, 20(4), 641–655.

Porter, E.J. (1986). Critical analysis of NANDA nursing diagnosis taxonomy I. *Image: Journal of Nursing Scholarship*, 18(4), 136–139.

Potter, M.L. and Bockenhauer, B.J. (2000). Implementing Orlando's nursing theory: A pilot study. *Journal of Psychosocial Nursing and Mental Health Services*, 38(3), 14–21.

Redes, S. and Lunney, M. (1997). Validation by school nurses of the Nursing Intervention Classification for computer software. *Computers in Nursing*, 15(6), 333–338.

Roberts, S.L., Johnson, L.H., and Keely, B. (1999). Fostering hope in the elderly congestive heart failure patient in critical care. *Geriatric Nursing*, 20(4), 195–199.

Scahill, L. (1991). Nursing diagnosis vs goal-oriented treatment planning in inpatient child psychiatry. *Image: Journal of Nursing Scholarship*, 23, 95–98.

Shamansky, S.L. and Yanni, C.R. (1983). In opposition to nursing diagnosis: A minority opinion. *Image: Journal of Nursing Scholarship*, 19(4), 184–185.

Sieleman, J. (1999). Utilization of nursing diagnoses in Iowa child health specialty clinics. *Nursing Diagnosis*, 10(3), 113–120.

Simon, J.M. (1998). Nursing theories and nursing diagnoses: How are they related? *Nursing Diagnosis*, 9(1), 3–4.

Sundin-Huard, D. and Fahy, K. (1999). Moral distress, advocacy and burnout: Theorizing the relationships. *International Journal of Nursing Practice*, 5(1), 8–13.

Taylor, S.G. (1991). The structure of nursing diagnosis from Orem's theory. *Nursing Science Quarterly*, 4(1), 24–32.

Thompson, C. (1999). A conceptual treadmill: The need for "middle ground" in clinical decision making theory in nursing. *Journal of Advanced Nursing*, 30(5), 1222–1229.

Tilley, J.D., Gregor, F.M., and Thieson, V. (1987). The nurses' role in patient education: Incongruent perceptions among nurses and patients. *Journal of Advanced Nursing*, 12, 291–391.

Titler, M.G., Bulechek, G.M., and McCloskey, J.C. (1996). Use of the nursing interventions classification by critical care nurses. *Critical Care Nurse*, 16(4), 45–54.

Tribotti, S., Lyons, N., Blackburn, S., Stein, M., and Withers, J. (1988). Nursing diagnosis for the postpartum woman. *Journal of Obstetric, Gynecologic, and Neonatal Nursing*, 17, 410–416.

Tripp-Reimer, T., Woodworth, G., McCloskey, J.C., and Bulechek, G. (1996). The dimensional structure of nursing interventions. *Nursing Research*, 45(1), 10–17.

Turkoski, B. (1988). Nursing diagnosis in print, 1950–1985. *Nursing Outlook*, 36(3), 142–144.

Turley, J.P. (1997). Developing informatics as a discipline. *Studies in Health Technologies and Informatics*, 46, 69–74.

Watson, R. and Lea, A. (1997). The Caring Dimensions Inventory (CDI): Content validity, reliability and scaling. *Journal of Advanced Nursing*, 25(1), 87–94.

Weber, P., Lovis, C.C., Michel, P.A., and Baud, R. (1997). Collection of nursing minimum data set (NMDS) could benefit from medical encoding experiences. *Studies in Health Technologies and Informatics*, 46, 263–268.

Wesorick, B. (1995). Moving nursing diagnosis from theory to reality. In M.J. Rantz et al. (Eds.), *Classification of nursing diagnoses: Proceedings of the eleventh conference, North American Nursing Diagnosis Association*, p. 249.

Whitley, G.G. (1997). Three phases of research in validating nursing diagnoses. *Western Journal of Nursing Research*, 19(3), 379–399.

Woodtli, A. (1995). Mixed incontinence: A new nursing diagnosis? *Nursing Diagnosis*, 6(4), 135–142.

Wooldridge, J.B., Brown, O.F., and Herman, J. (1993). Nursing diagnosis: The central theme in nursing knowledge. *Nursing Diagnosis*, 4, 50–55.

10. Theory and Education

Aggleton, P. and Chalmers, H. (1987). Models of nursing, nursing practice and nursing education. *Journal of Advanced Nursing*, 12(5), 573–581.

Algase, D.L., Newton, S.E., and Higgins, P.A. (2001). Nursing theory across curricula: A status report from midwest nursing schools. *Journal of Professional Nursing*, 17(5), 248–255.

Allen, D. (1997). Nursing, knowledge and practice. *Journal of Health Services Research and Policy*, 2(3), 190–193.

Anderko, L., Uscian M., and Robertson, J.F. (1999). Improving client outcomes through differentiated practice: A rural nursing center model. *Public Health Nursing*, 16(3), 168–175.

Armitage, G. (1998). Analysing childhood: A nursing perspective. *Journal of Child Health Care*, 2(2), 66–71.

Arthur, D., Chan, H.K., Fung, W.Y., Wong, K.Y., and Yeung, KW. (1999). Therapeutic communication strategies used by Hong Kong mental health nurses with their Chinese clients. *Journal of Psychiatric and Mental Health Nursing*, 6(1), 29–36.

Arvay, M., Banister, E., Hoskins, M., and Snell A. (1999). Women's lived experience of conceptualizing the self: Implications for health care practice. *Health Care for Women International*, 20(4), 363–380.

Ashmore, R. and Banks, D. (1997). Student nurses perceptions of their interpersonal skills: A re-examination of Burnard and Morrison's findings. *International Journal of Nursing Studies*, 34(5), 335–345.

Attewell, A. (1998). Florence Nightingale's relevance to nurses. *Journal of Holistic Nursing*, 16(2), 281–291.

Backman, K. and Kyngas, H.A. (1999). Challenges of the grounded theory approach to a novice researcher. *Nursing and Health Sciences*, 1(3), 147–153.

Baer, E.D. (1987). "A cooperative venture" in pursuit of professional status: A research journal for nursing. *Nursing Research*, 36(1), 18–25.

Baker, C. (1999). From chaos to order: A nursing-based psycho-education program for parents of children with attention-deficit hyperactivity disorder. *Canadian Journal of Nursing Research*, 31(2), 71–75.

Barker, P., ...kson, S., and Stevenson, C. (1999). The need for psychiatric nursing: ...a multidimensional theory of caring. *Nursing Inquiry*, 6(2), 103–111.

Barker, ...Tow...kson, S., and Stevenson, C. (1999). What are psychiatric nurses needed ...eloping a theory of essential nursing practice. *Journal of Psychiatric and ...Health Nursing*, 6(4), 273–282.

Ba...W., Jr., Rhodes, R.S., and Dufour, C.A. (1998). Predictors of success on the ...X-RN among baccalaureate nursing students. *Nursing and Health Care Per...ives*, 19(3), 132–137.

...M. (1999). Research in midwifery—The relevance of a feminist theoretical ...nework. *Journal of the Australian College of Midwives*, 12(2), 6–10.

...y, J. (1997). Nurse Miss Sahib: Colonial culture-bound education in India and ...anscultural nursing. *Journal of Transcultural Nursing*, 9(1), 14–19.

..., C. (1987). Nursing theory for undergraduates. *Nursing Outlook*, 35(4), 189–192.

...on, A. and Latter, S. (1998). Implementing health promoting nursing: The integration of interpersonal skills and health promotion. *Journal of Advanced Nursing*, 27(1), 100–107.

...rragan, L. (1998). Nursing practice draws upon several different ways of knowing. *Journal of Clinical Nursing*, 7(3), 209–217.

...Bevis, E.O. (1989, February). Curriculum building in nursing: A process (Publication No. 15–227, pp. i-xx, 1–282). New York: National League for Nursing.

Booth, K., Kenrick, M., and Woods, S. (1997). Nursing knowledge, theory and method revisited. *Journal of Advanced Nursing*, 26(4), 804–811.

Boykin, A. and Schoenhofer. S. (1997). Reframing outcomes: enhancing personhood. *Advanced Practice Nursing Quarterly*, 3(1), 60–65.

Brooks, E.M. and Thomas, S. (1997). The perception and judgment of senior baccalaureate student nurses in clinical decision making. *Advances in Nursing Science*, 19(3), 50–69.

Brown, R. (2000). Describing a model of nursing as a focus for psychiatric nursing care. *International Journal of Psychiatric Nursing Research*, 6(1), 670–682.

Brown, S.J. (1999). Student nurses' perceptions of elderly care. *Journal of the National Black Nurses Association*, 10(2), 29–36.

Buerhaus, P.I. and Norman, L. (2001). It's time to require theory and methods of quality improvement in basic and graduate nursing education. *Nursing Outlook*, 49(2), 67–69.

Bunkers, S.S. (2001). Teaching-learning processes. On global health and justice: A nursing theory-guided perspective. *Nursing Science Quarterly*, 14(4), 297.

Bunkers, S.S. (2002). Teaching-learning processes. Nursing theory-guided models for teaching-learning. *Nursing Science Quarterly*, 15(2), 117.

*Burgess, G. (1978). The personal development of the nursing student as a conceptual framework. *Nursing Forum*, 17(1), 96–102.

Burks, K.J. (2001). Intentional action. *Journal of Advanced Nursing*, 34(5), 668–675.

Cain, P. (1999). Respecting and breaking confidences: Conceptual, ethical and educational issues. *Nurse Education Today*, 19(3), 175–181.

Cash, K. (1997). Social epistemology, gender and nursing theory. *International Journal of Nursing Studies*, 34(2), 137–143.

Cave, P. (1998). Nursing knowledge: The role of Plato in wounc... *Nursing Standard,* 13(11), 40–43.

Cessario, L. (1987). Utilization of board gaming for conceptual m... f nursing. *Journal of Nursing Education,* 26(4), 167–169.

Chick, N. and Paull, D. (1988). Collaboration between nurse educa... stralia and New Zealand extends educational opportunities for nurses. *Inte... Journal of Nursing Studies,* 25(4), 279–286.

Chinn, P.L. (1988). Knowing and doing [Editorial]. *Advances in Nursin...* ...(3), vii-viii.

Christmyer, C.S., Catanzariti, P.M., Langford, A.M., and Reitz, J.A. (1988)... gap: Theory to practice—Part I, Clinical applications. *Nursing Manage...* 42–43, 46–48, 50.

Clarke, D.J. and Holt, J. (2001). Philosophy: A key to open the door to critica... *Nurse Education Today,* 21(1), 71–78.

Clifford, C. (1997). Nurse teachers and research. *Nurse Education Today,* 17(2), 1...

Cohen, S.S. and Milone-Nuzzo, P. (2001). Advancing health policy in nursing edu... through service learning. *Advances in Nursing Science,* 23(3), 28–40.

Colodny, A. (1997). Spinal cord injury nurses in action: Partners in practice. *SCI N... ing,* 14(3), 79–82.

Conley, V.M. (1998). Beyond knowledge deficit to a proposal for information-seeki... behaviors. *Nursing Diagnosis,* 9(4), 129–135.

Cudmore. J. (1998). Keep with it. *Nursing Times,* 94(23), 78–79.

Curtin, L.L. (1987). Education and licensure: Once more into the breach [Editorial]. *Nursing Management,* 18(5), 9–10.

Cutcliffe, J.R. and Goward, P. (2000). Mental health nurses and qualitative research methods: A mutual attraction? *Journal of Advanced Nursing,* 31(3), 590–598.

Davies, C., Welham, V., Glover, A., Jones, L., and Murphy, F. (1999). Teaching in practice. *Nursing Standard,* 13(35), 33–38.

Dawson, P.J. (1997). Comment on: *Journal of Psychiatric and Mental Health Nursing* (1996), 3(1), 7–12. A reply to Kevin Gournay's "Schizophrenia: A review of the contemporary literature and implications for mental health nursing theory, practice and education." *Journal of Psychiatric and Mental Health Nursing,* 4(1), 1–7.

Dawson, P.J. (1997). Is there anyone in there? Psychiatric nursing meets biological psychiatry. *Nursing Inquiry,* 4(3), 167–175.

Dean, J.M. and Mountford, B. (1998). Innovation in the assessment of nursing theory and its evaluation: A team approach. *Journal of Advanced Nursing,* 28(2), 409–418.

DeGroot, H.A., Ferketich, S.L., and Larson, P.J. (1987). Theory development in a non-university service setting. *Journal of Nursing Administration,* 17(4), 38–44.

DeMong, N.C. and Assie-Lussier, L.L. (1999). Continuing education: An aspect of staff development relating to the nurse manager's role. *Journal for Nurses in Staff Development,* 15(1), 19–22.

Derdiarian, A. (1979). Education: A way to theory construction in nursing. *Journal of Nursing Education,* 18(2), 36–47.

Derstine, J.B. (1989). The development of theory-based practice by graduate students in rehabilitative nursing. *Rehabilitation Nursing,* 14(2), 88–89.

DiBartolo, M.C. (1998). Philosophy of science in doctoral nursing education revisited. *Journal of Professional Nursing,* 14(6), 350–360.

Dickoff, J. and James, P. (1970). Beliefs and values: Bases for curriculum design. *Nursing* Research, 19(5), 415–427.

Diekelmann, N. (1988). Curriculum revolution: A theoretical and philosophical mandate for change (Publication No. 15–2224, pp. 137–157). New York: National League for Nursing.

Dougal, J. and Gonterman, R. (1999). A comparison of three teaching methods on learning and retention. *Journal for Nurses in Staff Development,* 15(5), 205–209.

Dowie, S. and Park, C. (1988). Relating nursing theory to students' life experiences. *Nurse Education Today,* 8(4), 191–196.

Downs, F.S. (1988). Doctoral education: Our claim to the future. *Nursing Outlook,* 36(1), 18–20.

Driver, J. and Campbell, J. (2000). An evaluation of the impact of lecturer practitioners on learning. *British Journal of Nursing,* 9(5), 292–300.

Dudley-Brown, S.L. (1997). The evaluation of nursing theory: A method for our madness. *International Journal of Nursing Studies,* 34(1), 76–83.

Duff, V. (1989). Perspective transformation: The challenge for the RN in the baccalaureate program. *Journal of Nursing Education,* 28(1), 38–39.

Duffy, K. and Scott, P.A. (1998). Viewing an old issue through a new lens: A critical theory insight into the education-practice gap. *Nurse Education Today,* 18(3), 183–189.

Duldt, B.W. (1995). Nursing process: The science of nursing in the curriculum. *Nurse Educator,* 20, 24–29.

Durgahee, T. (1998). Facilitating reflection: From a sage on stage to a guide on the side. *Nurse Education Today,* 18(2), 158–164.

Edmond, C.B. (2001). A new paradigm for practice education *Nurse Education Today,* 21(4), 251–259.

Edwards, S.D. (1998). The art of nursing. *Nursing Ethics,* 5(5), 393–400.

Elcock. K. (1998). Lecturer practitioner: A concept analysis. *Journal of Advanced Nursing,* 28(5), 1092–1098.

Emden, C. (1998). Conducting a narrative analysis. *Collegian,* 5(3), 34–39.

Emden, C. and Young, W. (1987). Theory development in nursing: Australian nurses advance global debate. *Australian Journal of Advanced Nursing,* 4(3), 22–40.

Fawcett, J. (1985). Theory: Basis for the study and practice of nursing education. *Journal of Nursing Education,* 24(6), 226–229.

Fealy, G.M. (1997). The theory-practice relationship in nursing: An exploration of contemporary discourse. *Journal of Advanced Nursing,* 25(5), 1061–1069.

Fernandez, E. (1997). Just "doing the observations": Reflective practice in nursing. *British Journal of Nursing,* 6(16), 939–943.

Fielding, R.G. and Llewelyn, S.P. (1987). Communication in nursing may damage your health and enthusiasm: Some warnings. *Journal of Advanced Nursing Science,* 12(3), 281–290.

Fishel, A.H. (1998). Nursing management of anxiety and panic. *Nursing Clinics of North America,* 33(1), 135–151.

Fitzpatrick, J.J. (1987). Use of existing nursing models. *Journal of Gerontological Nursing,* 13(9), 8–9.

Fletcher, J. (1997). Do nurses really care? Some unwelcome findings from recent research and inquiry. *Journal of Nursing Management,* 5(1), 43–50.

Ford-Gilboe, M., Campbell, J., and Berman, H. (1995). Stories and numbers: Coexistence without compromise. *Advances in Nursing Science,* 18(1), 14–26.

Fowler, J. and Chevannes, M. (1998). Evaluating the efficacy of reflective practice within the context of clinical supervision. *Journal of Advanced Nursing,* 27(2), 379–382.

Francis, D., Owens, J., and Tollefson, J. (1998). "It comes together at the end": The impact of a one-year subject in Nursing Inquiry on philosophies of nursing. *Nursing Inquiry,* 5(4), 268–278.

Frank, B. (1994). Teaching nursing theory: A walk around the golf course. *Nurse Educator,* 19, 26–27.

Funnell. C. (1999). Empathy in the clinical context. *Contemporary Nurse,* 8(4), 142–145.

Gagan, M.J., Badger, T.A., and de Leon Baker, M. (1999). Nurse practitioner interventions for domestic violence. *Clinical Excellence in Nurse Practice,* 3(5), 273–278.

Gaines, C. (1999) Clearing up the "concept fog". *Journal of the Association of Black Nursing Faculty in Higher Education,*10(2), 52–53.

Gassner, L.A, Wotton, K., Clare, J., Hofmeyer, A., and Buckman, J. (1999). Evaluation of a model of collaboration: Academic and clinician partnership in the development and implementation of undergraduate teaching. *Collegian,* 6(3), 14–21.

Geanellos, R. (1998). Hermeneutic philosophy. Part II: A nursing research example of the hermeneutic imperative to address forestructures/pre-understandings. *Nursing Inquiry,* 5(4), 238–247.

Goode, H. (1998). The theory-practice gap and student nurses. *Journal of Child Health Care,* 2(2), 86–90.

Gordon, N.S. (1998). Influencing mental health nursing practice through the teaching of research and theory: A personal critical review. *Journal of Psychiatric and Mental Health Nursing,* 5(2), 119–128.

Gormley, K.J. (1997). Practice write-ups: An assessment instrument that contributes to bridging the differences between theory and practice for student nurses through the development of core skills. *Nurse Education Today,* 17(1), 53–57.

Graham, L. (1979). The development of a useful conceptual framework in curriculum design. *Nursing Papers Perspective in Nursing,* 9(3), 84–92.

Greenwood, J. (1988). More considerations concerning the application of nursing models to curricula: A reply to Lorraine Smith. *Nurse Education Today,* 8(4), 187–190.

Greenwood, J. (1998). Establishing an international network on nurses' clinical reasoning. *Journal of Advanced Nursing,* 27(4), 843–847.

Greenwood, J. (2000). Critical thinking and nursing scripts: The case for the development of both. *Journal of Advanced Nursing,* 31(2), 428–436.

Haddock. J. (1997). Reflection in groups: Contextual and theoretical considerations within nurse education and practice. *Nurse Education Today,* 17(5), 381–385.

Hagey, R. MacKay RW. (2000). Qualitative research to identify racialist discourse: Tow equity in nursing curricula. *International Journal of Nursing Studies*, 37(1), 45

A. (1987). An analysis of senior nursing students' immediate responses to ed patients. *Journal of Advanced Nursing*, 12(4), 451–461.

1979, April). Current trends in the use of conceptual frameworks in nursing tion. *Journal of Nursing Education*, 18(4), 26–29.

.E. (1997). Learning through reflection in the community: The relevance of on's theories of coaching to nursing education. *International Journal of Nursing Studies*, 34(2), 103–110.

, C.E. (1997). The helping relationship in the community setting: The relevance f Rogerian theory to the supervision of Project (2000) students. *International Journal of Nursing Studies* 34(6), 415–419.

s, S. (1998). Intuition and the coronary care nurse. *Nursing in Critical Care*, 3(3), 130–133.

ncock, P. (1999). Reflective practice—Using a learning journal. *Nursing Standard*, 13(17). 37–40.

Happell, B. (1998). Psychiatric nursing: Has it been forgotten in contemporary nursing education? *Nurse Educator*, 23(6), 9–10.

Harrison, J., Saunders, M.E., and Sims, A. (1977). Integrating theory and practice in modular schemes for basic nursing education. *Journal of Advanced Nursing*, 2, 503–519.

Hart, M.A. and Foster, S.N. (1998). Self-care agency in two groups of pregnant women. *Nursing Science Quarterly*, 11(4), 167–171.

Hartley, L.A. (1988). Congruence between teaching and learning self-care: A pilot study. *Nursing Science Quarterly*, 1(4), 161–167.

Hartrick, G. (1998). A critical pedagogy for family nursing. *Journal of Nursing Education*, 37(2), 80–84.

Heinrich, K. (1989). Growing pains: Faculty stages in adopting a nursing model. *Nurse Educator*, 14(1), 3–4, 29.

Heinrich, K.T., Robinson, C.M., and Scales, M.E. (1998). Support groups: An empowering, experiential strategy. *Nurse Educator*, 23(4), 8–10.

Heslop, L. (1998). A discursive exploration of nursing work in the hospital emergency setting. *Nursing Inquiry*, 5(2), 87–95.

Heye, M.L. and Goddard. L. (1999). Teaching pain management: How to make it work. *Journal for Nurses in Staff Development*, 15(1), 27–36.

Hill, PF. (1998). Assessing the competence of student nurses. *Journal of Child Heal Care*, 2(1), 25–30.

Hilz, L.M. (2000). The informatics nurse specialist as change agent. Application innovation-diffusion theory. *Computers in Nursing*, 18(6), 272–278.

Hisama, K.K. (1999). Towards an international theory of nursing. *Nursing and H Sciences*, 1(2), 77–81.

Holland, S. (1999). Teaching nursing ethics by cases: A personal perspective. *N Ethics*, 6(5), 434–436.

Hurlock-Chorostecki, C. (1999). Holistic care in the critical [illegible]etting: Application of a concept through Watson's and Orem's theories of nu[illegible] *of the Canadian Association of Critical Care Nurses / CAC[illegible] Official Journal* [illegible]), 20–25.

Hyrkas, K., Koivula, M., and Paunonen, M. (1999). Clinical supervi[illegible]rsing in the 1990s—Current state of concepts, theory and research. *Journ[illegible]ing Management*, 7(3), 177–187.

Jaarsma, T., Halfens, R., Senten, M., Abu Saad, H.H., and Dracup, K. [illegible]lop-ing a supportive-educative program for patients with advanced hea[illegible] Orem's general theory of nursing. *Nursing Science Quarterly*, 11(2), [illegible]

Jacobs-Kramer, M.K. and Huether, S.E. (1988). Curricular considerations in nursing theory. *Journal of Professional Nursing*, 4(5), 373–380.

Jacobson, S. (1987). Studying and using conceptual models of nursing. *Imag[illegible] of Nursing Scholarship*, 19(2), 78–82.

Jameton, A. and Fowler, M.D. (1989). Ethical inquiry and the concept of re[illegible] *Advances in Nursing Science*, 11(3), 11–24.

Johnson, S.E. (1989). A picture is worth a thousand words: Helping students visu[illegible] a conceptual model. *Nurse Educator*, 14(3), 21–24.

Johnstone, M.J. (1999). Reflective topical autobiography: An under utilised interpret[illegible] research method in nursing. *Collegian*, 6(1), 24–29.

Jones, K.N. (1999). Reflection: An alternative to nursing models. *Professional Nurse*, 14(12), 853–855.

Jordan, S. (1998). From classroom theory to clinical practice: Evaluating the impact of a post-registration course. *Nurse Education Today*, 18(4), 293–302.

Karmels, P. (1993). Conundrum game for nursing theorists Neuman, King, and Johnson. *Nurse Educator*, 18(6), 8–9.

Kathol, D.D., Geiger. M.L., and Hartig, J.L. (1998). Clinical correlation map. A tool for linking theory and practice. *Nurse Educator*, 23(4), 31–34.

Kennedy, D. and Barloon, L.F. (1997). Managing burnout in pediatric critical care: The human care commitment. *Critical Care Nursing Quarterly*, 20(2), 63–71.

Ketefian, S. and Redman, R.W. (1997). Nursing science in the global community. *Image: Journal of Nursing Scholarship*, 29(1), 11–15.

Khatib, H.M. and Ford, S. (1999). The virtual theory-practice gap. *Journal of Child Health Care*, 3(2), 36–38.

Kim, H.S. (1999). Critical reflective inquiry for knowledge development in nursing practice. *Journal of Advanced Nursing*, 29(5), 1205–1212.

[illegible]ng, I.M. (1997). King's theory of goal attainment in practice. *Nursing Science Quarterly*, 10(4), 180–185.

[illegible]czyk, R.M. (1997). Teaching ethics: Effect on moral development. *Nursing Ethics*, [illegible]), 57–65.

[illegible]n, L.J., Tamblyn, R., and Kuypers, J.A. (1987). A model to guide development and [illegible]ation of multiple nursing theories. *Journal of Advanced Nursing*, 12(4), 523–529.

[illegible]ulx-Girouard, L., Lovitt, S., Katz, C.B., and Kennelly, P. (1997). A public [illegible]rsing model. *Public Health Nursing*, 14(2), 81–91.

[illegible]n, Y., Dellasega, C., and Salerno, F. (1999). Changing clinical practice [illegible]arch: The case of delirium. *Clinical Nursing Research*, 8(3), 235–250.

Landers, M.G. (2000). The theory-practice gap in nursing: The role of the nurse teacher. *Journal of Advanced Nursing*, 32(6), 1550–1556.

Lait, M.E. (2000). The place of nursing history in an undergraduate curriculum. *Nurse Education Today*, 20(5), 395–400.

Landers, M.G. (2000). The theory-practice gap in nursing: The role of the nurse teacher. *Journal of Advanced Nursing*, 32(6), 1550–1556.

Landrum, B.J. (1998). Marketing innovations to nurses. Part 1: How people adopt innovations. *Journal of Wound, Ostomy, and Continence Nursing*, 25(4), 194–199.

Lauder, W. (1994). Beyond reflection: Practical wisdom and the practical syllogism. *Nurse Education Today*, 14(2), 91–98.

Lauder, W., Reynolds, W., and Angus, N. (1999). Transfer of knowledge and skills: Some implications for nursing and nurse education. *Nurse Education Today*, 19(6), 480–487.

Lawrence, S.A. and Lawrence, R.M. (1983). Curriculum development: Philosophy, objectives, and conceptual framework. *Nursing Outlook*, 31(3), 160–163.

Leininger, M. (1997). Transcultural nursing research to transform nursing education and practice: 40 years. *Image: Journal of Nursing Scholarship*, 29(4), 341–347.

Leininger, M.M. (1997). Transcultural nursing as a global care humanizer, diversifier, and unifier. *Hoitotiede*, 9(5), 219–225.

Liaschenko, J. and Fisher, A. (1999). Theorizing the knowledge that nurses use in the conduct of their work. *Scholarly Inquiry for Nursing Practice*, 13(1), 29–41.

Linscott, J., Spee, R., Flint, F., and Fisher, A. (1999). Creating a culture of patient-focused care through a learner-centered philosophy. *Canadian Journal of Nursing Leadership*, 12(4), 5–10.

Lo, R. and Brown, R. (1999). The importance of theory in student nurses' psychiatric practicum. *International Journal of Psychiatric Nursing Research*, 5(1), 542–552.

Logsdon, M.C. and Ford, D. (1998). Service-learning for graduate students. *Nurse Educator*, 23(2), 34–37.

Long, G., Grandis, S., and Glasper, E.A. (1999). Investing in practice: enquiry- and problem-based learning. *British Journal of Nursing*, 8(17), 1171–1174.

Lott, J.W. and Hoath, S.B. (1998). Neonatal skin: The ideal nursing interface. *Journal of Pediatric Nursing*, 13(5), 302–306.

Luna, L. (1998). Culturally competent health care: A challenge for nurses in Saudi Arabia. *Journal of Transcultural Nursing*, 9(2), 8–14.

MacGregor, J. and Dewar, K. (1997). Opening up the options: Making the inflexible into a flexible framework. *Nurse Education Today*, 17(5), 502–507.

Mariano, C. (2002). Crisis theory and intervention: A critical component of nursing education. *Journal of the New York State Nurses Association*, 33(1), 19–24.

Markovic, M. (1997). From theory to perioperative practice with Parse. *Canadian Operating Room Nursing Journal*, 15(1), 13–19.

Martin, S.R. (1997). Agricultural safety and health: Principles and possibilities for nursing education. *Journal of Nursing Education*, 36(2), 74–78.

Masters, M. (1988). Nursing theory: An electric approach in baccalaureate education. *Kansas Nurse*, 63(12), 1–2.

Mavundla, T.R. (2000). Professional nurses' perception of nursing mentally ill people in a general hospital setting. *Journal of Advanced Nursing*, 32(6), 1569–1578.

McCance, T.V., McKenna, H.P., and Boore, J.R. (1999). Caring: Theoretical perspectives of relevance to nursing. *Journal of Advanced Nursing*, 30(6), 1388–1395.

McEwen, M. (2000). Teaching theory at the master's level: Report of a national survey of theory instructors. *Journal of Professional Nursing*, 16(6), 354–361.

McGrath, B.B. (1998). Illness as a problem of meaning: moving culture from the classroom to the clinic. *Advances in Nursing Science*, 21(2), 17–29.

McHolm, F.A. and Geib, K.M. (1998). Application of the Neuman Systems Model to teaching health assessment and nursing process. *Nursing Diagnosis*, 9(1), 23–33.

McKenna, H.P. (1997). Theory and research: A linkage to benefit practice. *International Journal of Nursing Studies*, 34(6), 431–437.

McLaughlin, C. (1997). The effect of classroom theory and contact with patients on the attitudes of student nurses towards mentally ill people. *Journal of Advanced Nursing*, 26(6), 1221–1228.

McLoughlin, A. (1997). The "F" factor: Feminism forsaken? *Nurse Education Today*, 17(2), 111–114.

McMahon, R. (1988). The "24-hour reality orientation" type of approach to the confused elderly: A minimum standard for care. *Journal of Advanced Nursing*, 13(6), 693–700.

McVicar, A. and Clancy, J. (1998). Homeostasis: A framework for integrating the life sciences. *British Journal of Nursing*, 7(10), 601–607.

Meleis, A.I. and May, K.M. (1981). Nursing theory and scholarliness in the doctoral program. *Advances in Nursing Science*, 4(1), 31–41.

Meleis, A.I. and Price, M. (1988). Strategies and conditions for teaching theoretical nursing: An international perspective. *Journal of Advanced Nursing*, 13, 592–604.

Meleis, A.I., Wilson, H.S., and Chater, S. (1980). Toward scholarliness in doctoral dissertations: An analytical model. *Journal of Research in Nursing and Health*, 3, 115–124.

Miller, S.K. (1999). Nurse practitioners in the county correctional facility setting: Unique challenges and suggestions for effective health promotion. *Clinical Excellence in Nurse Practice*, 3(5), 268–272.

Minicucci, D.S. (1998). A review and synthesis of the literature: The use of presence in the nursing care of families. *Journal of the New York State Nurses Association*, 29(3–4), 9–15.

Mohr, W.K. and Naylor, M.D. (1998). Creating a curriculum for the 21st century. *Nursing Outlook*, 46(5), 206–212.

Mulholland, J. (1997). Assimilating sociology: critical reflections on the "sociology in nursing" debate. *Journal of Advanced Nursing*, 25(4), 844–852.

Neal, L.J. (1997). The rehabilitation nursing paradigm: Implications for home care. *Caring*, 16(2), 66–68.

Neal, L.J. (1999). Facilitating the growth of nursing staff case management in PPS. *Caring*, 18(10), 46–48.

Nolan, M. and Tolson, D. (2000). Gerontological nursing. 1: Challenges nursing older people in acute care. *British Journal of Nursing*, 9(1), 39–42.

Nolan, M. and Tolson, D. (2000). Gerontological nursing. 5: Realizing the future potential. *British Journal of Nursing*, 9(5), 272–274.

Nolan, M., Lundh, U., and Tishelman, C. (1998). Nursing's knowledge base: Does it have to be unique? *British Journal of Nursing*, 7(5), 270–276.

Northrup, D.T. and Cody, W.K. (1998). Evaluation of the human becoming theory in practice in an acute care psychiatric setting. *Nursing Science Quarterly*, 11(1), 23–30.

Olsson, H.M. and Gullberg, M.T. (1987). Nursing education: A valuation of theoretical and practical sections of the education. Expectations and knowledge of the nurse role. *Vardi i Norden*, 7(13), 412–416.

Padgett, S.M. (2000). Benner and the critics: Promoting scholarly dialogue. *Scholarly Inquiry for Nursing Practice*, 14(3), 249–266.

Penney, W. and Warelow, P.J. (1999). Understanding the prattle of praxis. *Nursing Inquiry*, 6(4), 259–268.

Peplau, H.E. (1997). Peplau's theory of interpersonal relations. *Nursing Science Quarterly*, 10(4), 162–167.

Pepler, C. (1977). The practical aspects of using a conceptual framework. *Nursing Papers*, 9(3), 93–101.

Perry, B. (1998). Beliefs of eight exemplary oncology nurses related to Watson's nursing theory. *Canadian Oncology Nursing Journal*, 8(2), 97–107.

Phillips, R., Donald, A., Mousseau-Gershman, Y., and Powell, T. (1998). Applying theory to practice—The use of "ripple effect" plans in continuing education. *Nurse Education Today*, 18(1), 12–19.

Pierson, W. (1998). Reflection and nursing education. *Journal of Advanced Nursing*, 27(1), 165–170.

Potter, M.L. and Bockenhauer, B.J. (2000). Implementing Orlando's nursing theory: A pilot study. *Journal of Psychosocial Nursing and Mental Health Services*, 38(3), 14–21.

Priest, H. and Roberts, P. (1998). Assessing students' clinical performance. *Nursing Standard*, 12(48), 37–41.

Punton, S. (1989). King's fund nursing development. The Oxford experience. *Nursing Standard*, 3(22), 27–28.

Purdy. M. (1997). Humanist ideology and nurse education. 1. Humanist educational theory. *Nurse Education Today*, 17(3), 192–195.

Rafael, A.R. (2000). Watson's philosophy, science, and theory of human caring as a conceptual framework for guiding community health nursing practice. *Advances in Nursing Science*, 23(2), 34–49.

Rajabally, M. (1977). Frankly speaking. Nursing education: Another tower of Babel. *Canadian Nurse*, 73(9), 30–31.

Ray. M.A. (1997).Consciousness and the moral ideal: A transcultural analysis of Watson's theory of transpersonal caring. *Advanced Practice Nursing Quarterly*, 3(1), 25–31.

Ream, E. and Richardson, A. (1999). Comment in *Oncology Nursing Forum* (2000), 27(3), 425–426. From theory to practice: Designing interventions to reduce fatigue in patients with cancer. *Oncology Nursing Forum*, 26(8), 1295–1303.

Reid, B., Allen, A.F., Gauthier, T., and Campbell, H. (1989). Solving the Orem mystery: An educational strategy. *Journal of Continuing Education in Nursing*, 20(3), 108–110.

Rogers, M.E. (1989). Creating a climate for the implementation of a nursing conceptual framework. *Journal of Continuing Education in Nursing*, 20(3), 112–116.

Rolfe, G. (1997). Beyond expertise: Theory, practice and the reflexive practitioner. *Journal of Clinical Nursing*, 6(2), 93–97.

Rosanoff, N. (1999). Intuition comes of age: Workplace applications of intuitive skill for occupational and environmental health nurses. *Official Journal of the American Association of Occupational Health Nurses,* 47(4), 156–162.

Ross, M.M., Bourbonnais, F.F., and Carroll, G. (1987). Curricular design and the Betty Neuman systems model: A new approach to learning. *International Nursing Review,* 34(3), 75–79.

Roy, C. (1979). Relating nursing theory to education: A new era. *Nurse Educator,* 4(2), 16–21.

Rutty, J.E. (1998). The nature of philosophy of science, theory and knowledge relating to nursing and professionalism. *Journal of Advanced Nursing,* 28(2), 243–250.

Sadala, M.L. (1999). Taking care as a relationship: A phenomenological view. *Journal of Advanced Nursing,* 30(4), 808–817.

Sakalys, J.A. (2002). Literary pedagogy in nursing: A theory-based perspective. *Journal of Nursing Education,* 41(9), 386–392.

Sanford, R.C. (2000). Caring through relation and dialogue: A nursing perspective for patient education. *Advances in Nursing Science,* 22(3), 1–15.

Scammell, J. and Miller, S. (1999). Back to basics: Exploring the conceptual basis of nursing. *Nurse Education Today,* 19(7), 570–577.

Scanlan, J.M. and Chernomas, W.M. (1997). Developing the reflective teacher. *Journal of Advanced Nursing,* 25(6), 1138–1143.

Schmieding, N.J. and Waldman, R.C. (1997). Gastric decompression in adult patients. Survey of nursing practice. *Clinical Nursing Research,* 6(2), 142–155.

Schultz, E.D. (1998). Academic advising from a nursing theory perspective. *Nurse Educator,* 23(2), 22–25.

Selanders, L.C. (1998). Florence Nightingale: The evolution and social impact of feminist values in nursing. *Journal of Holistic Nursing,* 16(2), 227–243.

Severinsson, E.I. (1998). Bridging the gap between theory and practice: A supervision programme for nursing students. *Journal of Advanced Nursing,* 27(6), 1269–1277.

Shriver, C.B. and Scott-Stiles, A. (2000). Health habits of nursing versus non-nursing students: A longitudinal study. *Journal of Nursing Education,* 39(7), 308–314.

Sills, G.M. (1998). Peplau and professionalism: The emergence of the paradigm of professionalization. *Journal of Psychiatric and Mental Health Nursing,* 5(3), 167–171.

Slaninka, S.C. (1999). Nursing theories: Creative teaching strategies make this course come alive. *Nurse Educator,* 24(3), 40–43.

Smith, A. (1998). Learning about reflection. *Journal of Advanced Nursing,* 28(4), 891–898.

Smith, L.S. (1998). Concept analysis: Cultural competence. *Journal of Cultural Diversity,* 5(1), 4–10.

Sorrell, J.M. and Redmond, G.M. (1997). The lived experiences of students in nursing: Voices of caring speak of the tact of teaching. *Journal of Professional Nursing,* 13(4), 228–235.

Sortet, J.P. (1989). Incongruence in the nursing profession. *Nursing Management,* 20(5), 64–66, 68.

Spouse, J. (2001). Bridging theory and practice in the supervisory relationship: A sociocultural perspective. *Journal of Advanced Nursing,* 33(4), 512–522.

Stark, S., Cooke, P., and Stronach, I. (2000). Minding the gap: Some theory-practice disjunctions in nursing education research. *Nurse Education Today,* 20(2), 155–163.

Stein, K.F., Corte, C., Colling, K.B., and Whall, A. (1998). A theoretical analysis of Carper's ways of knowing using a model of social cognition. *Scholarly Inquiry for Nursing Practice,* 12(1), 43–60.

Stewart, K.E., DiClemente, R.J., and Ross, D. (1999). Adolescents and HIV: Theory-based approaches to education of nurses. *Journal of Advanced Nursing,* 30(3), 687–696.

Tanner, J. (1999). Problem based learning: An opportunity for theatre nurse education. *British Journal of Theatre Nursing,* 9(11), 531–536.

Thompson, J.M. (2001). Teaching tools. An icebreaker to introduce nursing theory. *Nurse Educator,* 26(1), 13–14.

Thorne, S.E., Kirkham, S.R. and Henderson, A. (1999). Ideological implications of paradigm discourse. *Nursing Inquiry,* 6(2), 123–131.

Tilley, S. (1999). Altschul's legacy in mediating British and American psychiatric nursing discourses: Common sense and the "absence" of the accountable practitioner. *Journal of Psychiatric and Mental Health Nursing,* 6(4), 283–295.

Timpka, T. (2000). The patient and the primary care team: A small-scale critical theory. *Journal of Advanced Nursing,* 31(3), 558–564.

Torres, G. and Yura, H. (1974). *Today's conceptual framework: Its relationship to the curriculum development process* (Publication No. 15–1529). New York: National League for Nursing.

Turnbull, J. (1999). Intuition in nursing relationships: The result of "skills" or "qualities?" *British Journal of Nursing,* 8(5), 302–306.

Turner, S.L. and Bentley, G.W. (1998). A meaningful health assessment course for baccalaureate nursing students. *Nursing Connections,* 11(2), 5–12.

Upton, D.J. (1999). How can we achieve evidence-based practice if we have a theory-practice gap in nursing today? *Journal of Advanced Nursing,* 29(3), 549–555.

Wainwright, P. (2000). Towards an aesthetics of nursing. *Journal of Advanced Nursing,* 32(3),750–756.

Walker, M.K. and Norby, R.B. (1987–1988). An essay on friendships of utility: Resolving the disalignment between nursing education and nursing service. *Nursing Forum,* 23(1), 30–35.

Warelow, P.J. (1997). A nursing journey through discursive praxis. *Journal of Advanced Nursing,* 26(5), 1020–1027.

Weingourt, R. (1998). Using Margaret A. Newman's theory of health with elderly nursing home residents. *Perspectives in Psychiatric Care,* 34(3), 25–30.

Wenzel, L.S., Briggs, K.L., and Puryear, B.L. (1998). Portfolio: Authentic assessment in the age of the curriculum revolution. *Journal of Nursing Education,* 37(5), 208–212.

Westbrook, L.O. and Schultz, P.R. (2000). From theory to practice: Community health nursing in a public health neighborhood team. *Advances in Nursing Science,* 23(2), 50–61.

White, S.J. (1997). Empathy: A literature review and concept analysis. *Journal of Clinical Nursing,* 6(4), 253–257.

Whitener, L.M., Cox, K.R., and Maglich, S.A. (1998). Use of theory to guide nurses in the design of health messages for children. *Advances in Nursing Science,* 20(3), 21–35.

Wilkinson, C., Peters, L., Mitchell, K., Irwin, T., McCorrie, K., and MacLeod, M. (1998). "Being there": Learning through active participation. *Nurse Education Today,* 18(3), 226–230.

Wilkinson, R.A. (1999). Triage in accident and emergency. 2: Educational requirements. *British Journal of Nursing,* 8(3), 165–168.

Williams, A.M. (1998). The delivery of quality nursing care: a grounded theory study of the nurse's perspective. *Journal of Advanced Nursing,* 27(4), 808–816.

Williams, R. (1999). Cultural safety—What does it mean for our work practice? *Australian and New Zealand Journal of Public Health* (1999), 23(2), 213–214. Comment in: *Australian and New Zealand Journal of Public Health,* 23(5), 552–553.

Willis, W.O. (1999). Culturally competent nursing care during the perinatal period. *Journal of Perinatal and Neonatal Nursing,* 13(3), 45–59.

Wilshaw, G. (1999). Perspectives on surviving childhood sexual abuse. *Journal of Advanced Nursing,* 30(2), 303–309.

Wissmann, J. L. (1994). Teaching nursing theory through an election campaign framework. *Nurse Educator,* 9, 21–23.

Wood, I. (1998). The effects of continuing professional education on the clinical practice of nurses: A review of the literature. *International Journal of Nursing Studies,* 35(3), 125–131.

Wynne, N., Brand, S., and Smith, R. (1997). Incomplete holism in pre-registration nurse education: The position of the biological sciences. *Journal of Advanced Nursing,* 26(3), 470–474.

Zoucha, R. and Husted, G.L. (2000). The ethical dimensions of delivering culturally congruent nursing and health care. *Issues in Mental Health Nursing,* 21(3), 325–340.

11. Theory and Administration

Allen, D. (1997). Nursing, knowledge and practice. *Journal of Health Services Research and Policy,* 2(3), 190–193.

Anderson, J.M. (1991). Reflexivity in fieldwork: Toward a feminist epistemology. *Image: Journal of Nursing Scholarship,* 23, 115–118.

Anderson, R.A., Dobal, M.T., and Blessing, B. (1992). Theory-based approach to computer skill development in nursing administration. *Computers in Nursing,* 10(4), 152–157.

August-Brady, M. (2000). Prevention as intervention. *Journal of Advanced Nursing,* 31(6), 1304–1308.

Barker, P. (1998). The future of the theory of interpersonal relations? A personal reflection on Peplau's legacy. *Journal of Psychiatric and Mental Health Nursing,* 5(3), 213–220.

Barker, P., Jackson, S., and Stevenson C. (1999). The need for psychiatric nursing: Towards a multidimensional theory of caring. *Nursing Inquiry,* 6(2), 103–111.

Barker, P., Jackson, S., and Stevenson C. (1999). What are psychiatric nurses needed for? Developing a theory of essential nursing practice. *Journal of Psychiatric and Mental Health Nursing,* 6(4), 273–282.

Barnes, M. (1999). Research in midwifery—The relevance of a feminist theoretical framework. *Journal of the Australian College of Midwives,* 12(2), 6–10.

Beck, C.T. (1982). The conceptualization of power. *Advances in Nursing Science*, 1, 1–17.

Beeber, L.S. (1998). Treating depression through the therapeutic nurse-client relationship. *Nursing Clinics of North America*, 33(1), 153–172.

Biley, F.C. and Freshwater, D. (1999). Trends in nursing and midwifery research and the need for change in complementary therapy research. *Complementary Therapies in Nursing and Midwifery*, 5(4), 99–102.

Blix, A. (1999). Integrating occupational health protection and health promotion: Theory and program application. *Journal of the American Association of Occupational Health Nurses*, 47(4), 168–171.

Bondas-Salonen, T. (1998). New mothers' experiences of postpartum care—A phenomenological follow-up study. *Journal of Clinical Nursing*, 7(2), 165–174.

Booth, K., Kenrick, M., and Woods, S. (1997). Nursing knowledge, theory and method revisited. *Journal of Advanced Nursing*, 26(4), 804–811.

Brennan, P.F. and Anthony, M.K. (2000). Measuring nursing practice models using Multi-Attribute Utility Theory. *Research in Nursing and Health*, 23(5), 372–382.

Brown, R. (2000). Describing a model of nursing as a focus for psychiatric nursing care. *International Journal of Psychiatric Nursing Research*, 6(1), 670–682.

Cash, K. (1997). Social epistemology, gender and nursing theory. *International Journal of Nursing Studies*, 34(2),137–143.

Chambers, M. (1998). Interpersonal mental health nursing: Research issues and challenges. *Journal of Psychiatric and Mental Health Nursing*, 5(3), 203–211.

Clark, J. (1998). The unique function of the nurse. *Nursing Standard*, 12(16), 39–42.

Clifford, C. (1997). Nurse teachers and research. *Nurse Education Today*, 17(2), 15–120.

Colodny, A. (1997). Spinal cord injury nurses in action: Partners in practice. *SCI Nursing*, 14(3), 79–82.

Crossan, F. and Robb, A. (1998). Role of the nurse: Introducing theories and concepts. *British Journal of Nursing*, 7(10), 608–612.

Cutcliffe, J.R. (2000). Methodological issues in grounded theory. *Journal of Advance*
Nursing, 31(6), 1476–1484.

DeGroot, H.A., Ferketich, S.L., and Larson, P.J. (1987). Theory development in a no
university service setting. *Journal of Nursing Administration*, 17(4), 38–44.

DeMong, N.C. and Assie-Lussier, L.L. (1999). Continuing education: An aspect of s
development relating to the nurse manager's role. *Journal of Nursing Staff D*
opment, 15(1), 19–22.

Dixon, E.L. (1999). Community health nursing practice and the Roy Adaptation M
Public Health Nursing, 16(4), 290–300.

Dorsey, K. and Purcell, S. (1987). Translating a nursing theory into a nursing
Geriatric Nursing, 8(3), 136–137.

Driver, J. and Campbell, J. (2000). An evaluation of the impact of lecturer pra
on learning. *British Journal of Nursing*, 9(5), 292–300.

Dunlap, K. (1998). The practice of nursing theory in the operating room. *T*
gical Nurse, 20(5), 18–22.

Dyson, M. (1999). Intensive care unit psychosis, the therapeutic nurse-pati
ship and the influence of the intensive care setting: Analyses of inte
tors. *Journal of Clinical Nursing*, 8(3), 284–290.

Engebretson, J. (1997). A multiparadigm approach to nursing. *Advances in Nursing Science*, 20(1), 21–33.

Fagerstrom, L. and Engberg, I.B. (1998). Measuring the unmeasurable: A caring science perspective on patient classification. *Journal of Nursing Management*, 6(3), 165–172.

Fawcett, J., Botter, M., Burritt, J., Crossly, J., and Frink, B. (1989). Conceptual models of nursing and organization theories. In B. Henry, C. Arndt, M. DiVincenti, and A. Marriner-Tomey (Eds.), *Dimensions of nursing administration: Theory, research, education, practice*. Boston: Blackwell Scientific Publications.

Fealy, G.M. (1999). The theory-practice relationship in nursing: The practitioners' perspective. *Journal of Advanced Nursing*, 30(1), 74–82.

Fielding, R.G. and Llewelyn, S.P. (1987). Communication training in nursing may damage your health and enthusiasm: Some warnings. *Journal of Advanced Nursing*, 12(3), 281–290.

Fishel, A.H. (1998). Nursing management of anxiety and panic. *Nursing Clinics of North America*, 33(1), 135–151.

Fisher, M.A. and Mitchell, G.J. (1998). Patients' views of quality of life: Transforming the knowledge base of nursing. *Clinical Nurse Specialist*, 12(3), 99–105 Comment in *Clinical Nurse Specialist* (1998) 12(3), 98.

Forchuk, C., Jewell, J., Schofield, R., Sircelj, M., and Valledor, T. (1998) From hospital to community: Bridging therapeutic relationships. *Journal of Psychiatric and Mental Health Nursing*, 5(3),197–202.

Fowler, J. and Chevannes, M. (1998). Evaluating the efficacy of reflective practice within the context of clinical supervision. *Journal of Advanced Nursing*, 27(2), 379–382.

Francis, D., Owens, J., and Tollefson, J. (1998). "It comes together at the end": The impact of a one-year subject in *Nursing Inquiry* on philosophies of nursing. *Nursing Inquiry*, 5(4), 268–278.

Fry, S.T. (1999). The philosophy of nursing. *Scholarly Inquiry in Nursing Practice*, 13(1), 5–15.

…gan, M.J., Badger, T.A., and de Leon Baker, M. (1999). Nurse practitioner interventions for domestic violence. *Clinical Excellence in Nurse Practice*, 3(5), 273–278.

…n, N.S. (1998). Influencing mental health nursing practice through the teaching …esearch and theory: A personal critical review. *Journal of Psychiatric and Men…ealth Nursing*, 5(2), 119–128.

…N. and Gottlieb, B. (1998). Evolutionary principles can guide nursing's future …nent. *Journal of Advanced Nursing*, 28(5), 1099–1105.

…999). Holism in the care of the allogeneic bone marrow transplant pop… of the nurse practitioner. *Holistic Nursing Practice*, 13(2), 20–27.

…. The helping relationship in the community setting: The relevance …ory to the supervision of Project (2000) students. *International …g Studies*, 34(6), 415–419.

…rtin, K. S., and Androwich, I. (1994). Informatics issues for nurs…*s in Nursing Science*, 16, 71–81.

…enti, M., and Marriner-Tomey, A. (Eds.). (1989). *Dimensions …n: Theory, research, education, practice*. Boston: Blackwell

Heslop, L. (1998) A discursive exploration of nursing work in the hospital emergency setting. *Nursing Inquiry*, 5(2), 87–95.

Hickey, G. and Kipping, C. (1998). Exploring the concept of user involvement in mental health through a participation continuum. *Journal of Clinical Nursing*, 7(1), 83–88.

Hicks, C. (1998). Barriers to evidence-based care in nursing: Historical legacies and conflicting cultures. *Journal of the Association of University Programs in Health Administration*, 11(3), 137–147.

Hilz, L.M. (2000). The informatics nurse specialist as change agent. Application of innovation-diffusion theory. *Computers in Nursing*, 18(6), 272–278.

Holland, S. (1999). Teaching nursing ethics by cases: A personal perspective. *Nursing Ethics*, 6(5), 434–436.

Hopkinson, J.B. and Hallett, C.E. (2001). Patients' perceptions of hospice day care: A phenomenological study. *International Journal of Nursing Studies*, 38(1), 117–125.

Hopton, J. (1997). Towards a critical theory of mental health nursing. *Journal of Advanced Nursing*, 25(3), 492–500.

Horrocks, S. (2000). Hunting for Heidegger: Questioning the sources in the Benner/Cash debate. *International Journal of Nursing Studies*, 37(3), 237–243.

Hyrkas, K., Koivula, M., and Paunonen, M. (1999). Clinical supervision in nursing in the 1990s—Current state of concepts, theory and research. *Journal of Nursing Management*, 7(3), 177–187.

Jaarsma, T., Halfens, R., Senten, M., Abu Saad, H.H., and Dracup, K. (1998). Developing a supportive-educative program for patients with advanced heart failure within Orem's general theory of nursing. *Nursing Science Quarterly*, 11(2), 79–85.

Jennings, B.M. and Meleis, A.I. (1988). Nursing theory and administrative practice: Agenda for the 1990s. *Advances in Nursing Science*, 10(3), 56–69.

Jorgenson, J. (1997). Therapeutic use of companion animals in health care. *Image: Journal of Nursing Scholarship*, 29(3), 249–254.

Keddy, B., Gregor, F., Foster, S., and Denney, D. (1999). Theorizing about nurses' work lives: The personal and professional aftermath of living with healthcare 'reform'. *Nursing Inquiry*, 6(1), 58–64.

King, I.M. (1997). King's theory of goal attainment in practice. *Nursing Science Quarterly*, 10(4), 180–185.

Kleinbeck, S.V. (2000). Dimensions of perioperative nursing for a national specialty nomenclature. *Journal of Advanced Nursing*, 31(3), 529–535.

Kulbok, P.A., Gates, M.F., Vicenzi, A.E., and Schultz, P.R. (1999). Focus on community: Directions for nursing knowledge development. *Journal of Advanced Nursing*, 29(5), 1188–1196.

Landers, M.G. (2000). The theory-practice gap in nursing: The role of the nurse teacher. *Journal of Advanced Nursing*, 32(6), 1550–1556.

Laurent, C.L. (2000). A nursing theory for nursing leadership. *Journal of Nursing Management*, 8(2), 83–87.

Lego, S. (1998). The application of Peplau's theory to group psychotherapy. *Journal of Psychiatric and Mental Health Nursing*, 5(3), 193–196.

LeVasseur, J.J. (1999). Toward an understanding of art in nursing. *Advances in Nursing Science*, 21(4), 48–63.

Linscott, J., Spee, R., Flint, F., and Fisher, A. (1999). Creating a culture of patient-focused care through a learner-centered philosophy. *Canadian Journal of Nursing Leadership*, 12(4), 5–10.

Machin, T. and Stevenson, C. (1997). Towards a framework for clarifying psychiatric nursing roles. *Journal of Psychiatric and Mental Health Nursing*, 4(2), 81–87.

Mackintosh, C. (2000). "Is there a place for 'care' within nursing?" *International Journal of Nursing Studies*, 37(4), 321–327.

Marck, P. (2000). Nursing in a technological world: Searching for healing communities. *Advances in Nursing Science,* 23(2), 62–81.

McGuire, E. (1999). Chaos theory. Learning a new science. *Journal of Nursing Administration*, 29(2), 8–9.

McKenna, B. and Roberts, R. (1999). Bridging the theory-practice gap. *Nursing New Zealand*, 5(2), 14–16.

McKenna, H. (1999). The role of reflection in the development of practice theory: A case study. *Journal of Psychiatric and Mental Health Nursing*, 6(2), 147–151.

McKenna, H.P. (1997). Theory and research: A linkage to benefit practice. *International Journal of Nursing Studies*, 34(6), 431–437.

Meleis, A.I. (1998). ReVisions in knowledge development: A passion for substance. *Scholarly Inquiry in Nursing Practice*, 12(1), 65–77.

Meleis, A.I. and Jennings, B.M. (1989). Theoretical nursing administration: Today's challenges, tomorrow's bridges. In B. Henry, C. Arndt, M. DiVincenti, and A. Marriner-Tomey (Eds.), *Dimensions of nursing administration: Theory, research, education, practice.* Boston: Blackwell Scientific Publications.

Miller, S.K. (1999). Nurse practitioners in the county correctional facility setting: Unique challenges and suggestions for effective health promotion. *Clinical Excellence in Nurse Practice*, 3(5), 268–272.

Minicucci, D.S. (1998). A review and synthesis of the literature: The use of presence in the nursing care of families. *Journal of the New York State Nurses Association*, 29(3–4), 9–15.

Mohr, W.K. and Naylor, M.D. (1998). Creating a curriculum for the 21st century. *Nursing Outlook*, 46(5), 206–212.

Monti, E.J. and Tingen, M.S. (1999) Multiple paradigms of nursing science. *Advances in Nursing Science*, 21(4), 64–80.

Mulholland, J. (1997). Assimilating sociology: Critical reflections on the 'sociology in nursing' debate. *Journal of Advanced Nursing*, 25(4), 844–852.

Neal, L.J. (1999). Facilitating the growth of nursing staff case management in PPS. *Caring*, 18(10), 46–48.

Neill, S.J. (1998). Developing children's nursing through action research. *Journal of Child Health Care*, 2(1), 11–15.

Nelson, S. (1997). Reading nursing history. *Nursing Inquiry*, 4(4), 229–236.

Nolan, M. and Tolson, D. (2000). Gerontological nursing. 1: Challenges nursing older people in acute care. *British Journal of Nursing*, 9(1), 39–42.

Northrup, D.T. and Cody, W.K. (1998). Evaluation of the human becoming theory in practice in an acute care psychiatric setting. *Nursing Science Quarterly*, 11(1), 23–30.

Nyberg, J. (1990). Theoretic explorations of human care and economics: Foundations of nursing administration practice. *Advances in Nursing Science*, 13(1), 74–84.

O'Connell, B., Rapley, P., and Tibbett, P. (1999). Does the nursing diagnosis form the basis for patient care? *Collegian*, 6(3), 29–34.

Parse, R.R. (1999). Nursing science: The transformation of practice. *Journal of Advanced Nursing*, 30(6), 1383–1387.

Penney, W. and Warelow, P.J. (1999). Understanding the prattle of praxis. *Nursing Inquiry*, 6(4), 259–268.

Peplau, H.E. (1997), Peplau's theory of interpersonal relations. *Nursing Science Quarterly*, 10(4), 162–167.

Phillips, R., Donald, A., Mousseau-Gershman, Y., and Powell, T. (1998). Applying theory to practice—The use of "ripple effect" plans in continuing education. *Nurse Education Today*, 18(1), 12–19.

Pierson, W. (1999). Considering the nature of intersubjectivity within professional nursing. *Journal of Advanced Nursing*, 30(2), 294–302.

Ray, M.A. (1997). The ethical theory of existential authenticity: The lived experience of the art of caring in nursing administration. *Canadian Journal of Nursing Research*, 29(1), 111–126.

Rogers, M.E. (1989). Creating a climate for the implementation of a nursing conceptual framework. *Journal of Continuing Education in Nursing*, 20(3), 112–116.

Rolfe, G. (1998). The theory-practice gap in nursing: From research-based practice to practitioner-based research. *Journal of Advanced Nursing*, 28(3), 672–679.

Rosanoff, N. (1999). Intuition comes of age: Workplace applications of intuitive skill for occupational and environmental health nurses. *Journal of the American Association of Occupational Health Nurses*, 47(4), 156–162.

Rosswurm, M.A. and Larrabee, J.H. (1999). A model for change to evidence-based practice. *Image: Journal of Nursing Scholarship*, 31(4), 317–322.

Rothrock, J.C. and Smith, D.A. (2000). Selecting the perioperative patient focused model. *Journal of the Association of periOperative Registered Nurses*, 71(5), 1030–1034.

Roy, C. (2000). A theorist envisions the future and speaks to nursing administrators. *Nursing Administration Quarterly*, 24(2), 1–12.

Rutty, J.E. (1998). The nature of philosophy of science, theory and knowledge relating to nursing and professionalism. *Journal of Advanced Nursing*, 28(2), 243–250.

Sanford, R.C. (2000). Caring through relation and dialogue: A nursing perspective for patient education. *Advances in Nursing Science*, 22(3), 1–15.

Scammell, J. and Miller, S. (1999). Back to basics: Exploring the conceptual basis of nursing. *Nurse Education Today*, 19(7), 570–577.

Scherer, P. (1988). Hospitals that attract (and keep) nurses. *American Journal of Nursing*, 88(1), 34–40.

Schmieding, N.J. (1988). Action process of nurse administrators to problematic situations based on Orlando's theory. *Journal of Advanced Nursing*, 13(1), 99–107.

Severinsson, E.I. (1999). Ethics in clinical nursing supervision—An introduction to the theory and practice of different supervision models. *Collegian*, 6(3), 23–28.

Sharp, K. (1998). The case for case studies in nursing research: The problem of generalization. *Journal of Advanced Nursing*, 27(4), 785–789.

Sheafor, M. (1991). Productive work groups in complex hospital units: Proposed contributions of the nurse executive. *Journal of Nursing Administration*, 21(5), 25–30.

Sills, G.M. (1998). Peplau and professionalism: The emergence of the paradigm of professionalization. *Journal of Psychiatric and Mental Health Nursing*, 5(3), 167–171.

Smith, M. and Cusack, L. (2000). The Ottawa Charter—From nursing theory to practice: Insights from the area of alcohol and other drugs. *International Journal of Nursing Practice*, 6(4), 168–173.

Smith, M.C. (1993). The contribution of nursing theory to nursing administration practice. *Image: Journal of Nursing Scholarship*, 25, 63–67.

Spouse, J. (2001). Bridging theory and practice in the supervisory relationship: A sociocultural perspective. *Journal of Advanced Nursing*, 33(4), 512–522.

Taylor, J.S. (1997). Nursing ideology: Identification and legitimation. *Journal of Advanced Nursing*, 25(3), 442–446.

Thorne, S.E., Kirkham, S.R., and Henderson, A. (1999). Ideological implications of paradigm discourse. *Nursing Inquiry*, 6(2), 123–131.

Tilley, S. (1999). Altschul's legacy in mediating British and American psychiatric nursing discourses: Common sense and the 'absence' of the accountable practitioner. *Journal of Psychiatric and Mental Health Nursing*, 6(4), 283–295.

Traynor, M. (1997). Postmodern research: No grounding or privilege, just free-floating trouble making. *Nursing Inquiry*, 4(2), 99–107.

Turner, S.L. and Bentley, G.W. (1998). A meaningful health assessment course for baccalaureate nursing students. *Nursing Connections*, 11(2), 5–12.

Upton, D.J. (1999). How can we achieve evidence-based practice if we have a theory-practice gap in nursing today? *Journal of Advanced Nursing*, 29(3), 549–555.

Verran, J.A. (1997). The value of theory-driven (rather than problem-driven) research. *Seminars for Nurse Managers*, 5(4), 169–172.

Verran, J.A. and Reid, P.J. (1987). Replicated testing of the nursing technology model. *Nursing Research*, 36(3), 190–194.

Ward, S.L. (1998). Caring and healing in the 21st century. *MCN, The American Journal of Maternal Child Nursing*, 23(4), 210–215.

Webster, J. and Cowart, P. (1999). An innovative professional nursing practice model. *Nursing Administration Quarterly*, 23(3), 11–16.

Westbrook, L.O. and Schultz, P.R. (2000). From theory to practice: Community health nursing in a public health neighborhood team. *Advances in Nursing Science*, 23(2), 50–61.

Wewers, M.E. and Lenz, E.R. (1987). Relapse among ex-smokers: An example of theory derivation. *Advances in Nursing Science*, 9(2), 44–53.

Williams, A.M. (1998). The delivery of quality nursing care: A grounded theory study of the nurse's perspective. *Journal of Advanced Nursing*, 27(4), 808–816.

Williams, R. (1999) Comment in *Australia New Zealand Journal of Public Health* (1999), 23(5), 552–553. Cultural safety—What does it mean for our work practice? *Australia and New Zealand Journal of Public Health*, 23(2), 213–214.

Wilshaw, G. (1999). Perspectives on surviving childhood sexual abuse. *Journal of Advanced Nursing*, 30(2), 303–309.

Wimpenny, P. and Gass, J. (2000). Interviewing in phenomenology and grounded theory: Is there a difference? *Journal of Advanced Nursing*, 31(6), 1485–1492.

Wood, I. (1998). The effects of continuing professional education on the clinical practice of nurses: A review of the literature. *International Journal of Nursing Studies*, 35(3), 125–131.

Woods, S. (1998). A theory of holism for nursing. *Medical Health Care Philosophy*, 1(3), 255–261.

Wuest, J. (2000). Negotiating with helping systems: An example of grounded theory evolving through emergent fit. *Qualitative Health Research*, 10(1), 51–70.

Yegdich, T. (1998). How not to do clinical supervision in nursing. *Journal of Advanced Nursing*, 28(1), 193–202.

Yegdich, T. (1999). Clinical supervision and managerial supervision: Some historical and conceptual considerations. *Journal of Advanced Nursing*, 30(5), 1195–1204.

Zerwekh, J.V. (2000). Caring on the ragged edge: Nursing persons who are disenfranchised. *Advances in Nursing Science*, 22(4), 47–61.

12. Theory Analysis and Critique: Factors Affecting the Acceptance of Scientific Theories

Acton, G.J., Irvin, B.L., and Hopkins, B A. (1991). Theory-testing research: Building the science. *Advances in Nursing Science*, 14(1), 52–61.

Acton, G.J., Irvin, B.L., Jensen, B.A., Hopkins, B.A. and Miller, E.W. (1997). Explicating middle-range theory through methodological diversity. *Advances in Nursing Science*, 19(3), 78–85.

Allan, J. and Hall, B. (1988). Challenging the focus on technology: A critique of the medical model in a changing health care system. *Advances in Nursing Science*, 10(3), 22–34.

Anderko, L., Uscian, M., and Robertson, J.F. (1999). Improving client outcomes through differentiated practice: A rural nursing center model. *Public Health Nursing*, 16(3), 168–175.

Andershed, B. and Ternestedt, B.M. (2001). Development of a theoretical framework describing relatives' involvement in palliative care. *Journal of Advanced Nursing*, 34(4), 554–562.

Annells, M. (1997). Grounded theory method, Part I: Within the five moments of qualitative research. *Nursing Inquiry*, 4(2), 120–129.

Arthur, D., Chan, H.K., Fung, W.Y., Wong, K.Y., and Yeung, K.W. (1999) Therapeutic communication strategies used by Hong Kong mental health nurses with their Chinese clients. *Journal of Psychiatric/Mental Health Nursing*, 6(1), 29–36.

Ashley, J.A. (1978). Foundations for scholarship: Historical research in nursing. *Advances in Nursing Science*, 1, 25–36.

Ashore, R. and Banks, D. (1997). Student nurses perceptions of their interpersonal skills: A re-examination of Burnard and Morrison's findings. *International Journal of Nursing Studies*, 34(5), 335–345.

Auvil-Novak, S.E. (1997). A middle-range theory of chronotherapeutic intervention for postsurgical pain. *Nursing Research*, 46(2), 66–71.

Baas, L.S., Fontana, J.A., and Bhat, G. (1997). Relationships between self-care resources and the quality of life of persons with heart failure: A comparison of treatment groups. *Progress in Cardiovascular Nursing,* 12(1), 25–38.

Backman, K. and Kyngas, H.A. (1999). Challenges of the grounded theory approach to a novice researcher. *Nursing and Health Sciences,* 1(3), 147–153.

Baker, C. (1999). From chaos to order: A nursing-based psycho-education program for parents of children with attention-deficit hyperactivity disorder. *Canadian Journal of Nursing Research,* 31(2), 71–75.

Barkley, T.W., Jr., Rhodes, R.S., and Dufour, C.A. (1998). Predictors of success on the NCLEX-RN among baccalaureate nursing students. *Nursing and Health Care Perspectives,* 19(3),132–137.

Barnum, B.J.S. (1994). Criteria for evaluating theories. In B.J.S. Barnum (Ed.), *Nursing theory: Analysis, application and evaluation* (4th ed.). Philadelphia: J.B. Lippincott.

Barrett, E.A. and Caroselli, C. (1998). Methodological ponderings related to the power as knowing participation in change tool. *Nursing Science Quarterly,* 11(1), 17–22.

Baumann, S.L. (1997). Contrasting two approaches in a community-based nursing practice with older adults: The medical model and Parse's nursing theory. *Nursing Science Quarterly,* 10(3), 124–130.

Beeman, P.B. and Waterhouse, J.K. (2001). NCLEX-RN performance: Predicting success on the computerized examination. *Journal of Professional Nursing,* 17(4), 158–165.

Bell, A., Horsfall, J., and Goodin. W. (1998). The Mental Health Nursing Clinical Confidence Scale: A tool for measuring undergraduate learning on mental health clinical placements. *Australian and New Zealand Journal of Mental Health Nursing,* 7(4), 184–190.

Bennett, J.A. (1997). A case for theory triangulation. *Nursing Science Quarterly,* 10(2), 97–102.

Bent, K.N. (1999) Seeking the both/and of a nursing research proposal. *Advances in Nursing Science,* 21(3), 76–89.

Berragan, L. (1998). Nursing practice draws upon several different ways of knowing. *Journal of Clinical Nursing,* 7(3), 209–217.

Blix, A. (1999). Integrating occupational health protection and health promotion: Theory and program application. *Journal of the American Association of Occupational Health Nurses,* 47(4), 168–171.

Bott, M. (1997). Embedded nursing practice: A case study. *Journal of the Canadian Association of Nephrology Nurses and Technicians,* 7(4), 25–26.

Boychuk Duchscher, J.E. (1999). Catching the wave: Understanding the concept of critical thinking. *Journal of Advanced Nursing,* 29(3), 577–583.

Bradshaw, A. (1995). What are nurses doing to patients? A review of theories of nursing past and present. *Journal of Clinical Nursing,* 4(2), 81–92.

Brennan, P.F. and Anthony, M. (2000). Measuring nursing practice models using Multi-Attribute Utility theory. *Research in Nursing and Health,* 23(5), 372–382.

Brooks, E.M. and Thomas, S. (1997). The perception and judgment of senior baccalaureate student nurses in clinical decision making. *Advances in Nursing Science,* 19(3), 50–69.

Brown, S.J. (1999). Student nurses' perceptions of elderly care. *Journal of National Black Nurses Association*, 10(2), 29–36.

Buchanan, B. (1987). Conceptual models: An assessment framework. *Journal of Nursing Administration*, 17(10), 22–26.

Burks, K.J. (2001). Intentional action. *Journal of Advanced Nursing*, 34(5), 668–675.

Cain, P. (1999). Respecting and breaking confidences: Conceptual, ethical and educational issues. *Nurse Education Today*, 19(3), 175–181.

Caris-Verhallen, W.M., Kerkstra, A., and Bensing, J.M. (1997). The role of communication in nursing care for elderly people: A review of the literature. *Journal of Advanced Nursing*, 25(5), 915–933.

Carson, M.G. and Mitchell, G.J. (1998). The experience of living with persistent pain. *Journal of Advanced Nursing*, 28(6), 1242–1248.

Chafetz, J.S. (1979). *A primer on the construction and testing of theories in sociology.* Itasca, IL: F.E. Peacock Publisher. (Especially note Chapter 8.)

Chinn, P.L. and Jacobs, M.K. (1987). *Theory and nursing: A systematic approach.* St. Louis, MO: C.V. Mosby.

Chinn, P.L. and Jacobs, M.K. (1983). The evaluation of theory. In P.L. Chinn and M.K. Jacobs (Eds.), *Theory and nursing: A systematic approach.* St. Louis: C.V. Mosby.

Clift, J. and Barrett, E. (1998). Testing nursing theory cross-culturally. *International Nursing Review*, 45(4), 123–126.

Conley, V.M. (1998). Beyond knowledge deficit to a proposal for information-seeking behaviors. *Nursing Diagnosis*, 9(4), 129–135.

Cooley, M.E. (1999). Analysis and evaluation of the Trajectory Theory of Chronic Illness Management. *Scholarly Inquiry for Nursing Practice*, 13(2), 75–95.

Copnell, B. (1998). Synthesis in nursing knowledge: An analysis of two approaches. *Journal of Advanced Nursing*, 27(4), 870–874.

Corner, J. (1997). Beyond survival rates and side effects: Cancer nursing as therapy. The Robert Tiffany Lecture. 9th International Conference on Cancer Nursing, Brighton, UK, August 1996 *Cancer Nursing*, 20(1), 3–11.

Cowley, S. and Billings, J.R. (1999). Resources revisited: Salutogenesis from a lay perspective. *Journal of Advanced Nursing*, 29(4), 994–1004.

Croom, S., Procter, S., and Couteur, A.L. (2000). Developing a concept analysis of control for use in child and adolescent mental health nursing. *Journal of Advanced Nursing*, 31(6), 1324–1332.

Crossan, F. and Robb, A. (1998). Role of the nurse: Introducing theories and concepts. *British Journal of Nursing*, 7(10), 608–612.

Davis, K. and Glass, N. (1999). Contemporary theories and contemporary nursing—Advancing nursing care for those who are marginalized. *Contemporary Nurse*, 8(2): 32–38.

Dawson, P.J. (1997). Is there anyone in there? Psychiatric nursing meets biological psychiatry. *Nursing Inquiry*, 4(3), 167–175.

Dean, J.M. and Mountfourd, B. (1998). Innovation in the assessment of nursing theory and its evaluation: A team approach. *Journal of Advanced Nursing*, 28(2), 409–418.

Deatrick, J.A., Knafl, K.A., and Murphy-Moore, C. (1999). Clarifying the concept of normalization. *Image: Journal of Nursing Scholarship*, 31(3), 209–214.

DeSantis, L. and Ugarriza, D.N. (2000). The concept of theme as used in qualitative nursing research. *Western Journal of Nursing Research*, 22(3), 351–372.

Dewey, J. (1958). *Experience and nature* (Rev. ed.). New York: Dover Publications.

Dierckx de Casterle, B., Roelens, A., and Gastmans, C. (1998). An adjusted version of Kohlberg's moral theory: Discussion of its validity for research in nursing ethics. *Journal of Advanced Nursing*, 27(4), 829–835.

Dijkstra, A., Buist, G., and Dassen, T. (1998) Operationalization of the concept of "nursing care dependency" for use in long-term care facilities. *Australian and New Zealand Journal of Mental Health Nursing*, 7(4), 142–151.

Dolan, K. (1997). Children in accident and emergency. *Accident and Emergency Nursing*, 5(2), 88–91.

Draper, P. (1993). A critique of Fawcett's "Conceptual models and nursing practice: The reciprocal relationship." *Journal of Advanced Nursing*, 18, 558–564.

Driver, J. and Campbell, J. (2000). An evaluation of the impact of lecturer practitioners on learning. *British Journal of Nursing*, 9(5), 292–300.

Dubos, R. (1963). *The cultural roots and social fruits of science.* Eugene, OR: University of Oregon Books.

Dudley-Brown, S.L. (1997). The evaluation of nursing theory: A method for our madness. *International Journal of Nursing Studies*, 34, 76–83.

Duffey, M. and Muhlenkamp, A.F. (1974). A framework for theory analysis. *Nursing Outlook*, 22(9), 570–574.

Duffy, M.E. (1994). Testing the theory of transcending options: Health behaviors of single parents. *Scholarly Inquiry for Nursing Practice*, 8, 191–282.

Eakes, G.G., Burke, M.L., and Hainsworth, M.A. (1998). Middle-range theory of chronic sorrow. *Image: Journal of Nursing Scholarship*, 30(2), 179–184.

Edwards, P. (Editor in Chief). (1967). *Pragmatic theory of truth: Pragmatism. The encyclopedia of philosophy* (Vol. 6). New York: Macmillan and Free Press.

Elcock, K. (1998). Lecturer practitioner: A concept analysis. *Journal of Advanced Nursing*, 28(5), 1092–1098.

*Ellis, R. (1968). Characteristics of significant theories. *Nursing Research*, 17(3), 217–222.

Emden, C. (1998). Conducting a narrative analysis. *Collegian*, 5(3), 34–39.

Evangelista, L.S. (1999). Compliance: A concept analysis. *Nursing Forum*, 34(1), 5–11.

Facione, N.C., Facione, P.A., and Sanchez, C.A. (1994). Critical thinking disposition as a measure of competent clinical judgment. The development of the "California Critical Thinking Disposition Inventory." *Journal of Nursing Education*, 33(8), 345–350.

Fagerstrom, L. and Engberg, I.B. (1998). Measuring the unmeasurable: A caring science perspective on patient classification. *Journal of Nursing Management*, 6(3), 165–172.

*Fawcett, J. (1980). A framework for analysis and evaluation of conceptual models of nursing. *Nurse Educator*, 5(6), 10–14.

Fawcett, J. (1989). *Analysis and evaluation of conceptual models of nursing* (2nd ed.). Philadelphia: F.A. Davis.

Fawcett, J., Watson, J,. Neuman, B., Walker, P.H., and Fitzpatrick, J.J. (2001). On nursing theories and evidence. *Journal of Nursing Scholarship*, 33(2),115–119.

Fealy, G.M. (1997). The theory-practice relationship in nursing: An exploration of contemporary discourse. *Journal of Advanced Nursing*, 25(5), 1061–1069.

Fernandez, E. (1997). Just "doing the observations": Reflective practice in nursing. *British Journal of Nursing*, 6(16), 939–943

Fisher, M.A. and Mitchell, G.J. (1998). Patients' views of quality of life: Transforming the knowledge base of nursing. *Clinical Nurse Specialist*, 12(3), 99–105. Comment in *Clinical Nurse Specialist* (1998), 12(3), 98.

Fitzpatrick, J. and Whall, A. (1989). *Conceptual models of nursing: Analysis and application* (2nd ed.). Bowie, MD: Robert J. Brady Co.

Forbes, D.A., King, K.M., Kushner, K.E , Letourneau, N.L., Myrick, A.F., and Profetto-McGrath, J. (1999). Warrantable evidence in nursing science. *Journal of Advanced Nursing*, 29(2), 373–379.

Forbes, M.A. (1999). Hope in the older adult with chronic illness: A comparison of two research methods in theory building. *Advances in Nursing Science*, 22(2), 74–87.

Forchuk, C., Jewell, J., Schofield, R., Sircelјm, M., and Valledor, T. (1998). From hospital to community: Bridging therapeutic relationships. *Journal of Psychiatric/Mental Health Nursing*, 5(3), 197–202.

Frank, P.G. (1954). The variety of reasons for the acceptance of scientific theories. *Scientific Monthly*, 79(3), 139–145.

Frank, P.G. (1956). The variety of reasons for the acceptance of scientific theories. In P.G. Frank (Ed.), *The validation of scientific theories*. Boston: Beacon Press.

Freshwater, D. (1998). From acorn to oak tree: A neoplatonic perspective of reflection and caring. *Australian Journal of Holistic Nursing*, 5(2), 14–19.

Gagan, M.J., Badger, T.A., and de Leon Baker, M. (1999), Nurse practitioner interventions for domestic violence. *Clinical Excellence in Nurse Practice*, 3(5), 273–278.

Gastaldo, D. and Holmes D. (1999). Foucault and nursing: A history of the present. *Nursing Inquiry*, 6(4), 231–240.

Geanellos, R. (2000). Exploring Ricoeur's hermeneutic theory of interpretation as a method of analysing research texts. *Nursing Inquiry*, 7(2), 112–119.

Goulet, C., Bell, L., St-Cyr, D., Paul, D., and Lang, A. (1998). A concept analysis of parent-infant attachment. *Journal of Advanced Nursing*, 28(5), 1071–1081.

Gramling, L.F., Lambert, V.A., and Pursley-Crotteau, S. (1998). Coping in young women: Theoretical retroduction. *Journal of Advanced Nursing*, 28(5), 1082–1091.

Greenwood. J. (1998). Establishing an international network on nurses' clinical reasoning. *Journal of Advanced Nursing*, 27(4), 843–847.

Gulzar, L. (1999). Access to health care. *Image: Journal of Nursing Scholarship*, 31(1), 13–19.

Gustafsson, G. and Andersson, L. (2001). "The Nine-Field Model" for evaluation of theoretical constructs in nursing. Part I: Development of a new model for nursing theory evaluation and application of this model to theory description of the SAUC model. *Theoria Journal of Nursing Theory*, 10(1), 10–33.

Gustafsson, G. and Andersson, L. (2001). "The Nine-Field Model" for evaluation of theoretical constructs in nursing. Part II: Application of the evaluation model to theory analysis, theory critique and theory support of the SAUC model. *Theoria Journal of Nursing Theory*, 10(2), 19–38.

Haas, B.K. (1999). Clarification and integration of similar quality of life concepts. *Image: Journal of Nursing Scholarship*, 31(3), 215–220.

Hall, B.A. (1997). Spirituality in terminal illness: An alternative view of theory. *Journal of Holistic Nursing*, 15(1), 82–96.

Hams, S.P. (1997). Concept analysis of trust: a coronary care perspective. *Intensive and Critical Care Nursing*, 13(6), 351–356.

Harden, J. (2000). Language, discourse and the chronotope: Applying literary theory to the narratives in health care. *Journal of Advanced Nursing*, 31(3), 506–512.

Hart, M.A. and Foster, S.N. (1998). Self-care agency in two groups of pregnant women. *Nursing Science Quarterly*, 11(4), 167–171.

Hartrick, G. (1998). A critical pedagogy for family nursing. *Journal of Nursing Education*, 37(2), 80–84.

Hall, B.A. (1997). Spirituality in terminal illness: An alternative view of theory. *Journal of Holistic Nursing*, 15(1), 82–96.

Hawley, P., Young, S., and Pasco, A.C. (2000). Reductionism in the pursuit of nursing science: (In)congruent with nursing's core values? *Canadian Journal of Nursing Research*, 32(2), 75–88.

Heinrich, K.T., Robinson, C.M., and Scales, M.E. (1998). Support groups: An empowering, experiential strategy. *Nurse Educator*, 23(4), 8–10.

Henly, S.J., Vermeersch, P.E., and Duckett, L.J. (1998). Model selection for covariance structures analysis in nursing research. *Western Journal of Nursing Research*, 20(3), 344–355.

Herth, K. (1998). Hope as seen through the eyes of homeless children. *Journal of Advanced Nursing*, 28(5), 1053–1062.

Heslop, L. (1997). The (im)possibilities of poststructuralist and critical social nursing inquiry. *Nursing Inquiry*, 4(1), 48–56.

Holmes, C.A. and Warelow, P.J. (1997). Culture, needs and nursing: A critical theory approach. *Journal of Advanced Nursing*, 25(3), 463–470.

Horsburgh, M.E. (1999). Self-care of well adult Canadians and adult Canadians with end stage renal disease. *International Journal of Nursing Studies*, 36(6), 443–453.

Hunk, M. (1981, November 16). Taking it: The scandal that rocked science. *This World, San Francisco Chronicle*, 16–19, 21.

Hyrkas, K., Koivula, M., and Paunonen, M. (1999). Clinical supervision in nursing in the 1990s—Current state of concepts, theory and research. *Journal of Nursing Management*, 7(3), 177–187.

Im, E.O. and Meleis, A.I. (1999). A situation-specific theory of Korean immigrant women's menopausal transition. *Image: Journal of Nursing Scholarship*, 31(4), 333–338.

Jacobs, M.K. (1986). Can nursing theory be tested? In P.L. Chinn (Ed.), *Nursing research methodology: Issues and implementation* (pp. 39–54). Rockville, MD: Aspen Systems.

Jacobson, S.F. (1987). Studying and using conceptual models of nursing. *Image: Journal of Nursing Scholarship*, 19(2), 78–82.

Johnstone, M.J. (1999). Reflective topical autobiography: An under utilised interpretive research method in nursing. *Collegian*, 6(1), 24–29.

Kaba, E., Th son, D.R., and Burnard, P. (2000). Coping after heart transplantation: A de e study of heart transplant recipients' methods of coping. *Journal of Nursing*, 32(4), 930–936.

Kapla 64). *The conduct of inquiry: Methodology of behavioral science.* San Ad : Chandler.

Geiger, M.L., and Hartig, J.L. (1998). Clinical correlation map: A tool for heory and practice. *Nurse Educator*, 23(4), 31–34.

K.H. (1998). Ready-to-wear: Discovering grounded formal theory. *Research sing and Health*, 21(2), 179–186.

Gregor, F., Foster, S., and Denney, D. (1999). Theorizing about nurses' work The personal and professional aftermath of living with healthcare "reform." *sing Inquiry*, 6(1), 58–64.

L.S. (1999). Evaluating change in quality of life from the perspective of the rson: Advanced practice nursing and Parse's goal of nursing. *Holistic Nursing ractice*, 13(4), 61–70.

H.S. (1999). Critical reflective inquiry for knowledge development in nursing practice. *Journal of Advanced Nursing*, 29(5), 1205–1212.

nbeck, S.V. (2000). Dimensions of perioperative nursing for a national specialty nomenclature. *Journal of Advanced Nursing*, 31(3), 529–535.

ight, M.M. (2000). Cognitive ability and functional status. *Journal of Advanced Nursing*, 31(6), 1459–1468.

Kuhn, T. (1977). *The essential tension: Selected studies in scientific tradition and change.* Chicago: University of Chicago Press. (Especially note Chapter 13.)

Langford, C.P., Bowsher, J., Maloney, J.P., and Lillis, P.P. (1997). Social support: A conceptual analysis. *Journal of Advanced Nursing*, 25(1), 95–100.

Laudan, L. (1977). Progress and its problems: Toward a theory of scientific growth. Berkeley, CA: University of California Press.

LeBlanc, R.G. (1997). Definitions of oppression. *Nursing Inquiry*, 4(4), 257–261.

Lee, M.B. (1999). Power, self-care and health in women living in urban squatter settlements in Karachi, Pakistan: A test of Orem's theory. *Journal of Advanced Nursing*, 30(1), 248–259.

Lee, P. (1998). An analysis and evaluation of Casey's conceptual framework. *International Journal of Nursing Studies*, 35(4), 204–209.

Lego, S., (1998). The application of Peplau's theory to group psychotherapy. *Journal of Psychiatric/Mental Health Nursing*, 5(3), 193–196.

Lerdal, A. (1998). A concept analysis of energy: Its meaning in the lives of three individuals with chronic illness. *Scandinavian Journal of Caring Sciences*, 12(1), 3–10.

Levesque, L., Ricard, N., Ducharme, F., Duquette, A., and Bonin, J.P. (1998). Empirical verification of a theoretical model derived from the Roy adaptation model: Findings from five studies. *Nursing Science Quarterly*, 11(1), 31–39.

Levine, M.E. (1995). The rhetoric of nursing theory. *Image: Journal of Nursing Scholarship*, 27(1), 11–14.

Liehr, P. and Smith, M.J. (1999). Middle range theory: Spinning research and practice to create knowledge for the new millennium. *Advances in Nursing Science*, 21(4), 81–91.

Linscott, J., Spee, R., Flint, F., and Fisher A. (1999). Creating a of patient-focused care through a learner-centered philosophy. *Canadian J of Nursing Leadership*, 12(4), 5–10.

Logan, J. and Jenny, J. (1997). Qualitative analysis of patients' w mechanical ventilation and weaning. *Heart and Lung*, 26(2), 140–147.

Long, A. and Slevin, E. (1999). Living with dementia: Communicatin son and her family. *Nursing Ethics*, 6(1), 23–36.

Lukkarinen, H. and Hentinen, M. (1997). Self-care agency and facto agency among patients with coronary heart disease. *International J per-ing Studies*, 34(4), 295–304.

Maggs-Rapport, F. (2000). Combining methodological approaches in researc phy and interpretive phenomenology. *Journal of Advanced Nursing*, 31(

Mahoney, J.S. and Engebretson, J. (2000). The interface of anthropology an guiding culturally competent care in psychiatric nursing. *Archives of Ps Nursing*, 14(4), 183–190.

Matas, K.E. (1997). Human patterning and chronic pain. *Nursing Science Qua* 10(2), 88–96.

Mavundla, T.R. (2000). Professional nurses' perception of nursing mentally ill peopl a general hospital setting. *Journal of Advanced Nursing*, 32(6), 1569–1578.

McCance, T.V., McKenna, H.P., and Boore, J.R. (1997). Caring: Dealing with a difficu concept. *International Journal of Nursing Studies*, 34(4), 241–248.

McCance, T.V., McKenna, H.P., and Boore, J.R. (1999). Caring: Theoretical perspectives of relevance to nursing. *Journal of Advanced Nursing*, 30(6), 1388–1395.

McCance, T.V., McKenna, H.P., and Boore, J.R. (2001). Exploring caring using narrative methodology: An analysis of the approach. *Journal of Advanced Nursing*, 33(3), 350–356.

McGrath, B.B. (1998). Illness as a problem of meaning: Moving culture from the classroom to the clinic. *Advances in Nursing Science*, 21(2), 17–29.

McHolm, F.A. and Geib, K.M. (1998). Application of the Neuman Systems Model to teaching health assessment and nursing process. *Nursing Diagnosis*, 9(1), 23–33.

McLaughlin C. (1997). The effect of classroom theory and contact with patients on the attitudes of student nurses towards mentally ill people. *Journal of Advanced Nursing*, 26(6), 1221–1228.

McQuiston, C.M. and Campbell, J.C. (1997). Theoretical substruction: A guide for theory testing research. *Nursing Science Quarterly*, 10(3), 117–123.

Meleis, A.I. (1983). A model for theory description, analysis, and critique. In N.L. Chaska (Ed.), *The nursing profession: A time to speak.* New York: McGraw-Hill.

Meleis, A.I. (1994). Theory testing and theory support: Principles, challenges, and a sojourn into the future. In B. Neuman (Ed.), *The Neuman systems model* (pp. 447–457). East Norwalk, CT: Appleton & Lange.

Meleis, A.I., Sawyer, L.M., Im, E.O., Hilfinger Messias, D.K., and Schumacher, K. (2000). Experiencing transitions: An emerging middle-range theory. *Advances in Nursing Science*, 23(1), 12–28.

Moore, B. (1954). Influence of political creeds on the acceptance of theories. *Scientific Monthly*, 79(3), 146–148.

Neill, S.J. (1998). Developing children's nursing through action research. *Journal of Child Health Care*, 2(1), 11–15.

Nuamah, I.F., Cooley, M.E., Fawcett, J., and McCorkle, R. (1999). Testing a theory for health-related quality of life in cancer patients: A structural equation approach. *Research in Nursing and Health*, 22(3), 231–242.

Olson, J. and Hanchett, E. (1997). Nurse-expressed empathy, patient outcomes, and development of a middle-range theory. *Image: Journal of Nursing Scholarship*, 29(1), 71–76.

Parse, R.R. (1987). *Nursing science: Major paradigms, theories, and critiques.* Philadelphia: W.B. Saunders.

Phillips, R., Donald, A., Mousseau-Gershman, Y., and Powell, T. (1998). Applying theory to practice—The use of "ripple effect" plans in continuing education. *Nurse Education Today*, 18(1), 12–19.

Pilkington, F.B. (1999). A qualitative study of life after stroke. *Journal of Neuroscience Nursing*, 31(6), 336–347.

Polk, L.V. (1997). Toward a middle-range theory of resilience. *Advances in Nursing Science*, 19(3), 1–13.

Rankin, S.H. and Weekes, D.P. (2000) Life-span development: A review of theory and practice for families with chronically ill members. *Scholarly Inquiry for Nursing Practice*, 14(4), 355–373.

Ray, M.A. (1997). Consciousness and the moral ideal: A transcultural analysis of Watson's theory of transpersonal caring. *Advanced Practice Nursing Quarterly*, 3(1), 25–31.

Reynolds, P.D. (1971). *A primer in theory construction.* Indianapolis, IN: Bobbs-Merrill.

Reynolds, W.J. (1997). Peplau' s theory in practice. *Nursing Science Quarterly*, 10(4), 168–170.

Richer, M.C. and Ezer, H. (2000). Understanding beliefs and meanings in the experience of cancer: A concept analysis. *Journal of Advanced Nursing*, 32(5), 1108–1115.

Riehl-Sisca, J.P. (1989). *Conceptual models for nursing practice* (3rd ed.). East Norwalk, CT: Appleton & Lange.

Rogan, F., Shmied, V., Barclay, L., Everitt, L., and Wyllie, A. (1997). "Becoming a mother"—Developing a new theory of early motherhood. *Journal of Advanced Nursing*, 25(5), 877–885.

Rolfe, G. (1998). The theory-practice gap in nursing: From research-based practice to practitioner-based research. *Journal of Advanced Nursing*, 28(3), 672–679.

Rolfe, G. (1999). The pleasure of the bottomless: Postmodernism, chaos and paradigm shifts. *Nurse Education Today*, 19(8), 668–672.

Rudner, R. (1954). Remarks on value judgments in scientific validation. *Scientific Monthly*, 79(3),1951–1953.

Ryles, S.M. (1999). A concept analysis of empowerment: Its relationship to mental health nursing. *Journal of Advanced Nursing*, 29(3), 600–607.

Scammell, J. and Miller, S. (1999). Back to basics: Exploring the conceptual basis of nursing. *Nurse Education Today*, 19(7), 570–577.

Schrag, C. (1967). Elements of theoretical analysis in sociology. In L. Gross (Ed.), *Sociological theory: Inquiries and paradigms.* New York: Harper & Row.

Severinsson, E.I. (1998). Bridging the gap between theory and practice: A supervision programme for nursing students. *Journal of Advanced Nursing*, 27(6), 1269–1277.

Sharp, K. (1998). The case for case studies in nursing research: The problem of generalization. *Journal of Advanced Nursing*, 27(4), 785–789.

Silva, M.C. (1986). Research testing nursing theory: State of the art. *Advances in Nursing Science*, 9(1), 1–11.

Silva, M.C. and Sorrell, J.M. (1992). Testing of nursing theory: Critique and philosophical expansion. *Advances in Nursing Science*, 14(4), 12–23.

Sim, J. (1998). Collecting and analysing qualitative data: Issues raised by the focus group. *Journal of Advanced Nursing*, 28(2), 345–352.

Sim, J. and Sharp, K. (1998). A critical appraisal of the role of triangulation in nursing research. *International Journal of Nursing Studies*, 35(1–2), 23–31.

Simko, L.C. (1999). Adults with congenital heart disease: Utilizing quality of life and Husted's nursing theory as a conceptual framework. *Critical Care Nursing Quarterly*, 22(3), 1–11.

Slaninka, S.C. (1999). Nursing theories: Creative teaching strategies make this course come alive. *Nurse Educator*, 24(3), 40–43.

Slusher, I.L. (1999). Self-care agency and self-care practice of adolescents. *Issues in Comprehensive Pediatric Nursing*, 22(1), 49–58.

Smith, L.S. (1998). Concept analysis: Cultural competence. *Journal of Cultural Diversity*, 5(1), 4–10.

Smith, M. and Cusack, L. (2000). The Ottawa Charter—From nursing theory to practice: Insights from the area of alcohol and other drugs. *International Journal of Nursing Practice*, 6(4), 168–173.

Spearman, S.A., Duldt, B.W., and Brown, S. (1993). Research testing theory: A selective review of Orem's self-care theory, 1986–1991. *Journal of Advanced Nursing*, 18, 1626–1631.

Stein, K.F., Corte, C., Colling, K.B., and Whall, A. (1998). A theoretical analysis of Carper's ways of knowing using a model of social cognition. *Scholarly Inquiry for Nursing Practice*, 12(1), 43–60.

Stewart, K.E., DiClemente, R.J., and Ross, D. (1999). Adolescents and HIV: Theory-based approaches to education of nurses. *Journal of Advanced Nursing*, 30(3), 687–696.

Thelander, B.L. (1997). The psychotherapy of Hildegard Peplau in the treatment of people with serious mental illness. *Perspectives in Psychiatric Care*, 33(3), 24–32.

Thibodeau, J. and MacRae, J. (1997). Breast cancer survival: A phenomenological inquiry. *Advances in Nursing Science*, 19(4), 65–74.

Thorne, S.E., Kirkham, S.R., and Henderson, A. (1999). Ideological implications of paradigm discourse. *Nursing Inquiry*, 6(2), 123–131.

Timpka, T. (2000). The patient and the primary care team: A small-scale critical theory. *Journal of Advanced Nursing*, 31(3), 558–564.

Torres, G. (1986). *Theoretical foundations of nursing*. Norwalk, CT: Appleton-Century-Crofts.

Upton, D.J. (1999). How can we achieve evidence-based practice if we have a theory-practice gap in nursing today? *Journal of Advanced Nursing*, 29(3), 549–555.

Villarruel, A.M. and Denyes, M.J. (1997). Testing Orem's theory with Mexican Americans. *Image: Journal of Nursing Scholarship*, 29(3), 283–288.

Walker, K.M. and Alligood M.R. (2001). Empathy from a nursing perspective: Moving beyond borrowed theory. *Archives of Psychiatric Nursing*, 15(3), 140–147.

Watson, J. (1981, July). Nursing's scientific quest. *Nursing Outlook*, 29(7), 413–416.

Webb, C. (1999). Analysing qualitative data: Computerized and other approaches. *Journal of Advanced Nursing*, 29(2), 323–330.

Webster, G., Jacox, A., and Baldwin, B. (1981). Nursing theory and the ghost of the received view. In M. Grace and N. McCloskey (Eds.), *Current issues in nursing*. Scranton, PA: Blackwell Scientific Publications.

West, P. and Isenberg, M. (1997). Instrument development: The Mental Health-Related Self-Care Agency Scale. *Archives of Psychiatric Nursing*, 11(3), 126–132.

Westbrook, L.O. and Schultz, P.R. (2000). From theory to practice: Community health nursing in a public health neighborhood team. *Advances in Nursing Science*, 23(2), 50–61.

White, S.J. (1997). Empathy: A literature review and concept analysis. *Journal of Clinical Nursing*, 6(4), 253–257.

Whitley, G.G. (1997). Three phases of research in validating nursing diagnoses. *Western Journal of Nursing Research*, 19(3), 379–399.

Widdershoven, G.A. (1999). Care, cure and interpersonal understanding. *Journal of Advanced Nursing*, 29(5), 1163–1169.

Wilkinson, C., Peters, L., Mitchell, K., Irwin, T., McCorrie, K., and MacLeod, M. (1998). "Being there": Learning through active participation. *Nurse Education Today*, 18(3), 226–230.

Wimpenny, P. and Gass, J. (2000). Interviewing in phenomenology and grounded theory: Is there a difference? *Journal of Advanced Nursing*, 31(6), 1485–1492.

Winstead-Fry, P. (Ed.). (1986). *Case studies in nursing theory*. New York: National League for Nursing.

Zetterberg, H.L. (1965). *On theory verification in sociology* (3rd ed.). New York: Bedminister Press.

Zoucha, R. and Husted, G.L. (2000). The ethical dimensions of delivering culturally congruent nursing and health care. *Issues in Mental Health Nursing*, 21(3), 325–340.

Zulkowski, K. (1998). Construct validity of Minimum Data Set items within the context of the Braden Conceptual Schema. *Ostomy/Wound Management*, 44(10), 36–40.

Nursing Theory and Theorists

13. Faye Abdellah

Abdellah, F.G. (1969). The nature of nursing science. *Nursing Research*, 18, 390–393.

*Abdellah, F.G. (1970). Overview of nursing research 1955–1968, Part 1. *Nursing Research*, 19, 6–17.

Abdellah, F.G. (1970). Overview of nursing research 1955–1968, Part 2. *Nursing Research*, 19, 151–162.

Abdellah, F.G. (1970). Overview of nursing research 1955–1968, Part 3. *Nursing Research*, 19, 239–252.

Abdellah, F.G. (1971). Evolution of nursing as a profession: Perspective on manpower development. *International Nursing Review*, 19, 119–235.

Abdellah, F.G. (1972). The physician-nurse team approach to coronary care. *Nursing Clinics of North America*, 7, 423–430.

Abdellah, F.G. (1976). Nurse practitioners and nursing practice. *American Journal of Public Health*, 66, 245–246.

Abdellah, F.G. (1976). Nursing's role in future health care. *AORN Journal*, 24(2), 236–240.

Abdellah, F.G. (1978). Long term care policy issues. *Annals of the American Academy of Political and Social Science*, 438, 22.

Abdellah, F.G. (1981). Nursing care of the aged in the United States of America. *Journal of Gerontological Nursing*, 7(11), 657–663.

Abdellah, F.G. (1982). The nurse practitioner 17 years later: Present and emerging issues. *Inquiry*, 19, 105–116.

Abdellah, F.G., Beland, I.L., Martin, A., and Matheney, R.V. (1973). *New directions in patient centered nursing: Guidelines for systems of service, education and research*. New York: Macmillan.

Abdellah, F.G., Foerst, H.V., and Chow, R.K. (1979). PACE: An approach to improving care to the elderly. *American Journal of Nursing*, 79, 1109–1110.

Abdellah, F.G. and Levine, R. (1957). Developing a measure of patient and personnel satisfaction with nursing care. *Nursing Research*, 5, 100–108.

Abdellah, F.G. and Levine, R. (1965). Aims of nursing research. *Nursing Research*, 14, 29–32.

Abdellah, F.G. and Levine, R. (1965). *Better patient care through nursing research*. New York: Macmillan.

Abdellah, F.G. and Levine, R. (1979). *Better patient care through nursing research* (2nd ed.). New York: Macmillan.

Alward, R.R. (1983). Patient classification systems: The ideal vs. reality. *Journal of Nursing Administration*, 13(2), 14–19.

Anderson, M.A., Pena, R.A., and Helms, L.B. (1998). Home care utilization by congestive heart failure patients: A pilot study. *Public Health Nursing*, 15(2), 146–162.

Avis, M. (1995). Valid arguments—A consideration of the concept of validity in establishing the credibility of research findings. *Journal of Advanced Nursing*, 22(6), 1203–1209.

Bergman, R., Stockler, R.A., Shavit, N., Sharon, R., Feinberg, D., and Danon, A. (1981). Role, selection and preparation of head nurses—I. *International Journal of Nursing Studies*, 18(2), 123–152.

Bergman, R., Stockler, R.A., Shavit, N., Sharon, R., Feinberg, D., and Danon, A. (1981). Role, selection and preparation of head nurses—III. *International Journal of Nursing Studies*, 18(4), 237–250.

Blegan, M.A., Goode, C.J., and Reed, L. (1998). Nurse staffing and patient outcomes. *Nursing Research*, 47(1), 43–50.

Brown, G.D. (1995). Understanding barriers to basing nursing practice upon research—A communication model approach. *Journal of Advanced Nursing*, 21(1), 154–157.

Chang, K. (1997). Dimensions and indicators of patients' perceived nursing care quality in the hospital setting. *Journal of Nursing Care Quality*, 11(6), 26–37.

Chow, R. (1969). Postoperative cardiac nursing research: A method for identifying and categorizing nursing action. *Nursing Research*, 18(1), 4–13.

Clarke, P.N., Pendry, N.C., and Kim, Y.S. (1997). Patterns of violence in homeless women. *Western Journal of Nursing Research*, 19(4), 490–500.

Copp, L.A. (1973). Professional change: Which trends do nurses endorse? *International Journal of Nursing Studies*, 10, 55–63.

Cornell, S.A. (1974). Development of an instrument for measuring quality of nursing care. *Nursing Research*, 23, 108–117.

Craig, S.L. (1980). Theory development and its relevance for nursing. *Journal of Advanced Nursing*, 5, 349–355.

Dickoff, J. and James, P. (1970). Beliefs and values: Bases for curriculum design. *Nursing Research*, 19, 415–427.

Ditzengerber, G.R., Collins, S.D., and Bartawright, S.A. (1995). Combining the roles of clinical nurse specialist and neonatal nurse practitioner—The experience in one academic tertiary care setting. *Journal of Perinatal and Neonatal Nursing*, 9(3), 45–52.

Downs, F.S. and Fitzpatrick, J.J. (1976). Preliminary investigation of the reliability and validity of a tool for the assessment of body position and motor activity. *Nursing Research*, 25, 404–408.

Dycus, D., Schmeiser, D., Taggart, F. and Yancey, R. (1989). Faye Glenn Abdellah: Twenty-one nursing problems. In A. Marriner-Tomey (Ed.), *Nursing theorists and their work* (2nd ed.). St. Louis, MO: C.V. Mosby.

Elms, R.R. (1972). Recovery room behavior and post-operative convalescence. *Nursing Research*, 21, 390–397.

Fairman, J. (2000). Economically practical and critically necessary? The development of intensive care at Chestnut Hill Hospital. *Bulletin of the History of Medicine*, 74(1), 80–106.

Fairman, J. and Kagan, S. (1999). Creating critical care: The case of the Hospital of the University of Pennsylvania, 1950–1965. *Advances in Nursing Science*, 22(1), 63–77.

Fiedler, I.G., Laud, P.W., Maiman, D.J., et al. (1999). Economics of managed care in spinal cord injury. *Archives of Physical Medicine and Rehabilitation*, 80(11), 1441–1449.

Fortinsky, R.H., Granger, C.V. and Seltzer, G.B. (1981). The use of functional assessment in understanding home care needs. *Medical Care*, 19(5), 489–497.

Goodwin, J.O. and Edwards, B.S. (1975). Developing a computer program to assist the nursing process: Phase I—From systems analysis to an expandable program. *Nursing Research*, 24, 299–305.

Gordon, M. (1980). Determining study topics. *Nursing Research*, 29, 83–87.

Gordon, M. and Sweeney, M.A. (1979). Methodological problems and issues in identifying and standardizing nursing diagnosis. *Advances in Nursing Science*, 2(1), 1–15.

Greaves, F. (1980). Objectively toward curriculum improvement in nursing education in England and Wales. *Journal of Advanced Nursing*, 5, 591–599.

Green, J.A. (1979). Science, nursing, and nursing science: A conceptual analysis. *Advances in Nursing Science*, 2(1), 57–64.

Grier, M.R. and Schnitzler, C.P. (1979). Nurses' propensity to risk. *Nursing Research*, 28(3), 186–190.

Hardy, L.K. (1982). Nursing models and research—A restricting view? *Journal of Advanced Nursing*, 7, 447–451.

Hill, J. (1997). Patient satisfaction in a nurse-led rheumatology clinic. *Journal of Advanced Nursing*, 25(2), 347–354.

Hisama, K.K. (2001). The acceptance of nursing theory in Japan: A cultural perspective. *Nursing Science Quarterly*, 14(3), 255–259.

Hlusko, D.L. and Nichols, B.S. (1996). Can you depend on your patient classification system? *Journal of Nursing Administration*, 26(4), 39–44.

Hunt, J. (2001). Research into practice: The foundation for evidence-based care. *Cancer Nursing*, 24(2), 78–87.

Jacob, G. and Bengel, J. (2000). The construct "patient satisfaction": A critical review. *Zeitschrift fur Klinische Psychologie Psychiatrie und Psychotherapie*, 48(3), 280–301.

Jennings, C.P. and Jennings, T.F. (1977). Containing costs through prospective reimbursement. *American Journal of Nursing*, 77, 1155–1159.

Jhandler, M.C. and Mason, W.H. (1995). Solution-focused therapy—An alternative approach to addictions nursing. *Perspectives in Psychiatric Care*, 31(1), 8–13.

Jones, P.E. (1979). A terminology for nursing diagnosis. *Advances in Nursing Science*, 2(1), 65–72.

King, I.M. (1968). A conceptual frame of reference for nursing. *Nursing Research*, 17, 27–31.

LaMontagne, L.L., Pressler, J.L., and Salisbury, M.H. (1996). Scholarly mission: Fostering scholarship in research, theory and practice. *N&HC Perspectives on Community*, 17(6), 298–302.

Lanara, V.A. (1976). Philosophy of nursing and current nursing problems. *International Nursing Review*, 23(2), 48–54.

Landi, F., Zuccala, G., Bernabei, R., et al. (1997). Physiotherapy and occupational therapy—A geriatric experience in the acute care hospital. *American Journal of Physical Medicine and Rehabilitation*, 76(1), 38–42.

Leke, J.T. (1978). Nigerian patients' perception of their nursing care needs. *Journal of Advanced Nursing*, 3, 181–187.

Majesky, S.J., Brester, M.H., and Nishio, K.T. (1978). Development of a research tool: Patient indicators of nursing care. *Nursing Research*, 27, 365–371.

McAuliffe, M.S. (1998). Interview with Faye G. Abdellah on nursing research and health policy. *Image: Journal of Nursing Scholarship*, 30(3), 215–219.

McSherry, R. (1997). What do registered nurses and midwives feel and know about research? *Journal of Advanced Nursing*, 25(5), 985–976.

McGilloway, F.A. (1980). The nursing process: A problem solving approach to patient care. *International Nursing Studies*, 17(2), 79–90.

McLane, A.M. (1978). Core competencies of masters-prepared nurses. *Nursing Research*, 27(1), 43–58.

Minckley, B.B. (1974). Physiological and psychological responses of elective surgical patients. *Nursing Research*, 23(5), 392–401.

Mulhall, A. (1996). Anthropology, nursing and midwifery: A natural alliance? *International Journal of Nursing Studies*, 33(6), 629–637.

Mulhall, A. (1997). Nursing research: Our world not theirs? *Journal of Advanced Nursing*, 25(5), 969–976.

Price, M.R. (1980). Nursing diagnosis: Making a concept come alive. *American Journal of Nursing*, 80(4), 668–671.

Regan, J.A. (1998). Will current clinical effectiveness initiatives encourage and facilitate practitioners to use evidence-based practice for the benefit of their clients? *Journal of Clinical Nursing*, 7(3), 244–250.

Riddlesperger, K.L., Beard, M., Flowers, D.L., et al. (1996). CINAHL: An exploratory analysis of the current status of nursing theory construction as reflected by the electronic domain. *Journal of Advanced Nursing*, 24(3), 599–606.

Rubenstein, L.Z. (1981). Specialized geriatric assessment units and their clinical implications. *Western Journal of Medicine*, 135(6), 497–502.

See, E.M. (1989). Abdellah's model for nursing: Twenty-one nursing problems. In J. Fitzpatrick and A. Whall (Eds.), *Conceptual models of nursing: Analysis and application* (2nd ed.). East Norwalk, CT: Appleton & Lange.

Sitzia, J. and Wood, N. (1997) Patient satisfaction: A review of issues and concepts. *Social Science and Medicine*, 45(12), 1829–1843.

Shi, L.Y., Samuels, M.E., Ricketts, T.C., et al. (1994). A rural-urban comparative-study of nonphysician providers in community and migrant health centers. *Public Health Reports*, 109(6), 809–815.

Stevens, B.J. (1971). Analysis of structural forms used in nursing curricula. *Nursing Research*, 20(5), 388–397.

Walker, C. and Deuble, H. (1968). A schema for analysis of accident prevention activities in public health nurses' records. *Nursing Research*, 17(5), 408–414.

Walker, L.O. (1971). Toward a clearer understanding of the concept of nursing theory. *Nursing Research*, 20(5), 428–435.

Wright, J. (1998). Female nurses' perceptions of acceptable female body size: An exploratory study. *Journal of Clinical Nursing*, 7(4), 307–315.

Ziff, M.A., Conrad, P., and Lachman, M.E. (1995). The relative effects of perceived personal control and responsibility on health and health-related behaviors in young and middle-aged adults. *Health Education Quarterly*, 22(1), 127–142.

14. Patricia Benner

Benner, P. (1991). The role of experience, narrative, and community in skilled ethical comportment. *Advances in Nursing Science*, 14(2), 13–28.

Benner, P. (1996). A response by P. Benner to K. Cash, "Benner and expertise in nursing: A critique." *International Journal of Nursing Studies*, 33(6), 669–674.

Benner, P. (1997). A dialogue between virtue ethics and care ethics. *Theoretical Medicine*, 18(1–2), 47–61.

Benner, P. (1997). Developing a language for nursing. [Article in German]. *Pflege*, 10(2), 67–71.

Benner, P., Tanner, C., and Chesla, C. (1991). From beginner to expert: Gaining a differentiated clinical world in critical care nursing. *Advances in Nursing Science*, 14(3), 13–28.

Benner, P.A. (1985). Quality of life: A phenomenological perspective on explanation, prediction, and understanding in nursing science. *Advances in Nursing Science*, 8(1), 1–14.

Benner, R. and Benner, P. (1991). Stories from the front lines. *Healthcare Forum Journal*, 34(4), 68–74.

Hofrocks, S. (2000). Hunting for Heidegger: Questioning the sources in the Benner/Cash debate. *International Journal of Nursing Studies*, 37(3), 237–243.

Padgett, S.M. (2000). Benner and the critics: Promoting scholarly dialogue. *Scholarly Inquiry for Nursing Practice*, 14(3), 249–271.

Paley, J. (2000). Asthma and dualism. *Journal of Advanced Nursing*, 31(6), 1293–1299.

Tanner, C.A., Benner, P., Chesla, C., and Gordon, D.R. (1993). The phenomenology of knowing the patient. *Image: Journal of Nursing Scholarship*, 25(4), 273–280.

Thompson, C. (1999). A conceptual treadmill: The need for "middle ground" in clinical decision making theory in nursing. *Journal of Advanced Nursing*, 30(5), 1222–1229.

15. Betty Jo Hadley

Hadley, B.J. (1967, April). The dynamic interactionist concept of role. *Journal of Nursing Education*, 6(2), 5–10, 24–25.

Hadley, B.J. (1969). Evolution of a conception of nursing. *Nursing Research*, 18(5), 400–406.

16. Beverly Hall

Artinian, B.M. (1983). Implementation of the intersystem patient-care model in clinical practice. *Journal of Advanced Nursing*, 8, 117–124.

Hall, B.A. (1975). Mutual withdrawal: The nonparticipant in a therapeutic community. *Perspectives in Psychiatric Care*, 14(2), 75–77.

Hall, B.A. (1975). Socializing patients into the psychiatric sick role. *Perspectives in Psychiatric Care*, 13, 123–129.

Hall, B.A. (1977). The effect of interpersonal attraction on the therapeutic relationship: A review and suggestion for further study. *Journal of Psychiatric Nursing*, 15(9), 18–23.

Hall, B.A. (1977). Occupational values and family perspectives: A comparison of pre-nursing and pre-medical women. *Communicating Nursing Research*, 8, 124–132.

*Hall, B.A. (1981). The change paradigm in nursing: Growth versus persistence. *Advances in Nursing Science*, 3(4), 1–6.

Hall, B.A., McKay, R.P., and Mitsunaga, B.K. (1971). Dimensions of role commitment: Career patterns of deans of nursing. *Communicating Nursing Research*, 4, 84–98.

Hall, B.A. and Mitsunaga, B.K. (1979). Education of the nurse to promote interpersonal attraction. *Journal of Nursing Education*, 18(5), 16–21.

Hall, B.A., Mitsunaga, B.K., and DeTornyay, R. (1981). Deans of nursing: Changing socialization patterns. *Nursing Outlook*, 29, 92–95.

Hall, B.A., von Endt, B., and Parker, G. (1981). A framework for measuring satisfaction of nursing staff. *Nursing Leadership*, 4(4), 29–33.

Mitsunaga, B.K. and Hall, B.A. (1979). Interpersonal attraction and perceived quality of medical-surgical care. *Western Journal of Nursing Research*, 1(1), 5–26.

*Murphy, S.A. and Hoeffer, B. (1983). Role of the specialties in nursing science. *Advances in Nursing Science*, 5(4), 31–39.

17. Mary Harms and Fred McDonald

Bailey, J.T., McDonald, F.J., and Harms, M.T. (1966). A new approach to curriculum development. *Nursing Outlook*, 14(7), 33–36.

Harms, M.T. and McDonald, F.J. (1966). A new curriculum design, Part III. *Nursing Outlook*, 14(9), 50–53.

Harms, M.T. and McDonald, F.J. (1966). The teaching-learning process, Part IV. *Nursing Outlook*, 14(10), 54–58.

McDonald, F.J. and Harms, M.T. (1966). A theoretical model for an experimental curriculum, Part II. *Nursing Outlook*, 14(8), 48–51.

18. Virginia Henderson

DeMeester, D., Lauer, T., Neal, S., and Williams, S. (1989). Virginia Henderson: Definition of nursing. In A. Marriner-Tomey (Ed.), *Nursing theorists and their work* (2nd ed.). St. Louis, MO: C.V. Mosby.

Fulton, J.S. (1987). Virginia Henderson: Theorist, prophet, poet. *Advances in Nursing Science*, 10(1), 1–17.

Furukawa, C.Y. and Howe, J.K. (1980) Virginia Henderson. In the Nursing Theories Conference Group, *Nursing theories: The base for professional nursing practice.* Englewood Cliffs, NJ: Prentice-Hall.

Henderson, V. (1964). The nature of nursing. *American Journal of Nursing*, 64(8), 62–68.

Henderson, V. (1966). *The nature of nursing*. New York: Macmillan.

Henderson, V. (1969). Excellence in nursing. *American Journal of Nursing*, 69(9), 2133–2137.

Henderson, V. (1978). The concept of nursing. *Journal of Advanced Nursing*, 3, 113–130.

Henderson, V. (1980). Preserving the essence of nursing in a technological age. *Journal of Advanced Nursing*, 5, 245–260.

Runk, J.A. and Quillin, S.I.M. (1989). Henderson's definition of nursing. In J.J. Fitzpatrick and A.L. Whall (Eds.), *Conceptual models of nursing: Analysis and application* (2nd ed.). Bowie, MD: Robert J. Brady Co.

19. Douglas Howland

Howland, D. (1963). Approaches to the systems problem, Part I. *Nursing Research*, 13, 172–174.

Howland, D. (1963). A hospital system model, Part II. *Nursing Research*, 12(4), 232–236.

Howland, D. (1966). Approach to nurse-monitor research. *American Journal of Nursing*, 66(3), 566–588.

Howland, D. and McDowell, W.E. (1964). The measurement of patient care: A conceptual framework. *Nursing Research*, 13(1), 4–7.

20. Dorothy Johnson

Adam, E. (1987). Nursing theory: What it is and what it is not. *Nursing Papers/Perspectives on Nursing*, 19(1), 5–14.

Auger, J.R. (1976). *Behavioral systems and nursing.* Englewood Cliffs, NJ: Prentice-Hall.

†Auger, J.R. and Dee, V. (1983). A patient classification system based on the behavioral system model of nursing: Part 1. *Journal of Nursing Administration,* 13, 38–43.

Botha, M.E. (1989). Theory development in perspective: The role of conceptual frameworks and models in theory development. *Journal of Advanced Nursing,* 14(1), 49–55.

†Broncatello, K.F. (1980). Auger in action: Application of the model. *Advances in Nursing Science,* 2(2), 13–23.

Clough, D.H. and Derdiarian, A. (1980). A behavioral checklist to measure dependence and independence. *Nursing Research,* 29(1), 55–58.

Conner, S., Magers, J., and Watt, J. (1989). Dorothy E. Johnson: Behavioral system model. In A. Marriner-Tomey (Ed.), *Nursing theorists and their work* (2nd ed.). St. Louis, MO: C.V. Mosby.

Cormack, D.F. and Reynolds, W. (1992). Criteria for evaluating the clinical and practical utility of models used by nurses. *Journal of Advanced Nursing,* 17(12), 1472–1478.

Damus, K. (1980). An application of the Johnson behavioral system model for nursing practice. In J.P. Riehl and C. Roy (Eds.), *Conceptual models for nursing practice.* New York: Appleton-Century-Crofts.

Dee, V. (1990). Implementation of the Johnson model: One hospital's experience. In M.E. Parker (Ed.), *Nursing theories in practice* (pp. 33–44). New York: National League for Nursing.

†Dee, V. and Auger, J.R. (1983). A patient classification system based on the behavioral system model of nursing: Part 2. *Journal of Nursing Administration,* 13, 18–23.

Derdiarian, A.K. and Clough, D. (1980). A behavioral checklist to measure dependence and independence. *Nursing Research,* 28, 55–58.

Derdiarian, A.K. (1981). Nursing conceptual frameworks: Implications for education, practice, and research. In D.L. Vredevoe et al. (Eds.), *Concepts of oncology nursing* (pp. 369–386). Englewood Cliffs, NJ: Prentice-Hall.

†Derdiarian, A.K. (1983). An instrument for theory and research development using the behavioral systems model for nursing: The cancer patient. Part I. *Nursing Research,* 32(4), 196–201.

Derdiarian, A.K. (1990). Effects of using systematic assessment instruments on patient and nurse satisfaction with nursing care. *Oncology Nursing Forum,* 17, 95–101.

Derdiarian, A.K. (1990). The relationships among the subsystems of Johnson's behavioral system model. *Image: Journal of Nursing Scholarship,* 22, 219–225.

Derdiarian, A.K. (1991). Effects of using a nursing model-based assessment instrument on quality of nursing care. *Nursing Administration Quarterly,* 15(3), 1–16.

Derdiarian, A.K. (1993). Application of the Johnson Behavioral System Model in nursing practice. In M.E. Parker (Ed.), *Patterns of nursing theories in practice* (pp. 285–298). New York: National League for Nursing.

Derdiarian, A.K. (1993). The Johnson Behavioral System Model: Perspectives for nursing practice. In M.E. Parker (Ed.), *Patterns of nursing theories in practice* (pp. 267–284). New York: National League for Nursing.

†Derdiarian, A. and Forsythe, A.B. (1983). An instrument for theory and research development using the behavioral systems model for nursing: The cancer patient, Part II. *Nursing Research,* 32(4), 260–267.

Fawcett, J. (1989). Johnson's behavioral system model. In J. Fawcett (Ed.), *Analysis and evaluation of conceptual models of nursing* (2nd ed.). Philadelphia: F.A. Davis.

Frey, M.A., Rooke, L., Sieloff, C., Messmer, P.R., and Kameoka, T. (1995). King's framework theory in Japan, Sweden, and the United States. *Image: Journal of Nursing Scholarship*, 27, 127–130.

Fruehwirth, S. (1989). An application of Johnson's behavioral model: A case study. *Journal of Community Health Nursing*, 6(2), 61–71.

†Grubbs, J. (1980). An interpretation of the Johnson behavioral system model for nursing practice. In J.P. Riehl and C. Roy (Eds.), *Conceptual models for nursing practice.* New York: Appleton-Century-Crofts.

Holaday, B. (1974). Achievement behavior in chronically ill children. *Nursing Research*, 23, 25–30.

†Holaday, B. (1980). Implementing the Johnson model for nursing practice. In J.P. Riehl and C. Roy (Eds.), *Conceptual models for nursing practice* (2nd ed.). New York: Appleton-Century-Crofts.

Holaday, B. (1981). Maternal response to their chronically ill infants' attachment behavior of crying. *Nursing Research,* 30(6), 343–347.

Holaday, B. (1981). The Johnson behavioral system model for nursing and the pursuit of quality health care. In G.E. Lasker (Ed.), *Applied systems and cybernetics* (Vol. 4). New York: Pergamon Press.

Holaday, B. (1982). Maternal conceptual set development: Identifying patterns of maternal response to chronically ill infant crying. *Maternal-Child Nursing Journal,* 11(1), 47–58.

Holaday, B. (1987). Patterns of interaction between mothers and their chronically ill infants. *Maternal-Child Nursing Journal,* 16, 29–45.

Holaday, B. (1997). Johnson's behavioral system model in nursing practice. In M.R. Alligood et al. (Eds.), *Nursing theory: Utilization and application* (pp 49–70). St. Louis, MO: Mosby Year Book.

*Johnson, D.E. (1959). The nature of a science of nursing. *Nursing Outlook,* 7(5), 291–294.

†Johnson, D.E. (1959). A philosophy of nursing. *Nursing Outlook*, 7(4), 198–200.

†Johnson, D.E. (1961). The significance of nursing care. *Nursing Outlook,* 61(11), 63–66.

Johnson, D.E. (1964). *Is there an identifiable body of knowledge essential to the development of a generic professional nursing program?* Paper presented at First Inter-university Faculty Work Conference Nursing Council, NEBHE, Stowe, VT.

Johnson, D.E. (1968). *One conceptual model of nursing.* Paper presented at Vanderbilt University, Nashville, TN.

*Johnson, D.E. (1968). Theory in nursing: Borrowed or unique. *Nursing Research*, 17(3), 206–209.

Johnson, D.E. (1974). Development of theory: A requisite for nursing as a primary health profession. *Nursing Research*, 23(5), 372–377.

†Johnson, D.E. (1980). The behavioral system model for nursing. In J.P. Riehl and C. Roy (Eds.), *Conceptual models for nursing practice* (2nd ed.). New York: Appleton-Century-Crofts.

Johnson, D.E. (1987). Evaluating conceptual models for use in critical care nursing practice. *Dimensions of Critical Care Nursing*, 6(4), 195–197.

Johnson, D.E. (1989). Some thoughts on nursing. *Clinical Nurse Specialist*, 3(1), 1–4.

Johnson, D.E. (1990). The behavioral system model for nursing. In M.E. Parker (Ed.), *Nursing theories in practice* (pp. 23–32). New York: National League for Nursing.

Johnson, D.E. (1992). The origins of the behavioral system model. In F.N. Nightingale, *Notes on nursing: What it is, and what it is not* (Commemorative edition, pp. 23–27). Philadelphia: J.B. Lippincott.

Karmels, P. (1993). Conundrum game for nursing theorists Neuman, King, and Johnson. *Nurse Educator*, 18(6), 8–9.

Lachicotte, J.L. and Alexander, J.W. (1990). Management attitudes and nurse impairment. *Nursing Management*, 21, 102–104, 106, 108, 110.

†Lovejoy, N.C. (1983). The leukemic child's perceptions of family behaviors. *Oncology Nursing Forum*, 10(4), 20–25.

Loveland-Cherry, C. and Wilkerson, S.A. (1989). Dorothy Johnson's behavioral system model. In J.J. Fitzpatrick and A.L. Whall (Eds.), *Conceptual methods of nursing: Analysis to application* (2nd ed.). Bowie, MD: Robert J. Brady Co.

Majesky, S.J., Brester, M.H., and Nishio, K.T. (1978). Development of a research tool: Patient indicators of nursing care. *Nursing Research*, 27, 365–371.

McCauley, K., Choromanski, J., and Liu, K. (1984). Learning to live with controlled ventricular tachycardia: Utilizing the Johnson model. *Heart and Lung*, 13(6), 633–638.

Newman, M.A. (1994). Theory for nursing practice. *Nursing Science Quarterly*, 7(4), 153–157.

†Porter, L.S. (1972). The impact of physical-physiological activity on infants' growth and development. *Nursing Research*, 21(3), 210–219.

Randell, B.P. (1992). Nursing theory: The 21st century. *Nursing Science Quarterly*, 5(4), 176–184.

†Rawls, A.C. (1980). Evaluation of the Johnson behavioral model in clinical practice. Report of a test and evaluation of the Johnson theory. *Image: Journal of Nursing Scholarship*, 12, 13–16.

Reynolds, W. and Cormack, D.F. (1991). An evaluation of the Johnson Behavioral System Model of Nursing. *Journal of Advanced Nursing*, 16(9), 1122–1130.

Roy, C. (1980). A case study viewed according to different models. In J.P. Riehl and C. Roy (Eds.), *Conceptual models for nursing practice*. New York: Appleton-Century-Crofts.

†Small, B. (1980). Nursing visually impaired children with Johnson's model as a conceptual framework. In J.P. Riehl and C. Roy (Eds.), *Conceptual models for nursing practice* (2nd ed.). New York: Appleton-Century-Crofts.

Wilkie, D. (1990). Cancer pain management: State-of-the-art care. *Nursing Clinics of North America*, 25, 331–343.

Wilkie, D.J., Lovejoy, N., Dodd, M., and Tesler, M. (1988). Cancer pain control behaviors: Description and correlation with pain intensity. *Oncology Nursing Forum*, 15(6), 723–731.

Wilkie, D.J., Lovejoy, N., Dodd, M., and Tesler, M. (1989). Pain control behaviors of patients with cancer. In S.G. Funk, E.M. Tornquist, M.T. Champagne, L.A. Copp, and R.A. Wiese (Eds.), *Key aspects of comfort: Management of pain, fatigue, and nausea*. New York: Springer-Verlag.

Wu, R. (1973). *Behavior and illness*. Englewood Cliffs, NJ: Prentice-Hall.

21. Imogene King

Ackermann, M., Brink, S., Clanton, J., Jones, C., Moody, S., Perlich, G., Price, D., and Prusinski, B. (1989). Imogene King: Theory of goal attainment. In A. Marriner-Tomey (Ed.), *Nursing theorists and their work* (2nd ed.). St. Louis: C.V. Mosby.

Aggleton, P. and Chalmers, H. (1990). Nursing models. King's model. *Nursing Times*, 86(1), 38–39.

Allan, N. (1999). Imogene King's goal attainment theory as the framework for nursing research. *Perspectives*, 23(2), 15–19.

Alligood, M.R. (2001). A theory of nursing empathy in King's Interacting Systems. *Tennessee Nurse*, 64(2), 18.

Archibong, U.E. (1999). Evaluating the impact of primary nursing practice on the quality of nursing care: A Nigerian study. *Journal of Advanced Nursing*, 29(3), 680–689.

Asay, M.K. and Osler, C.C. (Eds.) (1984). *Conceptual models of nursing. Applications in community health nursing.* Proceedings of the Eighth Annual Community Health Nursing Conference. Chapel Hill, NC: Department of Public Health Nursing, School of Public Health, University of North Carolina.

Astedt-Kurki, P., Friedemann, M.L., Paavilainen, E., et al. (2001). Assessment of strategies in families tested by Finnish families. *International Journal of Nursing Studies*, 38(1), 17–24.

Austin, J.K. and Champion, V.L. (1983). King's theory for nursing: Explication and evaluation. In P. Chinn (Ed.), *Advances in nursing theory development* (pp. 49–61). Rockville, MD: Aspen Systems.

Baumann, S.L. (2000). Family nursing: Theory-anemic, nursing theory-deprived. *Nursing Science Quarterly*, 13(4), 285–290.

Bradshaw, A. (1995). What are nurses doing to patients—A review of theories of nursing past and present. *Journal of Clinical Nursing*, 4(2), 81–92.

Bramlett, M.H., Gueldner, S.H., and Sowell, R.L. (1990). Consumer-centric advocacy: Its connection to nursing frameworks. *Nursing Science Quarterly*, 3(4), 156–161.

Brooks, E.M. and Thomas S. (1997). The perception and judgment of senior baccalaureate student nurses in clinical decision making. *Advances in Nursing Science,* 19(3), 50–69.

Brower, H.T. (1981). Social organization and nurses' attitudes toward older persons. *Journal of Gerontological Nursing*, 7, 293–298.

Brown, S.J. (1999). Student nurses' perceptions of elderly care. *Journal of the National Black Nurses Association,* 10(2), 29–36.

Brown, S.T. and Lee, B.T. (1980). Imogene King's conceptual framework: A proposed model for continuing nursing education. *Journal of Advanced Nursing*, 5(5), 467–473.

Bunting, S.M. (1988). The concept of perception in selected nursing theories. *Nursing Science Quarterly*, 1(4), 168–174.

Burney, M.A. (1992) King and Neuman: In search of the nursing paradigm. *Journal of Advanced Nursing,* 17(5), 601–603.

Byrne-Coker, E. and Schreiber, R. (1990). King at the bedside. *Canadian Nurse*, 86(1), 24–26.

Carter, K.F. and Dufour, L.I. (1994). King's theory: A critique of the critiques. *Nursing Science Quarterly*, 7(3), 128–133.

Clements, H. and Melby, V. (1998). An investigation into the information obtained by patients undergoing gastroscopy investigations. *Journal of Clinical Nursing*, 7(4), 333–342.

Daubenmire, M.J. and King, I.M. (1973). Nursing process models: A systems approach. *Nursing Outlook*, 21(8), 512–517.

Daubenmire, M.J. (1989). A baccalaureate nursing curriculum based on King's conceptual framework. In J. Riehl-Sisca (Ed.), *Conceptual models for nursing practice* (3rd ed.). Norwalk, CT: Appleton & Lange.

Douglas, T.S., Mann, N.H., and Hodge, A.L. (1998). Evaluation of preoperative patient education and computer-assisted patient instruction. *Journal of Spinal Disorders*, 11(1), 29–35.

DiNardo, P.B. (1989). Evaluation of the nursing theory of Imogene M. King. In J. Riehl-Sisca (Ed.), *Conceptual models for nursing practice* (3rd ed.). Norwalk, CT: Appleton & Lange.

Duldt, B.W. (1995). Integrating nursing theory and ethics. *Perspectives in Psychiatric Care*, 31(2), 4–10.

Elberson, K. (1989). Applying King's model to nursing administration. In B. Henry, C. Arndt, M. DiVincenti, and A. Marriner-Tomey (Eds.), *Dimensions of nursing administration: Theory, research, education, practice*. Boston: Blackwell Scientific Publications.

Fawcett, J. (1989). King's interacting systems framework. In J. Fawcett (Ed.), *Analysis and evaluation of conceptual models of nursing* (2nd ed.). Philadelphia: F.A. Davis.

Fontana, J.A. (1996). The emergence of the person-environment interaction in a descriptive study of vigor in heart failure. *Advances in Nursing Science*, 18(4), 70–82.

Frey, M.A. (1989). Social support and health: A theoretical formulation derived from King's conceptual framework. *Nursing Science Quarterly*, 138–148.

Frey, M.A. and Norris, D.(1997). King's systems framework and theory in nursing practice. In M.R. Alligood (Ed.), *Nursing theory: Utilization and application* (pp. 71–88). St. Louis, MO: Mosby Year Book.

Frey, M.A., Rooke, L., Sieloff, C., Messmer, P.R., and Kameoka, T. (1995). King's framework and theory in Japan, Sweden, and the United States. *Image: Journal of Nursing Scholarship*, 27(2), 127–130.

Frey, M.A., Sieloff, C.L. and Norris, D.M. (2002). King's conceptual system and theory of goal attainment: Past, present, and future. *Nursing Science Quarterly*, 15(2), 107–112.

Friedmann, M.L. (1989). The concept of family nursing. *Journal of Advanced Nursing*, 14, 211–216.

George, J.B. (1980). Imogene King. In The Nursing Theories Conference Group, *Nursing theories: The base for professional nursing practice*. Englewood Cliffs, NJ: Prentice-Hall.

Gonot, P.J. (1983). Imogene M. King: A theory for nursing. In J.J. Fitzpatrick and A.L. Whall (Eds.), *Conceptual models of nursing: Analysis and application*. Bowie, MD: Robert J. Brady Co.

Gonot, P.J. (1986). Family therapy as derived from King's conceptual model. In A.L. Whall (Ed.), *Family therapy for nursing. Four approaches*. Norwalk, CT: Appleton-Century-Crofts.

9). Imogene M. King's conceptual framework of nursing. In J.J. Fitzpatrick
Gonot, P.J. Whall (Eds.), *Conceptual models of nursing: Analysis and application* and Bowie, MD: Robert J. Brady Co.

(2nd King, I.M. (1988). King's general systems model: Application to cur- Gulit development. *Nursing Science Quarterly*, 1(3), 128–132.

.C. (1994). King's theory of goal attainment as a framework for managed care nentation in a hospital setting. *Nursing Science Quarterly*, 7(4), 170–173.

H E.S. (1990). Nursing models and community as client. *Nursing Science Quar-* 3(2), 67–72.

K.M. (1997). An oral contraceptive perception scale for female adolescents. *stern Journal of Nursing Research*, 19(4), 519–529.

K.M. (1999). Commentary on "An adolescent and young adult condom per- ption scale" —Response by Hanna. *Western Journal of Nursing Research*, 21(5), 33–634.

charurnkui, S. (1989). Comparative analysis of Orem's and King's theories. *Journal of Advanced Nursing*, 14, 365–372.

ıucharurnkui, S. and Vinya-nguag, P. (1991). Effects of promoting patients' participation in self-care on postoperative recovery and satisfaction with care. *Nursing Science Quarterly*, 4(1), 14–20.

lawks, J.H. (1991). Power: A concept analysis. *Journal of Advanced Nursing*, 16(6), 754–762.

Hilton, P.A. (1997). Theoretical perspectives of nursing: A review of the literature. *Journal of Advanced Nursing*, 26(6), 1211–1220.

Huch, M.H. (1991). Perspectives on health. *Nursing Science Quarterly*, 4(1), 33–40.

Huch, M.H. (1995). Nursing and the next millennium. *Nursing Science Quarterly*, 8(1), 38–44.

Husband, A. (1988). Application of King's theory of nursing to the care of the adult with diabetes. *Journal of Advanced Nursing*, 13(4), 484–488.

Janzen, S.K., Nelson, A., Nochturft, V., Quigley, P. (2001). James A. Haley's dedication to Dr. Imogene King, our link between theory and nursing services. *Florida Nurse*, 49(3), 21.

Karmels, P. (1993). Conundrum game for nursing theorists Neuman, King, and Johnson. *Nurse Educator*, 18(6), 8–9.

Kemppainen, J.K. (1990). Imogene King's theory: A nursing case study of a psychotic client with human immunodeficiency virus infection. *Archives of Psychiatric Nursing*, 4(6), 384–388.

Kenny, T. (1990). Erosion of individuality in care of elderly people in hospital—An alternative approach. *Journal of Advanced Nursing*, 15(5), 571–576.

King, I.M. (1964). Nursing theory: Problems and prospects. *Nursing Science*, 2, 394–403.

King, I.M. (1968). A conceptual frame of reference for nursing. *Nursing Research*, 17(1), 27–31.

King, I.M. (1971). *Toward a theory for nursing: General concepts of human behavior.* New York: John Wiley & Sons.

King, I.M. (1975). A process for developing concepts for nursing through research. In P.J. Verhonick (Ed.), *Nursing Research* (Vol. 1). Boston: Little, Brown.

King, I.M. (1976). The health care system: Nursing intervent. bsystem. In W.H. Werley et al. (Eds.), *Health research: The systems approac* York: Springer-Verlag.

King, I.M. (1978). USA: Loyola University of Chicago School of *Journal of Advanced Nursing,* 3, 390.

King, I.M. (1981). *A theory for nursing: Systems, concepts, process.* Ne Wiley & Sons.

King, I.M. (1983). The family coping with a medical illness. Analysis an King's theory of goal attainment. In I.W. Clements and F.B. Roberts *health: A theoretical approach to nursing care.* New York: John Wile

King, I.M. (1983). King's theory of nursing. In I.W. Clements and F.B. Ro *Family health: A theoretical approach to nursing.* New York: John Wile

King, I.M. (1984). Effectiveness of nursing care: Use of a goal oriented nursi in end stage renal disease. *American Association of Nephrology Nurses a nicians Journal,* 11(2), 11–17, 60.

King, I.M. (1984). Philosophy of nursing education: A national survey. *Western Jo of Nursing Research,* 6(4), 387–406.

King, I.M. (1987). Translating research into practice. *Journal of Neuroscience Nurs* 19(1), 44–48.

King, I.M. (1986). King's theory of goal attainment. In P. Winstead-Fry (Ed.), *Case studie in nursing theory.* New York: National League for Nursing.

King, I.M. (1987). King's theory of goal attainment. In R.R. Parse (Ed.), *Nursing science: Major paradigms, theories, and critiques.* Philadelphia: W.B. Saunders.

King, I.M. (1988). Concepts: Essential elements of theories. *Nursing Science Quarterly,* 1(1), 22–25.

King, I.M. (1989). King's systems framework and theory. In J. Riehl-Sisca (Ed.), *Conceptual models for nursing practice* (3rd ed.). Norwalk, CT: Appleton & Lange.

King, I.M. (1989). King's system framework for nursing administration. In B. Henry, C. Arndt, M. DiVincenti, and A. Marriner-Tomey (Eds.), *Dimensions of nursing administration: Theory, research, education, practice.* Boston: Blackwell Scientific Publications.

King, I.M. (1990). Health as the goal for nursing. *Nursing Science Quarterly,* 3(3), 123–128.

King, I.M. (1990). King's conceptual framework and theory of goal attainment. In M.E. Parker (Ed.), *Nursing theories in practice* (pp. 73–84). New York: National League for Nursing.

King, I.M. (1992). King's theory of goal attainment. *Nursing Science Quarterly,* 5(1), 19–26.

King, I.M. (1992). Window on general systems framework and theory of goal attainment. In M. O'Toole (Ed.). *Miller Keane encyclopedia and dictionary of medicine, nursing, and allied health* (p. 604). Philadelphia: W.B. Saunders.

King, I.M. (1994). Quality of life and goal attainment. *Nursing Science Quarterly,* 7(1), 29–32.

King, I.M. (1996). The theory of goal attainment in research and practice. *Nursing Science Quarterly,* 9(2), 61–66.

King, I.M. (1997). King's theory of goal attainment in practice. *Nursing Science Quarterly,* 10(4), 180–185.

Kim, I.M. and Whelton, B.J.B. (2001). Letters to the editor . . . "A nursing theory of personal system empathy: Interpreting a conceptualization of empathy in King's Interacting Systems." *Nursing Science Quarterly*, 14(1), 80–82.

Laben, J.K., Dodd, D., and Sneed, L. (1991). King's theory of goal attainment applied in group therapy for inpatient juvenile sexual offenders, maximum security state offenders, and community parolees, using visual aids. *Issues in Mental Health Nursing*, 12(1), 51–64.

Laitinen, P. and Isola, A. (1996). Promoting participation and informal caregivers in the hospital care of the elderly patient: Informal caregivers' perceptions. *Journal of Advanced Nursing*, 23(5), 942–947.

Larrabee, J.H., Engle, V.F., and Tolley, E.A. (1995). Predictors of patient-perceived quality. *Scandinavian Journal of Caring Sciences*, 9(3), 153–164.

Lawler, J., Dowswell, G., Hearn, J., et al. (1999). Recovering from stroke: A qualitative investigation of the role of goal setting in late stroke recovery. *Journal of Advanced Nursing*, 30(2), 401–409.

Lehna, C., Pfoutz, S., Peterson, T.G., et al. (1999). Nursing attire: Indicators of professionalism? *Journal of Professional Nursing*, 15(3), 192–199.

Leinonen, T.A., Leini-Kilpi, H. and Jouko, K. (1996). The quality of intraoperative nursing care: the patient's perspective. *Journal of Advanced Nursing*, 24(4), 843–852.

Lither, M. and Zilling, T. (2000). Pre- and postoperative information needs. *Patient Education and Counseling*, 40(1), 29–37.

Lowry, D.A. (1998). Issues of non-compliance in mental health. *Journal of Advanced Nursing*, 28(2), 280–287.

Magan, S. (1987). A critique of King's theory. In R.R. Parse (ed.), *Nursing science: Major paradigms, theories, and critiques*. Philadelphia: W.B. Saunders.

Martin, J.P. (1990). Male cancer awareness Impact of an employee education program. *Oncology Nursing Forum*, 17, 59–64.

Michota, S. (1995). A hospital-based skilled nursing facility—A special place to care for the elderly. *Geriatric Nursing*, 16(2), 64–66.

Moreira, T.M.M. and Araujo, T.L. (2002). The conceptual model of interactive open systems and the theory of goal attainment by Imogene King [Portuguese]. *Revista Latino-Americana de Enfermagem*, 10(1), 97–103.

Murray, R.L.E. and Baier, M. (1996). King's conceptual framework applied to a transitional living program. *Perspectives in Psychiatric Care*, 32(1), 15–19.

Norgan, G.H., Ettipio, A.M., and Lasome, C.E. (1995). A program plan addressing carpal tunnel syndrome: The utility of King's goal attainment theory. *Journal of the American Association of Occupational Health Nurses*, 43(8), 407–411.

Norris, D.M. and Hoyer, P.J. (1993). Dynamism in practice: Parenting within King's framework. *Nursing Science Quarterly*, 6(2), 79–85.

Paavilainen, E. and Astedt-Kurki, P. (1997). The client-nurse relationship as experienced by public health nurses: Toward better collaboration. *Public Health Nursing*, 14(3), 137–142.

Patistea, E. (1999). Nurses' perceptions of caring as documented in theory and research. *Journal of Clinical Nursing*, 8(5), 487–495.

Poroch, D. (1995). The effect of preparatory patient education on the anxiety and satisfaction of cancer patients receiving radiation therapy. *Cancer Nursing*, 18(3), 206–214.

Richard-Hughes, S. (1997). Attitudes and beliefs of Afro-Americans related to organ and tissue donation. *International Journal of Trauma Nursing*, 119–123.

Rooda, L.A. (1992). The development of a conceptual model for multicultural nursing. *Journal of Holistic Nursing*, 10(4), 337–347.

Rooke, L. (1995). Focusing on King's theory and systems framework in education by using an experiential learning model: A challenge to improve the quality of nursing care. In M.A. Frey and C. Sieloff (Eds.), *Advancing King's framework and theory for nursing* (pp. 278–293). Newbury Park, CA: Sage.

Rooke, L. and Norberg, A. (1988). Problematic and meaningful situations in nursing interpreted by concepts from King's nursing theory and four additional concepts. *Scandinavian Journal of Caring Sciences*, 2(2), 80–87.

Rosendahl, P.B. and Ross, V. (1982). Does your behavior affect your patient's response? *Journal of Gerontological Nursing*, 8, 572–575.

Ross, M.M., Hoff, L.A., and Coutu-Wakulczyk, G. (1998). Nursing curricula and violence issues. *Journal of Nursing Education*, 37(2), 53–60.

Schreiber, R. (1991). Psychiatric assessment "a la King." *Nursing Management*, 22(5), 90, 92, 94.

Shuldham, C. (1999). Pre-operative education—A review of the research design. *International Journal of Nursing Studies*, 36(2), 179–187.

Smith, M. (1988). King's theory in practice. *Nursing Science Quarterly*, 1(4), 145–146.

Sowell, R.L. and Lowenstein, A. (1994). King's theory as a framework for quality: Linking theory to practice. *Nursing Connections*, 7(2), 19–31.

Takahashi, T. (1992). Perspectives on nursing knowledge. *Nursing Science Quarterly*, 5(2), 86–91.

Temple, A. and Fawdry, K. (1992). King's theory of goal attainment. Resolving filial caregiver role strain. *Journal of Gerontological Nursing*, 18(3), 11–15.

Tritsch, J.M. (1998). Application of King's theory of goal attainment and the Carondelet St. Mary's case management model. *Nursing Science Quarterly*, 11(2), 69–73.

Uys, L. (1987). Foundational studies in nursing. *Journal of Advanced Nursing*, 12(3), 275–280.

Walker, K.M. and Alligood, M.R. (2001). Empathy from a nursing perspective: Moving beyond borrowed theory. *Archives of Psychiatric Nursing*, 15(3), 140–147.

West, P. (1991). Theory implementation: A challenging journey. *Canadian Journal of Nursing Administration*, 4(1), 29–30.

Williams, C. (1996). Patient-controlled analgesia: A review of the literature. *Journal of Clinical Nursing*, 5(3), 139–147.

Woods, E.C. (1994). King's theory in practice with elders. *Nursing Science Quarterly*, 7(2), 65–69.

22. Madeleine Leininger

Bodner, A. and Leininger, M. (1992). Transcultural nursing care values, beliefs, and practices of American (USA) gypsies. *Journal of Transcultural Nursing*, 4(1), 17–28.

Basuray, J. (1997). Nurse Miss Sahib: Colonial culture-bound education in India and transcultural nursing. *Journal of Transcultural Nursing*, 9(1), 14–19.

Carr, J.M. (1998). Vigilance as a caring expression and Leininger's theory of cultural care diversity and universality. *Nursing Science Quarterly*, 11(2), 74–78.

Chmielarczyk, V. (1991). Transcultural nursing: Providing culturally congruent care to the Hausa of Northwest Africa. *Journal of Transcultural Nursing*, 3(1), 15–19.

Cohen, J. A. (1991). Two portraits of caring: A comparison of the artists, Leininger and Watson. *Journal of Advanced Nursing*, 16, 899–909.

Fawcett, J. (2002). The nurse theorists: 21st century updates—Madeleine M. Leininger. *Nursing Science Quarterly*, 15(2), 131–136.

Horsburgh, M.E., and Foley D.M. (1990). The phenomena of care in Sicilian-Canadian culture: An ethnonursing case study. *Nursing Forum*, 25(3), 14–22.

Leininger, M. (1990). Leininger clarifies transcultural nursing [Letter; comment]. *International Nursing Review*, 37(6), 356.

Leininger, M. (1997). Transcultural nursing research to transform nursing education and practice: 40 years. *Image: Journal of Nursing Scholarship*, 29(4), 341–347.

Leininger, M. (2001). Response and reflections on Bruni's 1988 critique of Leininger's theory. *Collegian*, 8(1). 37–38.

Leininger, M. (2002). Culture care theory: A major contribution to advance transcultural nursing and practices. *Journal of Transcultural Nursing*, 13(3), 189–192.

Leininger, M.M. (1997). Transcultural nursing as a global care humanizer, diversifier, and unifier. *Hoitotiede*, 9(5), 219–225.

Luna, L. (1998). Culturally competent health care: A challenge for nurses in Saudi Arabia. *Journal of Transcultural Nursing*, 9(2), 8–14.

Luna, L.J. (1989). Transcultural nursing care of Arab Muslims. *Journal of Transcultural Nursing*, 1(1), 22–26.

McFarland, M.R. (1997). Use of cultural care theory with Anglo- and African-American elders in a long-term care setting. *Nursing Science Quarterly*, 10(4), 186–192.

Miller, J. (1997). Politics and care: A study of Czech Americans within Leininger's theory of culture care diversity and universality. *Journal of Transcultural Nursing*, 9(1), 3–13.

Morgan, M.G. (1992). Pregnancy and childbirth beliefs and practices of American Hare Krishna devotees within transcultural nursing. *Journal of Transcultural Nursing*, 4(1), 5–10.

Polaschek, N.R. (1998). Cultural safety: A new concept in nursing people of different ethnicities. *Journal of Advanced Nursing*, 27(3), 452–457.

Queiroz, M.V.O. and Pagliuca, L.M.F. (2001). The concept of transcultural nursing: The analysis of its development in a master's degree dissertation [Portuguese]. *Revista Brasileira de Enfermagem*, 54(4), 630–637.

Rosenbaum, J.N. (1989). Depression: Viewed from a transcultural nursing theoretical perspective. *Journal of Advanced Nursing*, 14(1), 7–12.

Spangler, Z. (1992). Transcultural care values and nursing practices of Philippine-American nurses. *Journal of Transcultural Nursing*, 4(2), 28–37.

Zoucha, R. and Husted, G.L. (2000). The ethical dimensions of delivering culturally competent congruent nursing and health care. *Issues in Mental Health Nursing*, 21(3), 325–340.

23. Myra Levine

Artigue, G.S., Foli, K.J., Johnson, T., Marriner-Tomey, A., Poat, M.C., Poppa, L.D., Woeste, R., and Zoretich, S.T. (1994). Myra Levine: Four conservation principles. In A. Marriner-Tomey (Ed.). *Nursing theorists and their work* (4th ed., pp. 199–210). St. Louis, MO: C.V. Mosby.

Bunting, S.M. (1988). The concept of perception in selected nursing theories. *Nursing Science Quarterly*, 1(4), 168–174.

†Esposito, C.H. and Leonard, M.K. (1980). Myra Estrin Levine. In The Nursing Theories Conference Group, *Nursing theories: The base for professional nursing practice* (pp. 150–163). Englewood Cliffs, NJ: Prentice-Hall.

Fawcett, J. (1989). Levine's conservation model. In J. Fawcett (Ed.), *Analysis and evaluation of conceptual models of nursing* (2nd ed.). Philadelphia: F.A. Davis.

Foli, K., Johnson, T., Marriner-Tomey, A., Poat, M., Poppa, L., Woeste, R., and Zoretich, S. (1989). Myra Estrin Levine: Four conservation principles. In A. Marriner-Tomey (Ed.), *Nursing theorists and their work* (2nd ed.), St. Louis, MO: C.V. Mosby.

Glass, J.L. (1989). Levine's theory of nursing: A critique. In J. Riehl-Sisca (Ed.), *Conceptual models for nursing practice* (3rd ed.). Norwalk, CT: Appleton & Lange.

Grindley, J. and Paradowski, M. (1991). Developing an undergraduate program using Levine's model. In K.M. Schaefer and J.B. Pond (Eds.), *Levine's conservation model: A framework for nursing practice* (pp. 199–208). Philadelphia: F.A. Davis.

†Hirschfeld, M.J. (1976). The cognitively impaired older adult. *American Journal of Nursing*, 76(12), 1981–1984.

†Levine, M.E. (1966). Adaptation and assessment: A rationale for nursing intervention. *American Journal of Nursing*, 66(11), 2450–2454.

Levine, M.E. (1966). Trophicognosis: An alternative to nursing diagnosis. In *Exploring progress in medical-surgical nursing practice* (pp. 55–70). New York: American Nurses' Association.

†Levine, M.E. (1967). The four conservation principles of nursing. *Nursing Forum*, 6(1), 45–59.

Levine, M. (1969). *Introduction to clinical nursing.* Philadelphia: F.A. Davis.

†Levine, M.E. (1969). The pursuit of wholeness. *American Journal of Nursing*, 69(1), 93–98.

†Levine, M.E. (1971). Holistic nursing. *Nursing Clinics of North America*, 6(2), 253–264.

†Levine, M.E. (1971). Time has come to speak of . . . health care. *AORN Journal,* 13, 37–43.

Levine, M.E. (1973). *Introduction to clinical nursing* (2nd ed.). Philadelphia: F.A. Davis.

Levine, M.E. (1977). Nursing ethics and the ethical nurse. *American Journal of Nursing*, 77(5), 845–849.

Levine, M.E. (1979). The science is spurious. *American Journal of Nursing*, 79(8), 1379–1383.

Levine, M.E. (1988). Antecedents from adjunctive disciplines: Creation of nursing theory. *Nursing Science Quarterly*, 1(1), 16–21.

Levine, M.E. (1988). Rationing health care [Letter}. *Nursing Outlook*, 36(6), 265.

Levine, M.E. (1989). Beyond dilemma. *Seminars in Oncology Nursing*, 5(2), 124–128.

Levine, M.E. (1989). The conservation principles: Twenty years later. In J. Riehl-Sisca (ed.), Conceptual models for nursing practice (3rd ed.). Norwalk, CT: Appleton & Lange.

Levine, M.E. (1989). Ethical issues in cancer care: Beyond dilemma. *Seminars in Oncology Nursing*, 5(2), 124–128.

Levine, M.E. (1989). The ethics of nursing rhetoric. *Image: Journal of Nursing Scholarship*, 21(1), 4–6.

Levine, M.E. (1989). The four conservation principles: Twenty years later. In J.P. Riehl-Sisca (Ed.), Conceptual models for nursing practice (3rd ed.). Norwalk, CT: Appleton & Lange.

Levine, M.E. (1989). Ration or rescue: The elderly patient in critical care. *Critical Care Nursing Quarterly*, 12(1), 82–89.

Levine, M.E. (1990). Conservation and integrity. In M.E. Parker (Ed.), *Nursing theories in practice* (pp. 189–202). New York: National League for Nursing.

Levine, M.E. (1995). The rhetoric of nursing theory. *Image: The Journal of Nursing Scholarship*, 27(1), 11–14.

Newport, M.A. (1984). Conserving thermal energy and social integrity in the newborn. *Western Journal of Nursing Research*, 6(2), 175–199.

Pieper, B.A. (1989). Levine's nursing model: The conservation principles. In J.J. Fitzpatrick and A.L. Whall (Eds.), *Conceptual models of nursing: Analysis and application* (2nd ed.). Bowie, MD: Robert J. Brady Co.

Pond, J.B. (1990). Application of Levine's conservation model to nursing the homeless community. In M.E. Parker (Ed.), *Nursing theories in practice* (pp. 203–216). New York: National League for Nursing.

Riehl, J.P. (1980). Nursing models in current use. In J.P. Riehl and C. Roy (Eds.), *Conceptual models for nursing practice* (2nd ed., pp. 393–398). New York: Appleton-Century-Crofts.

Schaefer, K.M. (1997). Levine's conservation model in nursing practice. In M.R. Alligood et al. (Eds.), *Nursing theory: Utilization and application* (pp. 89–107). St. Louis, MO: Mosby Year Book.

Taylor, J.W. (1974). Measuring the outcomes of nursing care. *Nursing Clinics of North America*, 9, 337–348.

Taylor, J.W. (1989). Levine's conservation principles: Using the model for nursing diagnosis in a neurological setting. In J. Riehl-Sisca (Ed.), *Conceptual models for nursing practice* (3rd ed.). Norwalk, CT: Appleton & Lange.

Tompkins, E.S. (1980). Effect of restricted mobility and dominance on perceived duration. *Nursing Research*, 29(6), 333–338.

24. Afaf Ibrahim Meleis

Dagenais, F. and Meleis, A.I. (1982). Professionalism, work ethic, and empathy in nursing: The nurse self-description form. *Western Journal of Nursing Research*, 4(4), 407–422.

Dracup, K., Meleis, A.I., Baker, C., and Edlefsen, P. (1984). Family-focused cardiac rehabilitation: A role supplementation program for cardiac patients and spouses. *Nursing Clinics of North America*, 19, 113–124.

Gaffney, K.F. (1992). Nursing practice model for maternal role sufficiency. *Advances in Nursing Science,* 15(2), 76–84.

Im, E.O. and Meleis, A.I. (1999). A situation-specific theory of Korean immigrant women's menopausal transition. *Image: Journal of Nursing Scholarship,* 31(4), 333–338.

Hall, J.M., Stevens, P.E., and Meleis, A.I. (1994). Marginalization: A guiding concept for valuing diversity in nursing knowledge development. *Advances in Nursing Science,* 16(4), 23–41.

Jones, P.S. and Meleis, A.I. (1993). Health is empowerment. *Advances in Nursing Science,* 15(3), 1–14.

Koniak-Griffin, D. (1993). Maternal role attainment. *Image: Journal of Nursing Scholarship,* 25, 257–262.

Mansell, D.M. and Porter-Chantemerle, K. (1979). *Conceptualization and measurement of a role supplementation program: The effect of role supplementation on career success of neophyte nurses.* MINH undergraduate psychiatric nursing training and demonstration project. Arizona State University, College of Nursing, Tempe, AZ.

Meleis, A.I. (1971). Self-concept and family planning. *Nursing Research,* 20, 229–236.

Meleis, A.I. (1974). Self-concept photographs: A research tool. *Videosociology,* 2(2), 46–62.

Meleis, A.I. (1975). Role insufficiency and role supplementation: A conceptual framework. *Nursing Research,* 24, 264–271.

Meleis, A.I. (1979). The graduate dilemma: The Kuwaiti experience. *International Journal of Nursing Studies,* 16, 337–343.

Meleis, A.I. (1986). Theory development and domain concepts. In P. Moccia (Ed.), *New approaches to theory development.* New York: National League for Nursing.

Meleis, A.I. (1990). Being and becoming healthy: The core of nursing knowledge. *Nursing Science Quarterly,* 3(3), 107–114.

Meleis, A. I. (1995). Theory testing and theory support: Principles, challenges, and a sojourn into the future. In Betty Neuman (Ed.), *The Neuman systems model* (pp. 447–457). Norwalk, CT: Appleton-Lange.

Meleis, A.I. (1998). ReVisions in knowledge development: A passion for substance. *Scholarly Inquiry in Nursing Practice,* 12(1), 65–77.

Meleis, A.I. and Burton, P. (1981). Educational innovations: A model. *International Journal of Nursing Studies,* 33–39.

Meleis, A.I. and Dagenais, F. (1981). Sex role identity and perception of professional self in graduates of three nursing programs. *Nursing Research,* 30, 162–167.

Meleis, A.I., Sawyer, L.M., Im, E.O., Hilfinger Messias, D.K. and Schumacher, K. (2000). Experiencing transitions: An emerging middle-range theory. *Advances in Nursing Science,* 23(1), 12–28.

Meleis, A.I. and Swendsen, L. (1975). Role supplementation: An empirical test of nursing intervention. *Nursing Research,* 24, 264–271.

Meleis, A.I., Swendsen, L., and Jones, D. (1980). Preventive role supplementation: A grounded conceptual framework. In M.H. Miller and B. Flynn (Eds.), *Current perspectives in nursing: Social issues and trends* (Vol. 2). St. Louis, MO: C.V. Mosby.

Meleis, A.I. and Trangenstein, P.A. (1994). Facilitating transitions: Redefinition of the nursing mission. *Nursing Outlook,* 42, 255–259.

Neves-Arruda, E.N., Larson, P.J., and Meleis, A.I. (1992). Comfort. Immigrant Hispanic cancer patients' views. *Cancer Nursing*, 15(6), 387–394.

Schumacher, K. and Meleis, A.I. (1994). Transitions: A central concept in nursing. *Image: Journal of Nursing Scholarship*, 26(2), 119–127.

Swendsen, L., Meleis, A.I., and Jones, D. (1978). Role supplementation for new parents: A role mastery plan. *MCN, The American Journal of Maternal Child Nursing*, 3(2), 84–91.

25. Betty Neuman

Aggleton, P. and Chalmers, H. (1989). Nursing models. Neuman's systems model. *Nursing Times*, 85(51), 27–29.

August-Brady, M. (2000). Prevention as intervention. *Journal of Advances in Nursing*, 31(6), 1304–1308.

Barnum, B.J.S. (1994). *Nursing theory: Analysis, application, and evaluation* (4th ed.). Philadelphia: J.B. Lippincott.

Beck, C.T. (1983). Parturients' temporal experiences during the phases of labor. *Western Journal of Nursing Research*, 5, 283–295.

Beddome, G. (1989). Application of the Neuman systems model to the assessment of community-as-client. In B. Neuman (Ed.), *The Neuman systems model* (2nd ed.). Norwalk, CT: Appleton & Lange.

Beitler, B., Tkachuck, B., and Aamodt, D. (1980). The Neuman model applied to health, mental health and medical-surgical nursing. In J.P. Riehl and C. Roy (Eds.), *Conceptual models of nursing practice*. New York: Appleton-Century-Crofts.

Benedict, M.B. and Sproles, J.B. (1982). Application of the Neuman model to public health nursing practice. In B. Neuman (Ed.), *The Neuman systems model. Application to nursing education and practice.* Norwalk, CT: Appleton-Century-Crofts.

Bergstrom, D. (1992). Hypermetabolism in multisystem organ failure: A Neuman systems perspective. *Critical Care Nursing Quarterly*, 15(3), 63–70.

Bertalanffy, L. (1968). *General system theory.* New York: George Braziller.

Biley, F. (1990). The Neuman model: An analysis. *Nursing*, 4(14), 25–28.

Black, P., Deeny, P., and McKenna, H. (1997). Sensoristrain: An exploration of nursing interventions in the context of the Neuman systems theory. *Intensive and Critical Care Nursing*, 13(5), 249–258.

Blank, J.J., Clark, L., Longman, A.J., and Atwood, J.R. (1989). Perceived home care needs of cancer patients and their caregivers. *Cancer Nursing*, 12(2), 78–84.

Bourbonnais, F.F. and Ross, M.M. (1985). The Neuman systems model in nursing. Course development and implementation. *Journal of Advanced Nursing*, 10(2), 117–123.

Bowman, A.M. (1997). Sleep satisfaction, perceived pain and acute confusion in elderly clients undergoing orthopaedic procedures. *Journal of Advanced Nursing*, 26(3), 550–564.

Breckenridge, D. (1989). Primary prevention as an intervention modality for the renal client. In B. Neuman (Ed.), *The Neuman systems model* (2nd ed.). Norwalk, CT: Appleton & Lange.

Brink, L.W., Neuman, B., and Wynn, J. (1992). Transport of the critically ill patient with upper airway obstruction. *Critical Care Clinics*, 8(3), 633–647.

Buchanan, B.R. (1987). Human environment interaction: A modification of the Neuman systems model for aggregates, families, and the community. *Public Health Nursing*, 4(1), 52–64.

Bunkers, S.S., Petardi, L.A., Pilkington, F.B., et al. (1996). Challenging the myths surrounding qualitative research in nursing. *Nursing Science Quarterly*, 9(1), 33–37.

Burke, M.E., Capers, C., O'Connell, R., Quinn, R., and Sinnott, M. (1989). Neuman-based nursing practice in a hospital setting. In B. Neuman (Ed.), *The Neuman systems model* (2nd ed.). Norwalk, CT: Appleton & Lange.

Burney, M.A. (1992). King and Neuman: In search of the nursing paradigm. *Journal of Advanced Nursing*, 17(5), 601–603.

Campbell, V. and Keller, K. (1989). The Betty Neuman health care systems model: An analysis. In J. Riehl-Sisca (Ed.), *Conceptual models for nursing practice* (3rd ed.). Norwalk, CT: Appleton & Lange.

Capers, C.F., O'Brien, C., Quinn, R., Kelly, R. and Fenerty, A. (1985). The Neuman systems model in practice. Planning phase. *Journal of Nursing Administration*, 15(5), 29–39.

Capers, C.F. and Kelly, R. (1987). Neuman's nursing process: A model of holistic care. *Holistic Nursing Practice*, 1(3), 19–26.

Caplan, G. (1964). *Principles of preventive psychiatry*. New York: Basic Books.

Caris-Verhallen, W.M.C.M., Kerkstra, A., and Bensing, J.M. (1997). The role of communication in nursing care for elderly people: A review of the literature. *Journal of Advanced Nursing*, 25(5), 915–933.

Chan, C.W.H. and Chang, A.M. (1999). Stress associated with tasks for family caregivers of patients with cancer in Hong Kong. *Cancer Nursing*, 22(4), 260–265.

Chardin, P.T. (1955). *The phenomena of man*. London: Collins.

Clark, J. (1982). Development of models and theories on the concept of nursing. *Journal of Advanced Nursing*, 7, 129–134.

Cody, A. (1996). Helping the vulnerable or condoning control within the family: Where is nursing? *Journal of Advanced Nursing*, 23(5), 882–886.

Cody, W.K. (1997). The many faces of change: Discomfort with the new. *Nursing Science Quarterly*, 10(2), 65–67.

Cody, W.K. (1998). Response: The threat of drowning in eclecticism. *Nursing Science Quarterly*, 11(3), 102–104.

Cornu, A. (1957). *The origins of Marxian thought*. Springfield, IL: Charles C. Thomas.

Craddock, R.B. and Stanhope, M.K. (1980). The Neuman health-care systems model: Recommended adaptation. In J.P. Riehl and C. Roy (Eds.), *Conceptual models of nursing practice*. New York: Appleton-Century-Crofts.

Cutcliffe, J.R. (1997). The nature of expert psychiatric nurse practice: A grounded theory study. *Journal of Clinical Nursing*, 6(4), 325–332.

Dale, M.L. and Savala, S.M. (1990). A new approach to the senior practicum. *Nursing Connections*, 3(1), 45–51.

Deloughery, G.W., Neuman, B.M., and Gebbie, K.M. (1970). Change in problem-solving ability among nurses receiving mental health consultation. *Communicating Nursing Research*, 3(3), 41–53.

Deloughery, G.W., Gebbie, K.M., and Neuman, B.M. (1974). Teaching organizational concepts to nurses in community mental health. *Journal of Nursing Education*, 13, 8–14.

Delunas, L.R. (1990). Prevention of elder abuse: Betty Neuman health care systems approach. *Clinical Nurse Specialist*, 4(1), 54–58.

Denyes, M.J., Neuman, B.M., and Villarruel, A.M. (1991). Nursing actions to prevent and alleviate pain in hospitalized children. *Issues in Comprehensive Pediatric Nursing*, 14(1), 31–48.

Drevdahl, D. (1999). Sailing beyond: Nursing theory and the person. *Advances in Nursing Science*, 21(4), 1–13.

Drew, L., Craig, D., and Beynon, C. (1989). The Neuman systems model for community health administration and practice: Provinces of Manitoba and Ontario, Canada. In B. Neuman (Ed.), *The Neuman systems model* (2nd ed.). Norwalk, CT: Appleton & Lange.

Dunn, S. and Trepanier, M. (1989). Application of the Neuman systems model to perinatal nursing. In B. Neuman (Ed.), *The Neuman systems model* (2nd ed.). Norwalk, CT: Appleton & Lange.

Easom, A. and Allbritton, G. (2000). Advanced practice nurses in nephrology. *Advances in Renal Replacement Therapy*, 7(3), 247–260.

Edwards, N., Bunn, H., Mei, W.C., et al. (1999). Building community health nursing in the People's Republic of China: A partnership between schools of nursing in Ottawa, Canada, and Tianjin, China. *Public Health Nursing*, 16(2), 140–145.

England, M. (1997). Self-coherence, emotional arousal and perceived health of adult children caring for a brain-impaired parent. *Journal of Advanced Nursing*, 26(4), 672–682.

Fagerstrom, L., Eriksson, K., and Engberg, I.B. (1998). The patient's perceived caring needs as a message of suffering. *Journal of Advanced Nursing*, 28(5), 978–987.

Fawcett, J. (1984). Neuman's systems model. In J. Fawcett (Ed.), *Analysis and evaluation of conceptual models of nursing*. Philadelphia: F.A. Davis.

Fawcett, J. (1989). Neuman's systems model. In J. Fawcett (Ed.), *Analysis and evaluation of conceptual models of nursing* (2nd ed.). Philadelphia: F.A. Davis.

Fawcett, J. (2001). The nurse theorists: 21st century updates—Betty Neuman. *Nursing Science Quarterly*, 14(3), 211–214.

Fawcett, J. and Giangrande, S.K.(2001). Neuman systems model-based research: An integrative review project. *Nursing Science Quarterly*, 14(3), 231–238.

Fawcett, J. and Gigliotti, E. (2001). Using conceptual models of nursing to guide nursing research: The case of Neuman systems model. *Nursing Science Quarterly*, 14(4), 339–345.

Field, P.A. (1987). The impact of nursing theory on the clinical decision making process. *Journal of Advanced Nursing*, 12(5), 563–571.

Flaskerud, J.H. and Halloran, E.J. (1980). Areas of agreement in nursing theory development. *Advances in Nursing Science*, 3(1), 1–7.

Fontana, J.A. (1996). The emergence of the person-environment interaction in a descriptive study of vigor in health failure. *Advances in Nursing Science*, 18(4), 70–82.

Foote, A.W., Piazza, D., and Schultz, M. (1990). The Neuman systems model: Application to a patient with a cervical spinal cord injury. *Journal of Neuroscience Nursing*, 22, 302–306.

Freshwater, D. (1999). Polarity and unity in caring: The healing power of symptoms. *Complementary Therapies in Nursing and Midwifery*, 5(5), 136–139.

Gebbie, K.M., Deloughery, G.W., and Neuman, B.M. (1970). Levels of utilization: Nursing specialists in community mental health. *Journal of Psychiatric Nursing*, 8, 37–39.

Gigliotti, E. (1997). Use of Neuman's lines of defense and resistance in nursing research: Conceptual and empirical considerations. *Nursing Science Quarterly*, 10(3), 136–143.

Gigliotti, E. (1999). Women's multiple role stress: Testing Neuman's flexible line of defense. *Nursing Science Quarterly*, 12(1), 36–44.

Gigliotti, E. (2001). Empirical tests of the Neuman systems model: Relational statement analysis. *Nursing Science Quarterly*, 14(2), 149–157.

Gigliotte, E. (2002). A theory-based clinical nurse specialist practice exemplar using Neuman's Systems Model and nursing's taxonomies. *Clinical Nurse Specialist*, 16(1), 10–16.

Goulet, C., Polomeno, V, and Harel, F. (1996). Canadian cross-cultural comparison of the High-Risk Pregnancy Stress Scale. *Stress Medicine*, 12(3), 145–154.

Haggart, M. (1993). A critical analysis of Neuman's systems model in relation to public health nursing. *Journal of Advanced Nursing*, 18, 1917–1922.

Hamilton, P. (1983). Community nursing diagnosis. *Advances in Nursing Science*, 5(3), 21–36.

Hanson, M.J.S. (1999). Cross-cultural study of beliefs about smoking among teenaged females. *Western Journal of Nursing Research*, 21(5), 635–647.

Harris, S., Hermiz, M., Meininger, M., and Steinkeler, S. (1989). Betty Neuman: Systems model. In A. Marriner-Tomey (Ed.), *Nursing theorists and their work* (2nd ed.). St. Louis: C.V. Mosby.

Hassell, J.S. (1996). Improved management of depression through nursing model application and critical thinking. *Journal of the American Academy of Nurse Practitioners*, 8(4), 161–166.

Heffline, M.S. (1991). A comparative study of pharmacological versus nursing interventions in the treatment of postanesthesia shivering. *Journal of Post Anesthesia Nursing*, 6(5), 311–320.

Henderson, B. (1978). Nursing diagnosis: Theory and practice. *Advances in Nursing Science*, 1(1), 75–83.

Herrick, C.A. and Goodykoontz, L. (1989). Neuman's systems model for nursing practice as a conceptual framework for a family assessment. *Journal of Child and Adolescent Psychiatric and Mental Health*, 2(2), 61–67.

Hiasma, K.K. (2001). The acceptance of nursing theory in Japan: A cultural perspective. *Nursing Science Quarterly*, 14(3), 255–259.

Higgins, P.A. and Moore, S.M. (2000). Levels of theoretical thinking in nursing. *Nursing Outlook*, 48(4), 179–183.

Hilton, P.A. (1997). Theoretical perspectives of nursing: A review of the literature. *Journal of Advanced Nursing*, 26(6), 1211–1220.

Hinds, C. (1990). Personal and contextual factors predicting patients' reported quality of life: Exploring congruency with Betty Neuman's assumptions. *Journal of Advanced Nursing*, 15(4), 456–462.

Hinton ...ker, P. and Raborn, M. (1989). Application of the Neuman model in nursing ...istration and practice. In B. Henry, C. Arndt, M. DiVincenti, and A. Marriner-...ey (Eds.), *Dimensions of nursing administration: Theory, research, education, ...ctice.* Boston: Blackwell Scientific Publications.

...n, S. and Winters, D.M. (1990). Theory based case management: High cervical ...inal cord injury. *Home Health Care Nurse*, 8, 25–33.

..., M.H. (1991). Perspectives on health. *Nursing Science Quarterly*, 4(1), 33–40.

...gelmann, J., Kenkel-Rossi, E., Klaasen, L., et al. (1996). Focus on spiritual well-being: Harmonious interconnectedness of mind-body-spirit—Use of the JAREL Spiritual Well-Being Scale—Assessment of spiritual well-being is essential to the health of individuals. *Geriatric Nursing*, 17(6), 262–265.

...ohn, W.S. (1998). Just what do we mean by community? Conceptualization from the field. *Health and Social Care in the Community*, 6(2), 63–70.

Johnson, E.D. (1989). In search of applications of nursing theories: The Nursing Citation Index. *Bulletin of the Medical Library Association*, 77(2), 176–184.

Johnson, M. (1983). Some aspects of the relation between theory and practice in nursing. *Journal of Advanced Nursing*, 8, 21–28.

Johnson, S.E. (1989). A picture is worth a thousand words: Helping students visualize a conceptual model. *Nurse Educator*, 14(3), 21–24.

Jones, P.S. (1978). An adaptation model for nursing practice. *American Journal of Nursing*, 78, 1900–1906.

Karmels, P. (1993). Conundrum game for nursing theorists Neuman, King, and Johnson. *Nurse Educator*, 18(6), 8–9.

Kaufman, J.E. (1996). Personal definitions of health among elderly people: A link to effective health promotion. *Family and Community Health*, 19(2), 58–68.

Kelley, J., Sanders, N., and Pierce, J. (1989). A systems approach to the role of the nurse administrator. In B. Neuman (Ed.), *The Neuman systems model* (2nd ed.). Norwalk, CT: Appleton & Lange.

Kim, H.S. (2000). An integrative framework for conceptualizing clients: A proposal for a nursing perspective in the new century. *Nursing Science Quarterly*, 13(1), 37–40.

Knight, J.B. (1990). The Betty Neuman Systems Model applied to practice: A client with multiple sclerosis. *Journal of Advanced Nursing*, 15(4), 447–455.

Lancaster, D. and Whall, A. (1989). The Neuman systems model. In J.J. Fitzpatrick and A.L. Whall (Eds.), *Conceptual models of nursing: Analysis and application* (2nd ed.). Norwalk, CT: Appleton & Lange.

Laschinger, H.K. and Duff, V. (1991). Attitudes of practicing nurses towards theory-based nursing practice. *Canadian Journal of Nursing Administration*, 4(1), 6–10.

Lebold, M. and Davis, L. (1980). A baccalaureate nursing curriculum based on the Neuman health-systems model. In J.P. Riehl and C. Roy (Eds.), *Conceptual models of nursing practice.* New York: Appleton-Century-Crofts.

Lillis, P. and Cora, V. (1989). A case study analysis using the Neuman nursing process format: An abstract. In B. Neuman (Ed.), *The Neuman systems model* (2nd ed.). Norwalk, CT: Appleton & Lange.

Lindell, M. and Olsson, H. (1991). Can combined oral contraceptives be made more effective by means of a nursing care model? *Journal of Advanced Nursing*, 16(4), 475–479.

Louis, M. (1989). An intervention to reduce anxiety levels for nurses ing with long-term care clients using Neuman's model. In J. Riehl-Sisca (Ed.), ptual mod-*els for nursing practice* (3rd ed.). Norwalk, CT: Appleton & Lang
Louis, M. (1995). The Neuman model in nursing research: An update. I euman (Ed.), *The Neuman systems model* (pp. 473–495). Norwalk, CT: App
Louis, M. and Koertvelyessy, A. (1989). The Neuman model in nursing B. Neuman (Ed.), *The Neuman systems model* (2nd ed.). Norwalk, CT: nge. Lange.
Lowry, L. and Jopp, M. (1989). An evaluation instrument for assessing an associat nursing curriculum based on the Neuman systems model. In J. Riehl-Sisca *Conceptual models for nursing practice* (3rd ed.). Norwalk, CT: Appleton & L
Lowry, L.W., Burns, C.M., Smith, A.A., et al (2000). Compete or complement? An in disciplinary approach to training health professionals. *Nursing and Health Ca Perspectives,* 21(2), 76–80.
Luker, K.A., Beaver, K., Leinster, S.J., et al. (1996). Meaning of illness for women with breast cancer. *Journal of Advanced Nursing,* 23(6), 1194–1201.
Marett, K.M., Gibbons, W.E., Memmott, R.J., et al. (1998). The organizational role of the clinical practice models in interdisciplinary collaborative practice. *Clinic Social Work Journal,* 26(2), 217–225.
May, K.M. and Hu, J. (2000). Caregiving and help seeking by mothers of low birthweight infants and mothers of normal birthweight infants. *Public Health Nursing,* 17(4), 273–279.
McHolm, F.A. and Geib, K.M. (1998). Application of the Neuman Systems Model to teaching health assessment and nursing process. *Nursing Diagnosis,* 9(1), 23–33.
McRae-Bergeron, C.E., May, L., Foulks, R.W., et al. (1999). A medical readiness model of health assessment or well-being in first-increment Air Combat Command medical personnel. *Military Medicine,* 164(6), 379–388.
Mohr, W.K. (1995). Multiple ideologies and their proposed roles in the outcomes of nurse practice settings—The for-profit psychiatric-hospital scandal as a paradigm case. *Nursing Outlook,* 43(5), 215–223.
Molassiotis, A. (1997). A conceptual mode of adaptation to illness and quality of life for cancer patients treated with bone marrow transplants. *Journal of Advanced Nursing,* 26(3), 572–579.
Moore, S.L. and Munro, M.F. (1990). The Neuman Systems Model applied to mental health nursing of older adults. *Journal of Advanced Nursing,* 15(3), 293–299.
Morales-Mann, E.T. and Kaitell, C.A. (2001). Problem-based learning in a new Canadian curriculum. Journal of Advanced Nursing, 33(1), 13–19.
Mrkonich, D.E., Hessian, M., and Miller, M. (1989). A cooperative process in curriculum development using the Neuman health care systems model. In J. Riehl-Sisca (Ed.), *Conceptual models for nursing practice* (3rd ed.). Norwalk, CT: Appleton & Lange.
Mrkonich, D., Miller, M., and Hessian, M. (1989). Cooperative baccalaureate education: The Minnesota intercollegiate nursing consortium. In B. Neuman (Ed.), *The Neuman systems model* (2nd ed.). Norwalk, CT: Appleton & Lange.
Mulhall, A. (1996). Cultural discourse and the myth of stress in nursing and medicine. *International Journal of Nursing Studies,* 33(5), 455–468.

Neal, J.E. (2001). Patient outcomes: A matter of perspective. *Nursing Outlook*, 49(2), 93–99.

Nelson, L., Hansen, M., and McCullagh, M. (1989). A new baccalaureate North Dakota-Minnesota nursing education consortium. In B. Neuman (Ed.), *The Neuman systems model* (2nd ed.). Norwalk, CT: Appleton & Lange.

Neufeld, A. (1983). Curriculum revision Making the process work. *Journal of Advanced Nursing*, 8, 213–220.

Neuman, B.M. (1974). The Betty Neuman health-care systems model: A total person approach to patient problems. In J.P. Riehl and C. Roy (Eds.), *Conceptual models for nursing practice*. New York: Appleton-Century-Crofts.

Neuman, B.M. (1980). The Betty Neuman health care systems model: A total person approach to patient problems. In J.P. Riehl and C. Roy (Eds.), *Conceptual models for nursing practice*. New York: Appleton-Century-Crofts.

Neuman, B.M. (1982). *The Neuman systems model. Application to nursing education and practice*. Norwalk, CT: Appleton-Century-Crofts.

Neuman, B.M. (1989). The Neuman systems model. In B. Neuman (Ed.), *The Neuman systems model* (2nd ed.). Norwalk, CT: Appleton & Lange.

Neuman, B.M. (1989). The Neuman nursing process format: Family case study. In J. Riehl-Sisca (Ed.), *Conceptual models for nursing practice* (3rd ed.). Norwalk, CT: Appleton & Lange.

Neuman, B. (1989). In conclusion-in transition. In B. Neuman (Ed.), *The Neuman systems model* (2nd ed.). Norwalk, CT Appleton & Lange.

Neuman, B.M. (1990). Health as a continuum based on the Neuman systems model. *Nursing Science Quarterly*, 3(3), 129–135.

Neuman, B. (1995). *The Neuman systems model*. Norwalk, CT: Appleton & Lange.

Neuman, B. (1996). The Neuman systems model in research and practice. *Nursing Science Quarterly*, 9(2), 67–70.

Neuman, B., Chadwick, P.L., Beynon, C.E., et al. (1997). The Neuman systems model: Reflections and projections. *Nursing Science Quarterly*, 10(1), 18–21.

Neuman, B., Newman, D.M.L., and Holder, P. (2000). Leadership-scholarship integration: Using the Neuman systems model for 21st century professional nursing practice. *Nursing Science Quarterly*, 13(1), 60–63.

Neuman, B.M. and Wyatt, M. (1980). The Neuman stress/adaptation systems approach to education for nurse administrators. In J.P. Riehl and C. Roy (Eds.), *Conceptual models of nursing practice*. New York: Appleton-Century-Crofts.

Neuman, B.M. and Wyatt, M. (1981). Prospects for change: Some evaluative reflections from one articulated baccalaureate program. *Journal of Nursing Education*, 20(1), 40–46.

Neuman, B.M. and Young, R.J. (1972). A model for teaching a total person approach to patient problems. *Nursing Research*, 21, 264–269.

Nosek, M.A. (1996). Wellness among women with physical disabilities. *Sexuality and Disability*, 14(3), 165–181.

Peternelj-Taylor, C.A. and Johnson, R. (1996). Custody and caring: Clinical placement of student nurses in a forensic setting. *Perspectives in Psychiatric Care*, 32(4), 23–29.

Pierce, J.D. and Hutton, E. (1992). Applying the new concepts of the Neuman Systems Model. *Nursing Forum*, 27(1), 15–18.

Polivka, B.J. (1996). Rural sex education: Assessment of programs and interagency collaboration. *Public Health Nursing,* 13(6), 425–433.

Putt, A. (1972). Entropy, evolution and equifinality in nursing. In J. Smith (Ed.), *Five years of cooperation to improve curricula in Western schools of nursing.* Boulder, CO: Western Interstate Commission for Higher Education.

Rafael, A.R.F. (2000). Watson's philosophy, science, and theory of human caring as a conceptual framework for guiding community health nursing practice. *Advances in Nursing Science,* 23(2), 34–49.

Randell, B.P. (1992). Nursing theory: The 21st century. *Nursing Science Quarterly,* 5(4), 176–184.

Reed, K. (1989). Family theory related to the Neuman systems model. In B. Neuman (Ed.), *The Neuman systems model* (2nd ed.). Norwalk, CT: Appleton & Lange.

Robichaud-Ekstrand, S. and Delisle, L. (1989). The Neuman model in medical-surgical settings. *Canadian Nurse,* 85(6), 32–35.

Ross, M. and Bourbonnais, F. (1985). The Betty Neuman systems model in nursing practice: A nursing study approach. *Journal of Advanced Nursing,* 10(3), 199–207.

Sabo, C.E. and Michael, S.R. (1996). The influence of personal message with music on anxiety and side effects associated with chemotherapy. *Cancer Nursing,* 19(4), 283–289.

Selye, H. (1950). *The physiology and pathology of exposure to stress.* Montreal, Canada: Acta.

Skillen, D.L., Anderson, M.C., and Knight, C.L. (2001). The created environment for physical assessment by case managers. *Western Journal of Nursing Research,* 23(1), 72–89.

Sipple, J. and Freese, B. (1989). Transition from technical to professional-level nursing education. In B. Neuman (Ed.), *The Neuman systems model* (2nd ed.). Norwalk, CT: Appleton & Lange.

Smith, M.C. (1989). Neuman's model in practice. *Nursing Science Quarterly,* 2(3), 116–117.

Sohier, R. (1989). Nursing care for the people of a small planet: Culture and the Neuman systems model. In B. Neuman (Ed.), *The Neuman systems model* (2nd ed.). Norwalk, CT: Appleton & Lange.

Sohier, R. (1997). Neuman's systems model in nursing practice. In M.R. Alligood et al. (Eds.), *Nursing theory: Utilization and application* (pp. 109–127). St. Louis, MO: Mosby Year Book.

Stepans, M.B.F. and Knight, J.R. (2002). Application of Neuman's framework: Infant exposure to environmental tobacco smoke. *Nursing Science Quarterly,* 15(4), 327–334.

Stewart, M., Brown, J.B., Donner, A., et al. (2000). The impact of patient-centered care on outcomes. *Journal of Family Practice,* 49(9), 796–804.

Story, E.L. and Ross, M.M. (1986). Family centered community health nursing and the Betty Neuman systems model. *Nursing Papers,* 18(2), 77–88.

Stranahan, S. (2001). Spiritual perception, attitudes about spiritual care, and spiritual care practices among nurse practitioners. *Western Journal of Nursing Research,* 23(1), 90–104.

Sullivan, J. (1986). Using Neuman's model in the acute phase of spinal cord injury. *Focus on Critical Care,* 13(5), 34–41.

Thorellekstrand, I. and Bjorvell, H. (1994). The VIPS-Model used by nursing students—Review of educational care plans. *Scandinavian Journal of Caring Sciences*, 8(4), 195–205.

Trepanier, M.J. (1989). Application of the Neuman systems model to perinatal nursing. In B. Neuman (Ed.), *The Neuman systems model* (2nd ed.). Norwalk, CT: Appleton & Lange.

Venable, J.F. (1980). The Neuman health-care systems model: An analysis. In J.P. Riehl and C. Roy (Eds.), *Conceptual models of nursing practice.* New York: Appleton-Century-Crofts.

Villarruel, A.M., Bishop, T.L., Simpson, E.M., et al. (2001). Borrowed theories, shared theories, and the advancement of nursing knowledge. *Nursing Science Quarterly*, 14(2), 158–163.

Whall, A.L. (1983). The Betty Neuman health care system model. In J.J. Fitzpatrick and A.L. Whall (Eds.), *Conceptual models of nursing: Analysis and application.* Bowie, MD: Robert J. Brady Co.

Wright, P.S., Piazza, D., Holcombe, J., and Foote, A. (1994). A comparison of three theories of nursing used as a guide for the nursing care of an 8-year-old with leukemia. *Journal of Pediatric Oncology Nursing*, 11(1), 14–19.

Ziemer, M.M. (1983). Effects of information on postsurgical coping. *Nursing Research*, 32, 282–287.

26. Margaret Newman

August-Brady, M. (2000). Prevention as intervention. *Journal of Advanced Nursing*, 31(6), 1304–1308.

Connor, M.J. (1998). Expanding the dialogue on praxis in nursing research and practice. *Nursing Science Quarterly*, 11(2), 51–55.

Endo, E. (1999). Comment in *Advances in Nursing Science*, 21(3), vii-viii. Pattern recognition as a nursing intervention with Japanese women with ovarian cancer. *Advances in Nursing Science* (1998), 20(4), 49–61.

Engle, V. (1989). Newman's model of health. In J.J. Fitzpatrick and A.L. Whall (Eds.), *Conceptual models of nursing: Analysis and application* (2nd ed.). Norwalk, CT: Appleton & Lange.

Field, L. and Newman, M. (1982). Clinical application of the unitary man framework: Case study analysis. In M.J. Kim and D.A. Moritz (Eds.), *Classification of nursing diagnosis* (pp. 249–263). New York: McGraw-Hill.

Ford-Gilboe, M.V. (1994). A comparison of two nursing models: Allen's developmental health model and Newman's theory of health as expanding consciousness. *Nursing Science Quarterly*, 7(3), 113–118.

Hall, B. (1980). Book review of *Theory Development in Nursing* by Margaret Newman. *Nursing Research*, 29(5), 311.

Hall, E.O.C. (1996). Husserlian phenomenology and nursing in a unitary-transformative program. *Vard I Norden Nursing Science and Research in the Nordic Countries*, 16(3), 4–8.

Hensley, D., Keffer, M., Kilgore-Keever, K., Langfitt, J., and Peterson, L. (1989). Margaret A. Newman: Model of health. In A. Marriner-Tomey (Ed.), Nursing theorists and their work (2nd ed.). St. Louis: C.V. Mosby.

Newman, M. (1984). Nursing diagnosis. *American Journal of Nursing*, 84(12), 1496–1499.

Newman, M. (1986). *Health as expanding consciousness.* St. Louis, MO: C.V. Mosby.

Newman, M. (1987). Aging as increasing complexity [Survey]. *Journal of Gerontological Nursing*, 13(9), 16–18.

Newman, M. (1987). Perception of time among Japanese inpatients. *Western Journal of Nursing Research*, 9(20), 299–300.

Newman, M. (1989). The spirit of nursing. *Holistic Nursing Practice*, 3(3), 1–6.

Newman, M.A. (1972). Time estimation in relation to gait tempo. *Perceptual Motor Skills*, 34, 359–366.

Newman, M.A. (1972). Nursing's theoretical evolution. *Nursing Outlook*, 20, 449–453.

Newman, M.A. (1976). Movement tempo and the experience of time. *Nursing Research*, 25(4), 273–279.

Newman, M.A. (1979). *Theory development in nursing.* Philadelphia: F.A. Davis.

Newman, M.A. (1981). The meaning of health. In G.E. Lasker (Ed.), *Applied systems research and cybernetics. Systems research in health care, biocybernetics and ecology* (Vol. 4, pp. 1739–1743). New York: Pergamon.

Newman, M.A. (1982). *Thoughts on Bohm's concept of implicate order and its meaning for nursing science.* Presented at the Nursing Theory Think Tank, Dallas, TX.

Newman, M.A. (1982). Time as an index of consciousness with age. *Nursing Research*, 31, 290–293.

Newman, M.A. (1982). What differentiates clinical research? *Image: Journal of Nursing Scholarship*, 14(3), 86–88.

Newman, M.A. (1983). *Health as expanding consciousness.* Proceedings of Seventh International Conference on Human Functioning. Wichita, KS: Biomedical Synergistics Institute.

Newman, M.A. (1983). Newman's health theory. In I. Clements and F. Roberts (Eds.), *Family health: A theoretical approach to nursing care* (pp. 161–175). New York: John Wiley & Sons.

Newman, M.A. (1995). Retrospective: Theory for nursing practice. In *A developing discipline: Selected works of Margaret Newman* (Publication No. 14–2671, pp. 273–285). New York: National League for Nursing.

Newman, M.A. (1994). Theory for nursing practice. *Nursing Science Quarterly*, 7, 153–157.

Newman, M.A. (1997). Experiencing the whole. *Advances in Nursing Science*, 20(1), 34–39.

Newman, M.A. and Gaudiano, J.K. (1984). Depression as an explanation for decreased subjective time in the elderly. *Nursing Research*, 33(3), 137–139.

Newman, M.A., Sime, A.M., and Corcoran-Perry, S.A. (1991). The focus of the discipline of nursing. *Advances in Nursing Science*, 14(1), 1–6.

Newman, M.A., Tompkins, E.S., Isenberg, M.A., Fitzpatrick, J.J., and Scott, D.W. (1980). Movement, time and consciousness: Parameters of health [Symposium]. Proceedings of Western Society for Research.

Nojima, Y., Oda, A., Nishii, H., Fukui, M., Seo, K., and Akiyoshi, H. (1987). Perception of time among Japanese inpatients. *Western Journal of Nursing Research*, 9(3), 288–300.

Picard, C. and Mariolis, T. (2002). Praxis as a mirroring process: Teaching psychiatric nursing grounded in Newman's health as expanding consciousness. *Nursing Science Quarterly*, 15(2), 1181–122.

Roy, C., Rogers, M.E., Fitzpatrick, J.J., Newman, M., and Orem, D.E. (1982). Nursing diagnosis and nursing theory. In M.J. Kim and D.A. Moritz (Eds.), *Classification of nursing diagnosis* (pp. 215–231). New York: McGraw-Hill.

Sarter, B. (1988). Philosophical sources of nursing theory. *Nursing Science Quarterly*, 1(2), 52–59.

Schlotzhauer, M. and Farnham, R. (1997). Newman's theory and insulin dependent diabetes mellitus in adolescence. *Journal of School Nursing*, 13(3), 20–23.

Weingourt, R. (1998). Using Margaret A. Newman's theory of health with elderly nursing home residents. *Perspectives in Psychiatric Care*, 34(3), 25–30.

Yamashita, M. (1997). Family caregiving Application of Newman's and Peplau's theories. *Journal of Psychiatric and Mental Health Nursing*, 4(6), 401–405.

Yamashita, M. (1998). Family coping with mental illness: A comparative study. *Journal of Psychiatric and Mental Health Nursing*, 5(6), 515–523.

Yamashita. M. (1998). Newman's theory of health as expanding consciousness: Research on family caregiving in mental illness in Japan. *Nursing Science Quarterly*, 11(3), 110–115.

Yamashita, M. and Tall, F.D. (1998). A commentary on Newman's theory of health as expanding consciousness. *Advances in Nursing Science*, 21(1), 65–75.

27. Florence Nightingale

Armstrong, D. (1983). The fabrication of nurse-patient relationships. *Social Science and Medicine*, 17(8), 457–460.

Attewell, A. (1998). Florence Nightingale's relevance to nurses. *Journal of Holistic Nursing*, 16(2), 281–291.

Barnard, K. and Neal, M.U. (1977). Maternal-child nursing research: Review of the past and strategies for the future. *Nursing Research*, 26, 193–200.

Boland, L. (1988). Five Nightingale theories spell success. *Today's Nurse*, 10(12), 18–21.

Bourgeois, M.J. (1975). The special nurse research fellow: Characteristics and trends. *Nursing Research*, 24, 184–188.

Brynes, M.A. (1982). Non-nursing functions: Nurses state their case. *American Journal of Nursing*, 82, 1089–1093.

Chinn, P.L. (1983). Editorial. *Advances in Nursing Science*, 6(1), ix-x.

Christoffel, T. (1976). Medical care evaluation: An old idea. *Journal of Medical Education*, 51(2), 83–88.

Cohen, I.B. (1984). Florence Nightingale. *Scientific America*, 250, 128–137.

Crow, R. (1982). How nursing and the community can benefit from nursing research. *International Journal of Nursing Studies*, 19(1), 37–45.

deGraaf, K., Marriner-Tomey, A., Mossman, C., and Slebodnik, M. (1989). Florence Nightingale: Modern nursing. In A. Marriner-Tomey (Ed.), *Nursing theorists and their work* (2nd ed.). St. Louis: C.V. Mosby.

Dennis, K.E. and Prescott, P.A. (1985). Florence Nightingale: Yesterday, today and tomorrow. *Advances in Nursing Science,* 7(2), 66–81.

Francis, G. (1980). Gesellschaft and the hospital: Is total care a misnomer? *Advances in Nursing Science,* 2(4), 9–13.

Francis, H.W. (1982). On gossips, eavesdroppers and peeping toms. *Journal of Medical Ethics,* 8, 134–143.

Goldwater, M. (1987). Like Florence Nightingale, we use the political system. *The American Nurse,* 19(2), 15.

Grier, B. and Grier, M. (1978). Contributions of the passionate statistician. *Research in Nursing and Health,* 1(3), 103–109.

Hays, J.D. (1989). Florence Nightingale and the India sanitary reforms. *Public Health Nursing,* 6(3), 152–154.

Henderson, V.A. (1978). The concept of nursing. *Journal of Advanced Nursing,* 3, 113–130.

Henderson, V.A. (1980). Preserving the essence of nursing in a technological age. *Journal of Advanced Nursing,* 5, 245–260.

Heistand, W.C. (1982). Nursing, the family and the "new" social history. *Advances in Nursing Science,* 4(3), 1–12.

Hughes, L. (1980). The public image of the nurse. *Advances in Nursing Science,* 2, 55–72.

Johnson, D.E. (1974). Development of theory: A requisite for nursing as a primary health profession. *Nursing Research,* 23(5), 372–377.

Kalish, B.J. and Kalish, P.A. (1983). Heroine out of focus: Media images of Florence Nightingale. Part I: Popular biographies and stage productions. *Nursing and Health Care,* 4, 181–187.

Kalish, B.J. and Kalish, P.A. (1983). Heroine out of focus: Media images of Florence Nightingale. Part II: Film, radio, and television dramatizations. *Nursing and Health Care,* 4, 181–187.

Kalish, P.A. and Kalish, B.J. (1982). The image of nurses in novels. *American Journal of Nursing,* 82, 1220–1224.

Keith, J.M. (1988). Florence Nightingale: Statistician and consultant epidemiologist. *International Nursing Review,* 35(5), 147–151.

Kelly, L.Y. (1976). Our nursing heritage: Have we renounced it? *Image: Journal of Nursing Scholarship,* 8(3), 43–48.

Kopf, E.W. (1978). Florence Nightingale as statistician. *Research in Nursing and Health,* 1(3), 93–102.

Kovacs, A.R. (1978). The personality of Florence Nightingale. *International Nursing Review,* 20, 78–81.

Macrae, J. (1995). Nightingale's spiritual philosophy and its significance for modern nursing. *Image: Journal of Nursing Scholarship,* 27, 8–10.

Matthews, C.A. and Gaul, A.L. (1979). Nursing diagnosis from the perspective of concept attainment and critical thinking. *Advances in Nursing Science,* 2(1), 17–26.

Monteiro, L. (1972). Research into things past: Tracking down one of Miss Nightingale's correspondents. *Nursing Research*, 21(5), 526–529.

Nightingale, F. (1992). *Notes on nursing* [Reprint of 1859 edition]. Philadelphia: J.B. Lippincott.

Novak, J.C. (1988). The social mandate and historical basis for nursing's role in health promotion. *Journal of Professional Nursing*, 4(2), 80–87.

Palmer, I.S. (1977). Florence Nightingale: Reformer, reactionary, researcher. *Nursing Research*, 26(2), 84–89.

Palmer, I.S. (1981). Florence Nightingale and international origins of modern nursing. *Image: Journal of Nursing Scholarship*, 13, 28–31.

Palmer, I.S. (1983). Nightingale revisited. *Nursing Outlook*, 31(4), 229–233.

Palmer, I.S. (1983). Origins of education for nurses. *Nursing Forum*, 22(3), 102–110.

Parker, P. (1977). Florence Nightingale First lady of administrative nursing. *Supervisor Nurse*, 8(3), 24–25.

Reed, P.G. and Zurakowski, T.L. (1983). Nightingale: A visionary model for nursing. In J.J. Fitzpatrick and A.L. Whall (Eds.), *Conceptual models of nursing: Analysis and application*. Bowie, MD: Robert J. Brady Co.

Reed, P.G. and Zurakowski, T.L. (1989). Nightingale revisited: A visionary model for nursing. In J.J. Fitzpatrick and A.L. Whall (Eds.), *Conceptual models of nursing: Analysis and application* (2nd ed.). Norwalk, CT: Appleton & Lange.

Rogers, P.S. (1972). Design for patient care. *International Nursing Review*, 19(3), 267–282.

Romano, C., McCormick, L.D., and McNeely, L.D. (1982). Nursing documentation: A model for a computerized data base. *Advances in Nursing Science*, 1(2), 43–56.

Schlotfeldt, R.M. (1977). Nursing research: Reflection of values. *Nursing Research*, 26(1), 4–9.

Schrock, R.A. (1977). On political consciousness in nurses. *Journal of Advanced Nursing*, 2, 41–50.

Seelye, A. (1982). Hospital ward layout and nurse staffing. *Journal of Advanced Nursing*, 7, 195–201.

Selanders, L.C. (1998). Florence Nightingale. The evolution and social impact of feminist values in nursing. *Journal of Holistic Nursing*, 16(2), 227–243.

Selanders, L.C. (1998). The power of environmental adaptation. Florence Nightingale's original theory for nursing practice. *Journal of Holistic Nursing*, 16(2), 247–263.

Seymer, L.R. (1960). One hundred years ago. *American Journal of Nursing*, 60, 658–661.

Smith, F.T. (1981). Florence Nightingale: Early feminist. *American Journal of Nursing*, 81, 1021–1024.

Tebbe, S. (1988). Nightingale's environmental theory—A 20th century reality. *Today's Nurse*, 10(8), 8–15.

Thompson, J.D. (1980). The passionate humanist: From Nightingale to the new nurse. *Nursing Outlook*, 28(5), 290–295

Torres, G. (1981). The nursing education administrator: Accountable, vulnerable and oppressed. *Advances in Nursing Science*, 3(3), 1–16.

Weiler, P.G. (1975). Health manpower dialectic: Physician, nurse, physician assistant. *American Journal of Public Health*, 65(8), 858–863.

Whittaker, E.W. and Olesen, V.L. (1967). Why Florence Nightingale? *American Journal of Nursing*, 67, 2338–2341.

Williams, B. (1965). Back to Florence Nightingale and Lawson Tait. *The Practitioner*, 194, 800–804.

Wolstenholme, G.E.W. (1970). Florence Nightingale: New lamps for old. *Proceedings of the Royal Society of Medicine*, 63, 1282–1288.

28. Dorothea Orem

Aggleton, P., and Chalmers, H. (1985). Models and theories: Orem's self care model (part 5). *Nursing Times*, 81(1), 36–39.

Ailinger, R.L. and Dear, M.R. (1993). Self-care agency in persons with rheumatoid arthritis. *Arthritis Care and Research*, 6(3), 134–140.

Aish, A.E. and Isenberg, M. (1996). Effects of Orem-based nursing intervention on nutritional self-care of myocardial infarction patients. *International Journal of Nursing Studies*, 33(3), 259–270.

Allan, J. (1988). Knowing what to weigh: Women's self care activities related to weight. *Advances in Nursing Science*, 11(1), 47–60

Allen, D. (2000). Negotiating the role of expert carers on an adult hospital ward. *Sociology of Health and Illness*, 22(2), 149–171.

†Allison, S.E. (1973). A framework for nursing action in a nurse-conducted diabetic management clinic. *Journal of Nursing Administration*, 3(4), 53–60.

Alteneder, R.R. (1998). Conceptualizing sexual health in cancer care—Commentary. *Western Journal of Nursing Research*, 20(6), 701–703.

Anastasio, C., McMahan, T., Daniels, A., Nicholas, P.K., and Paul-Simon, A. (1995). Self-care burden in women with human immunodeficiency virus. *Journal of the Association of Nurses in AIDS Care*, 6(3), 31–42.

Anderson, J.A. (2001). Understanding homeless adults by testing the theory of self-care. *Nursing Science Quarterly*, 14(1), 59–67.

Anderson, J.A. and Olnhausen, K.S. (1999). Adolescent self-esteem: A foundational disposition. *Nursing Science Quarterly*, 12(1), 61–67.

Anderson, S.B. (1992). Guillain-Barre syndrome: Giving the patient control. *Journal of Neuroscience Nursing*, 24(3), 158–162.

†Anna, D.J., Christensen, D.G., Hohn, S.A., Ord, L., and Wells, S.R. (1978). Implementing Orem's conceptual framework. *Journal of Nursing Administration*, 8(11), 8–11.

Arts, S., Kersten, H. and Kerkstra, A. (1996). The daily practice in home help services in the Netherlands: Instrument development. *Health and Social Care in the Community*, 4(5), 280–289.

Astedt-Kurki, P., Friedemann, M.L., Paavilainen, E., et al. (2001). Assessment of strategies in families tested by Finnish families. *International Journal of Nursing Studies*, 38(1), 17–24.

Autar, R. (1996). Nursing assessment of clients at risk of deep vein thrombosis (DVT): The Autar DVT scale. *Journal of Advanced Nursing*, 23(4), 763–770.

Backman, K. and Hentinen, M. (1999). Model for the self-care of home-dwelling elderly. *Journal of Advanced Nursing*, 30(3), 564–572.

Backscheider, J. (1971). The use of self as the essence of clinical supervision in ambulatory patient care. *Nursing Clinics of North America*, 6(4), 785–794.

†Backscheider, J.E. (1974). Self-care requirements, self-care capabilities, and nursing systems in the diabetic nurse management clinic. *American Journal of Public Health*, 64(12), 1138–1146.

Barnard, A. (1996). Technology and nursing: An anatomy of definition. *International Journal of Nursing Studies*, 33(4), 433–441.

Barnard, A. (1997). A critical review of the belief that technology is a neutral object and nurses are its master. *Journal of Advanced Nursing*, 16(1), 126–131.

Bartle, J. (1991). Nursing models: Caring in relation to Orem's theory. *Nursing Standard*, 5(37), 33–36.

Beach, E.K., Smith, A., Luthringer, L., et al. (1996). Self-care limitations of persons after acute myocardial infarction. *Applied Nursing Research*, 9(1), 24–28.

Behi, R. (1986). Look after yourself: Orem's self-care model. *Nursing Times*, 82(37), 35–37.

Bennett, J.A. (1995). Nurses' attitudes about acquired-immunodeficiency-syndrome care—What research tells us. *Journal of Professional Nursing*, 11(6), 339–350.

Bennett, J.A. (1997). A case for theory triangulation. *Nursing Science Quarterly*, 10(2), 97–102.

Bennett, J.G. (1980). Forward to the Symposium on the Self-care Concept in Nursing. *Nursing Clinics of North America*, 15(1), 129–130.

Berbiglia, V.A. (1991). A case study: Perspectives on a self-care deficit nursing theory-based curriculum. *Journal of Advanced Nursing*, 16(10), 1158–1163.

Berbiglia, V.A. (1997). Orem's self-care deficit theory in nursing practice. In M.R. Alligood, et al. (Eds.), *Nursing theory: Utilization and application* (pp. 129–152). St. Louis, MO: Mosby Year Book.

Bernhard, L. (1997). Self-care strategies of menopausal women. *Journal of Women and Aging*, 9(1–2), 77–89.

Bevan, M.T. (2000). Dialysis as "deus ex machina": A critical analysis of haemodialysis. *Journal of Advanced Nursing*, 31(2), 437–443.

Biehler, B.A.(1992). Impact of role-sets on implementing self-care theory with children. *Pediatric Nursing*, 18(1), 30–34.

Biley, F. and Dennerley, M. (1990). Orem's model: A critical analysis. *Nursing*, 4(13), 19–22.

Bliss-Holtz, J. (1996). Using Orem's theory to generate nursing diagnoses for electronic documentation. *Nursing Science Quarterly*, 9(3), 121–125.

Bliss-Holtz, J., Taylor, S.G., and McLaughlin, K. (1992). Nursing theory as a base for a computerized nursing information system. *Nursing Science Quarterly*, 5(3), 124–128.

Bonamy, C., Schultz, P., Graham, K., and Hampton, M. (1995). The use of theory-based nursing practice in the Department of Veterans' Affairs Medical Centers. *Journal of Nursing Staff Development*, 11(1), 27–30.

Bradshaw, A. (1995). What are nurses doing to patients—A review of theories of nursing past and present. *Journal of Clinical Nursing*, 4(2), 81–92

Bramlett, M.H., Gueldner, S.H., and Sowell, R.L. (1990). Consumer-centric advocacy: Its connection to nursing frameworks. *Nursing Science Quarterly*, 3(4), 156–161.

†Bromley, B. (1980). Applying Orem's self-care theory in enterostomal therapy. *American Journal of Nursing,* 80(2), 245–249.

†Buckwalter, K.C. and Kerfoot, K.M. (1982). Teaching patients self-care: A critical aspect of psychiatric discharge planning. *Journal of Psychiatric Nursing and Mental Health Services,* 20(5), 15–20.

Bunn, M.H., O'Connor, A.M., Tansey, M.S., et al (1997). Characteristics of clients with schizophrenia who express certainty or uncertainty about continuing treatment with depot neuroleptic medication. *Archives of Psychiatric Nursing,* 11(5), 238–248.

Burks, K.J. (1999). A nursing practice model for chronic illness. *Rehabilitation Nursing,* 24(5), 197–200.

Burks, K.J. (2001). Intentional action. *Journal of Advanced Nursing,* 34(5), 668–675.

Bussing, A. and Herbig, B. (1998). The challenges of a care information system reflecting holistic nursing care. *Computers in Nursing,* 16(6), 311–317.

Cade, N.V. (2001). Orem's self-care deficit theory applied to hypertensive people (Portuguese). *Revista Latino-Americana de Enfermagem,* 9(3), 43–50.

†Caley, J.M., Dirkensen, M., Engally, M., and Hennrich, M.L. (1980). The Orem self-care model. In J.P. Riehl and C. Roy (Eds.), *Conceptual models for nursing practice* (2nd ed.). New York: Appleton-Century-Crofts.

Cammermeyer, M. (1983). Growth model of self-care for neurologically impaired people. *Journal of Neurosurgical Nursing,* 15, 299–305.

Campbell, J.C. and Soeken, K.L. (1999). Women's responses to battering: A test of the model. *Research in Nursing and Health,* 22(1), 49–58.

Campbell, J.C. and Weber, N. (2000). An empirical test of a self-care model of women's responses to battering. *Nursing Science Quarterly,* 13(1), 45–53.

Campuzano, M. (1982). Self-care following coronary artery bypass surgery. *Focus on Critical Care,* 9(1), 55–56.

Caris-Verhallen, W.M.C.M., Kerkstra, A. and Bensing, J.M. (1997). The role of communication in nursing care for elderly people: A review of the literature. *Journal of Advanced Nursing,* 25(5), 915–933.

Carter, P.A. (1998). Self-care agency: The concept and how it is measured. *Journal of Nursing Measurement,* 6(2), 195–207.

†Chang, B.L. (1980). Evaluation of health care professionals in facilitating self-care: Review of the literature and a conceptual model. *Advances in Nursing Science,* 3(1), 43–58.

Chapman, P. (1984). Specifics and generalities: A critical examination of two nursing models . . . Orem's and Preisner's. *Nurse Educator Today,* 4(6), 141–144.

Chevannes, M. (1997). Nurses caring for families—Issues in a multiracial society. *Journal of Clinical Nursing,* 6(2), 161–167.

Clark, M. (1986). Application of Orem's theory of self-care: A case study. *Journal of Community Health Nursing,* 3(3), 127–135.

Clinton, J.F., Denyes, M.J., Goodwin, J.O., and Koto, E.M. (1977). Developing criterion measures of nursing care: Case study of a process. *Journal of Nursing Administration,* 7(7), 41–45.

Closson, B.L., Mattingly, L.J., Finne, K.M., and Larson, J.A. (1994). Telephone follow-up program evaluation: Application of Orem's self-care model. *Rehabilitation Nursing,* 19(5), 287–292.

Cody, W.K. (1996). Drowning in eclecticism. *Nursing Science Quarterly,* 9(3), 86–88.

Cody, W.K. (1997). The many faces of change: Discomfort with the new. *Nursing Science Quarterly*, 10(2), 65–67.

Cody, W.K. (2000). Paradigm shift or paradigm drift? A meditation on commitment and transcendence. *Nursing Science Quarterly*, 13(2), 93–102.

†Coleman, L.J. (1980). Orem's self-care concept of nursing. In J.P. Riehl and C. Roy (Eds.), *Conceptual models for nursing practice* (2nd ed., pp. 315–328). New York: Appleton-Century-Crofts.

Comley, A.L. (1995). A comparative analysis of Orem's self-care model and Peplau's interpersonal theory. *Journal of Advanced Nursing*, 20(4), 755–760.

Compton, P. (1989). Drug abuse, a self-care deficit. *Journal of Psychosocial Nursing*, 27(3), 22–26.

Craddock, R.B., Adams, P.F., Usui, W.M., et al. (1999). An intervention to increase use and effectiveness of self-care measures for breast cancer chemotherapy patients. *Cancer Nursing*, 22(4), 312–319.

Cull, V.V. (1996). Exposure to violence and self-care practices of adolescents. *Family and Community Health*, 19(1), 31–41.

Cutler, C.G. (2001). Self-care agency and symptom management in patients treated for mood disorder. *Archives of Psychiatric Nursing*, 15(1), 24–31.

Dahn, M.L.L. (1998). An innovative approach to appropriate resource utilization. *Nursing Economics*, 16(6), 317–319.

Dashiff, C. (1988). Theory development in psychiatric mental health nursing: An analysis of Orem's theory. *Archives of Psychiatric Nursing*, 2(6), 366–372.

Dashiff, C.J. (1992). Self-care capabilities in black girls in anticipation of menarche. *Health Care for Women International*, 13(1), 67–76.

Davidhizar, R. and Cosgray, R. (1990).The use of Orem's model in psychiatric rehabilitation assessment. *Rehabilitation Nursing*, 15(1), 39–41.

Decramer, M. Gosselink, R., Troosters, T., et al. (1997). Muscle weakness is related to utilization of health care resources in COPD patients. *European Respiratory Journal*, 10(2), 417–423.

Decurvas, L.H.O. and Campo, J.H.L. (1995). A program for the home care of patients with a symptomatic malignant terminal disease. *Cancer Nursing*, 18(5), 368–373.

DeGeest, S., Borgermans, L., Gemoets, H., et al. (1995). Incidence, determinants, and consequences of subclinical noncompliance with immunosuppressive therapy in renal transplant recipients. *Transplantation*, 59, 340–347.

Delbar, V. and Benor, D.E. (2001). Impact of a nursing intervention on cancer patients' ability to cope. *Journal of Psychosocial Oncology*, 19(2), 57–75.

Deng, X. and Xie, X. (2001). Apply Orem theory and theory of holistic nursing care to set up a nursing model for the aged in community [Chinese]. *Chinese Nursing Research*, 15(3), 173–174.

Denyes, M.J. (1982). Measurement of self-care agency in adolescents [Abstract]. *Nursing Research*, 31, 63.

Denyes, M.J. (1988). Orem's model used for health promotion: Directions from research. *Advances in Nursing Science*, 11(1), 13–21.

Denyes, M.J., Neuman, B.M., and Villarruel, A.M. (1991). Nursing actions to prevent and alleviate pain in hospitalized children. *Issues in Comprehensive Pediatric Nursing*, 14(1), 31–48.

Denyes, M.J., O'Connor, N., Oakley, D., and Ferguson, S. (1989). Integrating nursing theory, practice and research through collaborative research. *Journal of Advanced Nursing*, 14, 141–145.

Denyes, M.J., Orem, D.E., and SozWiss, G. (2001). Self-care: A foundational science. *Nursing Science Quarterly*, 14(1), 48–54.

†Dickson, G.L. and Lee-Villasenor, H. (1982). Nursing theory and practice: A self-care approach. *Advances in Nursing Science*, 5, 29–40.

Dijkstra, A., Buist, G., Moorer, P., et al (1999). Construct validity of the Nursing Care Dependency Scale. *Journal of Clinical Nursing*, 8(4), 380–388.

Dijkstra, A., Buist, G., Moorer, P., et al (2000). A reliability and utility study of the Care Dependency Scale. *Scandinavian Journal of Caring Sciences*, 14(3), 155–161.

Dijkstra, A., Sipsma, D. and Dassen, T. (1999). Predictors of care dependency in Alzheimer's disease after a two-year period. *International Journal of Nursing Studies*, 36(6), 487–495.

Dropkin, M.J. (1981). Development of a self-care teaching program for postoperative head and neck patients. *Cancer Nursing*, 103–106.

Dumas, L. (1991). The Orem's conceptual framework as a self determinant for the nursing profession. *Arctic Medical Research*, Supplement, 207.

Easton, K.L. (1993). Defining the concept of self-care. *Rehabilitation Nursing*, 18(6), 384–387.

Eben, J., Gashti, N., Nation, M., Marriner-Tomey, A., and Nordmeyer, S. (1989). Dorothea E. Orem: Self-care deficit theory of nursing. In A. Marriner-Tomey (Ed.), *Nursing theorists and their work* (2nd ed.). St. Louis: C.V. Mosby.

Emerson, J. and Enderby, P. (1996). Management of speech and language disorders in a mental illness unit. *European Journal of Disorders of Communication*, 31(3), 237–244.

England, M. (1996). Sense of relatedness and interpersonal network of adult offspring caregivers: Linkages with crisis, emotional arousal, and perceived health. *Archives of Psychiatric Nursing,* 10(2), 85–95.

England, M. (1997). Self-coherence, emotional arousal and perceived health of adult children caring for a brain-impaired parent. *Journal of Advanced Nursing*, 26(4), 672–682.

Estes, S.D. and Hart, M. (1993). A model for the development of the CNS role in adolescent health promotion self-care. *Clinical Nurse Specialist*, 7(3), 111–115.

Evers, G., Viane, A., Sermeus, W., et al (2000). Frequency of and indications for wholly compensatory nursing care related to enteral food intake: A secondary analysis of the Belgium National Nursing Minimum Data Set. *Journal of Advanced Nursing*, 32(1), 194–201.

Evers, G.C.M. (1997). Pseudo-opioid resistant pain. *Supportive Care in Cancer*, 5(6), 457–460.

Ewing, G. (1989). The nursing preparation of stoma patients for self-care. *Journal of Advanced Nursing,* 14, 41–420.

Faucett, J., Ellis, V., Underwood, P., Naqvi, A., and Wilson, D. (1990). The effect of Orem's self-care model on nursing care in a nursing home setting. *Journal of Advanced Nursing*, 15(6), 659–666.

Fawcett, J. (1984). Orem's self-care model. In J. Fawcett (Ed.), *Analysis and evaluation of conceptual models of nursing.* Philadelphia: F.A. Davis.

Fawcett, J. (1989). Orem's self-care model. In J. Fawcett (Ed.), *Analysis and evaluation of conceptual models of nursing* (2nd ed.). Philadelphia: F.A. Davis.

Fawcett, J. (2001). The nurse theorists: 21st-century updates—Dorothea E. Orem. *Nursing Science Quarterly,* 14(1), 34–38.

Fawdry, M.K., Berry, M.L., and Rajacich, D. (1996). The articulation of nursing systems with dependent care systems of intergenerational caregivers. *Nursing Science Quarterly,* 9(1), 22–26.

Feathers, R. (1989). Orem's self-care nursing theory. In J. Riehl-Sisca (Ed.), *Conceptual models for nursing practice* (3rd ed.). Norwalk, CT: Appleton & Lange.

Fenner, K. (1979). Developing a conceptual framework. *Nursing Outlook,* 27, 122–126.

Field, P.A. (1987). The impact of nursing theory on the clinical decision making process. *Journal of Advanced Nursing,* 12(5), 653–571.

Fitzgerald, S. (1980). Utilizing Orem's self-care nursing model in designing an educational program for the diabetic. *Topics in Clinical Nursing,* 2(2), 57–65.

Flensner, G. and Lindencrona, C. (2002). The cooling-suit: A study of ten multiple sclerosis patients' experiences in daily life. *Journal of Advanced Nursing,* 37(6), 541–550.

Fontana, J.A. (1996). The emergence of the person-environment interaction in a descriptive study of vigor in heart failure. *Advances in Nursing Science,* 18(4), 70–82.

Foster, P.C. and Janssens, N.P. (1980) Dorothea E. Orem. In The Nursing Theories Conference Group, *Nursing theories: The base for professional nursing practice.* Englewood Cliffs, NJ: Prentice-Hall.

Franklin, A. (2001). Orem's self-care model in practice. *Vision,* 7(13), 24–26.

Frey, M. A and Fox, M.A. (1990). Assessing and teaching self-care to youths with diabetes mellitus. *Pediatric Nursing,* 16, 597–800.

Furlong, S. (1996). Self-care: The application of a ward philosophy. *Journal of Clinical Nursing,* 5(2), 85–90.

Gaffney, K.F. and Moore, J.B. (1996). Testing Orem's theory of self-care deficit: Dependent care agent performance for children. *Nursing Science Quarterly,* 9(4), 160–164.

Garcia, M.A. and Castillo, L. (2000). Client categorization: A tool to assess nursing workloads. *Revista Medica de Chile,* 123(2), 177–183.

Gardulf, A., Bjorvell, H., Andersen, V., et al. (1995). Lifelong treatment with gammaglobulin for primary antibody deficiencies: The patients' experiences of subcutaneous self-infusions and home therapy. *Journal of Advanced Nursing,* 21(5), 917–927.

Geden, B. (1997). Theory based research and defining populations . . . Reprinted with permission from: Theory-based nursing process and produce: Using Orem's self-care deficit theory of nursing in practice, education, and research. *International Orem Society Newsletter,* 5(2), 6–9.

Geden, E. (1989). The relationship between self-care theory and empirical research. In J. Riehl-Sisca (Ed.), *Conceptual models for nursing practice* (3rd ed.). Norwalk, CT: Appleton & Lange.

Geden, E.A., Isaramalai, S.A., and Taylor, S.G. (2001). Self-care deficit nursing theory and the nurse practitioner's practice in primary care settings. *Nursing Science Quarterly,* 14(1), 29–33.

Glaven, K.A., Haynes, N., Jones, D.R., et al (1998). A military application of a medical self-care program. *Military Medicine,* 163(10), 678–681.

Good, M. (1995). A comparison of the effects of jaw relaxation and music on postoperative pain. *Nursing Research,* 44(1), 51–57.

Good, M. (1996). Effects of relaxation and music on postoperative pain: A review. *Journal of Advanced Nursing,* 24(5), 905–914.

Gormley, K.J. (1997). Practice write-ups: An assessment instrument that contributes to bridging the differences between theory and practice for student nurses through the development of core skills. *Nursing Education Today,* 17(1), 53–57.

Grant, M. and Hezekiah, J. (1996). Knowledge and beliefs about hypertension among Jamaican female clients. *International Journal of Nursing Studies,* 33(1), 58–66.

Greenfield, E. and Pace, J. (1985). Orem's self-care theory of nursing: Practical application to the end stage renal disease (ESRD) patient. *Journal of Nephrology Nursing,* 2(4), 187–193.

Griffiths, P. (1998). An investigation into the description of patients' problems by nurses using two different needs-based nursing models. *Journal of Advanced Nursing,* 28(5), 969–977.

Gulick, E.E. (2001). Emotional distress and activities of daily living functions in persons with multiple sclerosis. *Nursing Research,* 50(3), 147–154.

Haas, D.L. (1990). Application of Orem's Self-Care Deficit Theory to the pediatric chronically ill population. *Issues in Comprehensive Pediatric Nursing,* 13(4), 253–264.

Halfens, R.J.G., van Alphen, A., Hasman, A., et al. (1999). The effect of item observability, clarity and wording on patient/nurse ratings when using the ASA scale. *Scandinavian Journal of Caring Sciences,* 13(3), 159–164.

Hanchett, E.S. (1990). Nursing models and community as client. *Nursing Science Quarterly,* 3(2), 67–72.

Hanucharurnkui, S. and Vinya-nguag, P. (1991). Effects of promoting patients' participation in self-care on postoperative recovery and satisfaction with care. *Nursing Science Quarterly,* 4(1), 14–20.

Harris, J.K. (1980). Self-care is possible after delivery. *Nursing Clinics of North America,* 15(1), 191–194.

Harrison-Raines, K. (1993). Nursing and self-care theory applied to utilization review: Concepts and cases. *American Journal of Medical Quality,* 8(4), 197–199.

Hart, M.A. (1995). Orem's self-care deficit theory: Research with pregnant women. *Nursing Science Quarterly,* 8(3), 120–126.

Hart, M.A. and Foster, S.N. (1998). Self-care agency in two groups of pregnant women. *Nursing Science Quarterly,* 11(4), 167–171.

Hartley, L. (1988). Congruence between teaching and learning self care: A pilot study. *Nursing Science Quarterly,* 1(4), 161–167.

Hartweg, D.L. (1993). Self-care actions of healthy middle-aged women to promote well-being. *Nursing Research,* 42 (4), 221–227.

Hecker, E.J. (2000). Feria de Salud: Implementation and evaluation of a communitywide health fair. *Public Health Nursing,* 17(4), 247–256.

Higgins, P.A., and Moore, S.M. (2000). Levels of theoretical thinking in nursing. *Nursing Outlook,* 48(4), 179–183.

Hildebrandt, E. and Robertson, B. (1995). Self-care of older black adults in a South African community. *N&HC Perspectives on Community*, 16(3), 136–143.

Hiromoto, B.M. and Dungan, J. (1991). Contract learning for self-care activities. A protocol study among chemotherapy outpatients. *Cancer Nursing*, 14(3), 148–154.

Hisama, K.K. (2001). The acceptance of nursing theory in Japan: A cultural perspective. *Nursing Science Quarterly*, 14(3), 255–259.

Holzemer, W.L. (1992). Linking primary health care and self-care through case management. *International Nursing Review*, 39(3), 83–89.

Horsburgh, M.E. (1999). Self-care of well adult Canadians and adult Canadians with end stage renal disease. *International Journal of Nursing Studies*, 36(6), 443–453.

Horsburgh, M.E., Beanlands, H., Locking-Cusolito, H., et al. (2000). Personality traits and self-care in adults awaiting renal transplant. *Western Journal of Nursing Research*, 22(4), 407–430.

Huch, M.H. (1999). Welcome and introduction. *Nursing Science Quarterly*, 12(1), 80–83.

Huss, K., Salerno, M., and Huss, R.W. (1991). Computer-assisted reinforcement of instruction: Effects on adherence in adult atopic asthmatics. *Research in Nursing and Health*, 14(4)259–267.

Jaarsma, T., Abu-Saad, H.H., Dracup, K., et al. (2000). Self-care behaviour of patients with heart failure. *Scandinavian Journal of Caring Sciences*, 14(2), 112–119.

Jaarsma, T., Halfens, R., Senten, M., Abu-Saad, H.H., and Dracup, K. (1998). Developing a supportive-educative program for patients with advanced heart failure within Orem's general theory of nursing. *Nursing Science Quarterly*, 11(2), 79–85.

Jacobs, C.J. (1990). Orem's self-care model: Is it relevant to patients in intensive care? *Intensive Care Nursing*, 6(2), 100–103.

Jenny, J. (1991). Self-care deficit theory and nursing diagnosis: A test of conceptual fit. *Journal of Nursing Education*, 30(5), 227–232.

Jirovec, M.M. and Kasno, J. (1990). Self-care agency as a function of patient-environmental factors among nursing home residents. *Research in Nursing and Health*, 13(5), 303–309.

Johnston, R.L. (1983). Orem self-care model of nursing. In J.J. Fitzpatrick and A.L. Whall (Eds.), *Conceptual models of nursing: Analysis and application*. Bowie, MD: Robert J. Brady Co.

Johnston, R.L. (1989). Orem's self care model of nursing. In J.J. Fitzpatrick and A.L. Whall (Eds.), *Conceptual models of nursing: Analysis and application* (2nd ed.). Norwalk, CT: Appleton & Lange.

Jopp, M., Carroll, M.C., & Waters, L. (1993). Using self-care theory to guide nursing management of the older adult after hospitalization. *Rehabilitation Nursing*, 18(2), 91–94.

Joseph, L.S. (1980). Self-care and the nursing process. *Nursing Clinics of North America*, 15(1), 131–143.

†Karl, C.A. (1982). The effect of an exercise program on self-care activities for the institutionalized elderly. *Journal of Gerontological Nursing*, 8, 282–285.

Kaul, V., Khurana, S., and Munoz, S. (2000). Management of medication noncompliance in solid-organ transplant recipients. *BioDrugs*, 13(5), 313–326.

Kearney, B.Y. and Fleischer, B.J. (1979). Development of an instrument to measure exercise of self-care agency. *Research in Nursing and Health*, 2(1), 25–34.

Kim, H.S. (2000). An integrative framework for conceptualizing clients: A proposal for a nursing perspective in the new century. *Nursing Science Quarterly*, 13(1), 37–40.

King, C. (1980). The self-care, self-help concept. *Nurse Practitioner*, 5, 34–35.

Kinlein, M.L. (1977). *Independent nursing practice with clients.* Philadelphia: J.B. Lippincott.

Kinlein, M.L. (1977). Self-care concept. *American Journal of Nursing*, 77, 598–601.

Kinlein, M.L. (1978). Point of view on the front: Nursing and family and community health. *Family and Community Health*, 1, 57–68.

Krishnasamy, M. (1996). Social support and the patient with cancer: A consideration of the literature. *Journal of Advanced Nursing*, 23(4), 757–762.

Kulig, J.C. (2000). Community resiliency: The potential for community health nursing theory development. *Public Health Nursing*, 17(5), 374–85.

Kuriansky, J., Gurland, B., Fleiss, J., and Cowan, D. (1976). The assessment of self-care capacity in geriatric psychiatric patients by objective and subjective methods. *Journal of Clinical Psychology,* 32, 95–102.

Landau, J., Cole, R.E., Tuttle, J., et al (2000). Family connectedness and women's sexual risk behaviors: Implications for the prevention/intervention of STD/HIV infection. *Family Process,* 39(4), 461–475.

Lane, D.E. (1981). Self-medication of psychiatric patients. *Journal of Psychiatric Nursing and Mental Health Services*, 19, 27–28.

Langland, R.M. and Farrah, S.J. (1990). Using a self-care framework for continuing education in gerontological nursing. *Journal of Continuing Education in Nursing*, 21(6), 267–270.

Larrabee, J.H., Bolden, L.V., and Knight, M.R. (1998). The lived experience of patient prudence in health care. *Journal of Advanced Nursing*, 28(4), 802–808.

Laschinger, H.K. and Duff, V. (1991). Attitudes of practicing nurses towards theory-based nursing practice. *Canadian Journal of Nursing Administration*, 4(1), 6–10.

Lauder, W. (1999). A survey of self-neglect in patients living in the community. *Journal of Clinical Nursing*, 8(1), 95–102.

Lauder, W. (2001). The utility of self-care theory as a theoretical basis for self-neglect. *Journal of Advanced Nursing,* 34(4), 545–551.

Lee, M.B. (1999). Power, self-care and health in women living in urban squatter settlements in Karachi, Pakistan: A test of Orem's theory. *Journal of Advanced Nursing*, 30(1), 248–259.

Lee, P. (1998). An analysis and evaluation of Casey's conceptual framework. *International Journal of Nursing Studies*, 35(4), 204–209.

Levin, L.S. (1976). *Self-care: Lay initiatives in health.* New York: Neale Watson Academic Publications.

Levin, L.S. (1977). Forces and issues in the revival of interest in self-care: Impetus for redirection for health. *Health Education Monographs*, 5, 115–120.

Levin, L.S. (1978). Patient education and self-care: How do they differ? *Nursing Outlook*, 26(3), 170–175.

Ljungberg, C., Hanson, E., and Lovgren, M. (2001). A home rehabilitation program for stroke patients—A pilot study. *Scandinavian Journal of Caring Sciences*, 15(1), 44–53.

Logue, G.A. (1997). An application of Orem's theory to the nursing management of pertussis. *Journal of School Nursing*, 13(4), 20–25.

Lorensen, M., Holter, I., Evers, G., Isenberg, M.A., and Van Achterberg, T. (1991). Cross-cultural testing of the appraisal of self-care agency scale. *International Journal of Nursing Studies*, 30(1), 15–23.

Lukkarinen, H. and Hentinen, M. (1997). Self-care agency and factors related to this agency among patients with coronary heart disease. *International Journal of Nursing Studies*, 34(4), 295–304.

Lundgren, A. and Wahren, L.K. (1999). Effect of education on evidence-based care and handling of peripheral intravenous lines. *Journal of Clinical Nursing*, 8(5), 577–585.

Lundh, U., Soder, M., and Waerness, K. (1987). Nursing theories: A critical review. *Image: Journal of Nursing Scholarship*, 20(1), 36–40.

Lyte, G. and Jones, K. (2001). Developing a unified language for children's nurses, children and their families in the United Kingdom. *Journal of Clinical Nursing*, 10(1), 79–85.

Marland, G.R. (1999). Atypical neuroleptics: Autonomy and compliance? *Journal of Advanced Nursing*, 29(3), 615–622

McFarlane, E.A. (1980). Nursing theory: The comparison of four theoretical proposals. *Journal of Advanced Nursing*, 5, 3–9.

McBride, S.H. (1991). Comparative analysis of three instruments designed to measure self-care agency. *Nursing Research*, 40(1), 12–16.

McCaleb, A. and Edgil, A. (1994). Self-concept and self-care practices of healthy adolescents. *Journal of Pediatric Nursing*, 9(4), 233–238.

McCaughan, E.M. and Thompson, K.A. (2000). Information needs of cancer patients receiving chemotherapy at a day-case unit in Northern Ireland. *Journal of Clinical Nursing*, 9, 851–858.

McDermott, M.A. (1993). Learned helplessness as an interacting variable with self-care agency: Testing a theoretical model. *Nursing Science Quarterly*, 6(1), 28–38.

McGillivray, T. and Marland, G.R. (1999). Assisting demented patients with feeding: Problems in a ward environment. A review of the literature. *Journal of Advanced Nursing*, 29(3), 608–614.

McGraw, E., Barthel, H., and Arrington, M. (2000). A model for demand management in a managed care environment. *Military Medicine*, 165(4), 305–308.

McIntyre, K. (1980). The Perry model as a framework for self-care. *Nurse Practitioner*, 5(6), 34–37.

McLaughlin, K. (1993). Implementing self-care deficit nursing theory: A process of staff development. In M.E. Parker (Ed.), *Patterns of nursing theories in practice* (pp. 241–251). New York: National League for Nursing.

McQuiston, C.M. and Campbell, J.C. (1997). Theoretical substruction: A guide for theory testing research. *Nursing Science Quarterly*, 10(3), 117–123.

Melnyk, K.A.M. (1983). The process of theory analysis: An examination of the nursing theory of Dorothea E. Orem. *Nursing Research*, 32(3), 170–174.

Meriney, D.K. (1990). Application of Orem's conceptual framework to patients with hypercalcemia related to breast cancer. *Cancer Nursing*, 13(5), 316–323.

Michael, M.M. and Sewall, K.S. (1980). Use of the adolescent peer group to increase the self-care agency of adolescent alcohol abusers. *Nursing Clinics of North America*, 15, 157–176.

†Miller, J.F. (1980). The dynamic focus of nursing: A challenge to nursing administration. *Journal of Nursing Administration,* 10(1), 13–18.

†Miller, J.F. (1982). Categories of self-care needs of ambulatory patients with diabetes. *Journal of Advanced Nursing,* 7, 25–31.

Millio, N. (1977). Self-care in urban settings. *Health Education Monographs*, 5, 136–144.

Mitchell, G.J. (2001). Prescription, freedom, and participation: Drilling down into theory-based nursing practice. *Nursing Science Quarterly*, 14(3), 205–210.

Moore, J.B. (1993). Predictors of children's self-care performance: Testing the theory of self-care deficit. *Scholarly Inquiry for Nursing Practice*, 7(3), 199–212.

Moore, J.B. (1995). Measuring self-care practice of children and adolescents: Instrument development. *Maternal-Child Nursing Journal*, 23(3), 101–108.

Moore, J.B. and Pichler, V.H. (2000). Measurements of Orem's basic conditioning factors: A review of published research. *Nursing Science Quarterly*, 13(2), 137–142.

Morales-Mann, E.T. and Jiang, S.L. (1993). Applicability of Orem's conceptual framework: A cross cultural point of view. *Journal of Advanced Nursing*, 18(5), 737–741.

Morgan, S.A. and Dearduff, A. (1997). The cold clinic: A collaborative nursing effort to benefit students. *Journal of American College Health*, 46(1), 35–37.

Morse, W. and Werner, J. (1988). Individualization of patient care using Orem's theory. *Cancer Nursing*, 11(3), 195–202.

Mosher, R.B. (1998). The relationship of self-concept and self-care in children with cancer. *Nursing Science Quarterly*, 11(3), 116–122.

Mullin, V.I. (1980). Implementing the self-care concept in the acute care setting. *Nursing Clinics of North America,* 15(1), 177–190.

†Murphy, P.P. (1981). The hospice model and self-care theory. *Oncology Nursing Forum*, 8(2), 19–21.

Neal, J.E. (2001). Patient outcomes: A matter of perspective. *Nursing Outlook*, 49(2), 93–99.

Newell-Withrow, C. (2000). Health protecting and health promoting behaviors of African Americans living in Appalachia. *Public Health Nursing*, 17(5), 392–397.

Nilsson, U.B. and Willman, A. (2000). Evaluation of nursing documentation—A comparative study using the instruments NoGA(c) and Cat-ch-ing(c) after an educational intervention. *Scandinavian Journal of Caring Sciences*, 14(3), 199–206.

Noone, J. (1995). Acute pancreatitis: An Orem approach to nursing assessment and care. *Critical Care Nurse*, 15(4), 27–35.

Norris, C.M. (1979). Self-care. *American Journal of Nursing*, 79(3), 486–489.

Norris, M.K. (1991). Applying Orem's theory to the long-term care of adolescent transplant recipients. *American Nephrology Nurses Association Journal*, 18(1), 45–47, 53.

Nowakowski, L. (1980). Health promotion/self-care programs for the community. *Topics in Clinical Nursing*, 2, 21–27.

Nowicki, J.S. (1996). Health behaviors and the great depression. *Geriatric Nursing*, 17(5), 247–250.

Nursing Development Conference Group. (1973). *Concept formalization in nursing: Process and product.* Boston: Little, Brown.

Nursing Development Conference Group. (1979). *Concept formalization in nursing: Process and product* (2nd ed.). Boston: Little, Brown.

Oberle, K. and Allen, M. (2001). The nature of advanced practice nursing. *Nursing Outlook,* 49(3), 148–153.

Orem, D.E. (1959). *Guides for developing curriculae for the education of practical nurses.* Washington, DC: U.S. Department of Health, Education, and Welfare; Office of Education.

Orem, D.E. (1971). *Nursing: Concepts of practice.* New York: McGraw-Hill.

Orem, D.E. (1980). *Nursing: Concepts of practice* (2nd ed.). New York: McGraw-Hill.

Orem, D.E. (1983). The self-care deficit theory of nursing: A general theory. In I.W. Clements and F.B. Roberts (Eds.), *Family health: A theoretical approach to nursing care* (pp. 205–217). New York: John Wiley & Sons.

Orem, D.E. (1985). *Nursing: Concepts of practice* (3rd ed.). New York: McGraw-Hill.

Orem, D.E. (1987). Orem's general theory of nursing. In R.R. Parse (Ed.), *Nursing science: Major paradigms, theories, and critiques.* Philadelphia: W.B. Saunders.

Orem, D.E. (1988). The form of nursing science. *Nursing Science Quarterly,* 1(2), 75–79.

Orem, D.E. (1991). *Nursing: Concepts of practice* (4th ed.). St. Louis: C.V. Mosby.

Orem, D.E. (1995). *Nursing: Concepts of practice* (5th ed.). St. Louis: C.V. Mosby.

Orem, D.E. (1997). Views of human beings specific to nursing. *Nursing Science Quarterly,* 10(1), 26–31.

Orem, D.E. (2001). The utility of self-care theory as a theoretical basis for self-neglect. Response. *Journal of Advanced Nursing,* 34(4), 552–553.

Orem, D.E. and Taylor, S.G. (1986). Orem's general theory of nursing. In P. Winstead-Fry (Ed.), *Case studies in nursing theory.* New York: National League for Nursing.

Parse, R.R. (2000). Paradigms: A reprise *Nursing Science Quarterly,* 13(4), 275–276.

Patton, J.G., Conrad, M.A., and Kreidler M.C. (1995). Interdisciplinary faculty and student practice in a nurse-managed campus wellness program. *Nursing Connections,* 8(1), 27–35.

Payne, S., Hardey, M., and Coleman, P. (2000). Interactions between nurses during handovers in elderly care. *Journal of Advanced Nursing,* 32(2), 277–285.

Perrson, K., Svensson, P.G., and Ek, A.C. (1997). Breast self-examination: An analysis of self-reported practice. *Journal of Advanced Nursing,* 25(5), 886–892.

†Petrlik, J.C. (1976). Diabetic peripheral neuropathy. *American Journal of Nursing,* 76, 1794–1797.

Phillips, K.D. and Morris, J.H. (1998). Nursing management of anxiety in HIV infection. *Issues in Mental Health Nursing,* 19(4), 375–397.

Pickens, J.M. (1999). Living with serious mental illness: The desire for normalcy. *Nursing Science Quarterly,* 12(3), 233–239.

†Porter, D. and Shamian, J. (1983). Self-care in theory and practice. *Canadian Nurse,* 79(8), 21–23.

Priest, H.M. (1999). Psychological care in nursing education and practice: A search for definition and dimensions. *Nursing Education Today,* 19(1), 71–78.

Proot, I.M., Abu-Saad, H.H., de Esch-Janssen, W.P., et al (2000). Patient autonomy during rehabilitation: The experiences of stroke patients in nursing homes. *International Journal of Nursing Studies*, 37(3), 267–276.

Ramfelt, E., Langius, A., Bjorvell, H., et al. (2000). Treatment decision-making and its relation to the sense of coherence and the meaning of the disease in a group of patients with colorectal cancer. *European Journal of Cancer Care*, 9(3), 158–165.

Randell, B.P. (1992). Nursing theory: The 21st century. *Nursing Science Quarterly*, 5(4), 176–184.

Raven, M. (1988–1989). Application of Orem's self-care model to nursing practice in developmental disability. *Australian Journal of Advanced Nursing*, 6(2), 16–23.

Rawnsley, M.M. (1997). A case for theory triangulation—Response. *Nursing Science Quarterly*, 10(2), 103–106.

Reed, P.G. (1995). A treatise on nursing knowledge development for the 21st century—Beyond postmodernism. *Advances in Nursing Science*, 17(3), 70–84.

Reid, B., Allan, A., Gauthier, T., and Campbell, H. (1989). Solving the Orem mystery: An educational strategy. *Journal of Continuing Education in Nursing*, 20(3), 108–110.

Richardson, A. (1992). Studies exploring self-care for the person coping with cancer treatment: A review. *International Journal of Nursing Studies*, 29(2), 191–204.

Richardson, A. and Ream, E.K. (1997). Self-care behaviours initiated by chemotherapy patients in response to fatigue. *International Journal of Nursing Studies*, 34(1), 35–43.

Riehl-Sisca, J. (1989). Orem's general theory of nursing: An interpretation. In J. Riehl-Sisca (Ed.), *Conceptual models for nursing practice* (3rd ed.). Norwalk, CT: Appleton & Lange.

Roberts, C.S. (1982). Identifying the real patient problems. *Nursing Clinics of North America*, 17(3), 481–489.

Romine, S. (1986). Applying Orem's self-care to staff development. *Journal of Nursing Staff Development*, 2(2), 77–79.

Rosenbaum, J.N. (1986). Comparison of two theorists on care: Orem and Leininger. *Journal of Advanced Nursing*, 11, 409–419.

Ross, M.M., Carswell, A., Hing, M., et al (2001). Seniors' decision making about pain management. *Journal of Advanced Nursing*, 35(3), 442–451.

Roy, C. (1980). A case study viewed according to different models. In J.P. Riehl and C. Roy (Eds.), *Conceptual models for nursing practice* (2nd ed.). New York: Appleton-Century-Crofts.

Roy, C. (1995). Developing nursing knowledge—Practice issues raised from four philosophical perspectives. *Nursing Science Quarterly*, 8(2), 79–85.

Ruland, C.M. (1999). Decision support for patient preference-based care planning: Effects on nursing care and patient outcomes. *Journal of the American Medical Informatics Association*, 6(4), 304–312.

Russell, C.K., Bunting, S.M. and Gregory, D.M. (1997). Protective care-receiving: The active role of care-recipients. *Journal of Advanced Nursing*, 25(3), 532–540.

Sanford, R.C. (2000). Caring through relation and dialogue: A nursing perspective for patient education. *Advances in Nursing Science*, 22(3), 1–15.

Scammell, J. and Miller, S. (1999). Back to basics: Exploring the conceptual basis of nursing. *Nursing Education Today*, 19(7), 570–577.

Schottbaer, D., Fisher, L. and Gregory, C. (1995). Dependent care, caregiver burden, hardiness, and self-care agency of caregivers. *Cancer Nursing,* 18(4), 299–305.

Schuller, A. (1999). Aspects of autonomy-promoting elder care between individuals and organization. *Gruppendynamik,* 30(4), 353–363.

Schumacher, K.L. (1996). Reconceptualizing family caregiving: Family-based illness care during chemotherapy. *Research in Nursing and Health,* 19(4), 261–271.

Silva, M.C., Sorrell, J.M. and Sorrell, C.D. (1995). From Carper patterns of knowing to ways of being—An ontological philosophical shift in nursing. *Advances in Nursing Science,* 18(1), 1–13.

Slusher, I.L. (1999). Self-care agency and self-care practice of adolescents. *Issues in Comprehensive Pediatric Nursing,* 22(1), 49–58.

†Smith, M.C. (1979). Proposed metaparadigm for nursing research and theory development: An analysis of Orem's self-care theory. *Image: Journal of Nursing Scholarship,* 11(3), 75–79.

Smith, M.C. (1987). A critique of Orem's theory. In R.R. Parse (Ed.), *Nursing science: Major paradigms, theories, and critiques.* Philadelphia: W.B. Saunders.

Soderhamn, O. (1998). Self-care ability in a group of elderly Swedish people: A phenomenological study. *Journal of Advanced Nursing,* 28(4), 745–753.

Soderhamn, O., Evers, G. and Hamrin, E. (1996). A Swedish version of the Appraisal of Self-Care Agency (ASA) scale. *Scandinavian Journal of Caring Sciences,* 10(1), 3–9.

Soderhamn, O., Lindencrona, C., and Ek, A.C. (2000). Ability for self-care among home dwelling elderly people in a health district in Sweden. *International Journal of Nursing Studies,* 37(4), 361–368.

Spearman, S.A., Duldt, B.W., and Brown, S. (1993). Research testing theory: A selective review of Orem's self-care theory, 1986–1991. *Journal of Advanced Nursing,* 18(10), 1626–1631.

Storm, D. and Baumgartner, R. (1987). Achieving self-care in the ventilator-dependent patient: A critical analysis of a case study. *International Journal of Nursing Studies,* 24(2), 95–106.

†Sullivan, T.J. (1980). Self-care model for nursing. In *New directions for nursing in the '80s.* Kansas City, MO: American Nurses Association.

Taylor, S.G. (1988). Nursing theory and nursing process: Orem's theory in practice. *Nursing Science Quarterly,* 1(3), 111–119.

Taylor, S.G. (1991). The structure of nursing diagnosis from Orem's theory. *Nursing Science Quarterly,* 4(1), 24–32.

Taylor, S. G. (2001). A theory of dependent-care: A corollary theory to Orem's theory of self-care. Nursing Science Quarterly, 14(1), 39–47.

Taylor, S.G. (2001). Orem's general theory of nursing and families. *Nursing Science Quarterly,* 14(1), 7–9.

Taylor, S.G., Geden, E., Isaramalai, S., et al (2000). Orem's self-car deficit nursing theory: Its philosophic foundation and the state of the science. *Nursing Science Quarterly,* 13(2), 104–110.

Taylor, S.G. and Godfrey, N.S. (1999). The ethics of Orem's theory. *Nursing Science Quarterly,* 12(3), 202–207.

Taylor, S.G. and McLaughlin, K. (1991). Orem's general theory of nursing and community nursing. *Nursing Science Quarterly*, 4(4), 153–160.

Taylor, S.G., Renpening, K.E., Geden, E.A., et al. (2001). A theory of dependent-care: A corollary theory to Orem's theory of self-care. *Nursing Science Quarterly*, 14(1), 39–47.

Titus, S. and Porter, P. (1989). Orem's theory applied to pediatric residential treatment. *Pediatric Nursing*, 15(5), 465–468.

Ulbrich, S.L. (1999). Nursing practice theory of exercise as self-care. *Image: Journal of Nursing Scholarship*, 31(1), 65–70.

Underwood, P.R. (1980). Facilitating self-care. In P. Pothier (Ed.), *Psychiatric nursing* (pp. 115–144). Boston: Little, Brown.

Urbancic, J.C. (1992). Empowerment support with female survivors of childhood incest: Part I—Theories and research. *Archives of Psychiatric Nursing*, 6(5), 275–281.

Urbancic, J.C. (1992). Empowerment support with adult female survivors of childhood incest: Part II—Application of Orem's methods of helping. *Archives of Psychiatric Nursing*, 6(5), 282–286.

Utz, S.W. and Ramos, M.C. (1993). Mitral valve prolapse and its effects: A programme of inquiry within Orem's Self-Care Deficit Theory of Nursing. *Journal of Advanced Nursing*, 18(5), 742–751.

Utz, S.W., Shuster, G.F., 3rd, Merwin, E., & Williams, B. (1994). A community-based smoking-cessation program: Self-care behaviors and success. *Public Health Nursing*, 11(5), 291–299.

Uys, L. (1987). Foundational studies in nursing. *Journal of Advanced Nursing*, 12(3), 275–280.

Van Achterberg, T., Lorensen, M., Isenberg, M., Evers, G., Levin, E., and Philipsen, H. (1991). The Norwegian, Danish, and Dutch version of the appraisal of self-care agency scale: Comparing reliability aspects. *Scandinavian Journal of Caring Sciences*, 5(1), 1–8.

van der Scheuren, E., Kesteloot, K., and Cleemput, I. (2000). Federation of European Cancer Societies. Full Report. Economic evaluation in cancer care: Questions and answers on how to alleviate conflicts between rising needs and expectations and tightening budgets. *European Journal of Cancer*, 36(1), 13–36.

Vasquez, M.A. (1992). From theory to practice: Orem's self-care nursing model and ambulatory care. *Journal of Post Anesthesia Nursing*, 7(4), 251–255.

Villarruel, A.M. (1995). Mexican-American cultural meanings, expressions, self-care and dependent-care actions associated with experiences of pain. *Research in Nursing and Health*, 18(5), 427–436.

Villarruel, A.M., Bishop, T.L., Simpson, E.M., et al. (2001). Borrowed theories, shared theories, and the advancement of nursing knowledge. *Nursing Science Quarterly*, 14(2), 158–163.

Villarruel, A.M. and Denyes, M.J. (1991). Pain assessment in children: Theoretical and empirical validity. *Advances in Nursing Science*, 14(2), 32–41.

Villarruel, A.M. and Denyes, M.J. (1997). Testing Orem's theory with Mexican Americans. *Image: Journal of Nursing Scholarship*, 29(3), 283–288.

Walborn, K.A. (1980). A nursing model for hospice, primary and self-care. *Nursing Clinics of North America*, 15(1), 205–217.

Walker, D.M. (1993). A nursing administration perspective on use of Orem's Self-Care Deficit Nursing theory. In M.E. Parker (Ed.), *Patterns of nursing theories in practice* (pp. 252–263). New York: National League for Nursing.

Walker, L.O. and Grobe, S.J. (1999). The construct of thriving in pregnancy and postpartum. *Nursing Science Quarterly*, 12(2), 151–157.

Walton, J. (1985). An overview: Orem's self care deficit theory of nursing. *Focus Critical Care*, 12(1), 54–58.

Wang, C.Y. (1997). The cross-cultural applicability of Orem's conceptual framework. *Journal of Cultural Diversity*, 4(2), 44–48.

Wang, H.H. (2001). A comparison of two models of health-promoting lifestyle in rural elderly Taiwanese women. *Public Health Nursing*, 18(3), 204–211.

Wang, H.H. and Laffrey, S.C. (2001). A predictive model of well-being and self-care for rural elderly women in Taiwan. *Research in Nursing and Health*, 24(2), 122–132.

Watkins, G.R. (1995). Patient comprehension of gastroenterology (GI). Educational materials. *Gastroenterology Nursing*, 18(4), 123–127.

Webb, M. (2001). Integration of nursing theorists in community care practice. *Vision*, 7(13), 27–28.

Weinrich, S.P. (1990). Predictors of older adults' participation in fecal occult blood screening. *Oncology Nursing Forum*, 17(5), 715–720.

Wengstrom, Y, Haggmark, C., Strander, H., et al. (1999). Effects of a nursing intervention on subjective distress, side effects and quality of life of breast cancer patients receiving curative radiation therapy—A randomized study. *Acta Oncologica*, 38(6), 763–770.

Werlin, S.H., Schauffler, H.H., and Avery, C.H. (1977). Research and demonstration issues in self-care: Measuring the decline of medicocentricism. *Health Education Monographs*, 5(2), 161–181.

West, P. And Isenberg, M. (1997). Instrument development: The mental health-related self-care agency scale. *Archives of Psychiatric Nursing*, 11(3), 126–132.

Whelan, E. (1984). Analysis and application of Dorothea Orem's self-care practice model. *Journal of Nursing Education*, 24(6), 226–229.

Whitener, L.M., Cox, K.R., and Maglich, S.A. (1998). Use of theory to guide nurses in the design of health messages for children. *Advances in Nursing Science*, 20(3), 21–35.

Williams, P.D., Ducey, K.A., Sears, A.M., et al. (2001). Treatment type and symptom severity among oncology patients by self-report. *International Journal of Nursing Studies*, 38(3), 359–367.

Williams, S. and Ramos, M.C. (1993). Mitral valve prolapse and its effects: A program of inquiry within Orem's self-care deficit theory of nursing. *Journal of Advanced Nursing*, 18, 242–251.

Williams, S., Shuster, G.F. III, Merwin, E , and Williams, B. (1994). A community-based smoking cessation program: Self-care behaviors and success. *Public Health Nursing*, 11(5), 291–299.

Womack, S. (1997). The elderly in nursing homes: A special population. *Nurse Practitioner Forum*, 8(1), 32–35.

Woods, N. (1989). Conceptualizations of self-care: Toward health-oriented models. *Advances in Nursing Science*, 12(1), 1–13.

Wright, P.S., Piazza, D., Holcombe, J., and Foote, A. (1994). A comparison of three theories of nursing used as a guide for the nursing care of an 8-year-old child with leukemia. *Journal of Pediatric Oncology Nursing*, 11(1), 14–19.

Young, L. (1996). Spaces for famine: A comparative geographical analysis of famine in Ireland and the Highlands in the 1840s. *Transactions (Institute of British Geographers)*, 21(4), 666–680.

Zerull, L.M. (1999). Community nurse case management: Evolving over time to meet new demands. *Family and Community Health*, 22(3), 12–29.

29. Ida Orlando

Anderson, B.J., Mertz, H., and Leonard, R.C. (1965). Two experimental tests of a patient-centered admission process. *Nursing Research*, 14, 151–157.

Andrews, C.M. (1983). Ida Orlando's model of nursing. In J.J. Fitzpatrick and A.L. Whall (Eds.), *Conceptual models of nursing: Analysis and application.* Bowie, MD: Robert J. Brady Co.

Andrews, C.M. (1989). Ida Orlando's model of nursing practice. In J.J. Fitzpatrick and A.L. Whall (Eds.), *Conceptual models of nursing: Analysis and application* (2nd ed.). Norwalk, CT: Appleton & Lange.

Artinian, B.M. (1995). Risking involvement with cancer patients. *Western Journal of Nursing Research*, 17(3), 292–304.

Barnard, K.E. (1980). Knowledge for practice: Directions for the future. *Nursing Research*, 29(4), 208.

Barron, M.A. (1966). The effects varied nursing approaches have on patients' complaints of pain [Abstract]. *Nursing Research*, 15(1), 90–91.

Benoliel, J.Q. (1995). Multiple meanings of pain and complexities of pain management. *Nursing Clinics of North America,* 30(4), 583–596.

Blomqvist, K. and Hallberg, I.R. (2001). Recognising pain in order adults living in sheltered accommodations: The views of nurses and older adults. *International Journal of Nursing Studies*, 38(3), 305–318.

Bochnak, M.A. (1963). The effect of an automatic and deliberative process of nursing activity on the relief of patients' pain: A clinical experiment. *Nursing Research*, 12, 191–192.

Burssen, B. and Diers, D.K. (1964). Pseudo-patient centered orientations. *Nursing Forum*, 3(2), 38–50.

Cameron, J. (1963). An exploratory study of the verbal responses of the nurse-patient interactions. *Nursing Research*, 12, 192.

CarisVerhallen, W.M.C.M., Kerkstra, A., and Bensing, J.M. (1997). The role of communication in nursing care for elderly people. A review of the literature. *Journal of Advanced Nursing*, 25(5), 915–933.

Cody, W.K. (1996). Drowning in eclecticism. *Nursing Science Quarterly*, 9(3), 86–88.

Crane, M.D. (1980). Ida Jean Orlando. In The Nursing Theories Conference Group, *Nursing theories: The base for professional nursing practice.* Englewood Cliffs, NJ: Prentice-Hall.

Cutcliffe, J.R. and Goward, P. (2000). Mental health nurses and qualitative research methods: A mutual attraction? *Journal of Advanced Nursing*, 31(3), 590–598.

Diers, D.K. (1966). The nurse orientation system: A method for analyzing the nurse-patient interactions [Abstract]. *Nursing Research*, 15(1), 91.

Diers, D. (1970). Faculty research development at Yale. *Nursing Research*, 19(1), 64–71.

Dracup, K.A. and Breu, C.S. (1978). Using nursing research findings to meet the needs of grieving spouses. *Nursing Research*, 27(4), 212–216.

Dumas, R.G. (1963). Psychological preparation for surgery. *American Journal of Nursing*, 63(8), 52–55.

Dumas, R.G. and Leonard, R.C. (1963) The effect of nursing on the incidence of post-operative vomiting. *Nursing Research*, 12(1), 12–15.

Dye, M.C. (1963). A descriptive study of conditions conductive to an effective process of nursing activity. *Nursing Research*, 12, 194.

Dye, M.C. (1963). Clarifying patients' communication. *American Journal of Nursing*, 63(8), 56–59.

Dye, M., Orlando, I.J., and Dumas, R.G. (1963). Validating a theory of nursing practice. *American Journal of Nursing*, 63(8), 52–59.

Eisler, J., Wolfer, J., and Diers, D. (1972). Relationship between the need for social approval and postoperative recovery and welfare. *Nursing Research*, 21(5), 520–525.

Elder, R.G. (1963). What is the patient saying? *Nursing Forum*, 2(1), 25–37.

Elms, R.R. and Leonard, R.C. (1966). Effects of nursing approaches during admission. *Nursing Research*, 15(1), 39–48.

Fagerberg, I. and Ekman, S.L. (1997). First-year Swedish nursing students' experiences with elderly patients. *Western Journal of Nursing Research*, 19(2), 177–189.

Faust, C. (2002). Clinical outlook. Orlando's Deliberative Nursing Process Theory: A practice application in an extended care facility. *Journal of Gerontological Nursing*, 28(7), 14–18.

Forchuk, C. (1991). A comparison of the works of Peplau and Orlando. *Archives of Psychiatric Nursing*, 5(1), 38–45.

Forchuk, C. (1995). Uniqueness within the nurse-client relationship. *Archives of Psychiatric Nursing*, 9(1), 34–39.

Forchuk, C. and Dorsay, J.P. (1995). Hildegard-Peplau meets family systems nursing—Innovation in theory-based practice. *Journal of Advanced Nursing*, 21(1), 110–115.

Fitzpatrick, J. and Whall, A. (1983). *Conceptual models of nursing: Analysis and application.* Bowie, MD: Robert J. Brady Co.

Gilliss, S.L. (1976). Sleeplessness—Can you help? *Canadian Nurse*, 72(7), 32–34.

Gowan, N.I. and Morris, M. (1964). Nurses' responses to expressed patient needs. *Nursing Research*, 13, 68–71.

Graham, I. (1996). A presentation of a conceptual framework and its use in the definition of nursing development within a number of nursing development units. *Journal of Advanced Nursing*, 23(2), 260–266.

Haggerty, L.A. (1985). A theoretical model for developing students' communication skills. *Journal of Nursing Education*, 24(7), 296–298.

Haggerty, L.A. (1987). An analysis of senior nursing students' immediate response to distressed patients. *Journal of Advanced Nursing*, 12, 451–461.

Halloran, E.J. (1995). Guiding principles for nurse executives. *Journal of Nursing Administration*, 25(12), 5–6.

Hampe, S.O. (1975). Needs of grieving spouses in a hospital setting. *Nursing Research*, 24(2), 113.

Johnson, D.E. (1974). Development of theory: A requisite for nursing as a primary health profession. *Nursing Research*, 23(5), 372.

Johnson, J.E. (1999). Self-regulation theory and coping with physical illness. *Research in Nursing and Health*, 22(6), 435–448.

King, I.M. (1997). Reflections on the past and a vision for the future. *Nursing Science Quarterly*, 10(1), 15–17.

Kolcaba, K. (2001). Evolution of mid range theory of comfort for outcomes research. *Nursing Outlook*, 49(2), 86–92.

Kubsch, S.M. (1996). Conflict, enactment, empowerment: Conditions of independent therapeutic nursing intervention. *Journal of Advanced Nursing*, 23(1), 192–200.

Larson, P.A. (1977). Influence of patient status and health condition on nurse perceptions of patient characteristics. *Nursing Research*, 26(6), 416.

Lego, S. (1999). The one-to-one nurse-patient relationship. *Perspectives in Psychiatric Care*, 35(4), 4–23.

Leonard, R.C., Skipper, J.K., Jr., and Wodridge, P.J. (1967). Small sample field experiments for evaluating patient care. *Health Services Research*, 2(1), 47–60.

Marriner-Tomey, A., Mills, D., and Sauter, M. (1989). Ida Jean Orlando (Pelletier): Nursing process theory. In A. Marriner-Tomey (Ed.), *Nursing theorists and their work* (2nd ed.). St. Louis, MO: C.V. Mosby.

McCann, T.V. and Baker, H. (2001). Mutual relating: Developing interpersonal relationships in the community. *Journal of Advanced Nursing*, 34(4), 530–537.

McNaughton, D.B. (2000). A synthesis of qualitative home visiting research. *Public Health Nursing*, 17(6), 405–414.

Mertz, H. (1962). Nurse actions that reduce stress in patients. In *Emergency intervention by the nurse* (Monograph No. 1, pp. 10–14). New York: American Nurses Association.

Mohr, W.K. (1999). Deconstructing the language of psychiatric hospitalization. *Journal of Advanced Nursing*, 29(5), 1052–1059.

Morse, J.M., Bottorff, J.L., and Hutchinson, S. (1995). The paradox of comfort. *Nursing Research*, 44(1), 14–19.

Nagle, L.M. (1999). A matter of extinction or distinction. *Western Journal of Nursing Research*, 21(1), 71–82.

New England Board of Higher Education. (1977). *Mental health continuing education for associate degree nursing faculties: Project report.* Wellesley, MA: New England Board of Higher Education. NIH Training Grant No. 715 MH13182.

Orlando, I. (1961). *The dynamic nurse-patient relationship.* New York: G.P. Putnam's Sons.

Orlando, I. (1972). *The discipline and teaching of nursing process.* New York: G.P. Putnam's Sons.

Orlando, I. (1987). Nursing in the 21st century . . . alternate paths. *Journal of Advanced Nursing*, 12(4), 405–412.

Orlando, I. and Dugan, A.B. (1989). Independent and dependent path: The fundamental issue for the nursing profession. *Nursing and Health Care*, 10(2), 76–80.

Pascoe, E. (1996). The value to nursing research of Gadamer's hermeneutic philosophy. *Journal of Advanced Nursing*, 24(6), 1309–1314.

Peitchinis, J.A. (1972). Therapeutic effectiveness of counseling by nursing personnel. *Nursing Research*, 21(2), 138–148.

Pienschke, D. (1973). Guardedness or openness on the cancer unit. *Nursing Research*, 22(6), 484–490.

Potter, M. and Dawson, A. (2001). From safety contract to safety agreement. *Journal of Psychosocial Nursing and Mental Health Services*, 39(8), 38–45.

Potter, M.L. and Bockenhauer, B.J. (2000). Implementing Orlando's nursing theory: A pilot study. *Journal of Psychosocial Nursing and Mental Health Services*, 39(3), 14–21.

Rawnsley, M.M. (2000). Response to Kim's human living concept as a unifying perspective for nursing. *Nursing Science Quarterly*, 13(1), 41–44.

Reynolds, W.J. and Scott, B. (2000). Do nurses and other professional helpers normally display much empathy? *Journal of Advanced Nursing*, 31(1), 226–234.

Rosenthal, B.C. (1996). An interactionist's approach to perioperative nursing. *Journal of the Association of periOperative Registered Nurses*, 64(2), 254–260.

Rhymes, J. (1964). A description of nurse-patient interaction in effective nursing activity [abstract]. *Nursing Research*, 13(4), 365.

Schmieding, N.J. (1983). An analysis of Orlando's nursing theory based on Kuhn's theory of science. In P.L. Chinn (Ed.), *Advances in nursing theory development* (pp. 63–87). Rockville, MD: Aspen Systems.

Schmieding, N.J. (1984). Putting Orlando's theory into practice. *American Journal of Nursing*, 84(6), 759–761.

Schmieding, N.J. (1986). Orlando's theory. In P. Winstead-Fry (Ed.), *Case studies in nursing theory*. New York: National League for Nursing.

Schmieding, N.J. (1987). Face-to-face contacts: Exploring their meaning. *Nursing Management*, 18, 83–86.

Schmieding, N.J. (1987). Problematic situations in nursing: Analysis of Orlando's theory based on Dewey's theory of inquiry. *Journal of Advanced Nursing*, 12(4), 431–440.

Schmieding, N.J. (1988). Action process of nurse administrators to problematic situations based on Orlando's theory. *Journal of Advanced Nursing*, 13(1), 99–107.

Schmieding, N.J. (1990). Do head nurses include staff nurses in problem-solving? *Nursing Management*, 21(3), 58–60,

Schmieding, N.J. (1990). An integrative nursing theoretical framework. *Journal of Advanced Nursing*, 15(4), 463–467.

Schmieding, N.J. (1990). A model for assessing nurse administrators' actions. *Western Journal of Nursing Research*, 12(3), 293–306.

Schmieding, N.J. (1999). Reflective inquiry framework for nurse administrators. *Journal of Advanced Nursing*, 30(3), 631–639.

Sheafor, M. (1991). Productive work groups in complex hospital units: Proposed contributions of the nurse-executive. *Journal of Nursing Administration*, 21(5), 25–30.

Stevens, B.J. (1971). Analysis of structural forms used in nursing curricula. *Nursing Research*, 20(5), 388–397.

Theis, E.C. (1973). Book review of Ida J. Orlando's The discipline and teaching of nursing process. *Nursing Research*, 22(1), 73.

Thorellekstrand, I. and Bjorvell, H. (1994). The VIPS-Model used by nursing student—Review of educational care plans. *Scandinavian Journal of Caring Sciences*, 8(4), 195–204.

Tryon, P.A. (1962). The effect of patient participation in decision making on the outcome of a nursing procedure. In *Nursing and the patients' motivation* (Clinical Paper No. 19, pp. 14–18). New York: American Nurses Association.

Tryon, P.A. (1963). An experiment of the effect of patients' participation in planning the administration of a nursing procedure. *Nursing Research*, 12, 262–265.

Tryon, P.A. and Leonard, R.C. (1964). The effect of patients' participation on the outcome of a nursing procedure. *Nursing Forum*, 3(2), 79–89.

Varcoe, C. (1996). Disparagement of the nursing process: The new dogma? *Journal of Advanced Nursing*, 23(1), 120–125.

Vaughan, B. (1998). Developing nursing practice. *Journal of Clinical Nursing*, 7(3), 199–200.

Williamson, Y. (1978). Methodologic dilemmas in tapping the concept of patient needs. *Nursing Research*, 27(3), 172.

Wolfer, J. and Visintainer, M.A. (1975). Pediatric surgical patients' and parents' stress response and adjustment as a function of psychological preparation and stress-point nursing care. *Nursing Research*, 24(4), 244–255.

Wurzbach, M.E. (1996). Comfort and nurses' moral choices. *Journal of Advanced Nursing*, 24(2), 260–264.

30. Rosemarie Parse

Allchin-Petardi, L. (1998). Weathering the storm: Persevering through a difficult time. *Nursing Science Quarterly*, 11(4), 172–177.

Banonis, B. (1989). The lived experience of recovering from addiction: A phenomenological study. *Nursing Science Quarterly*, 2(1), 37–43.

Baumann, S.L. (1997). Contrasting two approaches in a community-based nursing practice with older adults: The medical model and Parse's nursing theory. *Nursing Science Quarterly*, 10(3), 124–130.

Bunkers, S.S. (1998). Considering tomorrow: Parse's theory-guided research. *Nursing Science Quarterly*, 11(2), 56–63.

Bunkers, S.S., Michaels, C., and Ethridge, P. (1997). Advanced practice nursing in community: Nursing's opportunity. *Advanced Practice Nursing Quarterly*, 2(4), 79–84.

Butler, M. (1988). Family transformation: Parse's theory in practice. *Nursing Science Quarterly*, 1(2), 68–74.

Butler, M.J. and Snodgrass, F.G. (1991). Beyond abuse: Parse's theory in practice. *Nursing Science Quarterly*, 4(2), 76–82.

Chrisman, M. and Riehl-Sisca, J. (1989). The systems-developmental-stress model. In J. Riehl-Sisca (Ed.), *Conceptual models for nursing practice* (3rd ed.). Norwalk, CT: Appleton & Lange.

Cody, W.K. and Mitchell, G.J. (1992). Parse's theory as a model for practice: The cutting edge. *Advances in Nursing Science*, 15(2), 52–65.

Cody, W.K. (2000). Parse's human becoming school of thought and families. *Nursing Science Quarterly*, 13(4). 281–284

Cowling, W.R. (1989). Parse's theory of nursing. In J.J. Fitzpatrick and A.L. Whall (Eds.), *Conceptual models of nursing: Analysis and application* (2nd ed.). Norwalk, CT: Appleton & Lange.

Daly, J., Mitchell, G.J., and Jonas-Simpson, C.M. (1996). The quality of life and the human becoming theory: Exploring discipline-specific contributions. *Nursing Science Quarterly*, 9(4), 170–174.

English, J. (1989). The systems-developmental-stress model in psychiatric nursing. In J. Riehl-Sisca (Ed.), *Conceptual models for nursing practice* (3rd ed.). Norwalk, CT: Appleton & Lange.

Freshwater, D. (1998). From acorn to oak tree: A neoplatonic perspective of reflection and caring. *Australian Journal of Holistic Nursing*, 5(2), 14–19.

Janes, N.M. and Wells, D.L. (1997). Elderly patients' experiences with nurses guided by Parse's theory of human becoming. *Clinical Nursing Research*, 6(3), 205–222.

Jonas-Simpson, C. (1997). Living the art of the human becoming theory. *Nursing Science Quarterly*, 10(4), 175–179.

Kelley, L.S. (1995). Parse's theory in practice with a group in the community. *Nursing Science Quarterly*, 8(3), 127–132.

Kim, M.S., Shin, K.R. and Shin, S.R (1998). Korean adolescents' experiences of smoking cessation: A prelude to research with the human becoming perspective. *Nursing Science Quarterly*, 11(3), 105–109.

Laschinger, H.K. and Duff, V. (1991). Attitudes of practicing nurses towards theory-based nursing practice. *Canadian Journal of Nursing Administration*, 4(1), 6–10.

Lee, R. and Schumacher, L. (1989). Rosemarie Rizzo Parse: Man-living-health. In A. Marriner-Tomey (Ed.), *Nursing theorists and their work* (2nd ed.). St. Louis, MO: C.V. Mosby.

Legault. F. and Ferguson-Pare, M. (1999). Advancing nursing practice: An evaluation study of Parse's theory of human becoming. *Canadian Journal of Nursing Leadership*, 12(1), 30–35.

Limandri, B.J. (1982). Review of "Man-living-health: A theory of nursing." *Western Journal of Nursing Research*, 4(1), 105–106.

Markovic, M. (1997). From theory to perioperative practice with Parse. *Canadian Operating Room Nursing Journal*, 15(1), 13–19.

Martin, P.J. (2000). Hearing voices and listening to those that hear them. *Journal of Psychiatric and Mental Health Nursing*, 7(2), 135–141.

Martin, M.L., Forchuk, C., Santopinto, M., & Butcher, H.K. (1992). Alternative approaches to nursing practice: Application of Peplau, Rogers, and Parse. *Nursing Science Quarterly*, 5(2), 80–85.

Mattice, M. (1991). Parse's theory of nursing in practice: A manager's perspective. *Canadian Journal of Nursing Administration*, 4(1), 11–13.

Melnechenko, K.L. (1995). Parse's theory of human becoming: An alternative guide to nursing practice for pediatric oncology nurses. *Journal of Pediatric Oncology Nursing*, 12(3), 122–127.

Michell, G.J. (1988). Man-living-health: The theory in practice. *Nursing Science Quarterly*, 1(3), 120–127.

Mitchell, G.J. (1990). The lived experience of taking life day-by-day in later life: Research guided by Parse's emergent method. *Nursing Science Quarterly*, 3(1), 29–36.

Mitchell, G.J. (1990). Struggling in change: From the traditional approach to Parse's theory-based practice. *Nursing Science Quarterly*, 3(4), 170–176.

Mitchell, G.J. (1992). Parse's theory and the multidisciplinary team: Clarifying scientific values. *Nursing Science Quarterly*, 5(3), 104–106.

Mitchell, G.J. (1994). Discipline-specific inquiry: The hermeneutics of theory-guided nursing research. *Nursing Outlook*, 42(5), 224–228.

Mitchell, G.J. and Cody, W.K. (1992). Nursing knowledge and human science: Ontological and epistemological considerations. *Nursing Science Quarterly*, 5(2), 54–61.

Mitchell, G.J. and Heidt, P. (1994). The lived experience of wanting to help another: Research with Parse's method. *Nursing Science Quarterly*, 7(3), 119–127.

Mitchell, G.J. and Pilkington, B. (1990). Theoretical approaches in nursing practice: A comparison of Roy and Parse. *Nursing Science Quarterly*, 3(2), 81–87.

Norris, J.R. (2002). One-to-one teleapprenticeship as a means for nurses teaching and learning Parse' theory of human becoming. *Nursing Science Quarterly*, 15(2), 143–149.

Northrup, D.T. and Cody, W.K. (1998). Evaluation of the human becoming theory in practice in an acute care psychiatric setting. *Nursing Science Quarterly*, 11(1), 23–30.

Parse, R.R. (1974). *Nursing fundamentals.* Flushing, NY: Medical Examination Publishers.

Parse, R.R. (1981). *Man-living-health: A theory of nursing.* New York: John Wiley & Sons.

Parse, R.R. (1987). *Nursing science: Major paradigms, theories, and critiques.* Philadelphia: W.B. Saunders.

Parse, R.R. (1987). Parse's man-living-health theory of nursing. In R.R. Parse (Ed.), *Nursing science: Major paradigms, theories, and critiques.* Philadelphia: W.B. Saunders.

Parse, R.R. (1987). The simultaneity paradigm. In R.R. Parse (Ed.), *Nursing science: Major paradigms, theories, and critiques.* Philadelphia: W.B. Saunders.

Parse, R.R. (1989). Man-living-health: A theory of nursing. In J. Riehl-Sisca (Ed.), *Conceptual models for nursing practice* (3rd ed.). Norwalk, CT: Appleton & Lange.

Parse, R.R. (1989). Essentials for practicing the art of nursing [Editorial]. *Nursing Science Quarterly*, 2(3), 111.

Parse, R.R. (1989). Making more out of less [Editorial]. *Nursing Science Quarterly*, 2(4), 155.

Parse, R.R. (1989). Parse's man-living-health model and administration of nursing service. In B. Henry, C. Arndt, M. DiVincenti, and A. Marriner-Tomey (Eds.), *Dimensions of nursing administration: Theory, research, education, practice*. Boston: Blackwell Scientific Publications.

Parse, R.R. (1989). Qualitative research: Publishing and funding [Editorial]. *Nursing Science Quarterly*, 2(1), 1–2.

Parse, R.R. (1990). Health: A personal commitment. *Nursing Science Quarterly*, 3(3), 136–140.

Parse, R.R. (1990). Nursing theory-based practice: A challenge for the 90s [Editorial]. *Nursing Science Quarterly,* 3(2), 53.

Parse, R.R. (1990). Parse's research methodology with an illustration of the lived experience of hope. *Nursing Science Quarterly*, 3, 9–17.

Parse, R.R. (1990). Promotion and prevention: Two distinct cosmologies [Editorial]. *Nursing Science Quarterly*, 3(3), 101.

Parse, R.R. (1991). Electronic publishing: Beyond browsing [Editorial]. *Nursing Science Quarterly*, 4(1), 1.

Parse, R.R. (1991). Growing the discipline of nursing [Editorial]. *Nursing Science Quarterly*, 4(4), 139.

Parse, R.R. (1991). Mysteries of health and healing: Two perspectives [Editorial]. *Nursing Science Quarterly*, 4(3), 93.

Parse, R.R. (1991). The right soil, the right stuff [Editorial]. *Nursing Science Quarterly*, 4(2), 47.

Parse, R.R. (1992). Nursing knowledge for the 21st century: An international commitment. *Nursing Science Quarterly*, 5(1), 8–12.

Parse, R.R. (1992). Human becoming: Parse's theory of nursing. *Nursing Science Quarterly*, 5(1), 35–42.

Parse, R.R. (1992). Moving beyond the barrier reef [Editorial]. *Nursing Science Quarterly*, 5(3), 97.

Parse, R.R. (1992). The performing art of nursing [Editorial]. *Nursing Science Quarterly*, 5(4), 147.

Parse, R.R. (1992). The unsung shapers of nursing science [Editorial]. *Nursing Science Quarterly*, 5(2), 47.

Parse, R.R. (1995). Building the realm of nursing knowledge. *Nursing Science Quarterly*, 8, 51.

Parse, R.R. (1996). The human becoming theory: Challenges in practice and research. *Nursing Science Quarterly*, 9(2), 55–60.

Parse, R.R. (1997). Transforming research and practice with the human becoming theory. *Nursing Science Quarterly*, 10(4), 171–174.

Parse, R.R. (1999). Nursing science: The transformation of practice. *Journal of Advanced Nursing*, 30(6), 1383–1387.

Parse, R.R., Coyne, A.B., and Smith, M.J. (1985). *Nursing research: Qualitative methods.* Bowie, MD: Robert J. Brady Co.

Phillips, J.R. (1987). A critique of Parse's man-living-health theory. In R.R. Parse (Ed.), *Nursing science: Major paradigms, theories, and critiques.* Philadelphia: W.B. Saunders.

Pilkington, F.B. (1999). A qualitative study of life after stroke. *Journal of Neuroscience Nursing*, 31(6), 336–347.

Pugliese, L. (1989). The theory of man-living-health: An analysis. In J. Riehl-Sisca (Ed.), *Conceptual models for nursing practice* (3rd ed.). Norwalk, CT: Appleton & Lange.

Quiquero, A., Knights, D., & Meo, C.O (1991). Theory as a guide to practice: Staff nurses choose Parse's theory. *Canadian Journal of Nursing Administration*, 4(1), 14–16.

Reed, P.G. (1983). Implications of the life-span developmental framework for well-being in adulthood and aging. *Advances in Nursing Science*, 6(1), 18–25.

Relf, M.V. (1997). Illuminating meaning and transforming issues of spirituality in HIV disease and AIDS: An application of Parse's theory of human becoming. *Holistic Nursing Practice*, 12(1), 1–8.

Sarter, B. (1988). Philosophy sources of nursing theory. *Nursing Science Quarterly*, 1(2), 52–59.

Smith, M.J. (1989). Research and practice application related to man-living-health. In J. Riehl-Sisca (Ed.), *Conceptual models for nursing practice* (3rd ed.). Norwalk, CT: Appleton & Lange.

Stanley, G.D. and Meghani, S.H. (2001). Reflections on using Parse's theory of human becoming in a palliative care setting in Pakistan. *Canadian Nurse*, 97(7), 23–25.

Walker, C.A. (1996). Coalescing the theories of two nurse visionaries: Parse and Watson. *Journal of Advanced Nursing*, 24(5), 988–996.

Winkler, S.J. (1983). Parse's theory of nursing. In J.J. Fitzpatrick and A.L. Whall (Eds.), *Conceptual models of nursing: Analysis and application.* Bowie, MD: Robert J. Brady Co.

31. Josephine Paterson and Loretta Zderad

Anderson, C. and Adamsen, L. (2001). Continuous video recording: A new clinical research tool for studying the nursing care of cancer patients. *Journal of Advanced Nursing*, 35(2), 257–267.

Baillie, L. (1996). A phenomenological study of the nature of empathy. *Journal of Advanced Nursing*, 24(6), 1300–1308.

Brouse, S.H. and Laffrey, S.C. (1989). Paterson and Zderad's humanistic nursing framework. In J.J. Fitzpatrick and A.L. Whall (Ed.), *Conceptual models of nursing: Analysis and application* (2nd ed.). Norwalk, CT: Appleton & Lange.

Cutcliffe, J.R. and Cassedy, P. (1999). The development of empathy in students on a short, skill based counselling course: A pilot study. *Nursing Education Today*, 19(3), 250–257.

Grevin, F. (1996). Posttraumatic stress disorder, ego defense mechanisms, and empathy among urban paramedics. *Psychological Reports*, 79(2), 483–495.

Hartrick, G. (1997). Relational capacity: The foundation for interpersonal nursing practice. *Journal of Advanced Nursing*, 26(3), 523–528.

Hartrick, G. (1999). Transcending behaviorism in communication education. *Journal of Nursing Education*, 38(1), 17–22.

Hopkinson, J.B. and Hallett, C.E. (2001). Patients' perceptions of hospice day care: A phenomenology study. *International Journal of Nursing Studies*, 38(1), 117–125.

Kleiman, S. (1986). Humanistic nursing: The phenomenological theory of Paterson and Zderad. In P. Winstead-Fry (Ed.), *Case studies in nursing theory.* New York: National League for Nursing.

Lego, S. (1999). The one-to-one nurse-patient relationship. *Perspectives in Psychiatric Care*, 35(4), 4–23.

Mason, T. and Patterson, R. (1990). A critical review of the use of Rogers' model within a special hospital: A single case study. *Journal of Advanced Nursing*, 15, 130–141.

McCance, C., Paterson, J.G., Nommo, A.W., and Hunter, D. (1987). Psychiatric geography: Where patients live and their use of services—A study of computerized mapping of case register data. *Health Bulletin*, 45(4), 197–210.

McQueen, A. (1997). The emotional work of caring, with a focus on gynaecological nursing. *Journal of Clinical Nursing*, 6(3), 233–240.

Olsen, D.P. (1997). When the patient causes the problem: The effect of patient responsibility on the nurse-patient relationship. *Journal of Advanced Nursing*, 26(3), 515–522.

Paterson, J.G. (1971). From a philosophy of clinical nursing to a method of nursology. *Nursing Research*, 20(2), 143–146.

Paterson, J.G. (1978). The tortuous way toward nursing theory. In J.G. Paterson (Ed.), *Theory development: What, why, how?* (Publication No. 15–1708, pp. 49–65). New York: National League for Nursing.

Paterson, J.G. and Zderad L.T. (1970–1971). All together through complementary syntheses the worlds of the many. *Image: Journal of Nursing Scholarship*, 4(3), 13–16.

Paterson, J.G. and Zderad, L.T. (1976). *Humanistic nursing*. New York: John Wiley & Sons.

Paterson, J.G. and Zderad, L.T. (1988). *Humanistic nursing* (Publication No. 41–2218, pp. i-iv, 1–129). New York: National League for Nursing.

Smyth, T. (1996). Reinstating the person in the professional: Reflections on empathy and aesthetic experience. *Journal of Advanced Nursing*, 24(5), 932–937.

White, S.J. (1997). Empathy: A literature review and concept analysis. *Journal of Clinical Nursing*, 6(4), 253–257.

Yegdich, T. (1999). On the phenomenology of empathy in nursing: Empathy or sympathy? *Journal of Advanced Nursing*, 30(1), 83–93.

Zderad, L.T. (1968). *A concept of empathy*. Unpublished doctoral dissertation, Georgetown University, Washington, DC.

Zderad, L.T. (1969). Empathetic nursing: Realization of a human capacity. *Nursing Clinics of North America*, 4, 655–662.

Zderad, L.T. (1970). Empathy: From cliche to construct. *Proceedings of the Third Nursing Theory Conference* (pp. 46–75). University of Kansas Medical Center Department of Nursing.

Zderad, L.T. (1978). From here and now to theory: Reflections on "how." In J.G. Paterson (Ed.), *Theory development: What, why, how?* (Publication No. 15–1708, pp. 35–48). New York: National League for Nursing.

32. Hildegard Peplau

Barker, P. (1998). The future of the theory of interpersonal relations? A personal reflection on Peplau's legacy. *Journal of Psychiatric and Mental Health Nursing*, 5(3), 213–220.

Beeber, L.S. (1998). Treating depression through the therapeutic nurse-client relationship. *Nursing Clinics of North America*, 33(1), 153–172.

Beeber, L.S. and Bourbonniere, M. (1998). The concept of interpersonal pattern in Peplau's theory of nursing. *Journal of Psychiatric and Mental Health Nursing*, 5(3), 187–192.

Carey, E.T., Noll, J., Rasmussen, L., Searcy, B., and Stark, N. (1989). Hildegard E. Peplau: Psychodynamic nursing. In A. Marriner-Tomey (Ed.), *Nursing theorists and their work* (2nd ed.). St. Louis, MO: C.V. Mosby.

Chambers, M. (1998). Interpersonal mental health nursing: Research issues and challenges. *Journal of Psychiatric and Mental Health Nursing*, 5(3), 203–211.

Feely, M. (1997). Using Peplau's theory in nurse-patient relations. *International Nursing Review*, 44(4), 115–120.

Forchuk, C. (1989). Establish a nurse-client relationship. *Journal of Psychosocial Nursing*, 27(2), 30–34.

Forchuk, C. (1991). A comparison of the works of Peplau and Orlando. *Archives of Psychiatric Nursing*, 5(1), 38–45.

Forchuk, C., Beaton, S., Crawford, L., Ide, L., Voorberg, N., and Bethune, J. (1989). Incorporating Peplau's theory and case management. *Journal of Psychosocial Nursing and Mental Health Services*, 27(2), 35–38.

Forchuk, C. and Dorsay, J.P. (1995). Hildegard Peplau meets family system nursing: Innovation in theory-based practice. *Journal of Advanced Nursing*, 21(1), 110–115.

Forchuk, C., Jewell, J., Schofield, R., Sircelj, M. and Valledor, T. (1998). From hospital to community: Bridging therapeutic relationships. *Journal of Psychiatric and Mental Health Nursing*, 5(3), 197–202.

Gregg, D.E. (1978). Hildegard E. Peplau: Her contributions. *Perspectives in Psychiatric Care*, 16(3), 118–121.

Haber, J. (2000). Hildegarde E. Peplau: The psychiatric nursing legacy of a legend. *Journal of the American Psychiatric Nurses Association*, 6(2), 56–62.

Lego, S. (1998). The application of Peplau's theory to group psychotherapy. *Journal of Psychiatric and Mental Health Nursing*, 5(3), 193–196.

Mahoney, J.S. and Engebretson, J. (2000). The interface of anthropology and nursing guiding culturally competent care in psychiatric nursing. *Archives of Psychiatric Nursing*, 14(4), 183–190.

Peden, A.R. (1998). The evolution of an intervention—The use of Peplau's process of practice-based theory development. *Journal of Psychiatric and Mental Health Nursing*, 5(3), 173–178.

Peplau, H. (1952). *Interpersonal relations in nursing*. New York: G.P. Putnam's Sons.

Peplau, H. (1967). Interpersonal relations and the work of the industrial nurse. *American Association of Industrial Nurses*, 15(11), 7–12.

Peplau, H. (1962). Interpersonal techniques: The crux of psychiatric nursing. *American Journal of Nursing*, 62(6), 50–54.

Peplau, H. (1963). Interpersonal relations and the process of adaptation. *Nursing Science*, 3, 272–279.

Peplau, H. (1964). *Basic principles of patient counseling*. Philadelphia: Smith Kline & French Laboratory.

Peplau, H. (1968). Operational definitions and nursing science. In L.T. Zderad and H.C. Belcher (Eds.), *Developing behavioral concepts in nursing*. Atlanta, GA: Southern Regional Education Board.

Peplau, H. (1968). Psychotherapeutic strategies. *Perspectives in Psychiatric Care*, 6(6), 264–270.

Peplau, H. (1969). Professional closeness . . . as a special kind of involvement with a patient, client, or family group. *Nursing Forum*, 8(4), 342.

Peplau, H. (1970). Changed patterns of practice. *Washington Street Journal of Nursing*, 42, 4–6.

Peplau, H. (1971). Communication in crisis intervention. *Psychiatric Forum*, 2, 1–7.

Peplau, H. (1974). Biography. *Nursing '74*, 4(2), 13.

Peplau, H. (1978). Psychiatric nursing: Role of nurses and psychiatric nurses. *International Nursing Review*, 25(2), 41–47.

Peplau, H. (1986). *Credentialing in nursing: Contemporary developments and trends: Internal vs. external regulation* [Pamphlet] (Publication No. G-172B, pp. 1–10). Kansas City, MO: American Nurses Association.

Peplau, H. (1987). Nursing science: A historical perspective. In R.R. Parse (Ed.), *Nursing science: Major paradigms, theories, and critiques*. Philadelphia: W.B. Saunders.

Peplau, H. (1988). The art and science of nursing: Similarities, differences, and relations. *Nursing Science Quarterly*, 1(1), 8–15.

Peplau, H. (1988). Future directions in psychiatric nursing from the perspective of history. *Journal of Psychosocial Nursing and Mental Health Services*, 27(2), 18–21, 25–28.

Peplau, H.E. (1991). *Interpersonal relations in nursing: A conceptual frame of reference for psychodynamic nursing*. New York: Springer. (Original work published 1952).

Peplau, H.E. (1997). Peplau's theory of interpersonal relations. *Nursing Science Quarterly*, 10(4), 162–167.

Price, B. (1998). Explorations in body image care: Peplau and practice knowledge. *Journal of Psychiatric and Mental Health Nursing*, 5(3), 179–186.

Reed, P.G. and Johnston, R.L. (1983). Peplau's nursing model: The interpersonal process. In J.J. Fitzpatrick and A.L. Whall (Eds.), *Conceptual models of nursing: Analysis and application*. Bowie, MD: Robert J. Brady Co.

Reed, P.G. and Johnston, R.L. (1989). Peplau's nursing model: The interpersonal process. In J.J. Fitzpatrick and A.L. Whall (Eds.), *Conceptual models of nursing: Analysis and application* (2nd ed.). Norwalk, CT: Appleton & Lange.

Reynolds, W.J. (1997). Peplau's theory in practice. *Nursing Science Quarterly*, 10(4), 168–170.

Roy, C. (1980). A case study viewed according to different models. In J.P. Riehl and C. Roy (Eds.), *Conceptual models for nursing practice* (2nd ed.). New York: Appleton-Century-Crofts.

Schafer, P. (1999). Working with Dave. Application of Peplau's interpersonal nursing theory in the correctional environment. *Journal of Psychosocial Nursing and Mental Health Services*, 37(9), 18–24.

Sills, G.M. (1978). Hildegard E. Peplau: Leader, practitioner, academician, scholar, theorist. *Perspectives in Psychiatric Care*, 16(3), 122–128.

Sills, G.M. (1998). Peplau and professionalism: The emergence of the paradigm of professionalization. *Journal of Psychiatric and Mental Health Nursing*, 5(3), 167–171.

Thelander, B.L. (1997). The psychotherapy of Hildegard Peplau in the treatment of people with serious mental illness. *Perspectives in Psychiatric Care*, 33(3), 24–32.

Thompson, L. (1986). Peplau's theory: An application to short-term individual therapy. *Journal of Psychological Nursing and Mental Health Service*, 24(8), 26–31.

Yamashita, M. (1997). Family caregiving: Application of Newman's and Peplau's theories. *Journal of Psychiatric and Mental Health Nursing*, 4(6), 401–405.

33. Martha Rogers

Aggleton, P. and Chalmers, H. (1984). Rogers' unitary field model. *Nursing Times*, 80(50), 35–39.

Alligood, M. (1989). Rogers's theory and nursing administration: A perspective on health and environment. In B. Henry, C. Arndt, M. DiVincenti, and A. Marriner-Tomey (Eds.), *Dimensions of nursing administration: Theory, research, education, practice.* Boston: Blackwell Scientific Publications.

Alligood, M.R. (1990). Rogers' theory: Research to practice. *Rogerian Nursing Science News,* 2(3), 2–3.

Armstrong, M.A. and Kelly, A.E. (1995). More than the sum of their parts: Martha Rogers and Hildegard Peplau. *Archives of Psychiatric Nursing,* 9(1), 40–44.

Banonis, B. (1989). The lived experience of recovering from addiction: A phenomenological study. *Nursing Science Quarterly,* 2(1), 37–43.

Barrett, E.A. (1989). A nursing theory of power for nursing practice: Derivation from Rogers' paradigm. In J. Riehl-Sisca (Ed.), *Conceptual models for nursing practice* (3rd ed.). Norwalk, CT: Appleton & Lange.

Barrett, E.A. (1990). The continuing revolution of Rogers' science-based nursing education. In E.A. Barrett (Ed.), *Visions of Rogers' science-based nursing* (pp. 303–317). New York: National League for Nursing.

Barrett, E.A. (1990). A measure of power as knowing participation in change. In O.L. Strickland and C.F. Waltz (Eds.), *Measurement in nursing outcomes* (pp. 159–175). New York: Springer.

Barrett, E.A. (1990). Visions of Rogers' science-based nursing. In E.A. Barrett (Ed.), *Visions of Rogers' science-based nursing* (pp. 31–44). New York: National League for Nursing.

Barrett, E.A. (1991). Space nursing. *Cutis,* 48(4), 299–303.

Barrett, E.A., Paletta, J., and Winstead-Fry, P. (1991). Transcultural exploration of measurement scales for the study of Rogers' science of unitary human beings. *Rogerian Nursing Science News,* 4(1), 6.

Barrett, K. (1972). Theoretical construct of the concepts of touch as they relate to nursing. *Nursing Research,* 21, 102–110.

Benedict, S.C. and Burge, J.M. (1990). The relationship between human field motion and preferred visible wavelengths. *Nursing Science Quarterly,* 3(2), 73–80.

Biley, F. (1990). Rogers' model: An analysis. *Nursing,* 4(15), 31–33.

Biley, F.C. (1992). The perception of time as a factor in Rogers' Science of Unitary Human Beings: A literature review. *Journal of Advanced Nursing,* 17(9), 1141–1145.

Biley, F.C. (1993). Energy fields nursing: A brief encounter of a unitary kind. *International Journal of Nursing Studies,* 30(6), 519–525.

Blair, C. (1979). Hyperactivity in children: Viewed within the framework of synergistic man. *Nursing Forum,* 18, 293–303.

Botha, M.E. (1989). Theory development in perspective: The role of conceptual frameworks and models in theory development. *Journal of Advanced Nursing,* 14(1), 49–55.

Bradshaw, A. (1995). What are nurses doing to patients—A review of theories of nursing past and present. *Journal of Clinical Nursing,* 4(2), 81–92.

Bramlett, M.H., Gueldner, S.H. and Sowell, R.L. (1990). Consumer-centric advocacy: Its connection to nursing frameworks. *Nursing Science Quarterly,* 3(4), 156–161.

Bultemeier, K. (1997). Rogers' science of unitary human beings in nursing practice. In M.R. Alligood et al. (Eds.), *Nursing theory: Utilization and application* (pp. 153–174). St. Louis, MO: Mosby Year Book.

Butcher, H.K. (1993). Kaleidoscoping in life's turbulence: From Seurat's art to Rogers' nursing science. In M.E. Parker (Ed.), *Patterns of nursing theories in practice* (pp. 183–198). New York: National League for Nursing.

Butcher, H.K. (1994). The unitary field pattern portrait method: Development of a research method for Rogers' science of unitary human beings. In M. Madrid and E.A. Barrett (Eds.), *Rogers' scientific art of nursing practice* (pp. 397–429, 430–435). New York: National League for Nursing.

Butcher, H.K. and Parker, N. (1988). Guided imagery within Rogers' science of unitary human beings: An experimental study. *Nursing Science Quarterly*, 1(3), 103–110.

Butcher, H.K. and Forchuk, C. (1992). The overview effect: The impact of space exploration on the evolution of nursing science. *Nursing Science Quarterly*, 5(3), 118–123.

Caggins, R.P. (1991). The Caggins Synergy Nursing Model. *ABNF Journal*, 2(1), 15–18.

Carboni, J.T. (1991). A Rogerian theoretical tapestry. *Nursing Science Quarterly*, 4(3), 130–136.

Carboni, J.T. (1995). Enfolding health-as-wholeness-and-harmony: A theory of Rogerian nursing practice. *Nursing Science Quarterly*, 8(2), 71–78.

Carboni, J.T. (1995). The Rogerian process of inquiry. *Nursing Science Quarterly*, 8(1), 22–37.

Caroselli, C. (1995). Power and feminism: A nursing science perspective. *Nursing Science Quarterly*, 8(3), 115–119.

Cerilli, K. and Burd, S. (1989). An analysis of Martha Rogers' nursing as a science of unitary human beings. In J. Riehl-Sisca (Ed.), *Conceptual models for nursing practice* (3rd ed.). Norwalk, CT: Appleton & Lange.

Clarke, P.L. (1986). Theoretical and measurement issues in the study of field phenomena. The human field and self actualization in healthy women. *Advances in Nursing Science*, 9(1), 29–39.

Compton, M.A. (1989). A Rogerian view of drug abuse: Implications for nursing. *Nursing Science Quarterly*, 2(2), 98–105.

Coulter, M.A. (1990). A review of two theories of learning and their application in the practice of nurse education. *Nurse Education Today*, 10(5), 333–338.

Dailey, J., Maupin, J., Satterly, M., Schnell, D., and Wallace, T. (1989). Martha E. Rogers: Unitary human beings. In A. Marriner-Tomey (Ed.), Nursing theorists and their work (2nd ed.). St. Louis, MO: C.V. Mosby.

Duffey, M. and Muhlenkamp, A.F. (1974). A framework for theory analysis. *Nursing Outlook*, 22(9), 570–574.

Egan, M. and Kadushin, G. (1997). Rural hospital social work: Views of physicians and social workers. *Social Work in Health Care*, 26(1), 1–23.

†Egbert, E. (1980, January). Concept of wellness. *Journal of Psychosocial Nursing and Mental Health Services*, 18(1), 9–12.

†Falco, S.M. and Lobo, M.L. (1980). Martha E. Rogers. In The Nursing Theories Conference Group. *Nursing theories: The base for professional nursing practice*. Englewood Cliffs, NJ: Prentice-Hall.

Fawcett, J. (1977). The relationship between identification and patterns of change in spouses' body image during and after pregnancy. *International Journal of Nursing Studies*, 14, 199–213.

Fawcett, J. (1984). Rogers' life process model. In J. Fawcett (Ed.), *Analysis and evaluation of conceptual models of nursing.* Philadelphia: F.A. Davis.

Ference, H. (1989). Comforting the dying: Nursing practice according to the Rogerian model. In J. Riehl-Sisca (Ed.), *Conceptual models for nursing practice* (3rd ed.). Norwalk, CT: Appleton & Lange.

Ference, H. (1989). Nursing science theories and administration. In B. Henry, C. Arndt, M. DiVincenti, and A. Marriner-Tomey (Eds.), *Dimensions of nursing administration: Theory, research, education, practice.* Boston: Blackwell Scientific Publications.

Field, L. and Newman, M. (1982). Clinical application of the unitary man framework: Case study analysis (1980). In M.J. Kim and D.A. Moritz (Eds.), *Classification of nursing diagnosis: Proceedings of the third and fourth national conference.* New York: McGraw-Hill.

Fisher, L. and Reichenbach, M. (1987–1988). From Tinkerbell to Rogers (how a fairy tale facilitated an understanding of Rogers' theory of unitary being). *Nursing Forum,* 13(1), 5–9.

Fitzpatrick, J.J. (1980). Patient's perception of time: Current research. *International Nursing Review*, 27, 148–153, 160.

Fitzpatrick, J.J. (1988). Theory based on Rogers' conceptual model. *Journal of Gerontological Nursing*, 14(9), 14–16.

Floyd, J.A. (1983). Research using Rogers' conceptual system: Development of a testable theorem. *Advances in Nursing Science*, 5(2), 37–48.

Forker, J.E. and Billing, C.V. (1989). Nursing therapeutics in a group encounter. *Archives of Psychiatric Nursing*, 3(2), 108–112.

Garon, M. (1992). Contributions of Martha Rogers to the development of nursing knowledge. *Nursing Outlook*, 40(2), 67–72.

Gill, B.P. and Atwood, J.R. (1981). Reciprocity and helicy used to relate mEGF and wound healing. *Nursing Research*, 30(2), 68–72.

Gioiella, E. (1989). Professionalizing nursing: A Rogers legacy. *Nursing Science Quarterly*, 2(2), 61–62.

Gjerberg, E. and Kjolsrod, L. (2001). The doctor-nurse relationship: How easy is it to be a female doctor co-operating with a female nurse? *Social Science and Medicine*, 52(2), 189–202.

Goldberg, W.G. and Fitzpatrick, J.J. (1980). Movement therapy with the aged. *Nursing Research*, 29(6), 339–346.

Green, C.A. (1998). Critically exploring the use of Rogers' Nursing Theory of Unitary Human Beings as a framework to underpin therapeutic touch practice. *European Nurse*, 3(3), 158–169.

Gudmunsen, A.M. (1995). Personal reflections on Martha E. Rogers. *Nursing and Healthcare Perspectives on Community,* 16(1), 36–37.

Gueldner, S. (1989). Applying Rogers's model to nursing administration: Emphasis on client and nursing. In B. Henry, C. Arndt, M. DiVincenti, and A. Marriner-Tomey

(Eds.), *Dimensions of nursing administration: Theory, research, education, practice*. Boston: Blackwell Scientific Publications.

Gueldner, S.H. (1994). Now she belongs to the ages. . . . A pandimensional tribute to the extraordinary life of Martha E. Rogers. *Reflections*, 20(2), 25.

Hallett, C.E. (1997). The helping relationship in the community setting: The relevance of Rogerian theory to the supervision of Project 2000 students. *International Journal of Nursing Studies*, 34(6), 415–419

Hanchett, E.S. (1990). Nursing models and community as client. *Nursing Science Quarterly*, 3(2), 67–72.

Heggie, J., Schoenmehl, P., Chang, M., and Grieco, C. (1989). Selection and implementation of Dr. Martha Rogers' nursing conceptual model in an acute care setting. *Clinical Nurse Specialist*, 3(3), 143–147.

Heidt, P. (1981). Effect of therapeutic touch on anxiety level of hospitalized patients. *Nursing Research*, 30(1), 32–37.

Heise, J.L. (1993). The valuing process. A vehicle for creating reality. *Journal of Holistic Nursing*, 11(1), 56–63.

Hektor, L.M. (1989). Martha E. Rogers: A life history. *Nursing Science Quarterly*, 2(2), 63–73.

Herdtner, S. (2000). Using therapeutic touch in nursing practice. *Orthopedic Nursing*, 19(5), 77–82.

Hill, L. and Oliver, N. (1993). Technique integration. Therapeutic touch and theory-based mental health nursing. *Journal of Psychosocial Nursing and Mental Health Services*, 31(2), 18–22.

Hosking, P. (1993). Utilizing Rogers' Theory of Self-Concept in mental health nursing. *Journal of Advanced Nursing*, 18(6), 980–984.

Huch, M.H. (1995). Nursing and the next millennium. *Nursing Science Quarterly*, 8(1), 38–44.

Huch, M.H. (1991). Perspectives on health. *Nursing Science Quarterly*, 4(1), 33–40.

Johnston, R.L., Fitzpatrick, J.J., and Donovan, M.J. (1982). Developmental stage: Relationship to temporal dimensions [Abstract]. *Nursing Research*, 31, 120.

†Katz, V. (1971). Auditory stimulation and developmental behavior of the premature infant. *Nursing Research*, 20(3), 196–201.

Kim, M.J. and Moritz, D.A. (Eds.). (1982). *Classification of nursing diagnosis: Proceedings of the third and fourth national conference*. New York: McGraw-Hill.

Kim, H.S. (1983). Use of Rogers' conceptual system in research: Comments. *Nursing Research*, 32(2), 89–91.

Kranzman, J. (1993). Use of computer technology in enterostomal therapy nursing. *Journal of Enterostomal Therapy Nursing*, 20(3), 116–120.

Krieger, D. (1975). Therapeutic touch: The imprimatur of nursing. *American Journal of Nursing*, 75(5), 784–787.

Krieger, D. (1976). Healing by the laying on of hands as a facilitator of bioenergetic change: The response of in-vivo human hemoglobin. *International Journal of Psychoenergetic Systems*, 1, 121–129.

Krieger, D. (1979). *Therapeutic touch: How to use your hands to help and heal*. Englewood Cliffs, NJ: Prentice-Hall.

Krieger, D., Peper, E., and Ancoli, S. (1979). Therapeutic touch: Searching for evidence of physiological change. *American Journal of Nursing*, 79, 660–662.

Laschinger, H.K. and Duff, V. (1991). Attitudes of practicing nurses towards theory-based nursing practice. *Canadian Journal of Nursing Administration*, 4(1), 6–10.

Leddy, S.K. (1995). Measuring mutual process: Development and psychometric testing of the Person-Environment Participation Scale. *Visions: Journal of Rogerian Nursing Science*, 3(1), 20–31.

Leksell, J.K., Johansson, I., Wibell, L.B., and Wikblad, K.F. (2001). Power and self-perceived health in blind diabetic and nondiabetic individuals. *Journal of Advanced Nursing*, 34(4), 511–519.

Lipp, A. (1998). An enquiry into a combined approach for nursing ethics. *Nursing Ethics*, 5(2), 122–138.

Macrae, J. (1979). Therapeutic touch in practice. *American Journal of Nursing*, 79, 664–665.

Madrid, M. and Winstead-Fry, P. (1986). Rogers's conceptual model. In P. Winstead-Fry, (Ed.), *Case studies in nursing theory*. New York: National League for Nursing.

Magan, S.J., Gibbon, E.J. and Mrozek, R. (1990). Nursing theory applications: A practice model. *Issues in Mental Health Nursing*, 11(3), 297–312.

Malinski, V.M. (1991). The experience of laughing at oneself in older couples. *Nursing Science Quarterly*, 4(2), 69–75.

Manhart, E.A. (1988). Using Rogers' science of unitary human beings in nursing practice. *Nursing Science Quarterly*, 50–51.

Manias, E. and Street, A. (2001). The interplay of knowledge and decision making between nurses and doctors in critical care. *International Journal of Nursing Studies*, 38(2), 129–140.

Martell, L.K. (1999). Maternity care during the post-World War II baby boom: The experience of general duty nurses. *Western Journal of Nursing Research*, 21(3), 387–404.

Mason, T. and Patterson, R. (1990). A critical review of the use of Rogers' model within a special hospital: A single case study. *Journal of Advanced Nursing*, 15(2), 130–141.

Matas, K.E. (1997). Human patterning and chronic pain. *Nursing Science Quarterly*, 10(2), 88–96.

McSherry, W. and Draper, P. (1998). The debates emerging from the literature surrounding the concept of spirituality as applied to nursing. *Journal of Advanced Nursing*, 27(4), 683–691.

Moccia, P. (1985). A further investigation of "Dialectical thinking as a means of understanding systems in development: Relevance to Rogers's Principles" [Commentary]. *Advances in Nursing Science*, 7(4), 33–38.

Newman, M.A. (1979). *Theory development in nursing*. Philadelphia: F.A. Davis.

Newman, M.A. (1994). Theory for nursing practice. *Nursing Science Quarterly*, 7(4), 153–157.

Newman, M.A., Sime, A.M., and Corcoran-Perry, S.A. (1991). The focus of the discipline of nursing. *Advances in Nursing Science*, 14(1), 1–6.

Overman, B. (1994). Lessons from the Tao for birthing practice. *Journal of Holistic Nursing*, 12(2), 142–147.

Parker, M. and Barry, C. (1999). Community practice guided by a nursing model. *Nursing Science Quarterly,* 12(2), 125–131.

Pesut, D.J. (1998). Matters of the mind, heart and soul. *Nursing Outlook,* 46(4), 154.

Phillips, J.R. (1989). Science of unitary human being: Changing research perspective. *Nursing Science Quarterly,* 2(2), 57–60.

Phillips, J.R. (1994). Martha E. Rogers' clarion call for global nursing research. *Nursing Science Quarterly,* 7(3), 100–101.

†Porter, L.S. (1972). The impact of physical-physiological activity on infant growth and development. *Nursing Research,* 21(3), 210–219.

Proctor, S., Wilcockson, J., Pearson P., et al. (2001). Going home from hospital: The carer/patient dyad. *Journal of Advanced Nursing,* 35(2), 206–217.

Quillin, S.I.M. and Runk, J.A. (1983). Martha Rogers' model. In J.J. Fitzpatrick and A.L. Whall (Eds.), *Conceptual models of nursing: Analysis and application.* Bowie, MD: Robert J. Brady Co.

Quillin, S.I.M. and Runk, J.A. (1989). Martha Rogers' unitary person model. In J.J. Fitzpatrick and A.L. Whall (Eds.), *Conceptual models of nursing: Analysis and application* (2nd ed.). Norwalk, CT: Appleton & Lange.

Quinn, J.F. (1979). One nurse's evolution as a healer. *American Journal of Nursing,* 79, 662–664.

Quinn, J.F. (1989). Therapeutic touch as energy exchange: Replication and extension. *Nursing Science Quarterly,* 2(2), 74–78.

Randell, B.P. (1992). Nursing theory: The 21st century. *Nursing Science Quarterly,* 5(4), 176–184.

Reed, P.G. (1991). Toward a nursing theory of self-transcendence: Deductive reformulation using developmental theories. *Advances in Nursing Science,* 13(4), 64–77.

Reeder, F. (1984). Philosophical issues in the Rogerian science of unitary human beings. *Advances in Nursing Science,* 6(2), 14–23.

Reeder, F. (1993). The science of unitary human beings and interpretive human science. *Nursing Science Quarterly,* 6(1), 13–24.

Rogers, M.E. (1963). Building a strong educational foundation. *American Journal of Nursing,* 63(6), 94–95.

Rogers, M.E. (1963). Some comments on the theoretical basis for nursing practice. *Nursing Science,* 63(1), 11–13, 60–61.

Rogers, M.E. (1964). *Reveille in nursing.* Philadelphia: F.A. Davis.

Rogers, M.E. (1969). *Nursing research: Relevant to practice?* Fifth Annual Research Conference of the American Nurses Association, pp. 352–359. Kansas City, MO: ANA.

†Rogers, M.E. (1970). *An introduction to the theoretical basis of nursing.* Philadelphia: F.A. Davis.

†Rogers, M.E. (1975). Euphemisms in nursing's future. *Image: Journal of Nursing Scholarship,* 7(2), 3–9.

†Rogers, M.E. (1980). Nursing: A science of unitary man. In J.P. Riehl and C. Roy (Eds.), *Conceptual models for nursing practice* (2nd ed.). New York: Appleton-Century-Crofts.

Rogers, M.E. (1980). *The science of unitary man* [Videotapes]. New York: Media for Nursing.

Rogers, M.E. (1981). Beyond the horizon. In N. Chaska (Ed.), *The nursing profession: A time to speak.* New York: McGraw-Hill.

Rogers, M.E. (1981). Science of unitary man: A paradigm for nursing. In G.E. Lasker (Ed.), *Applied systems and cybernetics* (Vol. IV, pp. 219–228). New York: Pergamon Press.

Rogers, M.E. (1983). *Nursing science: A science of unitary human beings.* Paper presented at the First National Rogerian Conference, New York University.

Rogers, M.E. (1983). Science of unitary human being: A paradigm for nursing. In I.W. Clements and F.B. Roberts (Eds.), *Family health: A theoretical approach to nursing care.* New York: John Wiley & Sons.

Rogers, M.E. (1987). Rogers's science of unitary human beings. In R.R. Parse (Ed.), *Nursing science: Major paradigms, theories, and critiques.* Philadelphia: W.B. Saunders.

Rogers, M.E. (1987). *Nursing research in the future* (Publication. No. 14–2203, pp. 121–123). New York: National League for Nursing.

Rogers, M.E. (1988). Nursing science and art: A prospective. *Nursing Science Quarterly,* 1(3), 99–102.

Rogers, M.E. (1989). Creating a climate for the implementation of a nursing conceptual framework. *Journal of Continuing Education in Nursing,* 20(3), 112–116.

Rogers, M.E. (1989). Nursing: A science of unitary human beings. In J. Riehl-Sisca (Ed.), *Conceptual models for nursing practice* (3rd ed.). Norwalk, CT: Appleton & Lange.

Rogers, M.E. (1990). Nursing: Science of unitary, irreducible, human beings: update 1990. In E.A. Barrett (Ed.), *Visions of Rogers' Science-Based Nursing* (pp. 5–11). New York: National League for Nursing.

Rogers, M.E. (1991). Nursing: Science of irreducible human and environmental energy fields [Glossary]. *Rogerian Nursing Science News,* 4(2), 6–7.

Rogers, M.E. (1992). Nursing science and the space age. *Nursing Science Quarterly,* 5(1), 27–34.

Rogers, M.E. (1994). Nursing science evolves. In M. Madrid and E.A. Barrett (Eds.), *Rogers' Scientific Art of Nursing Practice* (pp. 3–9). New York: National League for Nursing.

Rossi, L. and Krekeler, K. (1982). Small-group reactions to the theoretical framework "Unitary Man" (1980). In M.J. Kim and D.A. Moritz (Eds.), *Classification of nursing diagnosis: Proceedings of the third and fourth national conference.* New York: McGraw-Hill.

Roy, C. (1980). Rogers' theoretical basis of nursing. In J.P. Riehl and C. Roy (Eds.), *Conceptual models for nursing practice* (2nd ed.). New York: Appleton-Century-Crofts.

Safier, G. (1977). *Contemporary American leaders: An oral history.* New York: McGraw-Hill.

Sanchez, R. (1989). Empathy, diversity, and telepathy in mother-daughter dyads: An empirical investigation utilizing Rogers' conceptual framework. *Scholarly Inquiry for Nursing Practice,* 3(1), 29–51.

Sarter, B. (1988). *The stream of becoming: A study of Martha Rogers' theory.* New York: National League for Nursing.

Sarter, B. (1989). Some critical philosophical issues in the science of unitary human being. *Nursing Science Quarterly,* 3, 74–78.

Schodt, C. (1989). Parental-fetal attachment and couvade: A study of patterns of human-environment integrality. *Nursing Science Quarterly,* 2(2), 88–97.

Schneider, P.E. (1995). Focusing awareness: The process of extraordinary healing from a Rogerian perspective. *Visions: Journal of Rogerian Nursing Science,* 3(1), 32–43.

Sherman, D.W. (1997). Rogerian science: Opening new frontiers of nursing knowledge through its application in quantitative research. *Nursing Science Quarterly,* 10(3), 131–135.

Smith D.W. (1995). Power and spirituality in polio survivors: A study based on Rogers' science. *Nursing Science Quarterly,* 8(3), 133–139.

Smith, M.J. (1986). Human-environment process: A test of Rogers' principle of integrality. *Advances in Nursing Science,* 9(1), 21–28.

Smith, M.J. (1988). Testing propositions derived from Rogers' conceptual system. *Nursing Science Quarterly,* 1(2), 60–67.

Takahashi, T. (1992). Perspectives on nursing knowledge. *Nursing Science Quarterly,* 5(2), 86–91.

Tettero, I., Jackson, S. and Wilson, S. (1993). Theory to practice: Developing a Rogerian-based assessment tool. *Journal of Advanced Nursing,* 18(5), 776–782.

Timpka, T. (2000). The patient and the primary care team: A small-scale critical theory. *Journal of Advanced Nursing,* 31(3), 558–564.

Tudor, C.A., Keegan-Jones, L. and Bens, E.M. (1994). Implementing Rogers' science-based nursing practice in a pediatric nursing service setting. In M. Madrid and E.A. Barrett (Eds.), *Rogers' Scientific Art of Nursing Practice* (pp. 305–322). New York: National League for Nursing.

Uys, L.R. (1987). Foundational studies in nursing. *Journal of Advanced Nursing,* 12(3), 275–280.

Whall, A. (1987). A critique of Rogers's framework. In R.R. Parse (Ed.), *Nursing science: Major paradigms, theories, and critiques.* Philadelphia: W.B. Saunders.

†Whelton, B.J. (1979). An operationalization of Martha Rogers' theory throughout the nursing process. *International Journal of Nursing Studies,* 16, 7–20.

Yarcheski, A. and Mahon, N.E. (1991). An empirical test of Rogers' original and revised theory of correlates in adolescents. *Research in Nursing and Health,* 14(6), 447–455.

Yarcheski, A. and Mahon, N.E. (1995). Rogers' pattern manifestations and health in adolescents. *Western Journal of Nursing Research,* 17(4), 383–397.

In addition, the April 1979 volume of the *American Journal of Nursing* contains three articles on therapeutic touch based on Rogers' conceptual model.

34. Callista Roy

Aggleton, P. and Chalmers, H. (1984). The Roy adaptation model. *Nursing Times,* 80(40), 45–48.

Andrews, H. (1989). Implementation of the Roy adaptation model: An application of educational change research. In J. Riehl-Sisca, *Conceptual models for nursing practice* (3rd ed.). Norwalk, CT: Appleton & Lange.

Andrews, H.A. (1991). Overview of the self-concept mode. In C. Roy and H.A. Andrews (Eds.), *The Roy adaptation model: The definitive statement* (pp. 269–279). Norwalk, CT, Appleton & Lange.

Andrews, H. and Roy, C. (1986). *Essentials of the Roy adaptation model.* Englewood Cliffs, NJ: Prentice-Hall.

Araich, M. (2001). Roy's Adaptive Model: Demonstration of theory integration into process of care in coronary care unit. *Icus and Nursing Web Journal,* (7), 12.

Artinian, N.T. (1991). Stress experience of spouses of patients having coronary artery bypass during hospitalization and 6 weeks after discharge. *Heart and Lung,* 20, 52–59.

Artinian, N.T. (1992). Spouse adaptation to mate's CABG surgery: 1 year follow-up. *American Journal of Critical Care,* 1(2), 36–42.

Blue, C., Brubaker, K., Fine, J., Kirsch, M., Papazian, K., and Riester, C. (1989). Sister Callista Roy: Adaptation model. In A. Marriner-Tomey (Ed.), *Nursing theorists and their work* (2nd ed.). St. Louis, MO: C.V. Mosby.

†Brower, H.T. and Baker, D.J. (1976). Using the adaptation model in a practitioner curriculum. *Nursing Outlook,* 24(11), 686–689.

Bunting, S.B. (1988). The concept of perception in selected nursing theories. *Nursing Science Quarterly,* 1, 168–174.

Camooso, C., Green, M., and Reilly, P. (1981). Students' adaptation according to Roy. *Nursing Outlook,* 29, 108–109.

Clements, I.W. and Roberts, F.B. (Eds.). (1983). *Family health: A theoretical approach to nursing care.* New York: John Wiley & Sons.

Cottrell, B. and Shannahan, M. (1987). A comparison of fetal outcome in birth chair and delivery table births. *Nursing Research and Health,* 10, 239–243.

Craig, D.I. (1990). The adaptation to pregnancy of spinal cord injured women. *Rehabilitation Nursing,* 15(1), 6–9.

Dahlen, R. (1980). *Analysis of selected factors related to the elderly person's ability to adapt to visual prostheses following senile cataract surgery.* Doctoral dissertation, University of Maryland.

DiIorio, C. (1989). Application of the Roy model to nursing administration. In B. Henry, C. Arndt, M. DiVincenti, and A. Marriner-Tomey (Eds.), *Dimensions of nursing administration: Theory, research, education, practice.* Boston: Blackwell Scientific Publications.

Dixon, E.L. (1999). Community health nursing practice and the Roy Adaptation Model. *Public Health Nursing,* 16(4), 290–300.

Downey, C. (1974). Adaptation nursing applied to an obstetric patient. In J.P. Riehl and C. Roy (Eds.), *Conceptual models for nursing practice* (pp. 151–159). New York: Appleton-Century-Crofts.

Duffy, M.E. (1998). The concept of adaptation: Examining alternatives for the study of nursing phenomena. *Scholarly Inquiry in Nursing Practice,* 12(2), 163–176.

Dunn, H.C. and Dunn, D.G. (1997). The Roy Adaptation Model and its application to clinical nursing practice. *Journal of Ophthalmic Nursing and Technology,* 16(2), 74–78.

Duquette, A.M. (1997). Adaptation: A concept analysis. *Journal of School Nursing,* 13(3), 30–33.

†Farkas, L. (1981). Adaptation problems with nursing home application for elderly persons: An application of the Roy adaptation nursing model. *Journal of Advanced Nursing*, 6(5), 363–368.

Fawcett, J. (1981). Assessing and understanding the cesarean father. In C.F. Kehoe (Ed.), *The cesarean experience: Theoretical and clinical perspectives for nurses*. New York: Appleton-Century-Crofts.

Fawcett, J. (1981). Needs of cesarean birth parents. *Journal of Obstetric, Gynecologic, and Neonatal Nursing*, 10, 371–376.

Fawcett, J. (1984). Roy's adaptation model. In J. Fawcett (Ed.), *Analysis and evaluation of conceptual models of nursing*. Philadelphia: F.A. Davis.

Field, P.A. (1987). The impact of nursing theory on the clinical decision making process. *Journal of Advanced Nursing*, 12(5), 563–571.

Galbreath, J.G. (1980). Sister Callista Roy. In The Nursing Theories Conference Group. *Nursing theories: The base for professional nursing practice*. Englewood Cliffs, NJ: Prentice-Hall.

†Galligan, A.C. (1979). Using Roy's concept of adaptation to care for young children. *MCN, The American Journal of Maternal Child Nursing*, 4(1), 24–28.

Gless, P.A. (1995). Applying the Roy adaptation model to the care of clients with quadriplegia. *Rehabilitation Nursing*, 20(1), 11–16.

Goodwin, J.O. (1980). A cross-cultural approach to integrating nursing theory and practice. *Nurse Educator*, 5(6), 15–20.

Gordon, J. (1974). Nursing assessment and care plan for a cardiac patient. In J.P. Riehl and C. Roy (Eds.), *Conceptual models for nursing practice* (pp. 144–150). New York: Appleton-Century-Crofts.

Hallen, P. (1981). A holistic model of individual and family health based on a continuum of choice. *Advances in Nursing Science*, 3(4), 27–42.

Hamer, B.A. (1991). Music therapy: Harmony for change. *Journal of Psychosocial Nursing and Mental Health Services*, 29(12), 5–7.

Hanchett, E.S. (1990). Nursing models and community as client. *Nursing Science Quarterly*, 3, 67–72.

Harrison, L.L., Leeper, J.D., and Yoon, M. (1990). Effects of early parent touch on preterm infants' heart rates and arterial oxygen saturation levels. *Journal of Advanced Nursing*, 15, 877–885.

Hoch, C. (1987). Assessing delivery of nursing care. *Journal of Gerontological Nursing*, 13(1), 10–17.

Huch, M.H. (1987). A critique of the Roy adaptation model. In R.R. Parse (Ed.), *Nursing science: Major paradigms, theories, and critiques*. Philadelphia: W.B. Saunders.

Idle, B.A. (1978). SPAL: A tool for measuring self-perceived adaptation level appropriate for an elderly population. In E.E. Bauwens (Ed.), *Clinical nursing research: Its strategies and findings* (Monograph series No. 2). Indianapolis, IN: Sigma Theta Tau.

†Janelli, L.M. (1980). Utilizing Roy's adaptation model from a gerontological perspective. *Journal of Gerontological Nursing*, 6(3), 140–150.

†Jones, P.S. (1978). An adaptation model for nursing practice. *American Journal of Nursing*, 78(11), 1900–1906.

Kasemwatana, S. (1982). An application of Roy's adaptation model. *Thai Journal of Nursing*, 31(1), 25–46.

Kehoe, C.F. (1981). Identifying the nursing needs of the postpartum cesarean mother. In C.F. Kehoe (Ed.), *The cesarean experience: Theoretical and clinical perspectives for nurses.* New York: Appleton-Century-Crofts.

Kehoe, C.F. and Fawcett, J. (1981). An overview of the Roy adaptation model. In C.F. Kehoe (Ed.), *The cesarean experience: Theoretical and clinical perspectives for nurses.* New York: Appleton-Century-Crofts.

Kerr, M.E., Hoskins, L.M., Fitzpatrick, J.J., et al. (1992). Development of Definitions for Taxonomy II. *Nursing Diagnosis*, 3(2), 65–71.

Kim, H.S. (1993). Putting theory into practice: Problems and prospects. *Journal of Advanced Nursing*, 18, 1632–1639.

Kurek-Ovshinsky, C. (1991). Group psychotherapy in an acute inpatient setting: Techniques that nourish self-esteem. *Issues in Mental Health Nursing*, 12, 81–88.

Laros, J. (1977). Deriving outcome criteria from a conceptual model. *Nursing Outlook*, 25, 333–336.

Leuze, M., and McKenzie, J. (1987). Preoperative assessment: Using the Roy's adaptation model. *AORN Journal*, 46(6), 1126–1129, 1131–1134.

Levesque, L. (1980, October 22–24). Rehabilitation of the chronically ill elderly: A method of operationalizing a conceptual model for nursing. In R.C. MacKay and E.G. Zilm (Eds.), *Research for practice: Proceedings of the National Nursing Research Conference.* Halifax, Nova Scotia.

Levesque, L., Ricard, N., Ducharme, F., Duquette, A. and Bonin, J. (1998). Empirical verification of a theoretical model derived from the Roy Adaptation Model: Findings from five studies. *Nursing Science Quarterly*, 11(1), 31–39.

Lewis, F. et al. (1978). Measuring adaptation of chemotherapy patients. In J.C. Krueger, A.H. Nelson, and M. Opal (Eds.), *Nursing research: Development, collaboration, utilization.* Germantown, MD: Aspen Systems.

Lewis, F.M., Firsich, S.C., and Parsell, S. (1979). Clinical tool development for adult chemotherapy patients: Process and content. *Cancer Nursing*, 2(2), 99–108.

Limandri, B.J. (1986). Research and practice with abused women: Use of the Roy adaptation model as an explanatory framework. *Advances in Nursing Science*, 8(4), 52–61.

†Mastal, M.F. and Hammond, H. (1980). Analysis and expansion of the Roy adaptation model: A contribution to holistic nursing. *Advances in Nursing Science*, 2(4), 71–81.

†Mastal, M., Hammond, H., and Roberts, M. (1982). Theory into hospital practice: A pilot implementation. *Journal of Nursing Administration*, 12(6), 9–15.

Mengel, A., Sherman, S., Nahigian, E., and Coleman, I. (1989). Adaptation of the Roy model in an educational setting. In J. Riehl-Sisca (Ed.), *Conceptual models for nursing practice* (3rd ed.). Norwalk, CT: Appleton & Lange.

Morales-Mann, E.T. and Logan, M. (1990). Implementing the Roy model: Challenges for nurse educators. *Journal of Advanced Nursing*, 15, 142–147.

Norris, S., Campbell, L., and Brenkert, S. (1982). Nursing procedures and alterations in transcutaneous oxygen tension in premature infants. *Nursing Research*, 31(6), 330–336.

Nuamah, I.F., Cooley, M.E., Fawcett, J. and McCorkle, R. (1999). Testing a theory for health-related quality of life in cancer patients: A structural equation approach. *Research in Nursing and Health*, 22(3), 231–242.

Phillips, K.D. (1997). Roy's adaptation model in nursing practice. In M.R. Alligood, et al. (Eds.), *Nursing theory: Utilization and application* (pp. 175–200). St. Louis, MO: Mosby Year Book.

Pioli, C. and Sandor, J. (1989). The Roy adaptation model: An analysis. In J. Riehl-Sisca (Ed.), *Conceptual models for nursing practice* (3rd ed.). Norwalk, CT: Appleton & Lange.

Pollock, S.E., Frederickson, K., Carson, M.A., Massey, V.H., and Roy, C. (1994). Contributions to nursing science: Synthesis of findings from adaptation model research. *Scholarly Inquiry for Nursing Practice*, 8(4), 361–372.

Porth, C.M. (1977). Physiological coping: A model for teaching pathophysiology. *Nursing Outlook*, 25, 781–784.

Rambo, B. (1984). *Adaptation nursing: Assessment and intervention.* Philadelphia: W.B. Saunders.

Randell, B., Tedrow, M., and van Landingham, J. (1982). *Adaptation nursing: The Roy conceptual model applied.* St. Louis, MO: C.V. Mosby.

Roy, C. (1967). Role cues and mothers of hospitalized children. *Nursing Research*, 16(2), 178–182.

†Roy, C. (1970). Adaptation: A conceptual framework for nursing. *Nursing Outlook*, 18(3), 42–45.

†Roy, C. (1971). Adaptation: A basis for nursing practice. *Nursing Outlook*, 19(4), 254–257.

Roy, C. (1973). Adaptation: Implications for curriculum change. *Nursing Outlook*, 21(3), 163–168.

Roy, C. (1975). Adaptation framework. In *Curriculum innovation through framework application.* Loma Linda, CA: Loma Linda University.

Roy, C. (1975). The impact of nursing diagnosis. *AORN Journal*, 21(6), 1023–1030.

Roy, C. (1976). *Introduction to nursing: An adaptational model.* Englewood Cliffs, NJ: Prentice-Hall.

†Roy, C. (1976). The Roy adaptation model: Comment. *Nursing Outlook*, 24(11), 690–691.

Roy, C. (1977). *Decision-making by the physically ill and adaptation during illness.* Doctoral dissertation, University of California, Los Angeles.

Roy, C. (1978). The stress of hospital events: Measuring changes in level of stress. In M.V. Batey (Ed.), *Symposium on stress: Conference on communicating nursing research.* Boulder, CO: Western Interstate Commission on Higher Education.

Roy, C. (1979, December). Nursing diagnosis from the perspective of a nursing model. *Nursing Diagnosis Newsletter* (Vol. 6). St. Louis, MO: St. Louis School of Nursing.

†Roy, C. (1979). Relating nursing theory to education: A new era. *Nurse Educator*, 4(2), 16–21.

†Roy, C. (1980). The Roy adaptation model. In J.P. Riehl and C. Roy (Eds.), *Conceptual models for nursing practice* (2nd ed.). New York: Appleton-Century-Crofts.

Roy, C. (1981). *Introduction to nursing: An adaptation model.* Englewood Cliffs, NJ: Prentice-Hall.

Roy, C. (1981). A systems model of nursing care and its effect on the quality of human life. In *Proceedings of the International Congress on Applied Systems Research and Cybernetics*. London: Pergamon Press.

Roy, C. (1984). *Introduction to nursing: An adaptation model* (2nd ed.) Englewood Cliffs, NJ: Prentice-Hall.

Roy, C. (1983). The expectant family: Analysis and application of the Roy adaptation model. In I.W. Clements and F.B. Roberts (Eds.), *Family health: A theoretical approach to nursing care*. New York: John Wiley & Sons.

Roy, C. (1983). Roy adaptation model. In I.W. Clements and F.B. Roberts (Eds.), *Family health: A theoretical approach to nursing care*. New York: John Wiley & Sons.

Roy, C. (1983). Theory development in nursing: A proposal for direction. In N. Chaska (Ed.), *The nursing profession: A time to speak*. New York: McGraw-Hill.

Roy, C. (1984). *Introduction to nursing: An adaptation model* (2nd ed.). Englewood Cliffs, NJ: Prentice-Hall.

Roy, C. (1987). Response to "Needs of spouses of surgical patients: A conceptualization within the Roy adaptation model." *Scholarly Inquiry for Nursing Practice,* 1(1), 45–50.

Roy, C. (1987). Roy's adaptation model. In R.R. Parse (Ed.), *Nursing science: Major paradigms, theories, and critiques*. Philadelphia: W.B. Saunders.

Roy, C. (1988). An explication of the philosophical assumptions of the Roy adaptation model. *Nursing Science Quarterly,* 1(1), 26–34.

Roy, C. (1988). Human information processing. *Annual Review of Nursing Research*, 6, 237–262.

Roy, C. (1989). The Roy adaptation model. In J. Riehl-Sisca (Ed.), *Conceptual models for nursing practice* (3rd ed.). Norwalk, CT: Appleton & Lange.

Roy, C. (1991). The Roy adaptation model in nursing research. In C. Roy and H.A. Andrews (Eds.), *The Roy adaptation model: The definitive statement* (pp. 445–458). Norwalk, CT: Appleton & Lange.

Roy, C. (2000). A theorist envisions the future and speaks to nursing administrators. *Nursing Administration Quarterly,* 24(2), 1–12.

Roy, C. and Anway, J. (1989). Roy's adaptation model: Theories for nursing administration. In B. Henry, C. Arndt, M. DiVincenti, and A. Marriner-Tomey (Eds.), *Dimensions of nursing administration: Theory, research, education, practice*. Boston: Blackwell Scientific Publications.

Roy, C. and Andrews, H.A. (1991). *The Roy adaptation model: The definitive statement.* Norwalk, CT: Appleton & Lange.

Roy, C. and Corliss, C.P. (1993). The Roy adaptation model: Theoretical update and knowledge for practice. In M.E. Parker (Ed.), *Patterns of nursing theory in practice* (pp. 215–229). New York: National League for Nursing.

Roy, C. and McLeod, D. (1981). Theory of the person as an adaptive system. In C. Roy and S.L. Roberts (Eds.), *Theory construction in nursing: An adaptation model* (pp. 49–69). Englewood Cliffs, NJ: Prentice-Hall.

Roy, C. and Obloy, M. (1978). The practitioner movement: Toward a science of nursing. *American Journal of Nursing,* 78, 1698–1701.

Roy, C. and Roberts, S. (1981). *Theory construction in nursing: An adaptation model.* Englewood Cliffs, NJ: Prentice-Hall.

Roy, C.L. (1995). Developing nursing knowledge: Practice issues raised from four philosophical perspectives. *Nursing Science Quarterly,* 8(2), 79–85.

Sato, M. (1986). The Roy adaptation model. In P. Winstead-Fry (Ed.), *Case studies in nursing theory.* New York: National League for Nursing.

†Schmitz, M. (1980). The Roy adaptation model: Application in a community setting. In J.P. Riehl and C. Roy (Eds.), *Conceptual models for nursing practice* (2nd ed., pp. 193–206). New York: Appleton-Century-Crofts.

Silva, M.C. (1987). Needs of spouses of surgical patients: A conceptualization within the Roy adaptation model. *Scholarly Inquiry for Nursing Practice,* 1, 29–44.

Smith, M. (1988). Roy adaptation model in practice. *Nursing Science Quarterly,* 1(2), 97–98.

†Starr, S.L. (1980). Adaptation applied to the dying patient. In J.P. Riehl and C. Roy (Eds.), *Conceptual models for nursing practice* (2nd ed.). New York: Appleton-Century-Crofts.

Strohmyer, L.L., Noroian, E.L., Patterson, L.M., and Carlin, B.P. (1993). Adaptation six months after multiple trauma: A pilot study. *Journal of Neuroscience Nursing,* 25, 30–37.

Tiedman, M.E. (1983). The Roy adaptation model. In J.J. Fitzpatrick and A.L. Whall (Eds.), *Conceptual models of nursing: Analysis and application.* Bowie, MD: Robert J. Brady Co.

Tiedman, M.E. (1989). The Roy adaptation model. In J.J. Fitzpatrick and A.L. Whall (Eds.), *Conceptual models of nursing: Analysis and application* (2nd ed.). Norwalk, CT: Appleton & Lange.

†Wagner, P. (1976). The Roy adaptation model: Testing the adaptation model in practice. *Nursing Outlook,* 24(11), 682–685.

Wallace, C.L. (1993). Resources for nursing theories in practice. In M.E. Parker (Ed.), *Patterns of nursing theories in practice* (pp. 301–311). New York: National League for Nursing.

Whittemore, R. and Roy, C. (2002). Adapting to diabetes mellitus: A theory synthesis. *Nursing Science Quarterly,* 15(4), 311–317.

Woods, S.J. and Isenberg, M.A. (2001). Adaptation as a mediator of intimate abuse and traumatic stress in battered women. *Nursing Science Quarterly,* 14(3), 215–221.

Wright, P.S., Piazza, D., Holcombe, J., and Foote, A. (1994). A comparison of three theories of nursing used as a guide for the nursing care of an 8-year-old child with leukemia. *Journal of Pediatric Oncology,* 11(1), 14–19.

35. Joyce Travelbee

Barker, P. (2000). Reflections on caring as a virtue ethic within an evidence-based culture. *International Journal of Nursing Studies,* 37(4), 329–336.

Barker, P.J., Reynolds, W., and Ward, T. (1995). The proper focus of nursing—A critique of the caring ideology. *International Journal of Nursing Studies,* 32(4), 386–397.

Begat, I.B.E. and Severinsson, E.I. (2001). Nurses' reflections on episodes occurring during their provision of care—An interview study. *International Journal of Nursing Studies,* 38(1), 71–77.

Bennett, J. (1998). Fear of contagion: A response to stress? *Advances in Nursing Science,* 21(1), 76–87.

Bennett, J.A. (1995). Nurses' attitudes about acquired-immunodeficiency-syndrome care—What research tells us. *Journal of Professional Nursing,* 11(6), 339–350.

Bennett, J.A. (1997). A case for theory triangulation. *Nursing Science Quarterly,* 10(2), 97–102.

Bullough, V.L. and Bullough, B. (1997). Sex education in American nursing—A historical view. *Nursing History Review,* 5, 199–217.

Bunston, T., Mings, D., Mackie, A., et al (1995). Facilitating hopefulness: The determinants of hope. *Journal of Psychosocial Oncology,* 13(4), 79–103.

Cook, L. (1989). Nurses in crisis: A support group based on Travelbee's nursing theory. *Nursing and Health Care,* 10(4), 203–205.

Cutcliffe, J.R. and Goward, P. (2000). Mental health nurses and qualitative research methods: A mutual attraction? *Journal of Advanced Nursing,* 31(3), 590–598.

Dennison, S. (1995). An exploration of the communication that takes place between nurses and patients while cancer-chemotherapy is administered. *Journal of Clinical Nursing,* 4(4), 227–233.

Dewar, A.L. and Morse, J.M. (1995). Unbearable incidents—Failure to endure the experience of illness. *Journal of Advanced Nursing,* 22(5), 957–964.

Doona, M.E. (1979). *Travelbee's intervention in psychiatric nursing* (2nd ed.). Philadelphia: F.A. Davis.

Farrell, G.A. (2001). From tall poppies to squashed weeds: Why don't nurses pull together more? *Journal of Advanced Nursing,* 35(1), 26–33.

Frankel, V. (1963). *Man's search for meaning: An introduction to logotherapy.* New York: Washington Square Press.

Freihofer, P. and Felton, G. (1976). Nursing behaviors in bereavement: An exploratory study. *Nursing Research,* 25(5), 332–337.

Gadow, S. (1980). Introduction. In Spickor and S. Gadow (Eds.), *Nursing: Images and ideals—Opening dialogue with the humanities.* New York: Springer-Verlag.

Hawley, G. (1998). Facing uncertainty and possible death: the Christian patients' experience. *Journal of Clinical Nursing,* 7(5), 467–478.

Hertzberg, A. and Ekman, S.L. (2000). "We, not them and us?"—Views on the relationships and interactions between staff and relatives of older people permanently living in nursing homes. *Journal of Advanced Nursing,* 31(3), 614–622.

Hilton, P.A. (1997). Theoretical perspectives of nursing: A review of the literature. *Journal of Advanced Nursing,* 26(6), 1211–1220.

Hisama, K.K. (2001). The acceptance of nursing theory in Japan: a cultural perspective. *Nursing Science Quarterly,* 14(3). 255–259.

Hobble, W., Lansinger, T., and Magers, J. (1989). Joyce Travelbee: Human-to-human relationship. In A. Marriner-Tomey (Ed.), *Nursing theorists and their work* (2nd ed.). St. Louis, MO: C.V. Mosby.

Kitson, A.L. (1996). Does nursing have a future? *British Medical Journal,* 313(7072), 1647–1651.

Landmark, B.T., Strandmark, M., and Wahl, A.K. (2001). Living with newly diagnoses breast cancer: The meaning of existential issues—A qualitative study of 10 women with newly diagnosed breast cancer, based on grounded theory. *Cancer Nursing*, 24(3), 220–226.

Lego, S. (1999). The one-to-one nurse-patient relationship. *Perspectives in Psychiatric Care*, 35(4), 4–23.

McBride, M.A. (1967). Nursing approach, pain, and relief: An exploratory experiment. *Nursing Research*, 16(4), 337–341.

McCann, T.V. and Baker, H. (2001). Mutual relating: Developing interpersonal relationships in the community. *Journal of Advanced Nursing*, 34(4), 530–537.

Morse, J.M. (2001). Toward a praxis theory of suffering. *Advances in Nursing Science*, 24(1), 47–59.

Narayanasamy, A. (1999). Learning spiritual dimensions of care from a historical perspective. *Nursing Education Today*, 19(5), 386–395.

Nowak, K.B. and Wandel, J.C. (1998). The sharing of self in geriatric clinical practice: Case report and analysis. *Geriatric Nursing*, 19(1), 34–37.

Odling, G., Danielson, E., Christensen S.B., et al. (1998). Living with breast cancer: Caregivers' perceptions in a surgical ward. *Cancer Nursing*, 21(3), 187–195.

O'Gorman, S.M. (1998). Death and dying in contemporary society: An evaluation of current attitudes and the rituals associated with death and dying and their relevance to recent understandings of health and healing. *Journal of Advanced Nursing*, 27(6), 1127–1135.

Olsen, D.P. (1997). When the patient causes the problem: The effect of patient responsibility on the nurse-patient relationship. *Journal of Advanced Nursing*, 26(3), 515–522.

Pascoe, E. (1996). The value to nursing research of Gadamer's hermeneutic philosophy. *Journal of Advanced Nursing*, 24(6), 1309–1314.

Patistea, E. (1999) Nurses' perceptions of caring as documented in theory and research. *Journal of Clinical Nursing*, 8(5), 487–495.

Rawnsley, M.M. (1997). A case for theory triangulation—Response. *Nursing Science Quarterly*, 10(2), 103–106.

Ross, L. (1995). The spiritual dimension—Its importance to patients' health, well-being and quality-of-life and its implications for nursing practice. *International Journal of Nursing Studies*, 32(5), 457–468.

Rustoen, T. (1995). Hope and quality-of-life, two central issues for cancer patients—A theoretical analysis. *Cancer Nursing*, 18(5), 355–361.

Rustoen, T. and Hanestad, B.R. (1998). Nursing intervention to increase hope in cancer patients. *Journal of Clinical Nursing*, 7(1), 19–27.

Rustoen, T. and Wiklund, I. (2000). Hope in newly diagnosed patients with cancer. *Cancer Nursing*, 23(3), 214–219.

Rusteon, T., Wiklund, I., Hanestad, B.R., et al. (1998). Nursing intervention to increase hope and quality of life in newly diagnosed cancer patients. *Cancer Nursing*, 21(4), 235–245.

Sadala, M.L.A. (1999). Taking care as a relationship: A phenomenological view. *Journal of Advanced Nursing*, 30(4), 808–817.

Scanlon, C. and Weir, W.S. (1997). Learning from practice? Mental health nurses' perceptions and experiences of clinical supervision. *Journal of Advanced Nursing*, 26(2), 295–303.

Sloane, A. (1966). Review of "Interpersonal aspects of nursing" by J. Travelbee. *American Journal of Nursing,* 66(6), 77.

Smith, B.A. (1998). The problem drinker's lived experience of suffering: An exploration using hermeneutic phenomenology. *Journal of Advanced Nursing,* 27(1). 213–222.

Snowball, J. (1996). Asking nurses about advocating for patients: "Reactive" and "proactive" accounts. *Journal of Advanced Nursing,* 24(1), 67–75.

Stetler, C. (1977). Relationship of perceived empathy of nurses' communication. *Nursing Research,* 26(6), 432–438.

†Travelbee, J. (1963). What do we mean by "rapport?" *American Journal of Nursing,* 63(2), 70–72.

Travelbee, J. (1964). What's wrong with sympathy? *American Journal of Nursing,* 64(1), 68–71.

Travelbee, J. (1969). *Intervention in psychiatric nursing.* New York: Springer-Verlag.

Travelbee, J. (1971). *Interpersonal aspects of nursing* (2nd ed.). Philadelphia: F.A. Davis.

Travelbee, J. (1971). The nature of nursing. In J. Travelbee (Ed.), *Interpersonal aspects of nursing* (2nd ed., pp. 7–21). Philadelphia: F.A. Davis.

Tuck, I., Wallace, D., and Pullen, L. (2001). Spirituality and spiritual care provided by parish nurses. *Western Journal of Nursing Research,* 23(5), 441–453.

Webb, C. and Hope, K. (1995). What kind of nurses do patients want. *Journal of Clinical Nursing,* 4(2), 101–108.

Williams, A. (2001). A literature review on the concept of intimacy in nursing. *Journal of Advanced Nursing,* 33(5), 660–667.

Willis, W.O. (1999). Culturally competent nursing care during the perinatal period. *Journal of Perinatal and Neonatal Nursing,* 13(3), 45–59.

Wolff, I.S. (1966). Review of "Interpersonal aspects of nursing" by J. Travelbee. *Nursing Outlook,* 1504–1506

36. Jean Watson

Barker, P. and Reynolds, B. (1994). Watson's caring ideology: The proper focus of psychiatric nursing? *Journal of Psychosocial Nursing,* 32, 17–22.

Bennet, P., Porter, B., and Sloan, R. (1989). Jean Watson: Philosophy and science of caring. In A. Marriner-Tomey (Ed.), *Nursing theorists and their work* (2nd ed.). St. Louis, MO: C.V. Mosby.

Bevis, E.O. and Watson, J. (1989). *Toward a caring curriculum: A new pedagogy for nursing* (pp. iii-xix, 1–394). New York: National League for Nursing.

Boyd, C. and Mast, D. (1989). Watson's model of human care. In J.J. Fitzpatrick and A.L. Whall (Eds.), *Conceptual models of nursing: Analysis and application* (2nd ed.). Norwalk, CT: Appleton & Lange.

Bunkers, S.S., Michaels, C.and Ethridge, P. (1997). Advanced practice nursing in community: Nursing's opportunity. *Advanced Practice Nursing Quarterly,* 2(4), 79–84.

Burns, P. (1991). *Elements of spirituality and Watson's theory of transpersonal caring: Expansion of focus* (pp. 141–153). New York: National League for Nursing.

Carson, M.G. (1992). An application of Watson's theory to group work with the elderly. *Perspectives,* 16(4), 7–13.

Chipman, Y. (1991). Caring: Its meaning and place in the practice of nursing. *Journal of Nursing Education,* 30(4), 171–175.

Clayton, G. (1989). Research testing Watson's theory: The phenomena of caring in an elderly population. In J. Riehl-Sisca (Ed.), *Conceptual models for nursing practice* (3rd ed.). Norwalk, CT: Appleton & Lange.

Cohen, J.A. (1991). Two portraits of caring: A comparison of the artists, Leininger and Watson. *Journal of Advanced Nursing,* 16(8), 899–909.

Cooper, M.C. (1989). Gilligan's different voice: A perspective for nursing. *Journal of Professional Nursing,* 5(1), 10–16.

Fawcett, J. (2002). The nurse theorists: 21st century updates—Jean Watson. *Nursing Science Quarterly,* 15(3), 214–219.

Griffith, K.A. (1999). Holism in the care of the allogeneic bone marrow transplant population: Role of the nurse practitioner. *Holistic Nursing Practice,* 13(2), 20–27.

Jones, N., Kearins, J., and Watson, J. (1987). The human tongue show and observers willingness to interact: Replication and extensions. *Psychology Reports,* 60(3, Part 1), 759–764.

Kolcaba, K.Y. and Kolcaba, R.J. (1991). An analysis of the concept of comfort. *Journal of Advanced Nursing,* 16(11), 1301–1310.

Krysl, M. and Watson, J. (1988). Existential moments of caring: Facets of nursing and social support. *Advances in Nursing Science,* 10(2), 12–17.

Marckx, B. B. (1995). Watson's theory of caring: A model for implementation in practice. *Journal of Nursing Care Quality,* 9, 43–54.

Martin, L.S. (1991). Using Watson's theory to explore the dimensions of adult polycystic kidney disease. *American Nephrology Nurses Association Journal,* 18(5), 493–496, 499.

McCance, T.V., McKenna, H.P., and Boore, J.R. (1999). Caring: Theoretical perspectives of relevance to nursing. *Journal of Advanced Nursing,* 30(6), 1388–1395.

McKay, P., Rajacich, D., and Rosenbaum, J. (2002). Enhancing palliative care through Watson's carative factors. *Canadian Oncology Nursing Journal,* 12(1), 34–38.

Mendyka, B.E. (2000). Exploring culture in nursing: A theory-driven practice. *Holistic Nursing Practice,* 15(1). 32–41.

Mitchell, G.J. and Cody, W.K. (1992). Nursing knowledge and human science: Ontological and epistemological considerations. *Nursing Science Quarterly,* 5(2), 54–61.

Mullaney, J.A.B. (2000). The lived experience of using Watson's actual caring occasion to treat depressed women. *Journal of Holistic Nursing,* 18(2), 129–142.

Nelson-Marten, P., Hecomovich, K. and Pangle, M. (1998). Caring theory: A framework for advanced practice nursing. *Advanced Practice Nursing Quarterly,* 4(1), 70–77.

Norred, C.L. (2000). Minimizing preoperative anxiety with alternative caring-healing therapies. *Journal of the Association of periOperative Registered Nurses,* 72(5), 838–840.

Perry, B. (1998). Beliefs of eight exemplary oncology nurses related to Watson's nursing theory. *Canadian Oncology Nursing Journal,* 8(2), 97–107.

Piccinato, J.M. and Rosenbaum, J.N. (1997). Caregiver hardiness explored within Watson's Theory of Human Caring in Nursing. *Journal of Gerontological Nursing,* 23(10), 32–39.

Rafael, A.R. (2000). Watson's philosophy, science, and theory of human caring as a conceptual framework for guiding community health nursing practice. *Advances in Nursing Science*, 23(2), 34–49.

Ray, M.A. (1997). Consciousness and the moral ideal: A transcultural analysis of Watson's theory of transpersonal caring. *Advanced Practice Nursing Quarterly*, 3(1), 25–31.

Ryan, L. (1989). A critique of nursing: Human science and human care. In J. Riehl-Sisca (Ed.), *Conceptual models for nursing practice* (3rd ed.). Norwalk, CT: Appleton & Lange.

Shroeder, C. and Maeve, M.K. (1992). Nursing care partnerships at the Denver Nursing Project in Human Caring: An application and extension of caring theory in practice. *Advances in Nursing Science,* 15(2), 25–38.

Sithichoke-Rattan, N. (1989). A clinical application of Watson's theory. *Pediatric Nursing,* 15(5), 458–462.

Swanson, K.M. (1991)Empirical development of a middle range theory of caring. *Nursing Research,* 40(3), 161–166.

Walker, C.A. (1996). Coalescing the theories of two nurse visionaries: Parse and Watson. *Journal of Advanced Nursing,* 24(5), 988–996.

Watson, J. (1979). *Nursing: The philosophy and science of caring.* Boston: Little, Brown.

Watson, J. (1981). Conceptual systems of students, practitioners. *Western Journal of Nursing Research*, 3, 197–198.

Watson, J. (1981). The lost art of nursing. *Nursing Forum*, 20, 244–249.

Watson, J. (1981). Some issues related to a science of caring for nursing practice. In M. Leininger (Ed.), *Caring: An essential human need.* Thorofare, NJ: Charles Slack.

Watson, J. (1985). *Nursing: Human science and human care.* Norwalk, CT: Appleton-Century-Crofts.

Watson, J. (1987). *The dream curriculum* (Publication No. 15–2179, pp. 91–104.). New York: National League for Nursing

Watson, J. (1987). Nursing on the caring edge: Metaphorical vignettes. *Advances in Nursing Science,* 10(1), 10–18.

Watson, J. (1987). *The professional doctorate as an entry level into practice* (Publication No. 41–2199, pp. 41–47). New York: National League for Nursing

Watson, J. (1988). *An ethic of caring/curing/nursing qua nursing: Introduction* (Publication No. 15–2237, pp. 1–3). New York: National League for Nursing

Watson, J. (1988). *A case study: Curriculum in transition* (Publication No. 15–2224, pp. 1–8). New York: National League for Nursing.

Watson, J. (1988). Human caring as moral context for nursing education. *Nursing and Health Care,* 9(8), 422–425.

Watson, J. (1988). New dimensions of human caring theory. *Nursing Science Quarterly,* 1(4), 175–181.

Watson, J. (1988). *Nursing: Human science and human care. A theory of nursing* (Publication No. 15–2236, pp. 1–104). New York: National League for Nursing.

Watson, J. (1989). Watson's philosophy and theory of human caring. In J. Riehl-Sisca (Ed.), *Conceptual models for nursing practice* (3rd ed.). Norwalk, CT: Appleton & Lange.

Watson, J. (1990). Caring knowledge and informed moral passion. *Advances in Nursing Science,* 13(1), 15–24.

Watson, J. (2002). Intentionality and caring-healing consciousness: A practice of transpersonal nursing. *Holistic Nursing Practice*, 16(4), 12–19.

Watson, J. and Smith, M.C. (2002). Caring science and the science of unitary human beings: A transtheoretical discourse for nursing knowledge development. *Journal of Advanced Nursing*, 37(5), 452–461.

37. Ernestine Wiedenbach

Adamsen, L., Rasmussen, J.M. and Pedersen, L.S. (2001). "Brothers in arms": How men with cancer experience a sense of comradeship through group intervention which combines physical activity with information relay. *Journal of Clinical Nursing*, 10(4), 528–537.

Anderson, C. and Adamsen, L. (2001). Continuous video recording: A new clinical research tool for studying the nursing care of cancer patients. *Journal of Advanced Nursing*, 35(2), 257–267.

Bennett, A.M. and Foster, P.C. (1980). Ernestine Wiedenbach. In The Nursing Theories Conference Group, *Nursing theories: The base for professional nursing practice*. Englewood Cliffs, NJ: Prentice-Hall.

Burst, H.V. (1998). In memorium—Ernestine Widenbach, DNM, MA, FACNM. *Journal of Nurse-Midwifery,* 43(5), 361–362.

Burst, H.V. (2000). The circle of safety: A tool for clinical preceptors. *Journal of Midwifery and Women's Health,* 45(5), 408–410.

Clausen, J. et al. (1977). *Maternity nursing today*. New York: McGraw-Hill.

Danko, M., Hunt, N., Marich, J., Marriner-Tomey, A., McCreary, C., and Stuart, M. (1989). Ernestine Wiedenbach: The helping art of clinical nursing. In A. Marriner-Tomey (Ed.), *Nursing theorists and their work* (2nd ed.). St. Louis, MO: C.V. Mosby.

Dickoff, J., James, P., and Wiedenbach, E. (1968). Theory in a practice discipline. *Nursing Research*, 19(5), 415–427.

Diers, D. (1966). The nurse orientation system: A method for analyzing nurse-patient interactions. *Nursing Research*, 15(1), 91.

Dracup, K. and Breu, C. (1978). Using nursing research findings to meet the needs of grieving spouses. *Nursing Research*, 27(4), 212–216.

Dumas, R. and Leonard, R. (1963). The effect of nursing on the incidence of postoperative vomiting. *Nursing Research*, 12(1), 12–15.

Eisler, J., Wolfer, J.A., and Diers, D. (1972). Relationship between the need for social approval and postoperative recovery welfare. *Nursing Research*, 21(5), 520–525.

Elms, R.R. and Leonard, R.C. (1966). Effects of nursing approaches during admission. *Nursing Research*, 15(1), 37–48.

Flannery, J. and Van Gaasbeek, D.E. (1998). Factors of job satisfaction of the psychiatric clinical nurse specialist. *Nursing Connections*, 11(4), 27–36.

Hilton, P.A. (1997). Theoretical perspectives of nursing: A review of the literature. *Journal of Advanced Nursing*, 26(6), 1211–1220.

Larson, P.A. (1977). Nurse perception of client illness. *Nursing Research*, 26(6), 416–421.

Leonard, R.C., Skipper, J.K., and Woolridge, P.J. (1967). Small sample field experiments for evaluating patient care. *Health Services Research*, 2(1), 46–50.

Raleigh, E. (1983). Wiedenbach's model. In J.J. Fitzpatrick and A.L. Whall (Eds.), *Conceptual models of nursing: Analysis and application.* Bowie, MD: Robert J. Brady Co.

Raleigh, E. (1989). Wiedenbach's model of nursing practice. In J.J. Fitzpatrick and A.L. Whall (Eds.), *Conceptual models of nursing: Analysis and application* (2nd ed.). Norwalk, CT: Appleton & Lange.

Rickelman, B.L. (1971). Bio-psychosocial linguistics: A conceptual approach to nurse-patient interaction. *Nursing Research*, 20(5), 398–403.

Sharp, E.S. (1998). Ethics in reproductive health care: A midwifery perspective. *Journal of Nurse-Midwifery,* 43(3), 235–245.

Shields, D. (1978). Nursing care in labor and patient satisfaction. A descriptive study. *Journal of Advances in Nursing,* 3, 535–550.

Trivette, C.M., Dunst, C.J., Boyd, K., et al. (1996). Family-oriented program models, helpgiving practices, and parental control appraisals. *Exceptional Children*, 62(3), 237–248.

VandeVusse, L. (1997). Sculpting a nurse-midwifery philosophy—Ernestine Wiedenbach's influence. *Journal of Nurse-Midwifery,* 42(1), 43–48.

Villafuerte, A. (1996). Structured clinical preparation time for culturally diverse baccalaureate nursing students. *International Journal of Nursing Studies,* 33(2), 161–170.

Wallace, C.L. and Appleton, C. (1995). Nursing as the promotion of well-being—The client's experience. *Journal of Advanced Nursing,* 22(2), 285–289.

White, J. (1995). Patterns of knowing—Review, critique and update. *Advances in Nursing Science*, 17(4), 73–86.

Wiedenbach, E. (1962, June). *A concept of dynamic nursing: Philosophy, purpose, practice, and process*. A Conference on Maternal and Child Nursing, University of Pittsburg School of Nursing.

Wiedenbach, E. (1963). The helping art of nursing. *American Journal of Nursing*, 63(11), 54–57.

Wiedenbach, E. (1964). *Clinical nursing: A helping art.* New York: Springer-Verlag.

Wiedenbach, E. (1965). Family nurse practitioner for maternal and child care. *Nursing Outlook*, 13, 50–51.

Wiedenbach, E. (1968). Nurse's role in family planning: A conceptual base for practice. *Nursing Clinics of North America,* 3(2), 355–365.

Wiedenbach, E. (1969). *Meeting the realities in clinical teaching.* New York: Springer-Verlag.

Wiedenbach, E. (1970). Comment on beliefs and values: Basis for curriculum design. *Nursing Research*, 19(5), 427.

Wiedenbach, E. (1970). Nurses' wisdom in nursing theory. *American Journal of Nursing,* 70(5), 1057–1062.

Wiedenbach, E. (1973). The nursing process in maternity nursing. In J.P. Clausen et al. (Eds.), *Maternity nursing today*. New York: McGraw-Hill.

Wiedenbach, E. and Falls, C.E. (1978). *Communication: Key to effective nursing.* New York: Tiresias Press.

Wilmoth, T.A. and Elder, J.P. (1995). An assessment of research on breast-feeding promotion strategies in developing countries. *Social Science and Medicine,* 41(4), 579–594.

Wolfer, J. and Visintainer, M. (1975). Pediatric surgical patients' and parents' stress responses and adjustment. *Nursing Research*, 24(4), 244–255.

Paradigms That Have Influenced Nursing

38. Psychoanalytic Theory

Alexander, F. (1958). Unexplored areas in psychoanalytic theory and treatment. *Behavioral Sciences*, 3, 293–316.

Brams, J. (1968). From Freud to Fromm. *Psychology Today*, 1, 32–35, 64–65.

Brenner, C. (1973). *An elementary textbook of psychoanalysis*. Garden City, NY: International Universities Press.

Brill, A.A. (1922). *Psychoanalysis, its theories and practical application* (3rd ed.). Philadelphia: W.B. Saunders.

Brill, A.A. (1969). *Basic principles of psychoanalysis* (1921). Garden City, NY: Doubleday.

Burchard, E.M.L. (1960). Mystical and scientific aspects of the psychoanalytic theories of Freud, Adler, and Jung. *American Journal of Psychotherapy*, 15, 289–307.

Chertok, L. (1968). From Liebeault to Freud. *American Journal of Psychotherapy*, 22, 96–101.

Corsini, R. (1977). *Current personality theories*. Itasca IL: F.A. Peacock Publisher.

Desmonde, W.H., Mead, G.H., and Freud, S. (1957). American social psychology and psychoanalysis. *Psychoanalysis*, 4 & 5, 31–50.

Engel, G.L. (1980). The clinical application of the biopsychosocial model. *American Journal of Psychiatry*, 137(5), 535–544.

Engel, G.L. (1977, April). The need for a new medical model: A challenge for biomedicine. *Science*, 196, 129–135.

Fenichel, O. (1945). *The psychoanalytic theory of neurosis* (pp. 3–13). New York: W.W. Norton.

Fine, R. (1962). *Freud: A critical re-evaluation of his theories*. New York: McKay.

Fine, R. (1979). *A history of psychoanalysis*. New York: Columbia University Press.

Freedman, A., Kaplan, H., and Sadock, B. (1976). *Modern synopsis of comprehensive psychiatry* (2nd ed.). Baltimore: Williams & Wilkins.

Ford, D.H. and Urban, H.B. (1963). *Systems of psychotherapy: A comparative study*. New York: John Wiley & Sons.

Freud, S. (1924). *The complete introductory lectures on psychoanalysis*. New York: Pocket Books.

Freud, S. (1924). *A general introduction to psycho-analysis*. New York: Pocket Books.

Freud, S. (1925–1950). *Collected papers* (Vols. I-V). London: Hogarth.

Freud, S. (1938). *The basic writings of Sigmund Freud*. A.A. Brill (Ed.). New York: Random House.

Freud, S. (1946). *An autobiographical study* (1935), rev'd ed. London: Hogarth.

Freud, S. (1953–1955). *The standard edition of the complete psychological works* (24 Vols.). J. Strachey (Trans.). London: Hogarth.

Freud, S. (1954). *The origin of psychoanalysis: Letters to Wilhelm Fleiss*. E. Mosbacher and J. Strachey (Trans.), M. Bonaparte, A. Freud, and E. Dris (Eds.). New York: Basic Books.

Freud, S. (1957). *A general selection of the works of Sigmund Freud.* J. Rickman (Ed.). New York: Liveright.

Freud, S. (1959). *Beyond the pleasure principle.* J. Strachey (Trans.). New York: Bantam Books.

Freud, S. (1959). *Collected papers.* New York: Basic Books.

Freud, S. (1962). *The ego and the id.* J. Riviere and J. Strachey (Trans.). New York: W.W. Norton.

Freud, S. (1963). *Dora: An analysis of a case of hysteria.* P. Reiff (Ed.). New York: Macmillan.

Freud, S. (1965). *The interpretation of dreams.* J. Strachey (Ed.). New York: Avon Books.

Freud, S. (1965). *The psychopathology of everyday life.* New York: W.W. Norton.

Freud, S. (1966). *On the history of the psychoanalytic movement.* New York: W.W. Norton.

Freud, S. (1969). *An outline of psycho-analysis.* New York: W.W. Norton.

Glover, E. (1959). *Freud or Jung.* New York: W.W. Norton.

Goshen, C.E. (1952). The original case material of psychoanalysis. *American Journal of Psychiatry,* 108, 829–832.

Hall, C. (1954). *A primer of Freudian psychology.* New York: New American Library.

Hall, C.S. and Lindzey, G. (1970). *Theories of personality.* New York: John Wiley & Sons.

Janger J. (1968). *Theories of development.* New York: Holt, Rinehart & Winston.

Johnstone, R.L. (1982). Individual psychotherapy: Relationship of theoretical approaches to nursing conceptual models. In J.J. Fitzpatrick, A.L. Whall, R.L. Johnstone, and J.S. Floyd (Eds.), *Nursing models and their psychiatric mental health applications.* Bowie, MD: Robert J. Brady.

Jones, E. (1953, 1955, 1957). *The life and work of Sigmund Freud* (3 Vols.). New York: Basic Books.

Kardinar, A., Karush, A., and Ovesey, L. (1966). A methodological study of Freudian theory. *International Journal of Psychiatry,* 2, 489–544.

Kolb, L.C. (1977). *Modern clinical psychiatry.* Philadelphia: W.B. Saunders.

Krech, D. and Klein, G.S. (1966). *Theoretical models and personality theory.* New York: Greenwood Press.

Mahler, M. et al. (1975). *The psychological birth of the human infant.* New York: Basic Books.

Mehrabian, A. (1968). *An analysis of personality theories.* Englewood Cliffs, NJ: Prentice-Hall.

Munroe, R.L. (1955). *Schools of psychoanalytic thought.* New York: Dryden Press.

Murphy, G. (1956). The current impact of Freud upon psychology. *American Psychologist,* 11, 663–672.

Pervin, L.A. (1975). *Personality: Theory, assessment, and research.* New York: John Wiley & Sons.

Reiser, M.F. (1979). Psychosomatic medicine: A meeting ground for oriental and occidental medical theory and practice. *Psychotherapy Psychosomatics,* 31, 315–323.

Schmid, F. (1952). Freud's sociological thinking. *Bulletin of the Menninger Clinic,* 16, 1–13.

Shakow, N. and Rapaport, D. (1964). The influence of Freud on American psychology. *Psychological Issues,* 4, 1–243.

Shaw, M.E. and Costanzo, P.R. (1982). *Theories of social psychology* (2nd ed.). New York: McGraw-Hill.

Sherman, M.H. (1966). *Psychoanalysis in America.* Springfield, IL: Charles C. Thomas.

Sherwood, M. (1969). *The logic of explanation in psychoanalysis.* New York: Academic Press.

Stafford-Clark, D. (1967). *What Freud really said.* New York: Schoken Books.

Stone, I. (1971). *The passions of the mind.* New York: Doubleday.

Toman, W. (1960). *An introduction to psychoanalytic theory of motivation.* New York: Pergamon Press.

Turiell, E. (1967). An historical analysis of the Freudian conception of the superego. *Psychoanalytical Review,* 54, 118–140.

Waelder, R. (1960). *Basic theory of psychoanalysis.* New York: International Universities Press.

West, R. (1967). The social significance of the uncompleted father analysis of Sigmund Freud. *Psychotherapy Psychosomatics,* 15, 69.

Wolff, P.H. (1960). *The developmental psychologies of Jean Piaget and psychoanalysis.* New York: International University Press.

39. Symbolic Interaction

Allport, G.W. (1955). *Becoming: Basic considerations for a psychology of personality.* New Haven, CT: Yale University Press.

Banton, M. (1965). *Roles: An introduction to the study of social relations.* New York: Basic Books.

Benzies, K.M. and Allen, M.N. (2001). Symbolic interactionism as a theoretical perspective for multiple method research. *Journal of Advanced Nursing,* 33(4), 541–547.

Biddle, B.J. and Thomas, E.J. (1966). *Role theory: Concepts and research.* New York, John Wiley & Sons.

Blasi, A. (1972). Symbolic interactions as theory. *Sociology and Social Research,* 56(4), 453–455.

Blumer, H. (1966). Sociological implications of the thought of George Herbert Mead. *American Journal of Sociology,* 71, 535–544.

Blumer, H. (1969). *Symbolic interactionism: Perspective and method.* Englewood Cliffs, NJ: Prentice-Hall.

Blumer, H. (1980). Mead and Blumer: The convergent methodological perspectives of social behaviorism and symbolic interactionism. *American Sociological Review,* 45, 409–419.

Bower, F. and Jacobson, M.J. (1979). Family theories: Frameworks for nursing practice. In S.E. Archer and R. Fleshman (Eds.), *Community health nursing: Patterns and practice* (2nd ed.). North Scituate, MA: Duxbury Press.

Burr, W.R., Leigh, G.K., Day, R.D., and Constantine, J. (1979). Symbolic interaction and the family. In W.R. Burr, R. Hill, F.I. Nye, and I.L. Reiss, (Eds.): *Contemporary theories about the family, Vol 2: General theories/theoretical orientations.* New York: Free Press.

Charon, J. (1979). *Symbolic interaction.* Englewood Cliffs, NJ: Prentice-Hall.

Coser, L.A. (1971). George Herbert Mead, 1863–1931. In *Masters of sociological thought* (pp. 333–355). New York: Harcourt Brace Jovanovich.

Cottrell, L.S., Jr. (1942). The adjustment of the individual to his age and sex roles. *American Sociological Review,* 7, 617–620.

Gordon, C. and Gerzen, K.J. (1968). *The self in social interaction* (Vol. I). *Classic and contemporary perspectives.* New York: John Wiley & Sons.

Gordon, G. (1966). *Role theory and illness: A sociological perspective.* New Haven, CT: College and University Press.

Hammer, M.L. (1977). Symbols of aging as perceived by the young. *Journal of Gerontological Nursing,* 3(4), 17–18.

Hewitt, J. (1983). *Self and society: A symbolic interactionist social psychology* (3rd ed.). Boston: Allyn & Bacon.

Huber, J. (1973). Symbolic interaction as a pragmatic perspective: The bias of emergent theory. *American Sociological Review,* 38(2), 274–284.

Kuhn, M.H. (1964). Major trends in symbolic interaction theory in the past twenty-five years. *Sociological Quarterly,* 5, 61–84.

Laborde, J.M. (1979). Symbolism and gift-giving in family therapy. *Journal of Psychiatric Nursing,* 17(4), 32–35.

Linton, R. (1936). *The study of man.* New York: Appleton-Century-Crofts.

Manis, J.G. and Meltzer, B.N. (1972). *Symbolic interaction* (2nd ed.). Boston: Allyn & Bacon.

McPhail, C. and Rexroth, C. (1979). The divergent methodological perspectives of social behaviorism and symbolic interactionism. *American Sociological Review,* 44, 449–467.

Mead, G.H. (1937). *Mind, self and society.* Introduction by C.W. Morris. Chicago: University of Chicago Press.

Mead, G.H. (1956). *The social psychology of G.H. Mead.* Edited and with revised introduction by A. Strauss. Chicago: University of Chicago Press.

Meltzer, B.N. (1972). Mead's social psychology. In J.G. Manis and B.N. Meltzer (Eds.), *Symbolic interaction: A reader in social psychology* (2nd ed.). Boston: Allyn & Bacon.

Mowrer, O.H. (1960). *Learning theory and the symbolic process.* New York: John Wiley & Sons.

Porter, S.F. (1978). Interaction modeling: An educational strategy for new graduate leadership development. *Journal of Nursing Administration,* 8(4), 20–24.

Rickelman, B.L. (1971). Bio-psychosocial linguistics: A conceptual approach to nurse-patient interaction. *Nursing Research,* 20(5), 398–403.

Riehl, J.P. (1974). Application of interaction theory. In J.P. Riehl and C. Roy (Eds.), *Conceptual models for nursing practice.* New York: Appleton-Century-Crofts.

Rose, A. (1960). Incomplete socialization: Sociology and socialization. *Nursing Research,* 44, 244–250.

Rose, A. (Ed.). (1962). *Human behavior and social processes: An interactional approach.* Boston: Houghton-Mifflin.

Rose, A. (1974). A systematic summary of symbolic interaction theory. In J.P. Riehl and C. Roy (Eds.), *Conceptual models for nursing practice* (pp. 34–46). New York: Appleton-Century-Crofts.

Sarbin, T. (1954). Role theory. In G. Lindzey (Ed.), *Handbook of social psychology* (Vol. 1, pp. 223–258). Cambridge, MA: Addison-Wesley.

Sarbin, T. (1968). Role theory. In G. Lindzey and E. Aronson (Eds.), *Handbook of social psychology* (Vol. 1, 2nd ed., pp. 488–567). Cambridge, MA: Addison-Wesley.

Schroeder, K.A. (1981). Symbolic interactionism: A conceptual framework useful for nurses working with obese persons. *Image: Journal of Nursing Scholarship,* 13(3), 78–81.

Shibutani, T. (1961). *Society and personality.* Englewood Cliffs, NJ: Prentice-Hall.

Shott, S. (1979). Emotion and social life: A symbolic interactionist analysis. *American Journal of Sociology,* 84(2), 1317–1334.

Simmel, G. (1964). *The sociology of Georg Simmel.* K.H. Wolff (Ed., Trans.). New York: Free Press.

Strauss, A. (Ed.). (1956). *The social psychology of George H. Mead.* Chicago: University of Chicago Press.

Strauss, A. (1977). Sociological theories of personality. In R. Corsini (Ed.), *Current personality theories* (pp. 277–281). Itasca, IL: F.E. Peacock Publisher.

Strauss, A. and Fisher, B.M. (1978). *Interactionism (working paper).* University of California San Francisco and New York University.

Stryker, S. (1959). Symbolic interaction as an approach to family research. *Marriage Family Living,* 21, 111–119.

Turner, R.H. (1956). Role taking, role standpoint, and reference group behavior. *American Journal of Sociology,* 61, 316–328.

Turner, R.H. (1962). Role taking: Process vs. conformity. In A. Rose (Ed.), *Human behavior and social processes* (pp. 20–40) Boston: Houghton-Mifflin.

Turner, R.H. (1968). The self-conception in social interaction. In C. Gordon and K.J. Gergen (Eds.), *Self in social interaction.* New York: John Wiley & Sons.

Turner, R.H. (1978). *The structure of sociological theory* (2nd ed., Chap. 14–17). Homewood, IL: Dorsey Press.

40. Holism

Abbot, E.A. (1984). *Flatland: A romance of many dimensions.* New York: Signet.

Agan, R.D. (1987). Intuitive knowing as a dimension of nursing. *Advances in Nursing Science,* 10(1), 63–70.

Barnum, B.J.S. (1994). *Nursing theory: Analysis, application, and evaluation* (4th ed.). Philadelphia: J.B. Lippincott.

Bollinger, E. (2001). Applied concepts of holistic nursing. *Journal of Holistic Nursing,* 19(2), 212–214.

Drevdahl. D. (1999). Sailing beyond: Nursing theory and the person. *Advances in Nursing Science,* 21(4), 1–13.

Duhl, L. (1986). Health and the inner and outer self. *Journal of Humanistic Psychology,* 26(3), 46–61.

Flynn, P. (1980). *Holistic health.* Bowie, MD: Robert J. Brady Co.

Fuller, G. (1978). Holistic man and the science and practice of nursing. *Nursing Outlook,* 26(11), 700–704.

Hall, B. A. and Allan, J. D. (1994). Self in relation: A prolegomenon for holistic nursing. *Nursing Outlook*, 42(3), 110–116.

Harmon, W. and Rheingold, H. (1984). *Higher creativity: Liberating the unconscious for breakthrough insights*. Los Angeles: Jeremy P. Tarcher.

Holmes, C. A. (1990). Alternatives to natural science: Foundations for nursing. *International Journal of Nursing Studies*, 27, 187–198.

Kalischuk; R.G. and Davies, B. (2001). A theory of healing in the aftermath of youth suicide: Implications for holistic nursing practice. *Journal of Holistic Nursing*, 19(2), 163–186.

Kolcaba, R. (1997). The primary holisms in nursing. *Journal of Advanced Nursing*, 25(2), 290–296.

Mast, D. (1986). Effects of imagery. *Image: Journal of Nursing Scholarship*, 18(3), 118–120.

Morgan, A. (1998). Holism in nursing. *Australian Journal of Holistic Nursing*, 5(2), 32–35.

Mulholland, J. (1995). Nursing, humanism, and transcultural theory: The 'bracketing-out' of reality. *Journal of Advanced Nursing*, 22, 442–449.

Reed, P.G. (1998). A holistic view of nursing concepts and theories in practice. *Journal of Holistic Nursing*, 16(4), 415–419.

Schnect, K. (1985). Convergence, energy and optimal health. *Journal of Holistic Medicine*, 7(2), 178–193.

Smith, M. (1984). Transformation: The key to shaping nursing. *Image: Journal of Nursing Scholarship*, 16(1), 28–30.

Woods, S. (1998). A theory of holism for nursing. *Medicine, Health Care, and Philosophy*, 1(3), 255–261.

Yorks, L. and Sharoff, L. (2001). An extended epistemology for fostering transformative learning in holistic nursing education and practice. *Holistic Nursing Practice*, 16(1), 21–29.

41. Organizational Theory

Astley, W.G. (1985). Administrative science as socially constructed truth. *Administrative Science Quarterly*, 30, 497–513.

Daffe, R.L. (1986). *Organization theory and design* (2nd ed.). St. Paul, MN: West Publishing.

Hegyvary, S., Duxbury, M., Hall, R., Krueger, J., Lindeman, C., Scott, J., and Scott, W. (1987). *The evolution of nursing professional organizations: Alternative models for the future*. Kansas City, MO: American Academy of Nursing.

Jennings, B.M. and Meleis, A.I. (1988). Nursing theory and administrative nursing practice: Agenda for the 1990s. *Advances in Nursing Science*, 10(3), 56–69.

Kast, F.E. and Rosenzweig, J.E. (1985). The subject is organizations. In *Organization and management: A systems and contingency approach* (pp. 3–22). New York: McGraw-Hill.

Rakich, J., Longest, B., and Darr, K. (1985). *Managing health services organization* (2nd ed.). Philadelphia: W.B. Saunders.

Scott, W. (1987). The subject is organizations. In *Organizations: Rational, natural and open systems* (pp. 3–27). Englewood Cliffs, NJ: Prentice-Hall.

Roberts, S. (1980). Piaget's theory reapplied to the critically ill. *Advances in Nursing Science*, 2(2), 61–79.

Rowe, G.P. (1966). The developmental conceptual framework to the study of the family. In F.I. Nye and F.M. Berardo (Eds.), *Emerging conceptual frameworks in family analysis*. New York: Praeger.

Sanford, N. (1966). *Self and society: Social change and individual development*. New York: Atherton Press.

Schaie, W.K. (1977–1978). Toward a stage theory of adult cognitive development. *International Journal of Aging and Human Development*, 8(2), 129–138.

Schuster, C. (1980). *The process of human development*. Boston: Little, Brown.

Sheehy, G. (1976). *Passages: Predictable crises of adult life*. New York: E.P. Dutton.

Sullivan, C., Grant, M.Q., and Grant, J.D. (1957). The development of interpersonal maturity: Application to delinquency. *Psychiatry*, 20, 373–385.

Sullivan, H.S. (1953). *Interpersonal theory of psychiatry*. New York: W.W. Norton.

Thibaut, J.W. and Kelley, H.H. (1967). *The social psychology of groups, Part I: Dyadic Relationships*. New York: John Wiley & Sons.

Thomas, H. (1970). Theory of aging and cognitive theory of personality. *Human Development*, 13(1), 1–16.

Thomas, A. (1981). Current trends in development theory. *American Journal of Orthopsychiatry*, 51(4), 580–609.

Toffler, A. (1971). *Future shock*. New York: Bantam/Random House.

Troll, L.E. (1975). *Early and middle adulthood: The best is yet to be—Maybe*. Monterey, CA: Brooks/Cole.

Van Den Daele, L.D. (1975). Ego development and preferential judgment in life span perspective. In N. Datan and L.H. Ginsberg (Eds.), *Life-span developmental psychology*. New York: Academic Press.

Wadsworth, B.J. (1971). *Piaget's theory of cognitive development*. New York: David McKay Co.

Waechter, E.H. (1980). The developmental model. In M. Kalkman and A. Davis (Eds.). *New dimensions in mental health-psychiatric nursing* (2nd ed.). New York: McGraw-Hill.

Wahba, M. and Bridwell, L.G. (1976). Maslow reconsidered: A review of research on the need for hierarchy theory. *Organizational Behavior and Human Performance*, 15, 212–224.

Wolman, B.B. (Ed.). (1982) *Handbook of developmental psychology*. Englewood Cliffs, NJ: Prentice-Hall.

43. Systems Theory

Abbey, J.C. (1970). General system theory: A framework for nursing. In J. Smith (Ed.), *Improvement of curricula in schools of nursing through selection and application of care concepts of nursing: An interim report*. Boulder, CO: Western Interstate Commission for Higher Education.

Allport, G.W. (1960). The open system in personality theory. *Journal of Abnormal and Social Psychology*, 61, 310–21.

Altschul, A.T. (1978). A systems' approach to the nursing process. *Journal of Advanced Nursing*, 3(4), 333–340.

Barnum, B.J.S. (1994). *Nursing theory: Analysis, application, and evaluation* (4th ed.). Philadelphia, PA: J.B. Lippincott.

Battista, J.R. (1977). The holistic paradigm and general systems theory. *General Systems Yearbook*, 22, 65–71.

Beavers, W.R. (1977). Systems theory, family systems, and the self. In *Psychotherapy and growth: A family perspective* (pp. 19–41). New York: Brunner-Mazel.

Becht G. (1974, October). Systems theory, the key to holism and reductionism. *Bio Science*, 24(10), 569–578.

Bertalanffy, L. von. (1967). *Robots, men and minds.* Part 2. New York: George Braziller.

Bertalanffy, L. von. (1968). *General systems theory: Foundations, development application*, rev'd ed. New York: George Braziller.

Bertalanffy, L. von. (1969). General systems theory and psychiatry—An overview. In W. Gray et al. (Eds.). *General systems theory and psychiatry* (pp. 33–50). Boston: Little, Brown.

Bertalanffy, L. von. (1975). *Perspectives on general systems theory.* New York: George Braziller.

Black, M. (1961). *The social theories of Talcott Parsons: A critical examination.* Englewood Cliffs, NJ: Prentice-Hall.

Boulding, K.E. (1956). General systems theory—The skeleton of science. *Management Science*, 2, 197–208.

Brody, H. and Sobel, D.S. (1980). A systems view of health and disease. *Holistic Health Review*, 3(3), 163–178.

Broderick, C. and Smith, J. (1979). The general systems approach to family. In W.R. Burr (Ed.), *Contemporary theories about the family* (pp. 112–129). New York: Free Press.

Buckley, W. (1967). *Sociology and modern systems theory.* Englewood Cliffs, NJ: Prentice-Hall.

Bunge, M. (1977). General systems and holism. *General Systems Yearbook*, 22, 87–90.

Bunge, M. (1979). A systems concept of society; beyond individualism and holism. *General Systems Yearbook*, 24, 27–44.

Chin, R. (1961). The utility of system models and developmental models for practitioners. In W.G. Bennis, K.D. Benne and R. Chin (Eds.), *The planning of change.* New York: Holt, Rinehart & Winston.

Chinn, P.L. (1979). Practice oriented theory: Part 2. *Advances in Nursing Science*, 1(2), 41–52.

Chrisman, M. and Riehl, J. (1980). The system-developmental stress model. In J.P. Riehl and C. Roy (Eds.), *Conceptual models for nursing practice* (2nd ed.). New York: Appleton-Century-Crofts.

Churchman, C.W. (1968). *The systems approach.* New York: Dell.

Cummings, T.G. (Ed.). (1981). *Systems theory for organizational development.* New York: John Wiley & Sons.

Demerath, N.J. and Peterson, R.A. (Eds.). (1967). *System, change and conflict.* New York: Free Press.

Emery, F.E. (Ed.). (1969). *Systems thinking.* Middlesex, England: Penguin Books.

Ericson, R.F. (1979). Society for general systems research at twenty-five. What agenda for our second quarter century? *Behavioral Science,* 24(5), 225–237.

Gray, W. (1972). Bertalanffian principles as a basis for humanistic psychiatry. In E. Laszlo (Ed.), *The relevance of general systems theory.* New York: George Braziller.

Grinker, R.R. (Ed.). (1967). *Toward a unified theory of human behavior: An introduction to general systems theory,* rev'd ed. New York: Basic Books.

Hall, A.D. and Fagen, R.E. (1956). Definition of system. *General Systems Yearbook,* 1, 18–28.

Hamilton, G.A. (1979, January). Miller's living systems: A theory critique. *Advances in Nursing Science,* 1(2), 41–52.

Hazzard, M.E. (1971). An overview of systems theory. *Nursing Clinics of North America,* 6(3), 385–393.

Jantsch, E. (1970). Inter- and transdisciplinary university: A systems approach to education and innovation. *Policy Sciences,* 1, 403–428.

Kalmus, H. (Ed.). (1966). *Regulation and control in living systems.* New York: John Wiley & Sons.

Laszlo, E. (Ed.). (1972). *The relevance of general systems theory.* New York: George Braziller.

Laszlo, E. (1972). *The systems view of the world.* New York: George Braziller.

Laszlo, E. (1975). The meaning and significance of general systems theory. *Behavioral Science,* 20(1), 9–24.

Lilienfeld, R. (1978). *The rise of systems theory: An ideological analysis.* New York: John Wiley & Sons.

Maslow, A.H. (1970). *Motivation and personality* (2nd ed.). New York: Harper & Row.

Miller, J. (1965). Living systems: Basic concepts. *Behavioral Science,* 10, 193–237.

Parsons, T. (1951). *The social system.* London: Free Press of Glencoe.

Parsons. T. (1967). *Sociological theory and modern society.* New York: Free Press.

Pierce, L.M. (1972). Usefulness of a systems approach for problem conceptualization and investigation. *Nursing Research,* 21, 509–513.

Powers, P.S. and Girgenti, J.R. (1978). Analysis of a system. *Journal of Psychosocial Nursing and Mental Health Services,* 17–22.

Prigogine, I. and Stengers, I. (1984). *Order out of chaos.* New York: Bantam Books.

Rapoport, A. (1970). Modern systems theory—An outlook for coping with change. *General Systems Yearbook,* 15, 15–25.

Ritterman, M.K. (1977). Paradigmatic classification of family therapy theories. *Family Process,* 16(1), 29–48.

Rudolph, E. (1980). Defining the parameters of general living systems theory. *The Family,* 7(2), 83–91.

Shrode, W.A. and Voich, D. (1974). *Organization and management: Basic systems concepts.* Homewood, IL: R.D. Irwin.

Sills, G.M. and Hall, J.E. (1977). A general systems perspective for nursing. In J.E. Hall and B.R. Weaver (Eds.), *Distributive nursing practice: A systems approach to community health* (pp. 19–28). Philadelphia: J.B. Lippincott.

Somers, J.B. (1977). Purpose and performance: A system analysis of nurse staffing. *Journal of Nursing Administration,* 7, 4–9.

Stephen W.R. (1978). Toward a redefinition of action theory: Paying the cognitive element its due. *American Journal of Sociology,* 83(6), 1317–1349.

Sutherland, J.W. (1973). *A general systems philosophy for the social and behavioral sciences.* New York: George Braziller.

Tantsch, E. (1970). Inter- and transdisciplinary university: A systems approach to education and innovation. *Policy Sciences,* 1, 403–428.

Tashdjian, E. (1972). A systems approach to higher education with special reference to the core curriculum. *Policy Sciences,* 3, 219–33.

Weiner, N. (1948). *Cybernetics or control and communication in the animal and machine.* Paris: Herman and Cie.

Werley, H.H. et al. (Eds.). (1976). *Health research: The systems approach.* New York: Springer-Verlag.

44. Stress and Adaptation

Appley, M.H. (1971). *Adaptation-level theory: A symposium.* New York: Academic Press.

Auger, J.R. (1976). *Behavioral systems and nursing.* Englewood Cliffs, NJ: Prentice-Hall.

Bell, J.M. (1977). Stressful life events and coping methods in mental illness and wellness behaviors. *Nursing Research,* 26, 136–141.

Brower, H., Terri, F. and Baker, B.J. (1976). Using the adaptation model in a practitioner curriculum. *Nursing Outlook,* 24, 686–689.

Bruner, J. et al. (1966). *Studies in cognitive growth.* New York: John Wiley & Sons.

Coelho, G.V., Hamburg, D.A., and Adams, J.E. (1974). Introduction. In G.V. Coelho et al. (Eds.), *Coping and adaptation.* New York: Basic Books.

Cohen, F. and Lazarus, R. (1979). Coping with the stresses of illness. In G. Stine, F. Cohen, and N. Adler (Eds.), *Health psychology: A handbook.* San Francisco: Jossey-Bass.

Dobzhansky, T. (1962). *Mankind evolving.* New Haven, CT: Yale University Press.

Dobzhansky, T. (1967). Changing man. *Science,* 155, 409–415.

Dubos, R. (1965). Adaptation and its dangers. In *Man adapting* (pp. 254–280). New Haven, CT: Yale University Press.

Duffy, M.E. (1987). The concept of adaptation: Examining alternatives for the study of nursing phenomenon. *Scholarly Inquiry for Nursing Practice,* 3(1), 179–192.

Fagin, C. (1987). Stress: Implications for nursing research. *Image: Journal of Nursing Scholarship,* 19(1), 38–41.

Fielo, F.M.C. (1971). *Psychosocial nursing.* New York: Macmillan.

Folkman, S. and Lazarus, R. (1980). An analysis of coping in a middle-aged community sample. *Journal of Health and Social Behavior,* 21, 219–239.

Gossen, G. and Bush, H. (1979). Adaptation: A feedback process. *Advances in Nursing Science,* 1(4), 51–65.

Haan, N. (1969). A tripartite model of ego functioning values and clinical and research applications. *Journal of Nervous and Mental Disease,* 148, 14–30.

Hamburg, [illegible], Coelho, G.V.. and Adams, J.E. (1974). Coping and adaptation: Steps towa[illegible] synthesis of biological and social perspectives. In G.V. Coelho et al. (Eds.), [illegible]nd adaptation. New York: Basic Books.

Co[illegible] (1966). *Experience, structure and adaptability.* New York: Springer-Verlag.

Harve[illegible] (1959). Adaptation level theory. In S. Koch (Ed.), *Psychology: A study of a* [illegible] (Vol. 1, pp. 565–621). New York: McGraw-Hill.

Helso[illegible]. (1964). *Adaptation level theory* (Chap. 2). New York: Harper & Row.

[illegible] H. (1997). King's theory of goal attainment in practice. *Nursing Science Quar[illegible]y,* 10(4), 180–185.

[illegible] M. and Hammond, H. (1980). Analysis and expansion of the Roy adaptation [illegible]odel: A contribution to holistic nursing. *Advances in Nursing Science,* 2(4), 71–81.

[illegible]ley, B. et al. (1979). Myocardial infarct stress-of-transfer inventory: Development of a research tool. *Nursing Research.* 28(1), 4–10.

[illegible]ray, R. and Zentner, J. (1975). Application of adaptation theory to nursing. In R. Murray and J. Zentner (Eds.), *Nursing concepts for health promotion.* Englewood Cliffs, NJ: Prentice-Hall.

[illegible]urphy, J.F. (1971). *Adaptation as a unifying theory: Theoretical issues in professional nursing* (Chap. 4). New York: Appleton-Century-Crofts, Education Division.

Rabkin, J.G. and Struening, E.L. (1976). Life events, stress and illness. *Science,* 194, 1013–1020.

Redman, B.K. (1974). Why develop a conceptual framework? *Journal of Nursing Education,* 13, 2–10.

Riehl, J and Roy, C. (1974). *Conceptual models for nursing practice.* New York: Appleton-Century-Crofts.

Roy, C. (1971, April). Adaptation: A basis for nursing practice. *Nursing Outlook,* 21, 254–257.

Roy, C. (1973, March). Adaptation: Implications for curriculum change. *Nursing Outlook,* 21, 163–168.

Roy, C. (1974). The Roy adaptation model. In J. Riehl and C. Roy (Eds.), *Conceptual models for nursing practice.* New York: Appleton-Century-Crofts.

Sander, L.W. (1969). The longitudinal course of early mother-child interaction-cross-case comparison in a sample of mother-child pairs. In B.M. Foss (Ed.), *Determinants of infant behavior IV* (pp. 189–227). London: Methuen.

Scott, J. (1977, February). Stress and coping: A case for intervention. *Journal of Psychiatric Nursing and Mental Health Services,* 15, 14–17.

Scott, R. and Howard, A. (1970). Models of stress. In S. Levine and N. Scotch, (Eds.), *Social stress.* Chicago: Aldine.

Scott, D.W., Oberst, M., and Dropkin, M. (1980). A stress-coping model. *Advances in Nursing Science,* 3(1), 9–23.

Scott, D.W., Oberst, M. and Bookbinder, M. (1984). Stress-coping response to genitourinary carcinoma in men. *Nursing Research,* 32(6), 325–329.

Selye, H. (1950). *The physiology and pathology of exposure to stress.* Montreal, Canada: ACTA Medical Publishers.

Selye, H. (1950, June 17). Stress and the general adaptation syndrome. *British Medical Journal,* 1383–1392.

Selye, H. (1964). *From dream to discovery.* New York: McGra
Selye, H. (1965). The stress syndrome. *American Journal of N*
Selye, H. (1976). *The nature of adaptation. The stress of life* (
McGraw-Hill.
Spielberger, C.D. (1972). Anxiety as an emotional state. In *Anxiet*
theory and research (pp. 23–49). New York: Academic Press.
Stone, G., Cohen, F., and Adler, N. (1979). *Health psychology: A handb*
Jossey-Bass.
Thetford, W.N. and Schucman, H. (1971). Motivational factors and ada
In J.A. Downey and R.C. Darling (Eds.), *Physiological basis of rehab*
icine (pp. 353–371). Philadelphia: W.B. Saunders.
Vailliant, G.E. (1977). *Adaptation to life.* Boston: Little, Brown.
Wagner, P. (1976). Testing the adaptation model in practice. *Nursing O*
682–685.
Wild, B.S. and Hanes, C. (1976). A dynamic conceptual framework of generalize
tation to stressful stimuli. *Psychological Reports,* 37, 319–334.

45. Role Theory

Banton, M. (1965). *Roles: An introduction to the study of social relations.* New Yor
Basic Books.
Bem, S. (1975). Sex roles adaptability: One consequence of psychological androgeny. *Journal of Personality and Social Psychology,* 31(4), 634–43.
Berk, B.B. and Victor G. (1975). Selection vs. role occupancy as determinants of role-related attitudes among psychiatric aides. *Journal of Health and Social Behavior,* 16(2), 183–191.
Bertrand, A. (1972). *Social organization: A general systems of role theory perspective.* Philadelphia: F.A. Davis.
Biddle, B. and Thomas, E. (Eds.). (1966). *Role theory: Concepts and research.* New York: John Wiley & Sons.
Biddle, B.J. (1979). *Role theory: Expectations, identities, and behaviors.* New York: Academic Press.
Blasi, A.J. (1971–1972). Symbolic interactionism as theory. *Sociology and Social Research,* 56, 453–465.
Blumer, H. (1969). *Symbolic interactionism: Perspective and method.* Englewood Cliffs, NJ: Prentice-Hall.
Brouse, S.H. (1985). Effect of gender role identity patterns on self concept scores from later pregnancy to early post-partum. *Advances in Nursing Science,* 7(3), 32–48.
Bunch, B. and Zahra, D. (1976). Dealing with death: The unlearned role. *American Journal of Nursing,* 76(9), 1486–1488.
Burke, P.J. and Tully, J.C. (1977). The measurement of role identity. *Social Forces,* 54, 881–897.
Burr, W.R. (1972). Role transitions: A reformulation of theory. *Journal of Marriage and the Family,* 34, 407–416.

Conway, M.E. (1978). Theoretical approaches to the study of roles. In M. Hardy and M. Conway (Eds.), *Role theory: Perspectives for the health professional.* Norwalk, CT: Appleton-Century-Crofts.

Crossan, F. and Robb, A. (1998). Role of the nurse: Introducing theories and concepts. *British Journal of Nursing,* 7(10), 608–612.

Goffman, E. (1969). *Stigma.* Englewood Cliffs, NJ: Prentice-Hall.

Gordon, G. (1966). *Role theory and illness: A sociological perspective.* New Haven, CT: College and University Press.

Gross, N.C., Mason, W.S., and McEachern, A.W. (1958). *Explorations in role analysis: Studies of the school superintendency role.* New York: John Wiley & Sons.

Habeeb, M. and McLaughlin, F. (1977). Health care professional's role expectation and patient needs. *Nursing Research,* 26, 288–298.

Hadley, B.J. (1964). Nursing a la Weber. *Nursing Science,* 4, 95–110.

Hadley, B.J. (1967). The dynamic interactionist concept of role. *Journal of Nursing Education,* 2, 5–10.

Hardy, M. and Conway, M.E. (1989). *Role theory: Perspectives for health professionals.* New York: Appleton-Century-Crofts.

Heiss, J. (1976). *Family roles and interaction: An anthology* (2nd ed.). Chicago: Rand McNally.

Jones, S.L. (1976). Socialization vs. selection factors as sources of student definitions of the nurse role. *International Journal of Nursing Studies,* 13(3), 135–138.

Kassebaum, G. and Baumann, B. (1965). Dimension of the sick role in chronic illness. *Journal of Health and Human Behavior,* 6, 16–27.

Keller, N.S. (1973). The nurse's role: Is it expanding or shrinking? *Nursing Outlook,* 21, 236–240.

Levenstein, A. (1976). Role ambiguity in nursing. *Supervisor Nurse,* 7(6). 16–17.

Lewandowski, L.A. and Kramer, M. (1980). Role transformation of special care unit nurses: A comparative study. *Nursing Research,* 29(3), 170–179.

Lindersmith, A.R. and Strauss, A.L. (1968). Roles, role behavior and social structure. In A.R. Lindersmith, A.L. Strauss, and N.K. Denzin (Eds.), *Social psychology* (3rd ed., pp. 276–298). New York: Holt, Rinehart & Winston.

Lindersmith, A.R., Strauss, A.L., and Denzin, N. (1975). *Social psychology* (4th ed.). Hinsdale, IL: Dryden Press.

Meleis, A.I. (1975). Role insufficiency and role supplementation: A conceptual framework. *Nursing Research,* 24, 264–271.

Meleis, A.I. (1971). Self-concept and family planning. *Nursing Research,* 20, 299–236.

Meleis, A.I. and Swendsen, L.A. (1978). Role supplementation: An empirical test of a nursing intervention. *Nursing Research,* 27(1), 11–18.

Mercer, R.T. (1985). The process of role attainment over the first year. *Nursing Research,* 34, 198–204.

Miyamoto, F.S. (1963). The impact of research of different conceptions of role. *Sociological Inquiry,* 33, 144–123.

Miyamoto, F.S. and Dornbush, S. (1956). A test of the symbolic interactionist hypothesis of self-conception. *American Journal of Sociology,* 61, 399–403.

Morgan, W.R.B. (1975). Role theory: An attribution theory interpretation. *Sociometry,* 38, 429–444.

Morris, C.W. (Ed.). (1962). *Herbert Mead, 1863–1931. Mind, self and society from the standpoint of a social behaviorist.* Chicago: University of Chicago Press.

Murphy, J. (1968). Psychiatric nurses and their patients: A study of role perception of performance. *Communicating Nursing Research,* 1, 139–150.

Oda, D. (1977). Specialized role development, a three phase process. *Nursing Outlook,* 25(6), 374–377.

Plutchik, R., Conte, H.R., Wells, W., and Darasu, T.B. (1976). Role of the psychiatric nurse. *Journal of Psychiatric Nursing and Mental Health Services,* 14(9), 38–43.

Porter, S.F. (1978). Interaction modeling. *Journal of Nursing Administration,* 8, 20–24.

Robischon, P. and Scott, D. (1969). Role theory and its application in family nursing. *Nursing Outlook,* 17, 52–57.

Sarbin, T.R. (1954). Role theory. In G. Lindzey (Ed.), *Handbook of social psychology, Vol. 1. Theory and method* (pp. 223–258). Cambridge, MA: Addison-Wesley.

Sarbin, T.R. and Jones, D.S. (1955, September). An experimental analysis of role behavior. *Journal of Abnormal Social Psychology,* 51, 236–241.

Swendsen, L.A., Meleis, A.I., and Jones, D. (1978). Role supplementation for new parents—A role mastery plan. *MCN, The American Journal of Maternal Child Nursing,* 3, 84–91.

Thornton, R. and Nardi, P. (1975). The dynamics of role acquisition. *American Journal of Sociology,* 80, 870–885.

Turner, R.H. (1962). Role taking: Process vs. conformity. In A. Rose (Ed.), *Human behavior and social processes.* Boston: Houghton-Mifflin.

Turner, R.H. (1970). *Family interaction.* New York: John Wiley & Sons.

Turner, R.H. (1976). The real self from institution to impulse. *American Journal of Sociology,* 81(5), 989–1016.

Turner, R.H. (1978). The role and the person. *American Journal of Sociology,* 84, 1–23.

Turner, R.H. and Shosid, N. (1976). Ambiguity and interchangeability in role attribution: The effect of alter's response. *American Sociological Review,* 41, 993–1006.

Videbeck, R. and Bates, A. (1959). An experimental study of conformity to role expectations. *Sociometry,* 22(1).

Ward, C.R. (1986). The meaning of role strain. *Advances in Nursing Science,* 8(2), 39–49.

Weiss, S.J. (1983). Role differentiation between nurses and physician: Implications for nursing. *Nursing Research,* 32(3), 133–139.

46. Physiological Nursing Theory

Badgley, L.E. (1985). Therapeutic application of extra low frequency electromagnetic fields to living tissue. *Journal of Holistic Medicine,* 7(2), 135–144.

Carrieri, V.K., Lindsey, A.M., and West, C.M. (1986). *Physiological phenomena in nursing: Human responses to illness.* Philadelphia: W.B. Saunders.

Feldman, H.R. (1984). Psychological differentiation and the phenomenon of pain. *Advances in Nursing Science,* 6(2), 50–57.

Janson-Bjerklie, S., Broushey, H.D., Carrieri, V.K., and Lindsey, A.I. (1986). Emotionally triggered asthma as a predictor of airway response to suggestion. *Research in Nursing and Health*, 9, 43–59.

Janson-Bjerklie, S., Carrieri, V., and Hudes, M. (1986). The sensations of dyspnea. *Nursing Research*, 35(3), 154–159.

Longworth, J. (1982). Psychophysiological effects of slow stroke back massage in normotensive females. *Advances in Nursing Science*, 4(4), 44–61.

Ng, L. and McCormick, K. (1982). Position changes and their physiological consequences. *Advances in Nursing Science*, 4(4), 13–25.

47. Critical Theory and Hermeneutics

Baker, C., Norton, S., Young, P., and Ward, S. (1998). An exploration of methodological pluralism in nursing research. *Research in Nursing and Health*, 21(6), 545–555.

Bauman, Z. (1978). *Hermeneutics and society science.* New York: Columbia University Press.

Boutain, D.M. (1999). Critical nursing scholarship: Exploring critical social theory with African American studies. *Advances in Nursing Science*, 21(4), 37–47.

Browne, A.J. (2000). The potential contributions of critical social theory to nursing science. *Canadian Journal of Nursing Research*, 32(2), 35–55.

Bubner, R. et al. (Eds.). (1975). Theory and practice in the light of the hermeneutic-criticist controversy. *Cultural Hermeneutics*, 2, 237–377.

Bubner, R. et al. (1976). Is transcendental hermeneutics possible? In J. Manninen and R. Tuomela (Eds)., *Essays on explanation and understanding: Studies in the foundations of humanities and social sciences* (pp. 59–77). Boston: D. Reidel Publishing.

Butterfield, P.G. (1990). Thinking upstream: Nurturing a conceptual understanding of the societal context of health behavior. *Advances in Nursing Science*, 12(2), 1–8.

Dallmayr, W. (1972). Critical theory criticized: Habermas' knowledge and human interests and its aftermath. *Philosophy of Social Sciences,* 2, 211–229.

Duffy, K. and Scott, P.A. (1998). Viewing an old issue through a new lens: A critical theory insight into the education-practice gap. *Nurse Education Today,* 18(3), 183–189.

Ekstrom, D.N. and Sigurdsson, H.O. (2002). An international collaboration in nursing education viewed through the lens of critical social theory. *Journal of Nursing Education*, 41(7), 289–294.

Eriksson, K. (1997). Understanding the world of the patient, the suffering human being: The new clinical paradigm from nursing to caring. *Advanced Practice Nursing Quarterly*, 3(1), 8–13.

Floistad, G. (1973). Understanding hermeneutics. *Inquiry,* 16, 445–465.

Fraser, N. (1987). What's critical about critical theory? In S. Benhabib and D. Cornell (Eds.), *Feminism as critique* (pp. 31–55). Cambridge, England: Polity Press.

Frye, M. (1983). On being white: Thinking toward a feminist understanding of race and race supremacy. *The Politics of reality: Essays in feminist theory* (pp. 110–127). New York: Crossing Press.

Gadamer, H.G. (1975). Hermeneutics and social science. *Cultural Hermeneutics,* 2, 307–336.

Gadamer, H.G. (1976). *Philosophical hermeneutics.* D.E. Linge (Ed., Trans.). Berkeley/Los Angeles/London: University of California Press.

Geanellos, R. (1998). Hermeneutic philosophy. Part I: Implications of its use as methodology in interpretive nursing research. *Nursing Inquiry,* 5(3), 154–163.

Geanellos, R. (1998). Hermeneutic philosophy. Part II: A nursing research example of the hermeneutic imperative to address forestructures/pre-understandings. *Nursing Inquiry,* 5(4), 238–247.

Geanellos, R. (2000). Exploring Ricoeur's hermeneutic theory of interpretation as a method of analysing research texts. *Nursing Inquiry,* 7(2), 112–119.

Habermas, J. (1970). On systematically distorted communication. *Inquiry,* 13, 205–218.

Habermas, J. (1970). Towards a theory of communicative competence. *Inquiry,* 13, 360–375.

Habermas, J. (1971). *Knowledge and human interests.* Boston: Beacon Press.

Habermas, J. (1976). Theory and practice in a scientific society. In P. Connerton (Ed.), *Critical sociology* (pp. 331–347). New York: Penguin Books.

Habermas, J. (1977). *A review of Gadamer's Truth and Method.* In F.R. Dallmayr and T.H. McCarthy (Eds.), *Understanding and social inquiry* (pp. 335–363). Notre Dame, IN: University of Notre Dame Press.

Habermas, J. (1984). *The theory of communicative action, Vol. 2.* T. McCarthy (Trans.). Boston: Beacon Press.

Hegel, G.W.F. (1931). *The phenomenology of mind* (2nd ed.). Translated with an introduction and notes by J.B. Baillie. London/New York: Macmillan.

Heidegger, M. (1962). *Being and time.* J. MacQuarrie and E. Robinson (Trans.). London: SCM Press.

Held, D. (1980). *Introduction to critical theory.* Berkeley, CA: University of California Press.

Heslop, L. (1997). The (im)possibilities of poststructuralist and critical social nursing inquiry. *Nursing Inquiry,* 4(1), 48–56.

Holmes, C.A. and Warelow, P.J. (1997). Culture, needs and nursing: A critical theory approach. *Journal of Advanced Nursing,* 25(3), 463–470.

Holter, I.M. (1988). Critical theory: A foundation for the development of nursing theories. *Scholarly Inquiry for Nursing Practice,* 2, 223–232.

Hopton, J. (1997). Towards a critical theory of mental health nursing. *Journal of Advanced Nursing,* 25(3), 492–500.

Horkheimer, M. (1976). Traditional and critical theory. In P. Connerton (Ed.), *Critical sociology* (pp. 206–224). New York: Penguin Books.

Howard, R.J. (1982). *Three faces of hermeneutics: An introduction to current theories of understanding.* Berkeley, CA: University of California Press.

Koch, T. (1995). Interpretive approaches in nursing research: The influence of Husserl and Heidegger. *Journal of Advanced Nursing,* 21(5), 827–836.

Manias, E. and Street, A. (2000). Possibilities for critical social theory and Foucault's work: A toolbox approach. *Nursing Inquiry,* 7(1), 50–60.

Marshall, B.L. (1988). Feminist theory and critical theory. *Canadian Review of Sociology and Anthropology,* 25(2), 208–230.

Eisler, R. (1988). *The chalice and the blade: Our history, our future.* San Francisco: Harper & Row.

Eisenstein, Z. (1977). Developing a theory of capitalist patriarchy and socialist feminism. *The Insurgent Sociologist,* 7(3), 5–40.

Farganis, S. (1986). Social theory and feminist theory: The need for dialogue. *Sociological Inquiry,* 56(1), 50–68.

Flax, J. (1987). Postmodernism and gender relations in feminist theory. *Signs: Journal of Women in Culture and Society,* 12, 621–643.

Francis, B. (2000). Poststructuralism and nursing: Uncomfortable bedfellows? *Nursing Inquiry,* 7(1). 20–28.

Gilligan, C. (1982). *In a different voice: Psychological theory and women's development.* Cambridge, MA: Harvard University Press.

Georges, J.M. (2002). Suffering: Toward a contextual praxis. *Advances in Nursing Science,* 25(1), 79–86.

Grady, K. (1981). Sex bias in research design. *Psychology of Women Quarterly,* 5, 628–637.

Gray, D. P. (1995). A journey into feminist pedagogy. *Journal of Nursing Education,* 34, 77–81.

Hagell, E.I. (1989). Nursing knowledge: Women's knowledge. A sociological perspective. *Journal of Advanced Nursing,* 14(3), 226–233.

Hall, J.M. and Stevens, P.E. (1991). Rigor in feminist research. *Advances in Nursing Science,* 13(3), 16–29.

Harding, S. (1983). Common causes: Toward a reflexive feminist theory. *Women and Politics,* 3(4), 27–42.

Harding, S. (1986). *The science question in feminism.* Ithaca, NY: Cornell University Press.

Harding, S. (Ed.). (1987). *Feminism and methodology.* Bloomington, IN: Indiana University Press.

Harding, S. (1988). Feminism confronts the sciences: Reform and transformation. In C. Bridges and N. Wells (Eds.), *Proceedings of the fifth nursing science colloquium* (pp. 73–92). Boston: Boston University.

Hedin, B. (1986). Nursing, education, and emancipation: Applying the critical theoretical approach to nursing research. In P. Chinn (Ed.), *Nursing research methodology: Issues and implementation* (pp. 133–146). Rockville, MD: Aspen Systems.

Hedin, B. and Donovan, J. (1989). A feminist perspective on nursing education. *Nurse Educator,* 14(4), 8–13.

Henderson, D. (1997). Intersecting race and gender in feminist theories of women's psychological development. *Issues in Mental Health Nursing,* 18(5), 377–393.

Huntington, A.D. (2002). Working with women experiencing mid-trimester termination of pregnancy: The integration of nursing and feminist knowledge in the gynaecological setting. *Journal of Clinical Nursing,* 11(2), 273–279.

Jaggar, A. (1979). Political philosophies of women's liberation. In S. Bishop and M. Weinzweig (Eds.), *Philosophy and women.* Belmont, CA: Wadsworth.

Jaggar A. and Struhl, P.R. (1978). *Feminist frameworks: Alternative theoretical accounts of the relations between women and men.* New York: McGraw-Hill.

Jayaratne, T.E. (1983). The value of quantitative methodology for feminist research. In G. Bowles and R.D. Klein (Eds.), *Theories of Women's Studies* (pp. 140–161). Boston: Routledge & Kegan Paul.

Joseph, G.I. and Lewis, J. (1981). *Common differences: Conflicts in black and white feminist perspectives.* Boston: South End Press.

Karabenies, A., Miller, L., Nagel-Bamesberger, H., Rossiter, A., and Thompson, M. (1986). What makes a feminist social science? *Cassandra: Radical Feminist Nurses Newsjournal,* 4(1), 9–11.

Keddy, B., Sims, S.L., and Stern, P.N. (1996). Grounded theory as feminist research methodology. *Journal of Advanced Nursing,* 23(3), 448–453.

Keller, E.F. (1982). Feminism and science. In N.O. Keohane, M.Z. Rosaldo, and B.C. Gelpi (Eds.), *Feminist theory: A critique of ideology* (pp. 113–126). Chicago: University of Chicago Press.

Keller, E.F. (1983). *A feeling for the organism. The life and work of Barbara McClintock.* New York: W.H. Freeman.

Keller, E.F. (1985). *Reflections on gender and science.* New Haven, CT: Yale University Press.

Keohane, N.O., Rosaldo, M.Z., and Gelpi, B.C. (1981). *Feminist theory: A critique of ideology.* Chicago: University of Chicago Press.

Klein, R.D. (1983). How to do what we want to do: Thoughts about feminist methodology. In G. Bowles and R.D. Klein (Eds.), *Theories of women's studies* (pp. 88–104). Boston: Routledge & Kegan Paul.

Lengermann, P.M. and Niegrugge-Brantley, J. (1988). Contemporary feminist theory. In G. Ritzer (Ed.), *Contemporary sociological theory* (2nd ed.). New York: Alfred A. Knopf.

Longino, H.E. (1986). Can there be a feminist science? *Hypatia: Journal of Feminist Science.*

MacKinnon, C. (1982). Feminism, Marxism, method and the state: An agenda for theory. *Signs: Journal of Women in Culture and Society,* 7(3), 515–544.

MacPherson, K.I. (1983). Feminist methods: A new paradigm for nursing research. *Advances in Nursing Science,* 5(2), 17–25.

MacPherson, K.I. (1988). The missing piece: Women as partners in feminist research. *Advances in Nursing Science,* 5(2), 17–26.

Marshall, B.L. (1988). Feminist theory and critical theory. *Canadian Review of Sociology and Anthropology,* 25(2), 208–230.

Mason, D. J., Backer, B. A., and Georges, C. A. (1991). Toward a feminist model for the political empowerment of nurses. *Image: Journal of Nursing Scholarship,* 23, 72–77.

McLoughlin, A. (1997). The "F" factor: Feminism forsaken? *Nurse Education Today,* 17(2), 111–114.

Mies, M. (1983). Towards a methodology for feminist research. In G. Bowles and R. Klein (Eds.), *Theories of women's studies* (pp. 117–139). London: Routledge & Kegan Paul.

Moccia, P. (1988). A critique of compromise: Beyond the methods debate. *Advances in Nursing Science,* 10(4), 1–9.

Moraga, C. (1986). From a long line of vendidas: Chicanas and feminism. In T. de Lauretis (Ed.), *Feminist studies/critical studies* (Chap. 11). Bloomington, IN: Indiana University Press.

Oakley, A. (1981). Interviewing women: A contradiction in terms. In H. Roberts (Eds.), *Doing feminist research* (Chap. 2). New York: Routledge & Kegan Paul.

Parker, B. and McFarlane, J. (1991). Feminist theory and nursing: An empowerment model for research. *Advances in Nursing Science*, 13(3), 59–67.

Perry, P.A. (1994). Feminist empiricism as a method for inquiry in nursing. *Western Journal of Nursing Research*, 16, 480–494.

Reason, P. and Rowan, J. (1981). *Human inquiry: A sourcebook of new paradigm research*. New York: John Wiley & Sons.

Reinharz, S. (1983). Experimental analysis: A contribution to feminist research. In G. Bowles and R. Klein (Eds.), *Theories of women studies*. London: Routledge & Kegan Paul.

Roberts, H. (1981). *Doing feminist research*. London: Routledge & Kegan Paul.

Rose, H. (1983). Hand, brain, and heart: A feminist epistemology for the natural sciences. *Signs: Journal of Women in Culture and Society*, 9(1), 73–90.

Rose, H. (1986). Beyond masculinist realities: A feminist epistemology for the sciences. In R. Bleier (Ed.), *Feminist approaches to science*. New York: Pergamon Press.

Sampselle, C.M. (1990). The influence of feminist philosophy on nursing practice. *Image: Journal of Nursing Scholarship*, 22(4), 243–206.

Sherwin, S. (1987). Concluding remarks: A feminist perspective. *Health Care for Women International*, 8(4), 293–304.

Shields, L.E. (1995). Women's experiences of the meaning of empowerment. *Qualitative Health Research*, 5(1), 15–35.

Smith, D. (1974). Women's perspective as a radical critique of sociology. *Sociological Inquiry*, 44, 7–13.

Smith, D. (1990). *The conceptual practices of power: A feminist sociology of knowledge*. Toronto, Canada: University of Toronto Press.

Sohier, R. (1992). Feminism and nursing knowledge: The power of the weak. *Nursing Outlook*, 40, 62–66, 93.

Stacey, J. and Thorne, B. (1985). The missing feminist revolution in sociology. *Social Problems*, 32(4), 301–316.

Thomas, L.W. (1995). A critical feminist perspective of the health belief model: Implications for nursing theory, research, practice, and education. *Journal of Professional Nursing*, 11(4), 246–252.

Thompson, J.L. (1985). Practical discourse in nursing: Going beyond empiricism and historicism. *Advances in Nursing Science*, 7(4), 59–71.

Thompson, J.L. (1991). Exploring gender and culture with Khmer refugee women: Reflections on participatory feminist research. *Advances in Nursing Science*, 13(3), 30–48.

Tronto, J. (1987). Beyond gender difference to a theory of care. *Signs: Journal of Women in Culture and Society*, 12(4), 644–663.

Weedon, C. (1991). *Feminist practice and post-structuralist theory*. Cambridge, MA: Basil Blackwell.

Wuest, J. (1993). Removing the shackles: A feminist critique of noncompliance. *Nursing Outlook*, 41, 217–224.

Wuest, J. (1994). A feminist approach to concept analysis. *Western Journal of Nursing Research*, 16(5), 577–586.

Wuest, J. (1994). Professionalism and the evolution of nursing as a discipline: A feminist perspective. *Journal of Professional Nursing*, 10, 357–367.

Wuest, J. (2001). Precarious ordering: Toward a formal theory of women's caring. *Health Care for Women International,* 22(1/2), 167–193.

Middle-Range Theory

Acton, G.J., Irvin, B.L., Jensen, J.A., Hopkins, B.A., and Miller, E.W. (1997). Explicating middle-range theory through methodological diversity. *Advances in Nursing Science*, 19(3), 78–85.

Auvil-Novak, S.E. (1997). A middle-range theory of chronotherapeutic intervention for postsurgical pain. *Nursing Research*, 46(2), 66–71.

Chinn, P.L. (2001). Why middle-range theory? [Editorial]. *Advances in Nursing Science*, 19(3), viii.

Lenz, E.R. (1998). Beneath the surface: The role of middle-range theory for nursing research and practice: Part 2. Nursing practice. *Nursing Leadership Forum*, 3(2), 62–66.

Lenz, E.R., Pugh, L.C., Milligan, R.A., Gift, A., and Suppe, F. (1997). The middle range theory of unpleasant symptoms: An update. *Advances in Nursing Science*, 19(3), 14–27.

Meleis, A., Sawyer, L.M., Im, E., Messias, D.K.H., and Schumacher, K. (2000). Experiencing transitions: An emerging middle-range theory. *Advances in Nursing Science*, 23(1), 12–28.

Olsen, J. and Hanchett, E. (1997). Nurse-expressed empathy, patient outcomes, and development of middle-range theory. *Image: Journal of Nursing Scholarship*, 29(1), 71–76.

Polk, L.V. (1997). Toward a middle-range theory of resilience. *Advances in Nursing Science*, 19(3), 1–13.

Sanford, R.C. (2000). Caring through relation and dialogue: A nursing perspective for patient education. *Advances in Nursing Science*, 22(3), 1–15.

Smith, M.J. and Liehr, P. (1999). Attentively Embracing Story: A middle-range theory with practice and research implications. *Scholarly Inquiry for Nursing Practice*, 13(3), 187–204.

Video and Audio Tapes on Theory

49. Video Productions from the National League for Nursing

A Conversation with Virginia Henderson

Interview with Virginia Henderson about her life and work, conducted by Patricia Moccia.

Available from: NLN Customer Service, National League for Nursing, 350 Hudson Street, New York, NY 10014 (800) 669-9656, ext. 138, FAX (212) 989-3710. Send Internet e-mails (queries only) to: custserv@nln.org

Nursing in America: A History of Social Reform

Video that examines nursing's history of social reform while chronicling social, political, and economic influences that shaped American nursing.

Available from: NLN Customer Service, National League for Nursing, 350 Hudson Street, New York, NY 10014 (800) 669-9656, ext. 138, FAX (212) 989-3710. Send Internet e-mails (queries only) to: custserv@nln.org

Nursing Theory: A Circle of Knowledge

Video hosted by Patricia Moccia that examines issues related to philosophy of nursing science, particularly the relevance of nursing theory to practice. Features discussions with Patricia Benner, Virginia Henderson, Dorothea Orem, Martha Rogers, Callista Roy, and Jean Watson.

Available from: NLN Customer Service, National League for Nursing, 350 Hudson Street, New York, NY 10014 (800) 669-9656, ext. 138, FAX (212) 989-3710. Send Internet e-mails (queries only) to: custserv@nln.org

Theories at Work

Video hosted by Patricia Moccia about innovative applications of nursing theory in nurse-managed health care systems. Moccia visits centers of nursing practice around the country and talks with Dorothy Powell, Bernadine Lacey, Jean Watson, and Janet Quinn about their theory-based nursing care.

Available from: NLN Customer Service, National League for Nursing, 350 Hudson Street, New York, NY 10014 (800) 669-9656, ext. 138, FAX (212) 989-3710. Send Internet e-mails (queries only) to: custserv@nln.org

Therapeutic Touch: Healing through Human Energy Fields

A three-part video hosted by Janet F. Quinn. Part I explores the theoretical framework of therapeutic touch, defines key concepts, and highlights research studies documenting the clinical effectiveness of therapeutic touch. Part II explains the method nurses use in performing therapeutic touch, and Part III explores the clinical application of therapeutic touch in clinics, private practice, and hospitals.

Available from: NLN Customer Service, National League for Nursing, 350 Hudson Street, New York, NY 10014 (800) 669-9656, ext. 138, FAX (212) 989-3710. Send Internet e-mails (queries only) to: custserv@nln.org

Critical Thinking in Nursing: Lessons from Tuskegee

This video examines the story of nurse Eunice Rivers and the infamous Tuskegee Syphilis Study in which 400 African American men were left untreated for the disease as part of a government study. The presentation brings forth a number of social and ethical issues that warrant critical thinking among nurses. A companion book is also available.

Available from: NLN Customer Service, National League for Nursing, 350 Hudson Street, New York, NY 10014 (800) 669-9656, ext. 138, FAX (212) 989-3710. Send Internet e-mails (queries only) to: custserv@nln.org

A Conversation on Caring with Jean Watson and Janet Quinn

A video in which Jean Watson and Janet Quinn discuss the elements of caring.

Available from: NLN Customer Service, National League for Nursing, 350 Hudson Street, New York, NY 10014 (800) 669-9656, ext. 138, FAX (212) 989-3710. Send Internet e-mails (queries only) to: custserv@nln.org

A Guide to Applying the Art and Science of Human Care

A set of two videos in which Jean Watson gives an overview of her Theory of Human Science and Human Caring and a panel, moderated by Peggy Chinn, discusses the implementation of the caring model in diverse practice and educational settings.

Available from: NLN Customer Service, National League for Nursing, 350 Hudson Street, New York, NY 10014 (800) 669-9656, ext. 138, FAX (212) 989-3710. Send Internet e-mails (queries only) to: custserv@nln.org

The Power of Nursing

A discussion of the concept of power and of nurses' relation with health policy.

Available from: NLN Customer Service, National League for Nursing, 350 Hudson Street, New York, NY 10014 (800) 669-9656, ext. 138, FAX (212) 989-3710. Send Internet e-mails (queries only) to: custserv@nln.org

Nursing in America:Through a Feminist Lens

A video in which the issues of autonomy and control are compared in relation to nurses' historic struggle for independence and feminists' battle to empower women.

Available from: NLN Customer Service, National League for Nursing, 350 Hudson Street, New York, NY 10014 (800) 669-9656, ext. 138, FAX (212) 989-3710. Send Internet e-mails (queries only) to: custserv@nln.org

50. Video Productions from FITNE

The Nurse Theorists: Portraits of Excellence

Series of 16 videos about the lives and scholarly accomplishments of notable nurse theorists. Each video contains a biographical sketch of the theorist, an interview conducted by Jacqueline Fawcett, and a summary of the nursing theory. Videotapes include: (1) Virginia Henderson, "Definition of Nursing"; (2) Dorothy Johnson, "Behavioral Systems Model"; (3) Imogene King, "Interacting System Framework"; (4) Madeline Leininger, "Transcultural Nursing Care"; (5) Myra Levine, "The Conservative Model"; (6) Betty Neuman, "Neuman Systems Model"; (7) Florence Nightingale, "Special Edition"; (8) Dorothea Orem, "Self Care Framework"; (9) Ida Orlando Pelletier, "The Deliberative Nursing Process"; (10) Hildegard Peplau, "Interpersonal Relations in Nursing"; (11) Martha Rogers, "Science of Unitary Human Beings"; (12) Callista Roy, "The Adaptations Model of Nursing"; (13) Reva Rubin, "Theory of Maternal Identity"; (14) Jean Watson, "A Theory of Caring"; (15) Margaret Newman, "Health as Expanding Consciousness"; and (16) Rosemarie Parse, "Man-Living Health."

Available from: FITNE, 5 Depot Street, Athens, OH 45701, (614) 592-2511.

From Beginner to Expert: Clinical Knowledge in Critical Care Nursing

Dr. Patricia Benner and her research team discuss the methods and major findings of a study of clinical learning and skilled clinical judgment among critical care nurses, and the implications in terms of the process of becoming an expert nurse.

Available from: FITNE, 5 Depot Street, Athens, OH 45701, (614) 592-2511.

Adaptation Model in Practice

The application of Callista Roy's adaptation model, which promotes the biological, psychological and sociological aspects of patients in relation to a constantly changing environment, is demonstrated at two different health care institutions. Available from: FITNE, 5 Depot Street, Athens, OH 45701, (614) 592-2511.

Self-Care Framework Model in Practice

This video describes Dorothea Orem's self-care deficit nursing theory and presents case studies to demonstrate the application of the theory to nursing practice.

Available from: FITNE, 5 Depot Street, Athens, OH 45701, (614) 592-2511.

51. Video Productions from the Health Sciences Consortium

Care with a Concept

This program by Mary Hale and Gates Rhodes discusses the application of Dorothea Orem's self-care conceptual model in a pediatric rehabilitation center. As Orem's model is applied, nurse-managers are enabled to evaluate the effects of the nursing care rendered.

Available from: Health Sciences Consortium, 201 Silver Cedar Court, Chapel Hill, NC 27514-1517 (919) 942-8731, FAX (919) 942-3689.

52. Conference Videotapes

Nurse Theorist Conference 1985

Videotaped presentations include (1) Dorothea Orem, "Presentation"; (2) Hildegard Peplau, "Nursing Science: A Historical View"; and (3) "Panel Discussion with Theorists" with Dorothea E. Orem, Callista Roy, Imogene M. King, Martha E. Rogers, Rosemarie Rizzo Parse, and Hildegard E. Peplau.

Available from: Discovery International's Nurse Theorist Conferences, Veranda Communications, Inc., 4229 Taylorsville Road, Louisville, KY 40220, (502) 485-1484, FAX (502) 485-1482.

Nurse Theorist Conference 1987, Pittsburgh, PA

Videotaped presentations include (1) Hildegard Peplau, "Art and Science of Nursing: Similarities, Differences and Relations"; (2) Imogene King, "King's Theory"; (3) Rosemarie Parse, "Parse's Theory"; (4) Callista Roy, "Roy's Model"; (5) Martha Rogers, "Rogers' Framework"; (6) Jean Watson, "Watson's Model"; (7) Rozella Schlotfeldt, "Nursing Science in the 21st Century"; and (8) "Panel Discussion with Theorists."

Available from: Discovery International's Nurse Theorist Conferences, Veranda Communications, Inc., 4229 Taylorsville Road, Louisville, KY 40220, (502) 485-1484, FAX (502) 485-1482.

Nurse Theorist Conference 1989, Pittsburgh, PA

Videotaped presentations include (1) Afaf Meleis, "Being and Becoming Healthy: The Core of Nursing Knowledge"; (2) Betty Neuman, "Health as a Continuum in Neuman's Model"; (3) Rosemarie Parse, "Health as a Personal Commitment in Parse's Theory": (4) Martha Rogers, "Evolutionary Emergence: Infinite Potential";

(5) Nola Pender, "Expressing Health Through Beliefs and Actions"; (6) Imogene King, "Health as the Goal of Nursing in King's Theory"; and (7) "Panel Discussion with Theorists."

Available from: Discovery International's Nurse Theorist Conferences, Veranda Communications, Inc., 4229 Taylorsville Road, Louisville, KY 40220, (502) 485-1484, FAX (502) 485-1482.

Nurse Theorist Conference 1993, Pittsburgh, PA

Videotaped presentations include (1) Rosemarie Rizzo Parse, "Quality of Life and Becoming Human"; (2) Madeleine M. Leininger, "Quality of Life and Transcultural Nursing"; (3) Martha Rogers, "Quality of Life and the Science of Unitary Human Beings"; (4) Marlaine C. Smith, Cheryl Forchuk, Gail J. Mitchell, and Jacqueline Chapman, "Nursing Theory-based Practice and Research: A Glimpse of the Canadian Scene"; (4) Hildegard Peplau, "Quality of Life: An Interpersonal Perspective"; and (5) Imogene King, "Nursing and the Next Millennium" moderated by Marlaine C. Smith.

Available from: Discovery International's Nurse Theorist Conferences, Veranda Communications, Inc., 4229 Taylorsville Road, Louisville, KY 40220, (502) 485-1484, FAX (502) 485-1482.

53. Conference Audiotapes

Nursing Theory Congress 1986, Toronto, Canada

Audiotapes of plenary sessions by Betty Neuman, Imogene King, Callista Roy, Rosemarie Parse, Martha Rogers, and Myra Levine. Other audiotapes include (1) Moyra Allen, "A Developmental Health Model: Nursing as Continuous Inquiry"; (2) Patricia James and James Dickoff, "Overview of the Concept of Theoretical Pluralism"; (3) Bonnie Holaday, "Adaptation of Johnson's Framework"; (4) Susan Taylor, "Presenting Orem's Framework"; (5) Phyllis Kritek, "Impact of Nursing Theory on the Diagnostic Process"; and (6) Marian McGee, "Criteria for Selection and Use of a Nursing Model for Clinical Practice."

Available from: Audio Archives International, 100 West Beaver Creek, Unit 18, Richmond Hill, Ontario, Canada, L4B 1H4, (905) 889-6555.

Nursing Theory Congress 1988, Toronto, Canada

Audiotapes include (1) Carol Lindeman, "Nursing Theory: Elitism or Realism in 1988"; (2) Virginia Henderson, "Nursing Theory: A Historical Perspective"; (3) Jean Watson, "One Model or Many Models"; (4) Marjory Gordon, "Nursing Diagnosis: The Interface of Nursing Theory and Nursing Process"; (5) Rosemarie Parse, "Nursing Science as a Basis for Research"; (6) Phyllis Kritek and others, "Impact of Nursing Theory on the Profession"; and (7) Phyllis Kritek, "Agendas for the Future."

Available from: Audio Archives International, 100 West Beaver Creek, Unit 18, Richmond Hill, Ontario, Canada L4B 1H4, (905) 889-6555.

Nurse Theorist Conference 1985, Philadelphia, PA

Audiotapes include (1) Presentations by Dorothea Orem, Callista Roy, Imogene M. King, Martha E. Rogers, Rosemarie Rizzo Parse; (2) Hildegard Peplau, "Nursing Science: A Historical Overview"; (3) Mary Jane Smith, "Theorist: Dorothea E.

H

I

J

K

L

M

S

T

Subject Index

Page numbers followed by *f* indicate a figure: those followed by *t* indicate tabular material.

O